C000039652

A HISTORY OF LUMINAL
GASTROENTEROLOGY IN BRITAIN

To Maddy, Mark, James and Caroline

A HISTORY OF LUMINAL GASTROENTEROLOGY IN BRITAIN

THE INSIDE GUIDE

PETER DOWN

WATERY BOOKS

Copyright © Peter Down 2013
First published in 2013 by Watery Books
Broadwey House, Watery Lane, Weymouth, Dorset DT3 5QD
http://www.historyofgastroenterology.com

Distributed by Gardners Books, 1 Whittle Drive, Eastbourne, East Sussex,
BN23 6QH
Tel: +44(0)1323 521555 | Fax: +44(0)1323 521666

The right of Peter Down to be identified as the author of the work has
been asserted herein in accordance with the Copyright, Designs and
Patents Act 1988.

All rights reserved. This book is sold subject to the condition that it shall
not, by way of trade or otherwise, be lent, resold, hired out or otherwise
circulated without the publisher's prior consent in any form of binding
or cover other than that in which it is published and without a similar
condition including this condition being imposed on the subsequent
purchaser.

British Library Cataloguing in Publication Data
A catalogue record for this book is available from the British Library.

ISBN 978-0-9572504-0-6

Typeset by Amolibros, Milverton, Somerset
This book production has been managed by Amolibros
www.amolibros.com
Printed and bound by T J International Ltd, Padstow, Cornwall, UK

CONTENTS

LIST OF ILLUSTRATIONS

PREFACE

This book is intended for gastroenterologists, particularly those who would describe themselves as luminologists. It is an account of the contribution of British doctors to our knowledge of common gastrointestinal diseases, excluding the liver and pancreas.

The book is largely concerned with the nineteenth and twentieth centuries; in my view there is little that can be said about our understanding of intestinal diseases before the late eighteenth century. Until recently gastroenterology was considered part of general medicine and it is only in the last 30 years or so that it has been recognised as a specialty. At first doctors recorded their opinions in monographs based on their experience and knowledge of morbid anatomy. These men were generalists and wrote with authority but were prone to speculation. The rise in chemistry and physiology towards the end of the nineteenth century did little to curb their enthusiasm. During the twentieth century clinical and basic research became more critical, by which time authors were turning to scientific journals in which to publish their work. After the Second World War the need to "publish or perish" led to multi-authorship in an ever expanding number of journals. This has made it impossible for me to include the name of every gastroenterologist who has written a paper but the key players have been easy to select.

Although this is the story of British gastroenterology, the book includes contributions from workers in Europe, America and elsewhere. To omit them would not only detract from the story but be a gross injustice to their seminal work.

Historians will say that my approach has been old fashioned (with a heroic view) in dealing with the main characters and that I have not explained the historical or social context around them. This is true to an extent but in probing what we have learnt about diseases I have been inspired by the admirable words of Kipling's poem summarising the way we get most of our knowledge.

"I keep six honest serving men
(They taught me all I knew);
Their names are What and Why and When
And How and Where and Who."

Critics might also argue that the approach by character does not help the reader to follow the historical development of the study of a disease as the personal information is parallel and distracting. But my intention has not been to reveal anything new about gut diseases but merely to satisfy curiosity (my own at least) about who and how people made the discoveries they did. The more distinguished have generally received the most attention but others of equal merit may have been short-changed owing to my ignorance. For this I apologise and welcome help to redress such failings.

I hope readers will enjoy discovering the British contribution to gastroenterology as much as I have. One of the most useful parts of a history book is the index. With luck most people who have worked in the field will be there.

I want to record my appreciation to all those who have given me their time in the preparation of this book. In particular, I would like to mention Dr. Denis Gibbs, the notable medical historian, who has encouraged me from the beginning. He has taught me so much and has generously shared his encyclopaedic knowledge and his valuable library with me. In addition, he has given up much of his time to read and correct large sections of the manuscript. Thanks are also due to my friend, Dr John Ford, who fired my interest in medical history many years ago. Without their help this book would not have been written.

SECTION ONE

THE OESOPHAGUS

CHAPTER ONE

ACHALASIA

One morning in February 1908 a young physician parked his car in the front quadrangle of Guy's Hospital. It was a two-cylinder 10–12 Wolseley tourer and was probably the first car to enter the hallowed precincts of the hospital, doubtless raising eyebrows among senior medical staff, most of whom at that time drove to work in their carriages. The car belonged to Arthur Hurst (1879–1944), a man with boundless energy and enthusiasm, who had recently been elected to the staff at the early age of 27. He was highly gregarious and a year later was asked by Sir William Osler to be a founder member of the Association of Physicians. Nearly 30 years later he was to found the British Gastroenterological Club along similar lines to the Association of Physicians, which after his death became the British Society of Gastroenterology.

Hurst, whose family had the name of Hertz, trained at Magdalen College, Oxford and Guy's Hospital, qualifying in 1905. He was a good student and won the Treasurer's Gold Medals for clinical medicine and clinical surgery. Later, in his autobiography, he admitted that he was rather ashamed about the surgery medal he won because of his faculty of giving examiners the impression that he knew more than he really did. In fact he sold his medals and had replicas made in bronze, spending the large balance on books. After qualifying he was awarded a Radcliffe Travelling Fellowship of Oxford University. He spent some time in Europe before going to Boston where he met Walter B. Cannon (1871–1945), who had just been elected professor of physiology at Harvard. Hurst was deeply impressed by Cannon who, as an intern, had spent several years studying the movements of the stomach in cats using the exciting new discovery of X-rays.

On his return to Guy's Hospital in 1906 Hurst became demonstrator in physiology and was asked to take the revision class for the MB. In describing the act of swallowing he found it difficult to reconcile the old observations made by inserting rubber balloons into the human gullet with Cannon's recent work on cats, so he suggested to the students of

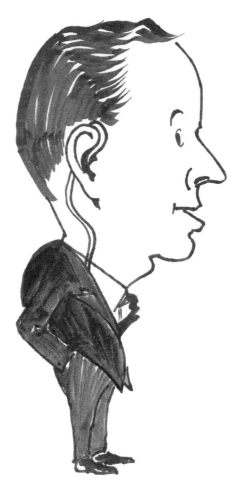

1 Arthur Hurst – Wind – is on the brain, not in the stomach nor round the heart.

the class that they should watch each other with the aid of the X-rays. They enthusiastically agreed, but the radiologist refused to cooperate, as he said his valuable apparatus had been bought for the examination of bones and was not meant for silly experiments such as he proposed to carry out. So Hurst applied to higher authority in the person of Dr.

(later Sir) Cooper Perry who was Superintendent as well as Physician of the hospital. He at once gave him permission to use the apparatus.[1]

Thus began a long series of investigations on the passage of food along the human alimentary tract, which he published in 1907.[2] The work was done under a constant barrage of insulting notes from the hospital radiologist who never ceased protest against the "bismuth orgies" (this was before the introduction of barium in 1912). Hurst did all his own examinations until 1914 and was particularly interested in the mechanism of swallowing. He saw several cases in which the oesophagus was dilated due to obstruction at its lower end, thought then to be caused by spasm of the lower oesophageal sphincter. However, he found that when the contents of the oesophagus had accumulated to a sufficient height, the weight of the column seemed able to force the lower sphincter and allow a certain amount of food to slip into the stomach. He showed that a rubber tube weighted with mercury passed easily into the stomach with no resistance whatever. Realising that the problem resulted from an absence of relaxation of the cardiac sphincter, he asked his friend, Cooper Perry, if he could think up a single word to express this. The next day Perry suggested achalasia of the cardia (alpha, absence of; chalsis, relaxation) and the name has been used ever since.[3]

No one understood the pathology underlying achalasia but in 1924 Hurst predicted that "the majority of cases are caused by progressive organic disease involving Auerbach's plexus".[4] In fact the following year Geoffrey Rake (1905–58), a medical student at Guy's Hospital, attended the autopsy on a patient who had died after surgery for a carcinoma of the tongue.[5] Besides the tongue cancer, the unfortunate man had a hypertrophied oesophagus, which Rake thought probably represented an early stage of achalasia. Encouraged by Adrian Stokes, then Professor of Pathology, and by Hurst himself, Rake looked carefully at the lower end of the oesophagus and found chronic inflammatory changes and degenerating ganglion cells in Auerbach's plexus.[6] While still a student, he went on to describe similar changes in several more patients with typical achalasia, none of whom had any ganglion cells in the plexus at all and precious few further up the oesophagus. This was an impressive piece of work and certainly helped to explain the mechanism of the disease, though the underlying cause remained a mystery. Rake was a shy, retiring, meticulous man with a severe stammer that made it impossible for him to consider clinical practice, but he was cut out for research. Soon after qualifying he emigrated to America where he had a distinguished career in microbiology and the development of antibiotics.

Hurst certainly deserves the credit for putting achalasia on the map, though a few cases had been described much earlier. None more remarkable than that by Thomas Willis (1620–75) in his *Pharmaceutice Rationalis* published in 1674, at the dawn of the new science in Britain, where an experimental approach to the study of nature was at last beginning to challenge centuries of Galenic learned medicine.[7]

> "No less will a very rare case of a certain man of Oxford shew, an almost perpetual vomiting to be stirred up by the shutting up of the left orifice. A strong man, and otherwise healthful enough, labouring for a long time with often vomiting, he was wont, very often, but not always, presently to cast up whatsoever he had eaten. At length the disease having overcome all remedies, he was brought into that condition, that growing hungry he would eat until the oesophagus was filled up to the throat, in the mean time nothing sliding down into the ventricle, he cast up raw (or crude) whatsoever he had taken in: when that no medicines could help and he languished away for hunger, and every day was in danger of death, I prepared an instrument for him like a rod, of a whale bone, with a little round button of sponge fixed to the top of it; the sick man having taken down meat and drink into his throat, presently putting this down in the oesophagus, he did thrust down into the ventricle, its orifice being opened, the food which otherwise would have come back again; and by this means he hath daily taken his sustenance for fifteen years and doth yet use the same machine, and is yet alive, and well, who would otherwise perish for want of food. Without doubt in this case the mouth of the stomach being always closed, either by a tumour or Palsie, nothing could be admitted into the ventricle unless it were violently opened."

Small wonder that Willis, a founder member of the Royal Society, "became so noted and so infinitely resorted to for his practice, that never any physician before went beyond him or got more money".[8]

Four further reports appeared during the nineteenth century that are worthy of mention. The first in 1821 came from Thomas Purton (1768–1833), a surgeon and botanist in Alcester, Warwickshire, who described an extraordinary 'Case of Distension of the Oesophagus, forming a Sac, extending from two inches below the Pharynx to the Cardiac Orifice of the Stomach'.[9] The victim, a blacksmith, suffered from intermittent obstruction and vomiting for twenty years before his death aged forty-three. He saw many medical men to no avail, including Sir Astley Cooper (1768–1841), the foremost surgeon of the day, who recommended a trial of bougies. Unfortunately they were so difficult to introduce and caused so much pain that they had to be abandoned.

In 1828 Herbert Mayo (1796–1852) described the fate of a young woman, Mary Blores aged 33, who had symptoms for ten years before her death from exhaustion.[10] For a month before admission she appeared to keep down nothing. She craved for food and drink, and seemed literally starving. A large oesophageal bougie passed readily into the stomach. She died, utterly exhausted, sixteen days after her admission. At autopsy the whole oesophagus except the lowest inch was greatly dilated and the lower extremity appeared healthy. Mayo was surgeon to the Middlesex Hospital and Professor of Comparative Anatomy at the Royal College of Surgeons, and is regarded as the father of the Middlesex Hospital medical school. Neither Purton nor Mayo offered an explanation for their cases.

Alexander Hannay, Professor of the Theory and Practice of Physic at Glasgow University, is generally said to have been the first to recognise the nature of the condition.[11] In 1833 he described a muscular man of 38 with progressive dysphagia for thirty years typical of achalasia. The patient's general health seemed to be unaffected and there was no obstruction on passing a probang. A bon viveur, he was little inclined to follow Hannay's remedy of temperance. Nonetheless he was fully aware of the obscurity of his case and frequently expressed his desire that for the sake of science he should be opened and the cause sought out. One night he went to a supper party where "he ate most heartily and drank as usual to excess". When he got home he fell asleep on a chair and was found dead the next morning, having fallen forward on his face and on his knees. At post mortem, his oesophagus was enormously dilated and full of food and required above eight gills of water to fill it, "and when so filled it looked like the arm of a person fifteen or sixteen years of age". Sections of the wall were reminiscent of a piece of sole or thick leather. There was no obstruction by tumour or constriction. The lungs were tuberculous but there was no evidence of aspiration. Hannay thought the man had probably died from apoplexy and considered that "a more harmless organic cause of dysphagia was difficult to imagine". Perceptively he argued that repeated attacks of inflammation had probably destroyed the muscular structure and contractile power of the oesophagus so swallowing was impaired.

In 1866 Sir Samuel Wilks (1824–1911), more of whom anon, showed what we would now regard as a typical specimen before the Pathological Society of London.[12] It was obtained at the post mortem examination of a man of 74 who had died of pneumonia. Since childhood there had been difficulty in swallowing solid food and he had been accustomed to regurgitate small quantities. He always ate slowly and washed down every bolus with a draught of fluid. Dr. Rootes of Ross, who had sent the specimen to Wilks, told him that his father, who had looked after the patient since 1812, had taken him 40 years before to Sir Astley Cooper, who had passed a bougie without difficulty into his stomach.

However, until the arrival of X-rays, the disease was misunderstood and only mentioned in textbooks under the general heading of dilatation. Osler in 1901 wrote in his famous textbook of medicine that spasm of the oesophagus was always hysterical even though death could follow it. A pioneer of oesophageal surgery, George Grey Turner (1877–1951) could not recall a case before the First World War, "but physicians were only too ready to speak of hysterical dysphagia and undoubtedly some examples of achalasia masqueraded under it".[13]

The management of achalasia has scarcely altered in over a century. Mercury-filled bougies were recommended by the great Viennese surgeon, Theodor Billroth (1829–94), and this was the method championed by Arthur Hurst, who first described it in 1913.[14] He would pass a series of bougies of increasing size at a single sitting during an X-ray examination, making the point that the largest met with as little resistance as the smallest. The patient was then taught to pass the largest bougie before each meal, leaving it in place for as nearly five minutes as possible. Gradually the frequency was reduced but the bougie was kept by the patient in case it was needed again. Though Hurst claimed excellent results, recurrence was inevitable and the technique had to be repeated indefinitely.

Alternatively the lower end could be stretched forcibly, and curiously the first man to try this was an obscure practitioner in Southport, James Cuningham Russel (1842–1915) who was surgeon to the Lancaster infirmary.[15] Russel recognised that the oesophagus could be obstructed by what he called a spasmodic stricture, and during the last decade of the nineteenth century, he devised a bag that could be expanded with air and used to dilate its lower end. Though the nature of achalasia was far from clear at the time, he wrote, in 1898, that "it should not be assumed that no stricture or spasm exists because none can be detected by a bougie, nor that stricture is not the cause of the symptoms because these persist after the largest possible bougies have been passed". Bearing in mind that this was before the discovery of X-rays, Russel was clearly a man with a cool head and considerable skill; "it is very easy to be deceived on the question as to whether (the instruments) have passed into the stomach or not; measurement of the length passed is not an infallible guide. In using the dilator I always pass it well below the point required, and then withdraw it until I judge it to be on the spot, before expanding." Unfortunately he died during the First World War when obituaries were preoccupied with those killed in action and I know little about him.

In America, Henry Plummer (1874–1937), the first physician to join the Mayo brothers in their new clinic, and best remembered for the Plummer-Vinson syndrome,* modified Russel's device and used water instead of air to inflate the bag. He reported forty cases treated successfully this way.[16] The patient first swallowed six yards of silk so that sufficient reached the intestine to prevent its withdrawal when pulled tight. An instrument was threaded over the silk, at the lower end of which there was a bag that was introduced into the sphincter. The bag was forcibly dilated by hydrostatic pressure. Hurst did not like this method because it was painful and carried a small risk of perforation, and this probably explains why it was neglected for many years in this country, but the long -term results were better than those obtained with his weighted tube.

In fact neither method was entirely satisfactory, which encouraged surgeons to try their hand. An early operation was digital dilatation through the opened stomach, which was first practised by Johann von Mikulicz (1850–1905), another pioneer gastric surgeon in Vienna and early pupil of Billroth.[17] This was never popular partly because it carried the risk of rupturing the oesophagus and partly because dilatation by

---

* Hypochromic anaemia, achlorhydria, atrophic gastritis, dysphagia and glossitis

balloon or bougie seemed just as good. Nonetheless Sir James Walton (1881–1955), a surgeon at the London Hospital, was an advocate of Mikulicz's method and reported complete cure in 68 per cent of his 39 cases though four died.[18] Walton, who was Surgeon to King George V and VI, was best known for his surgery on the biliary tract, and in retirement became a notable gemmologist.

The operation that gradually gained acceptance and is widely used today was devised in 1913 by Ernst Heller (1877–1964), a Leipzig surgeon.[19] He made a longitudinal incision through the muscular wall of the abdominal oesophagus, the operation being analogous with Ramstedt's (1867–1963) operation for congenital pyloric stenosis. He operated on sixteen patients with good results in twelve and no mortality. British surgeons were slow to adopt his procedure, though later Robert Rowlands (1874–1933), a leading surgeon at Guy's Hospital between the two World Wars, undertook the operation with excellent

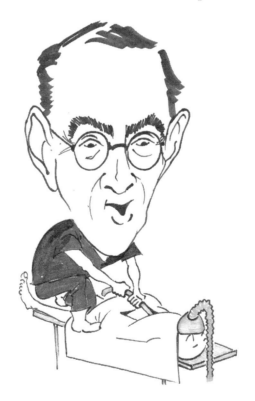

2 Grey Turner – Pull-through – oesophagectomy.

results, but he was unable to get his hand on many cases because Hurst treated most by dilatation.[20]

Earlier I mentioned Grey Turner, the great Geordie surgeon during the first half of the twentieth century and one of the first to tackle the oesophagus. He was influenced by Rutherford Morison (1853–1939), Professor of Surgery in Newcastle, who encouraged him to visit Vienna in 1912 where he met several surgeons from the Billroth school. After service in the RAMC during the First World War, he became consulting surgeon to the Royal Victoria Infirmary, Newcastle, and later Professor of Surgery in the University of Durham. In 1934, at the peak of his power, he had the courage to give up his position in Newcastle to become the first director of surgery at the new British Postgraduate Medical School at Hammersmith. He was particularly interested in cancer surgery, the repair of congenital defects of the urinary tract and of the diseased or damaged oesophagus. He was a small man with a large head and usually wore a bowler hat well down on the back of it. One of my favourite characters, he accepted the new but remembered the old, and this made him a valuable teacher, advisor and leader. Many honours came his way but he never received any civil decoration. His citation for knighthood was, I have read, not supported by the then President of the Royal College of Surgeons.[21]

Grey Turner visited the Mayo Clinic in 1906 and was impressed by Plummer's hydrostatic dilator, which he believed (correctly as it turned out) to be superior to Hurst's mercury-loaded bougies. But he realised that dilatation was not a cure and tried several surgical procedures over the years, while at the same time emphasising the importance of a temporary gastrostomy as a life-saving measure in emaciated patients. In 1920 he made one of his first major excursions into the realm of aggressive intrathoracic surgery on a lad of nineteen with severe achalasia, which he later described in his Bigelow memorial lecture delivered in Boston.[22]

"The patient was miserably thin and ill and very much depressed, for as he was too weak to work he was looked upon as more or less of an encumbrance in his family, who rather grudged him the necessary sustenance. All kinds of treatment had been meted out before he came under my care, and he was only too willing to grasp at any method that held out even the remotest prospect of relief. Assisted by Mr. George A. Mason* who was then my house surgeon, I opened the left chest,

* George Mason (1901–71), thoracic surgeon, Royal Infirmary, Newcastle-upon-Tyne.

explored and mobilised the dilated oesophagus, incised the diaphragm, drew up the stomach and made an anastomosis by direct suture. Convalescence was rather stormy and was marked by a temporary and unexplained paresis of the whole left arm. But eventually recovery was complete and the lad was able to take ordinary food like the other members of his family and soon to resume his occupation. Two and a half years later he was unfortunately knocked down by a motor car and died of his injuries. By the most fortunate coincidence I happened to be enquiring about his progress at that particular time and heard promptly of his demise. An enlightened coroner made it possible to arrange for a postmortem examination and to secure the specimen, which showed the anastomosis large enough to admit the forefinger and beautifully healed."

Subsequently he did a further six oesophago-gastrostomies but from below the diaphragm. This was before the days of antibiotics, modern anaesthesia, blood transfusion and other modern restorative methods, so presumably he preferred to avoid the added risks of entering the thoracic cavity. Nonetheless the sub-diaphragmatic approach was extremely difficult and he turned increasingly to cardioplasty. In his hands Heller's cardiomyotomy was unsatisfactory with recurrent dysphagia so he preferred to carry out a complete cardioplasty.[23]

Unfortunately though oesophago-gastrostomy and cardioplasty certainly helped dysphagia, both operations were plagued by a serious complication that was just beginning to be recognised – reflux oesophagitis. This was highlighted by two of the country's foremost oesophageal surgeons after the Second World War, Norman Barrett and Dick Franklin.

Pasty Barrett (1903–79) as he was perversely known at Eton, because of his somewhat florid complexion, was one of the pioneers of thoracic surgery and, apart from a visit to the Mayo Clinic as a Rockefeller Travelling Fellow, spent all his professional life at St. Thomas's Hospital. For several years he carried out oesophago-gastrostomy on patients with cardiospasm (achalasia), which he found was relatively easy to perform provided that he used a transthoracic approach. None of his patients died and convalescence was smooth. Franklin (1906–91) also trained at St. Thomas's Hospital but moved to the Postgraduate Medical School at Hammersmith in 1935 to be first assistant to Grey Turner. Obviously influenced by the great man, he submitted patients with achalasia to Turner's preferred operation, cardioplasty.

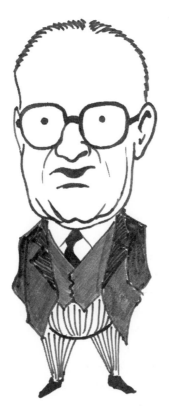

3 Barrett – Achalsia may be rare, my boy, but what are you going to do about it?

Barrett and Franklin knew each other well and soon realised that their patients were not doing well. In 1949 they joined forces to highlight the inevitable and disastrous consequences of destroying the lower oesophageal sphincter.[24] All their patients developed reflux oesophagitis with pain, bleeding and anaemia, which occasionally was extremely difficult to manage; one poor man who had an oesophago-gastrostomy in 1946 subsequently needed a laparotomy, followed by a further exploration through the chest, and yet another thoracotomy with formation of an ileo-jejunal bypass, not to mention over 100 transfusions, before he died from a gastro-jejunal fistula that caused an acute ulcer to rupture into his pericardium. In abandoning both oesophago-gastrostomy and cardioplasty, Barrett and Franklin strongly recommended conservative treatment by which they meant efficient dilatation of the lower oesophagus, preferably with a hydrostatic dilator akin to Plummer's instrument; "the swallowing of mercury bougies is, or should be, a thing of the past." If this failed, an operation that did not interfere with the competency of the cardia must be done, "and the success which follows Heller's procedure rests upon this cardinal point".

Hitherto, with the exception of Arthur Hurst and his colleagues at Guy's Hospital, the surgeons had monopolised the oesophagus. By the middle of the twentieth century thoracotomy was commonplace and oesophageal surgery relatively safe. The thoracic surgeon could rely on X-rays and the new technique of cine-radiography to diagnose motility disorders such as achalasia, and if necessary he could examine the oesophagus with a rigid endoscope under general anaesthetic. There was little for the physician to do.

Yet despite the help of X-rays, exactly how the oesophagus behaved during the act of swallowing was a matter of keen debate. In particular no one could agree on the existence of a sphincter at the lower end of the oesophagus; most accepted that something was preventing reflux but the pathologists were never able to demonstrate an anatomical sphincter. It was this controversy that rekindled interest among physicians. Clinical physiology was still the driving force in medical research and oesophageal motility was an ideal subject for study.

Nowhere was this better seen than at St. Thomas's Hospital during the 1950s under the leadership of Professor Peter Sharpey-Shafer (1908–63) whose enthusiasm was revolutionising research at the hospital. His reader in medicine at the time was Antony Dornhorst (1915–2003) whose primary interest lay in chest disease but easily strayed into the oesophagus. Dornhorst was highly talented and later became Professor of Medicine at St. George's Hospital; he could be prickly and lived up to his Dutch name meaning thornbush. Another member of Sharpey-Shafer's clique was Benjie Pierce (1913–88), a much-loved radiologist who was also on the staff of the Brompton Hospital where with George Simon he made interpretation of the humble chest X-ray a work of art. Pierce was interested in gastrointestinal radiology and collaborated with Dornhorst and a delightful Canadian surgeon at St. Thomas's, George Kent Harrison (1907–87) to study what happened in the normal oesophagus during swallowing.[25] They measured oesophageal pressures in students using manometers fitted to fine polythene tubes. The studies were elegant and certainly showed the well known propulsive wave down the oesophagus, but Dornhorst could not explain what prevented reflux.

He was unable to find evidence for a sphincter and all he could suggest was a valve mechanism formed by heaping up of the muscularis mucosa.

The riddle of the lower oesophageal sphincter mechanism was finally solved by two American investigators working independently, Franz Ingelfinger (1910–80) in Boston and Charles Code (1910–97) at the Mayo Clinic in Rochester, Minnesota. They were contemporaries with considerable respect for one another. Ingelfinger, who emigrated to the United States from Germany in childhood, graduated from Harvard Medical School in 1936 and four years after qualification was appointed chief of gastroenterology at the Evans Memorial Hospital at Boston. For many years he studied intestinal motility and later became the legendary editor of the *New England Journal of Medicine*. Code was a distinguished physiologist and able to take advantage of the huge experience of achalasia at the Mayo Clinic. In recognition of his work he was later asked to deliver the inaugural Arthur Hurst lecture to the British Society of Gastroenterology on "Alimentary motor activity and electrical correlates". During the 1950s both men, using slightly different recording techniques, showed conclusively that there was a segment of increased pressure in the lower oesophagus at the gastro-oesophageal junction. During a swallow, this segment relaxed just ahead of the peristaltic wave sweeping down the oesophagus and quickly contracted again with its arrival.[26]

Ingelfinger and Code went on to show that in patients with achalasia, the normal propulsive peristaltic wave was lost throughout the body of the oesophagus and the lower oesophageal sphincter failed to relax just as Arthur Hurst had originally suggested. They each presented a summary of their work at the International Congress of Gastroenterology held in July 1956 in London.[27/28] This gathering, organised by Thomas Hunt (1901–80) a founder member of the British Society of Gastroenterology, attracted gastroenterologists from far and wide though many from Britain were surgeons rather than physicians; gastroenterology was still in its infancy at the time. Indeed some probably did not think of themselves as gastroenterologists at all such as John Trounce (1920–2007).

Trounce was a general physician at Guy's Hospital with an interest in pharmacology and is probably best remembered to a generation of medical students for his co-authorship of a popular medical textbook known as "Houston, Joiner and Trounce". However, early in his career he followed up the work of Geoffrey Rake and studied the autonomic nerve supply to the oesophagus.[29/30] He obtained strips of tissue from patients undergoing surgery for achalasia and showed that the body of the oesophagus had lost its cholinergic innervation whereas the cardia of the oesophagus still retained some nervous activity. Trounce presented his findings at the London Congress and they neatly complemented the physiological studies of Ingelfinger and Code.

Among the delegates at the congress were two young physicians, Brian Creamer and Michael Atkinson, who were in no doubt that their future lay in the field of gastroenterogy. Creamer (1926–2005) qualified at St. Thomas's Hospital where he spent most of his working life. In 1954–5 he was a research fellow at the Mayo Clinic with Charles Code and his colleague Arthur Olsen, a professor of medicine, and became intimately involved in their research on the oesophageal abnormalities in achalasia.[31] On his return to St. Thomas's Hospital, he repeated Dornhorst's original oesophageal study but this time managed to demonstrate the lower oesophageal sphincter.[32] Whereas Dornhorst had filmed students drinking a cup of barium, which swept unimpeded into the stomach, Creamer asked them to swallow individual mouthfuls, which were held up momentarily by the sphincter. He then abandoned research on the oesophagus and turned his attention to the small intestine, as we shall see later.

Michael Atkinson (born 1925) on the other hand will be remembered for his work on the oesophagus. He received his training at University College Hospital and in 1951 was Registrar to John Hawksley (1903–93) who had started a gastroenterological service there. He learnt to use the semi-flexible Hermon Taylor gastroscope and consolidated his technique while he was Registrar to Sheila Sherlock at the Hammersmith Hospital under the tutelage of Francis Avery Jones. In 1955–6 he was one of the first British graduates to be a research fellow, or "fingerling" as they were known, on Ingelfinger's unit in Boston. The work on oesophageal motility fired his interest in the oesophagus, which stayed with him for the rest of his career. On his return to University College Hospital he worked with Norman (Tom) Rowlands (1912–2003) and David Edwards (1920–2001) and applied the manometric methods he had learnt in America to show that the function of the lower oesophageal sphincter was crucial in preventing reflux in patients with hiatus hernia.[33] After his appointment as lecturer in medicine at Leeds in 1957, he demonstrated that gastro-oesophageal reflux after cardiomyotomy was proportional

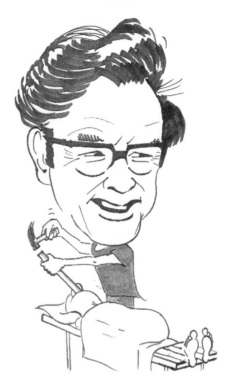

4 Atkinson – Introducing his tube.

to the degree of sphincteric function left by the surgeon, though some patients with no sphincter did not develop symptoms of reflux.[34] This made him realise that there must be another factor helping to prevent reflux, most probably a mechanical valve effect as the oesophagus passed through the diaphragm.

For many years after the Second World War most patients with achalasia were treated by cardiomyotomy, largely because, as we have seen, the oesophagus belonged to the surgeon. Admittedly the likes of Barrett and Franklin recommended forceful dilatation of the lower oesophageal sphincter, but most surgeons were afraid that they would perforate the oesophagus with this method and preferred the safer Heller's type procedure. But with the increasing use of flexible endoscopes during the 1970s, physicians found themselves entranced by the oesophagus and tentatively began to dilate strictures themselves. They were greatly encouraged when in 1983 Michael Atkinson, now a physician at the University Hospital, Nottingham, reported that he had treated 63 patients with achalasia by pneumatic dilatation safely and effectively.[35] Only one patient had a perforation, only a third needed further dilatation and none developed reflux. In his view dilatation was the treatment of choice in achalasia, reserving surgical cardiomyotomy for the failures. In Britain this is now standard practice.

The most sinister complication of achalasia that has been recognised for many years is cancer of the oesophagus.

CHAPTER TWO

CANCER OF THE OESOPHAGUS

In 1901, William Osler wrote that cancer of the oesophagus was not an uncommon disease, yet in a lecture delivered in 1943, George Grey Turner said that some members of the profession thought that cancer of the oesophagus was so infrequent that it was hardly worth considering.[36] The likelihood is that most doctors at the time were preoccupied by infectious disease of one sort or another and that cancer was only just beginning to have an impact as a disease that could be treated. The need for early and accurate diagnosis began to assume great importance, though with its dismal prognosis cancer of the oesophagus was not a priority. The fact that diagnosis of oesophageal cancer was relatively simple was small comfort when even palliative treatment had so little to offer.

Osler wrote from personal experience but was also able to draw on a considerable literature. John Hunter (1728–93), the father of modern scientific surgery in Britain, who always tried to explain his observations, noted that scirrhus (i.e. hard or malignant) ulcers usually affected the upper and lower oesophagus.[37] This was where the oesophagus was narrowest and at risk of injury by the passage of anything sharp or hard. Anyone with an oesophagus predisposed to scirrhus who swallowed such an irritant might develop a scirrhus ulcer. His dissections were later beautifully illustrated and described by his nephew and protégé, Mathew Baillie (1761–1823) in his book, *The Morbid Anatomy of Some of the Most Important Parts of the Human Body,* published in 1793. Hunter may have been wrong about the distribution of oesophageal cancer but he was years ahead of his time and, even today, the best we can say is that certain irritants such as cigarette smoke may trigger the disease in genetically determined individuals.

Another early description came from the pen of a remarkable Edinburgh physician, John Abercrombie (1780–1844), who carried out his own autopsies. In his book, *Pathological and Practical Researches on Diseases of the Stomach, the Intestinal Canal, the Liver, and Other Viscera of the Abdomen*, he describes a man aged 60 "who had been liable for many months to difficulty in swallowing, which had at different times been better and worse, and sometimes entirely removed for a week at a time; but he was now emaciated to a great degree.[38] By the probang (probe) an obstruction was felt about the middle of the oesophagus; and under treatment directed to this in the usual manner, he seemed to improve considerably in swallowing. But his strength continued to sink, and he died after a few weeks. On inspection (at post mortem), there was a slight contraction about the middle of the oesophagus, two inches in extent, without any thickening of its coats. The cardiac orifice was compressed by a tumour the size of a walnut, situated on the outside of the oesophagus, or rather confined under its external membranous covering, without any other disease of the parts". Abercrombie does not say what the usual manner of treatment was but it was almost certainly a liquid diet. I have written in greater detail about Hunter, Baillie and Abercrombie in the chapter on peptic ulcer.

By the middle of the nineteenth century the nature of cancer was coming to light as people looked at tissue sections under the microscope and saw small undifferentiated cells for the first time. This was quickly passed on to medical students by their teachers. One of the most popular lecturers of his time was Sir Thomas Watson (1792–1882) PRCP whose series of lectures on the "Principles and Practice of Physic at King's College, London" ran to five editions. In lecture No 64 on asthma and diseases of the oesophagus (lumped together), he describes a dilated oesophagus with cancerous degeneration of the cardiac orifice of the stomach.[39] He stressed the importance of examining the gullet, which was frequently overlooked; "we are apt, in such cases, to satisfy ourselves with ascertaining the gastric disease, without carefully examining that part of the alimentary canal which lies above". He concludes on a sombre note; "for maladies like these medicine has no cure. Opiates may give comfort, and promote euthanasia: and that is all".

Lecturing to medical students at St. Thomas's Hospital, William Brinton (1823–67), of whom more later, adopted a less nihilistic approach and extolled the merits of enemata as a way to administer food and medicines. "Those who have had the gloomy duty of battling with all the resources of their art against the starvation gradually inflicted by obstructive cancer of the oesophagus, must have been occasionally struck by the length of time to which life can sometimes be protracted, by a sedulous adoption of this plan of nourishing the system. In spite of what seems to be perfect occlusion of the oesophagus, and even in spite of that additional extenuation which is produced by the cancerous cachexia, or by secondary cancerous deposits in the lungs or liver, the patient may sometimes be kept alive day after day – one might almost say week after week – by such alimentation only."[40] He used milk, raw eggs, cod-liver oil, strong unsalted beef tea, wine, and in extreme cases even diluted brandy or opium, and emphasised that enemata should be reduced to the smallest possible size. "The ingestion of liquids may be best accomplished by external applications; such as wet bandages around the arms and legs, and prolonged fomentation or immersion of these limbs in tepid water (to which milk may be sometimes added with great advantage)." Quite what the patient made of all this is not, to my knowledge, recorded, but Brinton was clearly aware that life could be prolonged if nourishment was possible.

Meanwhile William Beaumont's experiments on Alexis St. Martin in the 1820s and 1830s had shown that a gastric fistula was compatible with life, and in 1837 a Norwegian military surgeon, Egeberg, suggested that it should be possible to make "an opening into the cavity of the stomach either for injecting a sufficient quantity of food or for attacking an oesophageal stricture from below". Gradually, after the introduction of anaesthesia in 1846 and antiseptic surgery in the late 1860s, several surgeons attempted to fashion a gastrostomy without success until in 1875 a surgeon at St. Thomas's Hospital, Sydney Jones (1831–1913), had the first recovery.[41] Jones was a quick and brilliant operator, considered by many to be the best of his day in London, and he was receptive to new ideas and techniques. His patient, a man aged 67, was fed through the gastrostomy tube on the sixth day and died of bronchitis and haemorrhage from his oesophageal cancer forty days after the operation.

Thereafter the variety of methods suggested for opening the stomach was almost bewildering. Unfortunately the technique was ill understood by many who simply opened the stomach and anastomosed the opening directly to the abdominal wall, which allowed gastric juice to dribble onto the surface of the abdomen. The skin was digested, the pain was described as unendurable, and the patient welcomed death as a relief from suffering. Fortunately by the end of the nineteenth century, European surgeons had perfected the formation of a valvular orifice, like an inverted ink-bottle, so that fluid could be introduced into the stomach but was unable to escape from it, and this was soon adopted by British surgeons.

Though gastrostomy was a great advance and fulfilled a useful place for several decades, it did not protect the patient from choking and spluttering on his saliva and obviously he could swallow nothing. The concept of inserting a tube down the oesophagus was appealing and had been attempted unsuccessfully as early as 1845 by a Belgian surgeon, Leroy d'Etoilles, using a short tube made of decalcified ivory.[42] In Britain Sir Morell Mackenzie (1837–92) was among the first to toy with the idea. Mackenzie was a notable laryngologist who came to grief when, in 1887, he failed to diagnose laryngeal cancer in no less a patient than Crown Prince Frederick the Noble, heir to the throne of the newly created German Empire. Vilified by the Germans Mackenzie gained further notoriety when he published a book in his defence and was censured by the Royal College of Physicians, after which he resigned his membership. His story highlights how in the nineteenth century the laryngologist was a physician, skilled in examination of the larynx with a light and a mirror – indirect laryngoscopy – and adept at the manipulation of instruments under mirror control yet not allowed to perform external operations. The general surgeon on the other hand could not examine the larynx with a mirror so he acted on the advice of the laryngologist. Only in the twentieth century did the throat surgeon incorporate the skills of the laryngologist.

Even so Victorian surgeons, particularly those who embraced Listerism early, were frequently called upon to tackle tumours of the throat, many of which obstructed the upper oesophagus. Excision was impossible but some inserted rubber tubes. One was John Croft (1833–1905), surgeon to St. Thomas's Hospital, best known for his plaster of Paris splint. He managed to pass a long tube (not unlike a Ryle's tube) through the mouth of two patients, which they "wore" for 149 and 108 days respectively before death.[43] Food was simply poured down the tube. Another was Arthur Durham (1833–95) at Guy's Hospital, a graceful surgeon noted for his invention of a lobster-tailed tracheotomy tube. His patient wore a tube through the mouth for more than four months though it was uncomfortable, causing pain and irritation in the throat.[44] This inspired Sir Charters Symonds (1852–1932), then Assistant Surgeon to Guy's Hospital, a post that carried responsibility for the throat department, to devise a short tube only six inches long that could be pushed through the stricture and left within the oesophagus. At first he fixed the tube to a boxwood funnel with German silver wire. Later he tried ivory and silver instead of boxwood and eventually had the tube and funnel made as one in gum elastic. He would use repeated bouginage until the patient could no longer swallow solids. Thereafter the short tube was introduced for a week or two and could be removed by means of a piece of silk attached to the ear to be cleaned or replaced by a larger one as necrosis "dilated" the stricture.[45] When complete obstruction supervened the tube was replaced by a long tube or a gastrostomy was fashioned. He managed to help one lady, aged 43, who was 6 months pregnant, through her pregnancy and a further 5 months beyond. Symonds was later knighted for his services during the First World War. In fact few adopted his tube because it was inserted blindly with a significant risk of perforation, and it was almost forgotten until revived by Sir Henry Souttar in 1924.

Souttar (1875–1964) was an inventive surgeon with a double first in mathematics from Oxford, where he also studied engineering. Three years after qualifying, while still on the house, he wrote an article in the *British Medical Journal* on the gastroscope and its uses. After distinguished service during the First World War he resumed civilian practice as surgeon to the London Hospital where he gained a great reputation as teacher, clinician and fearless operator. By this time, cancer of the oesophagus was recognised as a common and desperate disease with an annual mortality of roughly 1,600 in England and Wales. The diagnosis could be confirmed by X-rays and oesophagoscopy at which he was an expert. Gastrostomy was in Souttar's opinion a miserable option for the patient "who regarded it as the invention of the devil, leaving him an invalid, kept alive by artificial feeding and debarred from the exercise of a function without which life was not worth living".[46] So he adapted Symonds' method using a coiled metallic tube with an enlarged funnel; he pushed the tube through the tumour under direct vision over a guidewire using the oesophagoscope and a special introducer. In his hands the results were good and he virtually abandoned gastrostomy. Others used it with varying success but the tube often worked loose and migrated into the stomach, especially with growths at the cardia. Furthermore the risk of creating a false passage was still high. Souttar had many interests including the physics of radium and he wrote extensively on this subject, but he is probably best known today for performing the first mitral valvotomy on a girl of 15 in 1925; it would be 22 years before that operation was repeated.

After the Second World War a variety of plastic materials became available and several new tubes appeared. Hitherto they had been pushed through the obstruction either blindly or with the aid of an oesophagoscope, but in 1956 two Frenchmen, Mousseau and Barbin introduced their method of pulling the tube into position through a temporary gastrostomy.[47] This was much safer than the push method but the tube was long and thin so only fluids were possible. It also irritated the oesophageal mucosa causing ulceration and obstruction above its funnel. This led Roger Celestin (born 1925), a research registrar in the department of surgery at the Hammersmith Hospital, to rethink the whole design of oesophageal tubes in the late 1950s.

Celestin was born in Mauritius and like his father won a scholarship to study medicine at University College Hospital, London. Unlike his father, he did not return home but decided to pursue a career in surgery in Britain. At the Hammersmith Hospital he came under the influence of Dick Franklin (1906–91), one of the leading oesophageal surgeons of the time, and soon realised that even in the best hands the results of oesophagectomy for cancer were appalling. The need for an effective, well tolerated tube remained as great as ever.

With Franklin's encouragement, Celestin looked carefully at the distortion of the oesophagus caused by cancer using wax casts. Patients swallowed the wax on the way to theatre and it was removed during oesophagectomy. Comparison of the cast with pictures obtained by cine-radiography showed that even patients with total dysphagia had a lumen of at least four millimetres at the narrowest point. He managed to construct a polythene bougie that could safely negotiate and dilate the lumen. He also modified the funnel of the Mousseau-Barbin tube so that it did not ulcerate the oesophagus. The tube worked well; patients found that they could eat anything provided that they chewed their food thoroughly and they were unaware of the tube's presence.[48]

News of his work spread quickly even before he had had time to publish; during the Victor Negus lecture at the Royal National Throat,

Nose and Ear Hospital, Golden Square in 1958, his chief, Franklin, showed a slide in which he referred to the Celestin tube. Next day the telephone did not stop ringing, and the tube was widely adopted transforming the palliative care of oesophageal cancer.

Celestin was later appointed gastro-intestinal surgeon at Frenchay Hospital, Bristol, where he later introduced a successful, carrot-shaped bougie for dilating oesophageal strictures.[49]

Unfortunately the need for laparotomy and gastrotomy to pull the tube through the oesophagus had its disadvantages. Most patients were old and debilitated and in 1971 Jack Collis (1911–2003), an experienced thoracic surgeon at Queen Elizabeth Hospital, Birmingham reported a disheartening hospital mortality of 31 per cent among his cases undergoing Mousseau-Barbin intubation.[50] Others found the same.

Meanwhile Michael Atkinson had left Leeds in 1962 to take up a post in general medicine in Worcester, where he maintained his interest in gastroenterology once a week as an associate physician in Trevor Cooke's unit in Birmingham. Here he met Collis and shared his dismay at the high mortality from laparotomy and intubation for malignant strictures in the oesophagus.

By now Atkinson was a highly competent endoscopist and one of the first people in Britain to handle the new fibreoptic forward-viewing oesophagoscope that was revolutionising the difficult and dangerous technique of oesophagoscopy. He moved to Nottingham in 1973 and spurred on by the high mortality from intubation decided to re-explore the possibility of endoscopic intubation with the flexible endoscope using the old push technique, thereby avoiding the need for laparotomy.[51] The results were very encouraging; he found that he was usually able to pass the flexible endoscope through a malignant stricture and assess its extent before intubation though sometimes the stricture needed dilating first. Then he passed a modified Celestin tube mounted on an introducer over a guide wire in much the same way as Souttar had done years before. During the development of the "Atkinson tube" he was ably assisted by his senior registrar, Roger Ferguson (born 1946), who had been introduced to the technique of endoscopy by Atkinson when he was his registrar in Worcester.[52] Ferguson moved to the Wirral Hospital and was succeeded by Alan Ogilvie (born 1950) now at Northampton; and Michael Dronfield (born 1946) now in Peterborough.[53] The group showed that palliative endoscopic intubation was remarkably safe and effective; patients were delighted to be able to swallow again and most of them could be managed at home during their final illness.

For twenty years plastic stents were widely used until superseded by self-expanding metal stents developed in America. These are easier to insert and less likely to perforate the oesophagus but cannot be removed should the need arise.

The prognosis of cancer of the oesophagus was so poor that most surgeons were deterred from aggressive surgery for many years. Souttar, writing in 1927, believed that these tumours were, and never could be, amenable to direct surgical attack, except in cases so rare as to be of no practical importance. Yet the only prospect of cure was radical surgery and occasionally a striking success was reported. Supreme among these must be a patient operated upon in 1909 by Arthur Evans (1872–1950), surgeon to the Westminster Hospital and laryngologist to many music hall and opera singers. The case is so incredible as to be almost the stuff of fiction by H. G. Wells (1866–1946), who actually taught Evans biology when he was not writing his stories.

A lady aged 40 presented with dysphagia in 1909 due to a large malignant mass in the lower pharynx and upper oesophagus. Evans advised against operation but later succumbed to her entreaties. After a preliminary gastrostomy, he opened the neck anteriorly and excised what he could, leaving her with a fistula in the neck and a tracheostomy. Examining the specimen he found that he had sectioned the oesophagus too near the growth (squamous cell carcinoma) so he retrieved the oesophageal stump and removed another inch – which was as far as his fingers could reach within the thorax. Later he tidied up the fistula and connected it to the gastrostomy with a long rubber empyema tube that the lady hid beneath her blouse. After some initial trouble with the tube she prospered and put on weight. In 1932 she wrote "I am thankful to say I am very well. I have to be careful not to take a cold, and if I do a bit too much the tube chafes the entrance to the stomach, and I have to rest a day; but I really lead a normal life. I often go into B – for a day's shopping and lunch at a restaurant – so the swallowing tube acts well. No one seems to notice my whisper."[54] She was still alive and in good health in 1943, 32 years after the operation.

Surgeons were afraid to attack the oesophagus across the pleural cavity for several reasons; for example it was thought, on the basis of animal experiments, that a large opening in the chest wall would cause mediastinal displacement, cardiac flutter and death. There were also worries about pleural infection, which would be disastrous, and a third concern was the inability to control ventilation (this was before the days of positive pressure anaesthesia).

Yet as early as 1913, a New York surgeon, Franz Torek (1861–1938), caused almost a sensation in the profession when he successfully removed the oesophagus for carcinoma by the transthoracic route.[55] The patient enjoyed good health until her death from pneumonia fourteen years later without any sign of recurrence.

Torek's case was an inspiration to surgeons such as Grey Turner, who spent years after the First World War hoping to emulate him. But he was fearful of the transthoracic approach and preferred his collo-abdominal or pull-through method. This involved opening the abdomen to free the lower end of the gullet and opening the neck to free the upper end. Then, working from above downwards in the neck, and from below upwards in the abdomen, the oesophagus was freed and pulled out. Eventually, in 1933, he had his first success after "several encouraging failures".[56] He managed to remove the whole of the thoracic oesophagus and to restore the power of swallowing by the construction of an antethoracic gullet. This type of gullet was first devised in 1904 by Jean Roux, the "Tiger of Lausanne", long before the days of thoracotomy. He brought a loop of mobilised small intestine up under the skin of the chest to about the level of the clavicle and joined it to the oesophageal stump.[57] As a young man Grey Turner had watched Roux operating and been profoundly influenced by his meticulous attention to detail.[58]

Unfortunately successes were few and progress was hampered during the late 1930s by the shadow of the Second World War. However, in America surgical energy refused to be fettered, and by 1940 John Garlock (1896–1965), another surgeon from New York, had reported six successful operations using Torek's thoracic approach.[59]

Though surgeons now felt at home with thoracotomy for lung diseases, this did not yet include the oesophagus. Its position – in the very lifeline of the thorax – made its removal by this route formidable. Apart from the technical demands on the surgeon, the patients were often old and frail, and blood transfusion, modern anaesthesia and antibiotics, to say nothing of intravenous feeding, were still in their infancy. The cases described by Garlock, and a further two by Dick Franklin at the

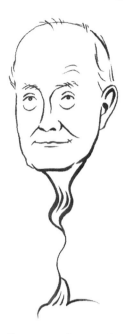

5 Franklin – Congenital oesophageal – atresia.

Hammersmith Hospital in 1942 (encouraged by Grey Turner) were notable chiefly for the fact that these men managed to remove the oesophagus at all.[60] No attempt was made to restore continuity of the gut within the thorax; instead an external artificial oesophagus was constructed from rubber tubes, and this miserable arrangement demanded exceptional co-operation from the patient, assuming he lived long enough to use it. Successful surgery merely implied that the patient had survived the operation and was able to leave hospital, but most were dead within two years.

In fact Grey Turner and others realised that it must be better to restore the functional capacity of the original oesophagus than to supplant it with an extrathoracic tube, however ingeniously this might be constucted. He predicted that restoration in situ by anastomosis to the fundus of the stomach mobilised into the chest would be the method of choice. Indeed this was already a reality for tumours at the lower end of the oesophagus. A Japanese surgeon, Ohsawa, as far back as 1933 had managed to excise a growth, mobilising the stomach upwards after extending his abdominal incision into the thorax.[61] In 1938 surgeons in America carried out the first successful thoracotomy to remove a growth from the cardia and rejoin the stomach to the oesophagus in the lower chest (oesophagogastrostomy).[62]

Others soon followed and in Britain Vernon Thompson (1905–95), a surgeon at the London Hospital and the London Chest Hospital, had the first success in 1941.[63] The next year Russell Brock (1903–80), later Lord Brock, of Guy's Hospital and cardiac surgery fame, published a case.[64] As they were skilled thoracic surgeons this was almost to be expected but the third man to report a case was a little known general practitioner surgeon in Guildford, Gerald Steele (1903–46). Steele was educated at University College Hospital where he won several prizes and the gold medal at the University of London MB, BS examination. After settling in general practice at Guildford he was appointed surgeon to St. Luke's Hospital in 1928, the year he became a Fellow of the Royal College of Surgeons. He performed his successful operation in 1943,[65] but sadly just three years later he became severely depressed after his wife's death, and took poison.

Surgeons now knew that they could at last tackle tumours in the distal oesophagus through a left-sided thoracotomy, drawing the stomach through the diaphragm and anastomosing it to the cut end of the oesophagus. But neoplasms further up the oesophagus presented them with a much greater challenge, being far less accessible, and many felt that radiotherapy was the better option. Admittedly a few eminent British surgeons had managed to remove the whole oesophagus using Torek's original approach from the left side of the chest, including Tudor Edwards (1890–1946), an operator of supreme skill at the Westminster Hospital,[66] and Philip Allison (1907–74), the first thoracic surgeon in Leeds,[67] but none of their patients survived more than a few months and there was no question of replacing the oesophagus with anything but a rubber tube. The snag was that though left-sided thoracotomy provided reasonable access to the oesophagus it left the surgeon with a very difficult gastric anastomosis, if indeed this was contemplated. However, Franklin had shown with his cases in 1942 that it was in fact perfectly feasible to remove the whole oesophagus through a right-sided thoracotomy, and it was this that paved the way for the first successful oesophagogastric anastomoses for cancer of the middle oesophagus by two London surgeons working quite independently of each other.

Remarkably both men worked in municipal hospitals. The first was a Welshman, Ivor Lewis (1895–1982), who was never on the staff of a great teaching hospital nor was he a Fellow of the Royal College of Surgeons. After several years as a surgeon in Plymouth he moved to the North Middlesex Hospital in 1933 where he established his reputation as a thoracic surgeon. In 1939 he accomplished the first successful pulmonary embolectomy, which remained unequalled for many years. During the war he performed half a dozen oesophagectomies and found that recurrence was likely to occur early and always before he had time to reconstruct the oesophagus. The wretched patient not only underwent a formidable operation but had the added misery of a gastrostomy and an additional stoma in the neck discharging several ounces of saliva on their chest wall every day. Determined to find a way around this problem he took himself to the postmortem room and showed by repeated dissections of the cadaver that the whole of the distal oesophagus could be removed through the right pleura (as Franklin had shown). Further dissections showed that if the stomach was mobilised it could be brought up through the enlarged hiatus and the fundus could be actually brought up as far as the apex of the pleura. So it seemed to him possible not only to remove the oesophagus, but to complete the operation by an oesophagogastrostomy at any level demanded. His first patient, a 66-year-old metal-polish worker, presented with a malignant stricture in the mid oesophagus in August 1944.[68] Surgery went as planned and the operation took just over three hours. Recovery was uneventful and eighteen months later he was well with a good appetite and able to eat anything without discomfort. For this pioneering work Lewis was appointed as a Hunterian professor and elected a Fellow of the Royal College of Surgeons in 1948. A key factor in his success was his wife, Nancie, who was his expert anaesthetist for many years.

The second surgeon, Norman Tanner (1906–82), also made his name in the developing municipal hospital service and became senior resident surgeon at St. James's Hospital, Balham, in 1939. He remained on the staff there until his retirement, by which time Balham was a household name among surgeons. Early on the facilities were appalling and a visiting surgeon once said that he had never seen better gastric surgery done in such primitive conditions. In 1944 Tanner developed an almost identical operation for removing carcinoma of the oesophagus as Lewis performed[69] and this quickly became known as the Lewis-Tanner procedure. Many honours came his way including his election as President of the British Society of Gastroenterology in 1968.

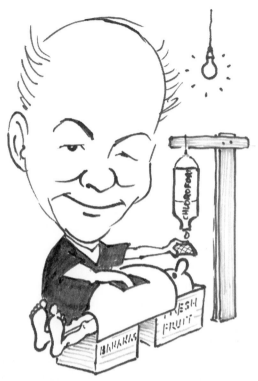

6 Tanner – Few resources and appalling facilities.

Suddenly an air of optimism replaced the previous pessimism. Oesophagectomy, which provided the only hope of cure, was now feasible and with experience the high operative mortality began to fall. Thoracic surgeons throughout the land tackled the problem with some success and by 1949 Allison in Leeds was reporting that 33 per cent of his cases were still alive two years after their operation.[70] This was impressive but tempered by the fact that more than half his patients were inoperable in the first place and the operative mortality was about twenty per cent. Moreover the number of patients with middle or upper oesophageal cancer surviving more than five years after resection was infinitesimal. Many physicians and surgeons remained sceptical about radical surgery and advised simple palliation with an oesophageal tube or radiotherapy. Radiotherapy was championed by David Smithers (1908–95), later Sir David, who found that nine per cent of all his cases treated at the Royal Marsden Hospital were alive after two years.[71] In particular patients with cancer in the upper oesophagus fared better after radiotherapy than surgery.

Smithers' findings prompted Jack Collis (1911–2003) in Birmingham to defend the case for surgery. During the first decade after the Second World War Collis saw over 300 patients with carcinoma of the oesophagus and his results were remarkably similar to Allison's.[72] Particularly gratifying was his operative mortality that fell as his surgical experience increased, and even patients discovered at operation to be incurable felt better if their tumour was excised. He found that patients with middle or lower oesophageal tumours were three times more likely to be alive in two years after surgery than after radiotherapy. This encouraged most surgeons to continue radical excision as often as possible, and an extension of the Lewis-Tanner operation was devised by Kenneth McKeown (1912–95), yet another surgeon at a non-teaching hospital.[73]

As a young man McKeown had served in the Royal Army Medical Corps as a surgical specialist. After the war he was appointed lecturer in surgery in Grey Turner's department at the Hammersmith Hospital where he came under the influence of the experienced and practical Dick Franklin (1906–91). In 1950 he moved to the Darlington Memorial Hospital in Yorkshire where he developed a new consultant surgical service supported by general practitioner anaesthetists. Fired by his experience at the Hammersmith, McKeown began to operate on patients with oesophageal cancer. Though a general surgeon, he had dealt with many gunshot wounds of the chest during the war and felt at home with thoracotomy. Gradually he took on more difficult tumours in the mid-oesophagus, perfecting the Lewis-Tanner technique. He was concerned by the risk of leaks from the anastomosis with their procedure and added a third cervical phase of his own, which made it safer. It was a long operation, so after freeing up the stomach through an opening in the abdomen (phase one), he insisted on a tea break. Next he dissected out the oesophagus through a right-sided thoracotomy (phase two), and had a further tea break. Finally he opened the neck and pulled up the oesophagus and stomach through the opening. He then excised the diseased oesophagus and completed a simple anastomosis between the oesophageal stump and the stomach (phase three). By now he was probably ready for a gin and tonic. This operation brought McKeown international fame and he was awarded a Hunterian professorship in 1972. He always thought of himself as a general surgeon and in his memoirs, *A Tale of Two Citadels*, he recalls how, soon after his appointment in 1950, he removed the colon from a lady with severe colitis. The patient recovered but could not contemplate a permanent ileostomy and attempted suicide, so reluctantly he agreed to join her diseased rectum to the small bowel. To his astonishment she did very well, bore two children and was still alive 40 years later. This may have been the first case of ileo-rectal anastomosis carried out for ulcerative colitis (see under colitis, page 73).[74]

Oesophagectomy was now the standard treatment for cancer of the oesophagus in spite of its having the highest mortality of any operation routinely performed and the fact that the majority of patients were incurable. Why was this? Surgeons argued that excision offered the best, if not the only, chance of a cure and often the full extent of the disease only became apparent at operation, when it was still reasonable, they said, to carry out some form of palliative surgery or by-pass procedure. They were highly competent operators, took pride in their handicraft and managed to convince themselves that major surgery of this nature was worth a try. Several published their results, which certainly demonstrated their surgical prowess but they frequently failed to comment on the long-term survival of their patients. In contrast, radiotherapy, which can be highly effective for squamous cell cancer, was reserved for people thought to be inoperable or too frail to withstand surgery, and inevitably the results were disappointing.

But there were misgivings among the more conservative surgeons who were anxious to avoid an unnecessary procedure, which carried its own risk of death. One was Richard Earlam (born 1934), a thoracic surgeon at the London Hospital, who had long been interested in oesophageal disease having worked with Dr. F. Henry Ellis Jr., a surgeon at the Mayo Clinic, in 1966. Earlam could see that the results of surgery were dreadful but realised that if he wanted to change the climate of opinion he needed to produce compelling evidence to support his views. No two surgeons reported their results in quite the same way so he had to pool the figures from a very large number of studies before drawing any conclusions. Wherever possible he excluded adenocarcinoma of the lower oesophagus, which he regarded as a different disease (cancer of the stomach). Eventually with the help of his Brazilian research assistant, Cunha-Melo, he reviewed over 84,000 patients treated worldwide between 1960 and 1980 and managed to calculate what happened to any 100 patients in a community.[75] The figures were stark and brought home the grim message. No fewer than 58 would be operated upon, only 39 would have their tumour resected and 13 of these would die in hospital. Of the 26 who went home after resection only 9 would be alive at the end of two years.

At the same time Earlam looked at the figures for radiotherapy and despite the fact that this treatment was generally used for those patients with extensive disease or those who were unfit for surgery, he found that the two-year survival was eight per cent, and of course there was no operative mortality.[76]

This was uncomfortable news for the more aggressive surgeons for two reasons. Firstly one third of the patients undergoing thoracotomy had widespread cancer that was beyond resection. Clearly better ways were needed to find out if a tumour was resectable before subjecting people to surgery. As it happened Earlam's survey was carried out in 1980 just as CT scanning was being introduced, and this has undoubtedly helped to identify many of the tumours that are inoperable. Then a decade later endoscopic ultrasound appeared, which gave crucial information about the size and invasiveness of oesophageal cancers. As a result the number of patients undergoing futile thoracotomies has fallen dramatically.

Secondly Earlam's study highlighted that on the face of it there was nothing to choose between major surgery and radiotherapy. What was needed was a prospective controlled trial comparing the two treatments. Accordingly a Medical Research Council working party on oesophageal cancer was formed with Earlam as chairman to run a trial. The country's thoracic surgeons agreed to contribute 400 patients with operable squamous cell carcinoma of the oesophagus each year. Radiotherapy would be compared with surgery and survival would be assessed at one, three and five years.[77] The trial began in 1986 but had to be abandoned after two years when only 40 patients had been recruited. The surgeons had changed their minds and felt unable to give up their patients. Some even suggested that Earlam could not, or would not, operate and to this day the trial has not been done and probably never will be.

CHAPTER THREE

BARRETT'S OESOPHAGUS

For years doctors have tried to find out why people get cancer of the oesophagus. The disease is often so advanced at presentation that until the cause is known and can be prevented, the prognosis is unlikely to improve. There is no evidence for a strong genetic component though 50 years ago, in 1954, Cyril Clarke (1907–2000), doyen of medical genetics in Liverpool, and Richard McConnell (1920–2003), a gastroenterologist particularly interested in genetics, described a remarkable family in which no fewer than six members had carcinoma of the oesophagus.[78] This strongly suggested dominant inheritance, but the finding could have been due to chance. However, shortly afterwards, they found a second family in which twelve cases of carcinoma of the oesophagus had occurred. Both families lived in Liverpool and a century earlier both had originated in the same district of the city. They were probably related, in which case eighteen cases of oesophageal cancer had occurred in three generations.[79] The victims all had keratosis of the hands and feet known as tylosis, which is inherited as Mendelian dominant. This particular form of tylosis is very rare, and now known to be strongly associated with carcinoma of the oesophagus.

As the case for a genetic component was weak, clinicians looked at possible environmental factors, and it has long been known for example that heavy smokers are prone to cancer of the oesophagus, presumably from the irritant effect of tobacco on squamous epithelium. By the same token, as mentioned above, cancer occasionally occurs as a complication of achalasia of the cardia. This was first observed in 1872 by Hilton Fagge (1838–83), physician to Guy's Hospital, who was to die after a long illness at the early age of 45, just before the completion of his textbook, *The Principle and Practice of Medicine*, which was published posthumously and ran to four editions. Fagge described and illustrated a carcinoma commencing within a dilated oesophagus in a man of 84 who had had difficulty in swallowing for 40 years.[80]

The association was so rare that it was not until 1930 that Arthur Hurst and Geoffrey Rake first noticed it.[81] They came across three patients in all of whom the diagnosis was overlooked including a man of 43 who had been admitted to Guy's Hospital in the last stages of malignant cachexia. He gave a history of some disability in swallowing for many years but his whole story was very vague. Secondary nodules of carcinoma were felt in the right tibia and elsewhere, but the primary tumour was not found before death, which occurred within four days. At autopsy a greatly dilated oesophagus was found characteristic of achalasia. The oesophagus was found to contain quantities of decomposing, fluid food debris. The mucous membrane was severely inflamed and had many epithelial warts scattered on its surface, one of which had become malignant. They thought that the papillomas or warts arose as a response to repeated irritation from putrifying food and that occasionally these turned malignant.

Even after the Second World War only 28 cases of oesophageal carcinoma complicating achalasia had been reported, and many believed that the association was pure chance. However, in the early 1970s Ronald Belsey (1910–2008) showed that the development of the two diseases in the same patient was more than coincidence.[82] Belsey was an energetic surgeon with a forceful personality; he qualified at St. Thomas's Hospital and was appointed thoracic surgeon in Bristol in 1946, where he became one of the pioneers in oesophagectomy and hiatus hernia repair. After 25 years he had operated upon nearly 200 patients with cancer of the oesophagus and nine of these arose in patients with achalasia, far more than could be put down to chance. However, achalasia was a rare condition accounting for very few cases of cancer, whereas Barrett's oesophagus, another pre-cancerous condition, was not.

Norman Barrett (1903–79) was an influential but modest man and would be the first to agree that the famous eponym called after him was a fluke. When he wrote about peptic ulcer of the oesophagus in 1950 his intention was to distinguish it from reflux oesophagitis, with which it was easily confused. In this he was undoubtedly successful but unfortunately he argued that the ulcer was simply a gastric ulcer occurring in stomach pulled into the chest by a congenitally short oesophagus. At first he did not believe that the lower oesophagus was lined by ectopic gastric mucosa. For those who appreciate eponyms as I do, the name Barrett's ulcer seems more justified than Barrett's oesophagus.

In 1900 all inflammatory conditions affecting the gullet were considered as varieties of oesophagitis but in 1906 Wilder Tileston (1875–1919), a New Haven physician, drew attention to peptic ulcer of the oesophagus, which he said exactly simulated chronic gastric ulcer.[83] In his four autopsies the ulcer lay in the oesophagus but the mucosa was gastric in type, which he assumed to be ectopic. His work excited little attention because no one was particularly interested in the oesophagus, radiology was still in its infancy and oesophagoscopy was a dangerous and difficult technique. The condition went unrecognised in Britain for many years until 1929, when two important publications appeared. The first came from Chevalier Jackson (1865–1958), the legendary laryngologist from Philadelphia, who was a master with the rigid oesophagoscope. In the course of 42 years he had seen 21 active ulcers and 67 scars of healed ulcers in a personal series of 4,000 oesophagoscopies.[84] Obviously this relatively benign condition was being overlooked by clinicians. The second publication was by Matthew Stewart (1885–1956) and Stanley Hartfall (1899–1982) in Leeds who reported the death of a man from perforation of an oesophageal ulcer.[85] Professor Stewart was an eminent pathologist, renowned for his work on peptic ulceration, but this was the first time that he had come across an ulcer in the oesophagus in the course of over 10,000 autopsies. The ulcer lay just above the gastro-oesophageal junction and was associated with heterotopic mucosa and he thought that regurgitation of the stomach contents was the cause. Hartfall was the medical registrar in Leeds (there was only one for the whole city at that time) and shortly afterwards he moved to Guy's Hospital as medical assistant to Arthur Hurst, before returning to Leeds as Professor of Therapeutics in 1936.

Hurst who had just collaborated with Stewart on their great monograph, *Gastric and Duodenal Ulcer*, was somewhat shaken by the fact that he had never seen or recognised an oesophageal ulcer himself. By this time he was senior physician at Guy's Hospital but spent most of his week in private practice at New Lodge Clinic, a nursing home in Windsor Great Park. Here, in conjunction with his long-standing friend and colleague P. J. Briggs, a skilful radiologist, and supported by a succession of residents from Guy's Hospital, he carried out much of his clinical research. Oesophageal ulcers were easy to miss clinically as for example was the case in Glasgow where a pathologist, Alexander Lyall, found eight chronic ulcers in 1,500 post mortem examinations between 1932 and 1936, none of which had been suspected in life. Lyall singled out one case with ectopic mucosa: "close examination of the mucous membrane in the region of the ulcer showed the presence of a remarkable state of affairs. The intact mucosa separating the lateral edges of the ulcer was found to be heterotopic gastric mucosa which extended as a tongue-shaped process of well-preserved tissue upwards from that of the fundus of the stomach...The mucosa bore a resemblance to that normally found towards the pyloric end of the stomach."[86]

Hurst and Briggs recognised their first case in 1933 and went on to diagnose fifteen more ulcers at New Lodge before the clinic was closed at the outbreak of the Second World War.[87] The diagnosis depended on a high index of suspicion, careful radiology and occasionally oesophagoscopy, though this was unreliable because spasm often prevented access to the ulcer itself. Hurst was in no doubt that the cause of these ulcers, which always lay above the cardiac sphincter, was gastric juice regurgitating through an incompetent cardia caused by a congenitally short oesophagus. He wondered about acid secretion from heterotopic gastric mucosa but this was impossible to detect with the oesophagoscope and unlikely to be important. Hurst reported this series of patients with the help of Robert Dick, his last RMO at New Lodge.[88] R. C. S. Dick (1917–2004) is best remembered for his outstanding skill as a rugby player. He was captain of the Guy's Hospital team and as a medical student represented his country, Scotland, for four years including 1938 when the team won the Triple Crown. After the war he emigrated to New Zealand. Hurst meanwhile had moved to Oxford during the Second World War, and within two years he was dead. He had asthma and died suddenly in an attack at the home of his friend, Lionel Hardy, in Birmingham in 1944.

Before the Second World War herniation of the stomach through the oesophageal hiatus was scarcely recognised in this country and on the rare occasion when it was found radiologists assumed that it was associated with congenital shortening of the oesophagus. Only a Berlin physician, Professor Gustav von Bergmann (1878–1955), believed that herniation was a common occurrence.[89] The hernia that he described was small and intermittent and could be demonstrated using a special

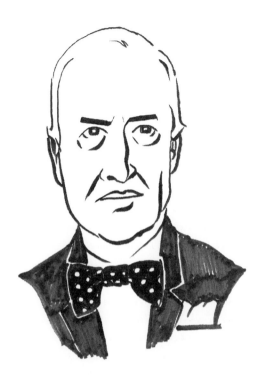

7 Allison – Not a man to be trifled with.

radiological technique. The oesophagus was of normal length and the tissues of the hiatus through which it passed were abnormally lax. But Bergmann's views attracted little attention in Britain because the hernia could be produced in half the elderly population if the abdomen was compressed and the patient tipped upside down. It was thought to be clinically unimportant and was ignored until Philip Allison (1907–74), the first and technically outstanding thoracic surgeon in Leeds, and his radiological colleague A. S. Johnstone, described seven patients with oesophageal ulcer in 1941.[90] They all had definite shortening of the oesophagus but Allison realised that this was not the predisposing cause. He believed that his patients had Bergmann's type of hernia, which he called a sliding hernia that they had acquired later in life.[91] This was not a congenital condition and the oesophagus became shortened by cicatricial contraction of the ulcer.

Allison continued his studies over the next decade and showed that the angle of the oesophagus as it passed through the diaphragm created a valve-like mechanism that helped to prevent reflux. If the hiatus was lax the stomach could slide through it and hang like a bell from the oesophagus eliminating the valve mechanism. If in addition the intrinsic cardiac sphincter was weak, reflux ensued. Most of his patients were refluxing gastric contents into the oesophagus and had oesophagitis. This in turn caused spasm or ulceration and scarring resulting in shortening of the oesophagus.[92]

By 1950 Allison had established an international reputation and was generally held to be a leader in his field. He had seen over 200 patients with hiatus hernia, only one of whom, in his opinion, had congenital shortening of the oesophagus, which he regarded as extremely rare.[93] Of the rest one third had a chronic oesophageal ulcer with stenosis, one third had superficial oesophagitis and the rest were normal. The surprisingly high proportion of patients with a stricture was to be expected in patients referred to a thoracic unit.

Allison believed that without surgical treatment the oesophagitis could progress to chronic ulceration, fibrosis and stricture formation. The hernia would no longer be reducible and a difficult resection of the stricture would be needed. Much better to repair the hernia early, and by 1950 he had tackled half the hernias of patients who had simple oesophagitis before they developed stenosis. He reduced the hernia using a thoracic approach and simply stitched up the hiatus. Initially his patients did well but recurrence was common and his operation was later abandoned in favour of some form of fundoplication.[94]

Allison's research stimulated widespread interest in hiatus hernia and the numbers rose rapidly as people began to look for it. At the Central Middlesex Hospital for example the radiologists found only 5 cases in 1947, but the number had risen to 61 by 1951. The condition naturally attracted the attention of several thoracic surgeons, none more so than Ronald Belsey in Bristol who devoted many years to anti-reflux surgery.[95] He developed a type of fundoplication procedure in which the distal oesophagus was partially invaginated into the stomach. This then acted as a substitute sphincter by compressing the lower oesophagus as intragastric pressure increased, thus preventing gastro-oesophageal reflux. The main drawback to his operation was that it required a thoracic approach and for this reason most surgeons preferred another type of fundoplication, devised by Nissen in Switzerland, that used the easier abdominal approach.[96] Incidentally it was Nissen who coined the term fundoplication.

In 1950 gastric and duodenal ulcer was a national scourge with ten per cent of the male population smitten by the disease and unable to work. The problem dominated the minds of most clinicians but now people who had not given the oesophagus a thought were suddenly confronted by this outbreak of oesophagitis. Was this the same condition as oesophageal ulcer described by Hurst and others? Were they about to witness an epidemic of peptic ulcers in the oesophagus with all the problems of bleeding and perforation for which they were notorious? It was to allay their concerns that Barrett attempted to clarify the matter.[97]

First he paid tribute to Allison's work and emphasised that the ulceration he was reporting was common and important and could best be described as reflux oesophagitis. He included the ulcers reported by Hurst in this group. So far so good. Next he put forward his view that the only true way to distinguish the oesophagus from the stomach was by the nature of its mucous membrane. If this was squamous it was oesophagus, if columnar it was stomach. It was as simple as that. If a patient had a congenitally short oesophagus the lower part of the gullet was in fact stomach even if it did not look like stomach anatomically. The cases reported by Tileston, Stewart and Hartfall, and Lyall were not, he suggested, peptic ulcers of the oesophagus at all but peptic ulcers of the stomach, which happened to lie in the chest because the oesophageal was congenitally short. Fortunately they were rare and of little clinical significance.

Allison was delighted with Barrett's coinage of the term reflux oesophagitis but took issue with him over his views of the oesophagus lined with gastric mucosa.[98] This was surely not stomach for three reasons. Firstly it had no peritoneal lining, secondly congenital short oesophagus was excessively rare, and thirdly the gastric mucosa was not true gastric mucosa because it did not contain oxyntic cells. To call this segment of the lower oesophagus stomach was merely replacing one confusion with another. He suggested that the abnormality, which from the outside looked like oesophagus and from the inside looked like stomach, should be referred to as "oesophagus lined with gastric mucous membrane". At the same time to avoid confusion he was happy to refer to the occasional ulcer occurring within this area as Barrett's ulcer.

So why did the condition of columnar-lined oesophagus become known as Barrett's oesophagus? The answer seems to be that Barrett was the first to distinguish the ulcer known as Barrett's ulcer and the fact that he modified his opinion considerably over the next few years and wrote and spoke extensively on the subject. Allison on the other hand wrote little further on the matter.

By the time he addressed the International Congress of Gastroenterology in London in 1956 Barrett had accepted Allison's view that congenital shortening of the oesophagus was rare and that the lower end was indeed lined by what appeared to be gastric mucous membrane.[99] He rebuffed those anxious to remind him that islets of ectopic gastric mucosa had been recognised for half a century by pointing out that these islets only occurred in the upper oesophagus and were quite different from the continuous, unbroken sheet of columnar epithelium spreading upward from the oesophagogastric junction that he was now describing.

Later in the same year he gave a lecture at the Mayo Clinic summarising his latest views, many of which hold good today.[100] The condition was probably the result of a failure of the embryonic lining of the gullet to achieve normal maturity but could conceivably be acquired by repeated reflux of digestive gastric juice, which would help to explain why it always involved the lower oesophagus. It was often but not always associated with a sliding hiatus hernia. Oesophagoscopy was the only way to make the diagnosis in the absence of complications such as oesophagitis, benign stricture, Barrett's ulcer or even an adenocarcinoma. Though many of the symptoms were shared with hiatus hernia, accurate diagnosis was important because of its unique complications.

It is easy to see why the simple eponym, Barrett's oesophagus, was preferred to the descriptive but long-winded columnar-lined lower oesophagus or worse, CLLO. However, for some years interest in the condition was limited; it was thought to be rare, only thoracic surgeons who were adept with a rigid oesophagoscope could recognise it and most treated it as a medical curiosity. Adenocarcinoma of the oesophagus arising in an area of ectopic mucosa was almost unheard of; Alan Carrie in Toronto described a case in 1950 but this came from ectopic mucosa in the upper end of the oesophagus. He reviewed the literature and likened the lesion to the unicorn in that many authors had described it, but only one had ever seen it.[101]

In fact Basil Morson and John Belcher described an adenocarcinoma of the mid-oesophagus that was removed by Mr. (later Sir) Thomas Holmes Sellors at the Middlesex Hospital in 1952.[102] The mucous membrane above the tumour was entirely squamous in type and the lining below the growth was entirely glandular. They also noted that the glandular membrane was more intestinal than gastric in appearance and contained many goblet cells. This was the first example of an adenocarcinoma definitely arising in Barrett's oesophagus, though it was several years before people were convinced of the risk. Only eight more cases had been recorded by 1970.

More convincing evidence came during the early 1970s from America and Switzerland, where surgeons noticed that more patients with Barrett's oesophagus were developing cancer than was expected. These reports coincided with the introduction of flexible fibreoptic endoscopy that was to transform the practice of gastroenterology. For the first time gastroenterologists everywhere began to see what Barrett had been describing all those years before. Workers in Boston identified a distinctive type of intestinal metaplasia that they called specialised columnar epithelium, which helped to clarify the histological diagnosis.[103] In Britain Christopher Stoddard (born 1948) a surgeon in Liverpool and David Day (born 1947) a pathologist confirmed these findings and suggested that this intestinal metaplasia was particularly prone to dysplasia, which in their view was the best indicator of potential malignant transformation.[104]

Once oesophagoscopy became widely available clinicians realised that Barrett's oesophagus was quite common, affecting perhaps ten per cent of patients with reflux oesophagitis, and therefore the most important predisposing factor for oesophageal adenocarcinoma yet known. Oddly enough an immediate difficulty was literally where to draw the line, how to define the oesophago-gastric junction, how in fact to decide if an individual had Barrett's or not. The diagnosis was straightforward in patients with long segments of columnar epithelium extending well into the middle or upper oesophagus but much more difficult in those with short segments of oesophageal columnar lining, particularly in the presence of a hiatal hernia and severe reflux oesophagitis. It was only too easy to make a false positive diagnosis of Barrett's oesophagus by taking specimens of columnar epithelium from the stomach by mistake. So during the 1980s several groups adopted arbitrary criteria for the diagnosis according to the length of the columnar lining; for example Stoddard included only patients who had more than five centimetres of oesophageal columnar lining in their studies.

Michael Atkinson in Nottingham did the same. In 1976 he established an endoscopic surveillance programme for Barrett's oesophagus taking at least five centimetres as the minimum length for the diagnosis. By 1990 he had 102 patients under regular observation.[105] Twelve of these developed dysplasia all of whom had a columnar-lined oesophagus at least eight centimetres long. This encouraged many clinicians to ignore columnar epithelium limited to the distal few centimetres of the oesophagus and to concentrate on patients with long segments of columnar epithelium. Inevitably some protested at this practice arguing that Barrett's oesophagus should include any that were lined by columnar epithelium, however short. A great debate ensued fuelled by the fact that adenocarcinoma of the gastro-oesophageal junction was increasing at an alarming rate. Gradually endoscopists lowered their threshold for the diagnosis and most accepted a minimum of three centimetres though purists maintained that any amount of intestinal metaplasia was abnormal and prone to adenocarcinoma.

Once it was realised that Barrett's oesophagus was caused by reflux, clinicians hoped that measures to prevent this might help the condition to regress. For several years anti-reflux surgery was the only realistic option but even the most enthusiastic surgeons in America had to admit that their results were on the whole disappointing. When H2–receptor antagonists were introduced patients were amazed at their effectiveness and more than half felt better after years of misery. At the time Barrett's oesophagus was still relatively unknown to most physicians; for example when Brian Cooper was research fellow with Professor Gil Barbezat in Dunedin, New Zealand, in 1984, he was surprised to come across so many cases. Cooper (born 1947) had been a gastroenterological trainee for ten years by this time illustrating just how small an impact the condition had made on physicians then. For example apart from two communications to the annual meeting of the British Society of Gastroenterology in York (one of which came from the Mayo Clinic), there was not a single article on Barrett's oesophagus published in *Gut* in 1983.

Cooper and Barbezat found Barrett's oesophagus in ten per cent of their patients with gastro-oesophageal reflux at endoscopy. They managed to collect 52 cases in six years, half of whom had oesophagitis, which responded well to an H2 receptor antagonist. Surprisingly few had a stricture and none had dysplasia or cancer though the follow-up period was short.[106]

A decade later the first proton pump inhibitor, omeprazole, appeared and it was soon apparent that this drug could suppress acid even more effectively than the H2–receptor antagonists. Two trials in Britain showed that it was particularly useful in oesophagitis. The first in 1990 was a multicentre study organised by Astra, the manufacturers of omeprazole. The main contributors to this trial were Colin Bate and Simon Wilkinson, gastroenterologists in Wigan and Gloucester respectively.[107] In the second trial, Paul Smith (born 1937), a gregarious gastroenterologist in Cardiff, Graeme Kerr (born 1935), a New Zealand-born physician in Shrewsbury, and Roy Cockel (born 1937), a gastroenterologist in Birmingham, joined forces to show convincingly that omeprazole prevented reflux-induced peptic strictures better than ranitidine, an H2–receptor antagonist.[108] They noted incidentally that at least ten per cent of their patients had Barrett's oesophagitis.

Where the H2-receptor antagonists had failed to improve Barrett's oesophagus the new proton pump inhibitors might succeed, and it was now that the Gloucester Royal Hospital of all unlikely places began to establish a reputation as one of the leading centres in oesophageal research in Britain. Since his appointment in 1970 Michael Gear (born 1933), a surgeon with vision and enthusiasm, had specialised in upper gastro-intestinal surgery and gastro-oesophageal reflux, becoming well-known for the repair of hiatus hernia with the Angel-Chick prosthesis. He was also one of the first to set up an open access endoscopy service.[109] In due course he was joined by Simon Wilkinson (born 1945), a gastroenterologist interested in oesophageal disease, and in 1988 by Neil Shepherd (born 1956), fresh from St. Bartholemew's Hospital, where he had been senior lecturer in histopathology specialising in diseases of the gut. Wilkinson had been one of the first to take part in trials of omeprazole, as we have just seen. Both he and Gear were seeing patients with Barrett's oesophagus and they naturally wondered if the drug could suppress acid sufficiently to reduce the columnar lining in these patients. With the help of their registrars, notably Stephen Gore (born 1959), now a gastroenterologist at Yeovil Hospital, and Christopher Healey (born 1960), now at Airdale Hospital, they treated 23 patients for two years.[110] To their delight the patients had significant regression of their columnar mucosa but the most striking change was the appearance of large squamous islands emerging within it. Shortly after the trial Wilkinson was lured to Derriford Hospital, Plymouth (partly attracted by the sea, as he was a keen sailor), where he has been experimenting with endoscopic anti-reflux procedures, and Gear retired from the NHS, but Shepherd and Wilkinson continued to coordinate their trial with the help of Stephen Gore for a further three years. Though the improvement was sustained, only one patient reverted to normal.[111] Shepherd realised that the squamous re-epithelialisation was superficial and was concealing underlying columnar mucosa, which could still pose a neoplastic risk. On the other hand eliminating gastric acid was helping the mucosa and reducing the risk of dysplasia.

Meanwhile Brian Cooper, now a gastroenterologist in Birmingham, had begun a similar trial in forty-seven patients, some of whom were followed up for six years. But whereas Wilkinson had used a high dose of omeprazole (40 milligrams daily), Cooper only gave the standard dose (20 milligrams daily) that was approved for maintenance treatment.[112] Again there was partial squamous re-epithelialisation with islands of normal mucosa in about half the patients, but this time no regression in the length of the Barrett's epithelium. Cooper agreed with the Gloucester group that despite the disappointing lack of regression, acid suppression seemed to reduce the number of patients developing dysplasia and was well worthwhile.

Until the 1990s any patient with high-grade dysplasia faced radical surgery in the form of oesophagectomy, which carried a significant mortality (five per cent or more) and a high morbidity. By this time many centres had set up screening programmes hoping to detect and treat dysplasia and early oesophageal cancer and so improve survival. Some did better than others. In Liverpool a large team of surgeons and physicians reviewed all the patients with Barrett's oesophagus seen between 1981 and 1992.[113] Many of the patients were unsuitable for screening because they were unfit for surgery in the first place. Five patients developed cancer that was early and operable, which the Liverpool team felt justified the programme, though it was very expensive. On the other hand in Leicester, Raymond Playford (born 1955), Professor of Gastroenterology, and his colleague Anthony Wicks (born 1941), a gastroenterologist, asked their registrar, Christopher Macdonald (born 1966), now a gastroenterologist in Carlisle, to review all the patients with Barrett's mucosa seen between 1984 and 1994. Only one patient with asymptomatic cancer was detected as a result of the screening programme and the Leicester group doubted the benefit of continuing their surveillance programme.[114] The great problem with screening was ensuring adequate and plentiful biopsies and expert interpretation by the pathologist. Unfortunately this was hard to achieve in many district hospitals with a mixed bag of endoscopists and general pathologists. Yet screening offered the only chance of detecting dysplasia and by now a promising new method of treating Barrett's dysplasia had arrived, namely endoscopic mucosal ablation.

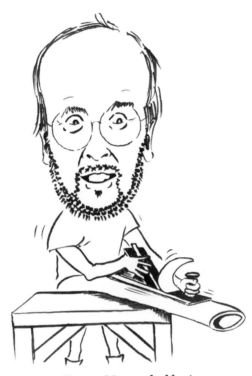

8 Barr – Mucosal ablation.

The attraction of ablating the mucosa, quite apart from avoiding surgery, was that it not only removed dysplastic mucosa and even some early cancers but also dealt with benign metaplastic (Barrett's) epithelium. Though the mucosa could be resected by a suck-and-cut technique most people preferred some form of laser ablation. In this country the man whose name became synonymous with this treatment was Hugh Barr (born 1954). Barr, a Liverpool graduate, decided to pursue a career as an upper gastrointestinal surgeon and like others was struck by the rapid increase in adenocarcinoma of the oesophagus that was occurring in Britain more than anywhere else. Barrett's oesophagus seemed to be the key and while Hunterian Professor with the Royal College of

Surgeons he worked with Steven Bown at the National Medical Laser Centre in London, experimenting on various ways to ablate the mucosa. In particular they used photothermal treatment successfully, but they also modified the technique of photodynamic therapy.[115] Patients were given a porphyrin precursor to drink, which was taken up by the cells of the gastrointestinal mucosa rendering them highly photosensitive. Subsequently light from a dye laser was applied endoscopically, which targeted the sensitised cells and destroyed them. The beauty of this method was that it was safe with no risk of perforating the oesophagus and could tackle large areas of mucosa.

In 1992 Barr was appointed upper gastrointestinal surgeon in Gloucester with Mike Gear. This was an inspired move for two reasons. First he could enjoy the histological expertise provided by Neil Shepherd that was so helpful in the interpretation of dysplasia, and second he was able to take advantage of the link being forged between Gloucester Hospital and Cranfield University, the recently upgraded Institute of Technology in the city. Barr became the first clinical professor and foundation dean of the new postgraduate medical school at Cranfield. With a series of PhD and MD students, Barr and Shepherd promoted the cause of mucosal ablation.[116] This treatment combined with acid suppression certainly slowed the onset of cancer of the oesophagus in some patients but many questions remained unanswered.[117] As Barr put it, ablation and re-epithelialisation of the mucosa was only "mowing the lawn, it was not paving the garden", in other words not all the abnormal mucosa was removed.

What we really need to know is why only a few patients with Barrett's oesophagus develop dysplasia. A genetic predisposition is the favourite explanation but until this is known regular screening for dysplasia, though flawed, is the best that can be offered. Unfortunately most people with Barrett's oesophagus go undetected and the vast majority of patients with adenocarcinoma of the oesophagus are unaware that they have Barrett's. So far the rewards have been few and bestowed infrequently but

"Delusion sweet thus tempts us on
Till all the leaves are like to one
Yet Hope looks back as heretofore
And smiling seems to say encore."

J. M. W. Turner

REFERENCES

Section One

1   *A Twentieth Century Physician, Being the Reminiscences of Sir Arthur Hurst*, 1949, Edward Arnold and Co., London

2   Hurst A., Morton C. J., Cook F., Cox A. N., Gardiner N., Schlesinger E. G., Todd A. H. 1907 The passage of food along the human alimentary canal. *Guy's Hosp. Reports.*, 61, 85–110

3   Hurst A. F. 1915 Achalasia of the cardia. *Quart. J. Med.* 8 300–308

4   Hurst A. F. 1924 *Essays and Addresses on Digestive and Nervous Diseases and on Addisons's Anaemia and Asthma*. Heinemann, London, p110

5   Rake G. W. 1926 A case of annular muscular hypertrophy of the oesophagus. *Guy's Hosp. Reports* 76 145–152

6   Rake G. W. 1927 On the pathology of achalasia of the cardia. *Guy's Hosp. Reports.* 77 141–150

7   Willis T. 1674 *Pharmaceutice Rationalis*. First English Translation London 1679 p23

8   Quoted by Bailey and Bishop in *Notable Names in Medicine and Surgery* 1946 p10

9   Purton T. 1821 An extraordinary case of distension of the oesophagus, forming a sac, extending from two inches below the pharynx to the cardiac orifice of the stomach. *London Med. and Physical Journal* XLV1 540–542

10 Mayo H. 1828 A case of dilated oesophagus. Letter, *Lond. Med. Gaz.* 3 121

11 Hannay A. J. 1833 An extraordinary dilatation (with hypertrophy?) of all the thoracic portions of the oesophagus causing dysphagia. *Edin. Med. & Surg. J.* XL 65–72

12 Wilks S. 1866 Dilatation of the oesophagus. *Trans. Path. Soc. London* 17 138–9

13 Turner G. Grey. 1946 *Injuries and Diseases of the Oesophagus*. Cassell and Co. Ltd, Chap 9, p65

.14 Hurst A. F. 1913 Discussion following Jordan's paper. *Brit. Med. J.* Oct 11th 915–918

15 Russel J. C. 1898 Diagnosis and treatment of spasmodic stricture of the oesophagus. *Brit. Med. J.* June 4th 1450–1451

16   Plummer H. S. 1908 Cardiospasm; with a report of forty cases *J.A.M.A.* 51 549–554

17   Mikulicz-Radecki, Johann von., 1882 uber gastroskopie und oesophagoskopie mit demonstration am lebenden. Verhard, d. Dent. *Gesellsch. F. Chir. XI Cong.* 30–38

18   Walton A. J. 1925 The surgical treatment of cardiospasm. *Brit. J. Surg.* 13 701–737

19   Heller E. 1914 Extra-mukosa cardioplastik beim chronischen cardiospasmus etc mittheil a. d. grenzgeb. *D. Med. U. Chir.* Lvii s 141–9

20   Hurst A. F., Rowlands R. P. 1924 Case of achalasia of the cardia relieved by operation. *Proceedings of the Royal Society of Medicine (clin. section)* xvii No. 10 45

21   McKeown K. C. 1994 in *A Tale of Two Citadels.* Pentland Press p104

22   Turner G. Grey. 1931 Some experiences in the surgery of the oesophagus. Bigelow Memorial Lecture *New England Journal of Medicine* 205: 657– 674

23   Turner G. Grey. 1946 *Injuries and Diseases of the Oesophagus.* Cassell and Co., Ltd. chap 9 p73

24   Barrett N. R., Franklin R. H., 1949 Concerning the unfavourable late results of certain operations performed in the treatment of cardiospasm. *Brit. J. Surg.* 37: 194–202

25   Dornhorst A. C., Kent Harrison. Pierce J. W., 1954 Observations on the normal oesophagus and cardia *Lancet* i 695–698

26   Kramer P., Ingelfinger F. J. 1949 Motility of the human esophags in control subjects and patients with esophageal disorders. *Amer. J. Med.* 7 168–174

27   Kramer P., Ingelfinger F. J., Atkinson M 1956 The motility and pharmacology of the esophagus in cardiospasm *Gastroenterologia* Basel 86 174–8

28   Fyke F. E., Code C. F., Schlegel J. F. 1956 The gastrooesophageal sphincter in healthy human beings *Gastroenterologia* Basel 86 135–150

29   Trounce J. R., Deuchar D. C., Kauntze R., Stevenson J. J., Thomas G. A. 1956 Observations on achalasia of the cardia. *Gastroenterologia* Basel 86: 178. Trounce J. R., Deuchar D. C., Kauntze R., Stevenson J. J., Thomas G. A. 1957 Observations on achalasia of the cardia. *Quart. J. Med. n.s.* 26 433–443

30   Ibid

31   Creamer B., Olsen A. M., Code C. F. 1957 The esophageal sphincter in achalasia of the cardia (cardiospasm) *Gastroenterology* 33 293–301

32   Creamer B., Pierce J. W. 1957 Observations on the gastro-oesophageal junction during swallowing and drinking *Lancet* 2 1309–12

33   Atkinson M., Edwards D. A. W., Honour A. J., Rowlands E. N. 1957 The oesophago-gastric sphincter in hiatus hernia. *Lancet* 2 1138–42

34   Atkinson M. 1959 The oesophago-gastric sphincter after cardiomyotomy. *Thorax* 14 125–131

35   Fellows I. W., Ogilvie A. L., Atkinson M. 1983 Pneumatic dilatation in achalasia. *Gut* 24 1020–23

36   Turner G. Grey. 1944–45 The George Haliburton Hume Memorial Lectures *Newcastle Medical J.* XXII

37 Baillie M. 1833 *The Morbid Anatomy of Some of the Most Important Parts of the Human Body.* 8th edition London p61

38 Abercrombie J. 1830 *Pathological and Practical Researches on Diseases of the Stomach, the Intestinal Canal, the Liver, and Other Viscera of the Abdomen.* Philadelphia Section 2 p87–88

39 Watson T. 1848 *Lectures on the Principles and Practice of Physic.* 3rd edition London Vol 2 Lecture 64 343–350

40 Brinton W. 1864 *Lectures on Diseases of the Stomach.* London. 2nd edition p174–5

41 Jones S. 1875 *St. Thos. Hosp. Reports.* Successful gastrostomy

42 Leroy d'Etoilles. 1845 in *De Lavacherie "De l'Oesophagectomie",* Bruxelles

43 Croft J. 1882 Relief of oesophageal malignancy by endotubation. Report of a case. *St. Thos. Hosp. Reports* 12: 45–53

44 Durham A. E. 1881 Carcinoma of the oesophagus. Gastrostomy. *Lancet* ii 872.

45 Symonds C. J. 1887 The treatment of malignant stricture of the oesophagus by tubage or permanent catheterism. *Brit. Med. J.* I 870–873

46 Souttar H. S. 1927 Treatment of carcinoma of the oesophagus: based on 100 personal cases and 18 post-mortem reports. *Brit. J. Surg.* 15 76–94

47 Mousseau M., Barbin J. et al. 1956 *Arch. Mal. Appar. Digest.* 45 208

48 Celestin L. R. 1959 Permanent intubation in inoperable cancer of the oesophagus and cardia. A new tube. *Ann. Roy. Coll. Surg. (Eng.)* 25 165–170

49 Celestin L. R., Campbell W. B. 1981 A new and safe system for oesophageal dilatation. *Lancet* i 74– 75

50 Collis J. L. 1971 Surgical treatment of carcinoma of the oesophagus and cardia *Brit. J. Surg.* 58 801–804

51 Atkinson M., Ferguson R. 1977 Fibreoptic endoscopic palliative intubation of inoperable oesophago-gastric neoplasms. *Brit. Med. J.* I 266–267

52 Atkinson M., Ferguson R., Parker G. C. 1978 Tube introducer and modified celestin tube for use in palliative intubation of oesophago-gastric neoplasms at fibreoptic endoscopy *Gut* 19 669–671

53 Ogilvie A. L. Dronfield M. W., Ferguson R., Atkinson M. 1982 Palliative intubation of oesophago-gastric neoplasms at fibreoptc endoscopy *Gut* 23 1060–67

54 Evans A. 1933 A rubber oesophagus. *Brit. J. Surg.* 20 388–392

55 Torek F. 1913 The first successful case of resection of the thoracic portion of the oesophagus for carcinoma. *Surg. Gynae. Obstet.* 16 614–617

56 Turner G. Grey. 1933 Excision of the thoracic oesophagus for carcinoma – with construction of an extrathoracic gullet. *Lancet* ii 1315–16

57 Kocher T. 1911 (trans. Styles) *Textbook of Operative Surgery.* London 5th edition

58 Turner G. Grey. 1946 *Injuries and Diseases of the Oesophagus.* Cassell & Co. Ltd. p91

59 Garlock J. 1940 Surgical treatment of carcinoma of the esophagus. *Arch. Surg.* 41 1184–1214

60 Franklin R. H. 1942 Two cases of successful removal of the thoracic oesophagus for carcinoma. *Brit. J. Surg.* 30 141–6

61 Ohsawa T. 1933 The surgery of the esophagus. *Arch. Jap. Surg.* 10 605–700

62   Adams W. E., Phemister D. B. 1938 Carcinoma of the lower thoracic esophagus: report of a successful resection and esophagogastrostomy. *J. Thorac. Surg.* 7 621–632

63   Thompson V. C. 1945 Successful resection for carcinoma of the lower end of the oesophagus with immediate oesophagogastrostomy. *Brit. J. Surg.* 32 377–380

64   Brock R. C. 1942 Cardio-oesophageal resection for tumour of the cardia. *Brit. J. Surg.* 30: 146–160

65   Steele G. H. 1943 Excision of oesophagus and oesophago gastrostomy *Lancet* ii 797– 798

66   Tudor Edwards A., Lee E. S. 1936 Extirpation of the oesophagus for carcinoma. *J. Laryngol. Otol.* 51 281–292

67   Allison P. R. 1942 Excision of oesophagus via a left thoracotomy *Brit. J. Surg.* 30: 132–141

68   Lewis I. 1946 The surgical treatment of carcinoma of the oesophagus. *Brit. J. Surg.* 34: 18–31

69   Tanner N. 1947 The present position of carcinoma of the oesophagus. *Postgrad. Med. J.* 23 109–139

70   Allison P. R., Borrie J. 1949 Bypass oesophagectomy for carcinoma. *Brit. J. Surg.* 37: 1–21

71   Smithers D. W. 1955 Radiotherapy for carcinoma of the oesophagus. *Brit. J. Radiol.* ns28: 554–564

72   Collis J. L. 1957 Carcinoma of the oesophagus; the case for surgical excision. *Lancet* ii 613–616

73   McKeown K. C. 1976 Total three-stage oesophagectomy for cancer of the oesophagus. *Brit. J. Surg.* 63 259–262

74   McKeown K. C. 1994 *A Tale of Two Citadels. Memoirs of a Surgeon and His Times.* The Pentland Press Ltd. Durham. ISBN 1–85821–208–1

75   Earlam R., Cunha-Melo J. R. 1980 Oesophageal squamous cell carcinoma. 1. A critical review of surgery. *Brit. J. Surg.* 67 381–390

76   Earlam R., Cunha-Melo J. R. 1980 Oesophageal squamous cell carcinoma. 2. A critical review of radiotherapy. *Brit. J. Surg.* 67 457–461

77   Earlam R. 1991 An MRC prospective randomised trial of radiotherapy versus surgery for operable squamous cell carcinoma of the oesophagus. *Ann. Roy. Coll. Surg. (Eng.)* 73 8–12

78   Clarke C. A., McConnell R. B. 1954 Six cases of carcinoma of the oesophagus occurring in one family. *Brit. Med. J.* ii 1137–38

79   Howel-Evans W., McConnell R. B., Clarke C. A., Sheppard P. M. 1958 Carcinoma of the oesophagus with keratosis palmaris et plantaris (tylosis). A study of two families. *Quart. J. Med.* 27 413–429

80   Fagge C. H. 1872 A case of simple stenosis of the oesophagus, followed by epithelioma. *Guy's Hosp. Reports* 17: 413– 421

81   Hurst A. H., Rake G. W. 1930 Achalasia of the cardia. *Quart. J. Med.* 23–508

82   Belsey R. H. R. 1972 Recent progress in oesophageal surgery. *Acta. Chir. Beg.* 71 230

83   Tilestone W. 1906 Peptic ulcer of the oesophagus. *Amer. J. Med. Sci.* 132 240–265

84   Jackson C. 1929 Peptic ulcer of the oesophagus. *J.A.M.A.* 92 369–372

85 Stewart M. J., Hartfall S. J. 1929 Chronic peptic ulcer of the oesophagus. *J. Path. Bact.* 32 9–14

86 Lyall A. 1937 Chronic peptic ulcer of the oesophagus: a report of 8 cases. *Brit. J. Surg.* 24 534–547

87 Briggs, P. J., Dick, R. C. S., Hurst, Sir A. 1939 Simple ulcer of the oesophagus and short oesophagus. *Proceedings of the Royal Society of Medicine* XXXII 11 1423–45

88 Dick R. C. S., Hurst A. 1942 Chronic peptic ulcer of the oesophagus and its association with congenitally short oesophagus and diaphragmatic hernia. *Quart. J. Med.* 11 105–120

89 von Bergmann G. 1932 *Funktionelle Pathologie,* Berlin p68

90 Johnstone A. S. 1941 Annotation *Lancet* ii 18

91 Allison P. R., Johnstone A. S., Royce G. B. 1943 Short oesophagus with simple peptic ulceration. *J. Thorac. Surg.* 12: 432– 457

92 Allison P. R. 1948 Peptic ulcer of the oesophagus. *Thorax* 3 20– 42

93 Allison P. R. 1951 Reflux esophagitis, sliding hiatus hernia, and the anatomy of repair. *Surg. Gynae. Obstet.* 92 419– 431

94 Allison P. R. 1973 Hiatus hernia: (A 20 year retrospective survey) *Annals of Surgery.* 178 273– 276

95 Skinner D. B., Belsey R. H. R. 1967 Surgical management of esophageal reflux and hiatus hernia: Long term results with 1,030 patients. *J. Thorac. Cardiovasc. Surg.* 53: 33– 54

96 Nissen R. 1961 Gastropexy and "Fundoplication" in surgical treatment of hiatus hernia. *Amer. J. Dig. Dis.* 6: 954– 961

97 Barrett N. R. 1950 Chronic peptic ulcer of the oesophagus and oesophagitis. *Brit. J. Surg.* 38 175–182

98 Allison P. R., Johnstone A. S. 1953 The oesophagus lined with gastric mucous membrane. *Thorax* 8 87–101

99 Barrett N. R. 1956 The oesophagus lined by columnar epithelium. *Gastroenterologia* 86 183–6

100 Barrett N. R. 1957 The lower oesophagus lined by columnar epithelium. *Surgery* 41 6 881–894

101 Carrie A. 1950 Adenocarcinoma of the upper end of the oesophagus arising from ectopic gastric epithelium. *Brit. J. Surg.* 37: 474.

102 Morson B. C., Belcher J. R. 1952 Adenocarcinoma of the oesophagus and ectopic gastric mucosa. *Brit. J. Cancer* 6 127–130

103 Paull A., Trier J. S., Dalton M. D., Camp R. C., Loeb P., Goyal R. K. 1976 The histologic spectrum of Barrett's oesophagus. *New England Journal of Medicine* 295 476–480

104 Rothery G. A., Patterson J. E., Stoddard C. J., Day D. W. 1986 Histological and histochemical changes in columnar lined (Barrett's) oesophagus *Gut* 27 1062–68

105 Iftikhar S. Y., James P. D., Steele R. J. C., Hardcastle J. D., Atkinson M. 1992 Length of Barrett's oesophagus: an important factor in the development of dysplasia and adenocarcinoma. *Gut* 33 1155–58

106   Cooper B. T., Barbezat G. O. 1987 Barrett's oesophagus: a clinical study of 52 patients. *Quart. J. Med. n.s.* 62 238 97–108

107   Bate C. M., Keeling P. W. N., O'Morain C., Wilkinson S. P. et al 1990 Comparison of omeprazole and cimetidine in reflux oesophagitis: symptomatic, endoscopic, and histological evaluations. *Gut* 31 968–972

108   Smith P. M., Kerr G. D., Cockel R. et al 1994 A comparison of omeprazole and ranitidine in the prevention of recurrence of benign oesophageal stricture. *Gastroenterology* 107 1312–18

109   Gear M. W. L., Wilkinson S. P. 1989 Open access upper alimentary endoscopy. *Brit. J. Hosp. Med.* 41 438–444

110   Gore S., Healy C. J., Sutton R., Eyre-Brook I. A., Gear M. W. L., Shepherd N. A., Wilkinson S. P. 1993 Regression of columnar lined (Barrett's) oesophagus with continuous omeprazole therapy. *Alimentary Pharmacology and Therapeutics* 7 623–628

111   Wilkinson S. P., Biddlestone L., Gore S., Shepherd N. A. 1999 Regression of columnar lined (Barrett's) oesophagus with omeprazole 40mg daily: results of 5 years of continuous therapy. *Alimentary Pharmacology and Therapeutics* 13 1205–09

112   Cooper B. T., Neumann C. S., Cox M. A., Iqbal T. H. 1998 Continuous treatment with omeprazole 20mg daily up to 6 years in Barrett's oesophagus. *Aliment. Pharmacol. Ther* 12 893–897

113   Wright T. A., Gray M.R., Morris A. I., Gilmore I. T. et al 1996 Cost effectiveness of detecting Barrett's cancer. *Gut* 39 574–579

114   MacDonald C. E., Wicks A. C., Playford R. J. 1997 Ten year experience of screening patients with Barrett's oesophagus in a University Teaching Hospital. *Gut* 41 303–307

115   Regula J. et al 1995 Photosensitisation and photodynamic therapy of oesophageal, duodenal, and clolrectal tumours using 5 aminolaevulinic acid induced protoporphyrin 1X – a pilot study *Gut* 36 67–75

116   Barr H., Shepherd N. A., Dix A., Roberts D. J. H., Tan W. C., Krasner N. 1996 Eradication of high-grade dysplasia in columnar-lined (Barrett's) oesophagus by photodynamic therapy with endogenously generated protoporphyrin 1X *Lancet* Vol 348 584–585

117   Barham C. P., Jones R. L., Biddlestone L. R., Hardwick R. H., Shepherd N. A., Barr H. 1997 Photothermal laser ablation of Barrett's oesophagus: endoscopic and histological evidence of squamous re-epithelialisation. *Gut* 41 281–284

SECTION TWO

THE STOMACH AND DUODENUM

CHAPTER FOUR

PEPTIC ULCER IN THE NINETEENTH CENTURY

Were it not for his ulcer John Buchan may not have written *The Thirty-nine Steps*. At the beginning of the First World War he became unwell and was advised that the choice lay between an operation or three months rest in bed. He chose to go to bed and to while away the hours he hatched the plot of his famous novel. I don't know how his ulcer was diagnosed but he may have had a barium meal.

The diagnosis of peptic ulcer is easy today (so simple in fact that we hardly need to bother with a careful history and examination), an endoscopy reveals all in a few minutes. But during the nineteenth century when the importance of gastric ulcer was first recognised the diagnosis was very difficult indeed and could only be proved if the unfortunate victim succumbed and underwent an autopsy. Before post mortems were freely available, how could anyone possibly single out an ulcer from the all pervading dyspepsia?

Recently I found myself staying for bed and breakfast in a residence called Fitz Manor, near Shrewsbury. I noticed some bound volumes on a shelf containing immaculate lecture notes in copperplate by a medical student. They were written in 1892 by Robert Craig Dun (1870–1941), who qualified in Edinburgh and later became a paediatric surgeon in Liverpool. After his retirement he went to live at Fitz Manor. I turned to his section on diseases of the stomach. The simple perforating ulcer of the stomach was described but there was no mention of duodenal ulcer. Pyloric stenosis was caused by cancer or excessive consumption of whisky. In 1892 abdominal surgery was in its infancy, X-rays were yet to be discovered and duodenal ulcer was virtually unknown. Yet gastric ulcer was well described as our friend

Craig Dun illustrates. Much of the credit for this belongs to William Brinton MD FRS.

Brinton (1823–67) was born at Kidderminster and became articled to the local surgeon at the age of seventeen. He trained with distinction at King's College, winning several prizes, subsequently becoming physician at the Royal Free Hospital as well as St. Thomas's Hospital. Inspired by the likes of Bright, Addison, and Hodgkin at Guy's Hospital he took every opportunity on the wards and in the post mortem room to study the underlying physiology and pathology of disease.

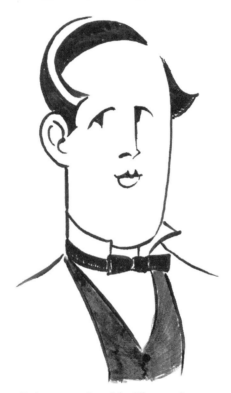

9   Brinton – A noble Thomas's man.

His interest in gastric disease was stimulated by the death of a close relative in 1843. He was impressed by how little was known about abdominal diseases "From that time," he wrote, "I have given to these maladies whatever attention could be justifiably devoted to a special group of diseases by a student and practitioner of physic in general."[1]

He began by pooling the records of 1,200 ulcer cases that had all been verified by careful necropsy, though the clinical details were usually meagre. Most of these had been published as scattered cases in various journals, but he also dug out the records from the metropolitan hospitals and museums. At the same time he spent twelve years studying 200 patients of his own whose symptoms convinced him that they had ulcers, though only a few of these came to post mortem. By comparing the clinical findings with the pathology he felt confident that he could reach a diagnosis of gastric ulcer. He published this work in 1857, a classic monograph entitled *The Symptoms, Pathology and Treatment of Ulcer of the Stomach*, in which he first reviewed the natural history of gastric ulcer then turned his attention to each symptom: pain, vomiting, haemorrhage, cachexia and perforation.[2]

His comments on the pain of gastric ulcer are remarkably astute, indeed they are repeated almost verbatim 100 years later by Thomas Hunt in Price's *Textbook of the Practice Medicine*.[3] Vomiting is common and often effortless, relieving the pain but frequently leading to the characteristic cachexia. Haemorrhage supports the diagnosis strongly and probably occurs in all cases to some extent, but unless severe can be overlooked by patient and doctor alike. Perforation is usually fatal.

He was particularly impressed by anterior perforating gastric ulcers in young females whom he identified as a special high-risk group. Many of these girls had amenorrhoea and were thought to be suffering from chlorosis or the green sickness.[4] This peculiar disease reached its heyday in the late nineteenth century. It affected teenage girls who were pale, weak, breathless and had a host of other problems including irregular menstrual periods. The name meant literally "a state of greenness" but no one knew whether this applied to the pale colour of these girls or their immaturity. It disappeared in the early twentieth century. Brinton certainly accepted chlorosis as a disease entity but thought the cachexia found in ulcer patients was distinct from it. Ulcers in common with other serious illnesses could suppress menstruation.

In making the diagnosis he suggests that a decided opinion can be reached by evaluation of some of these "chief symptoms" but cautions that many ulcers will be overlooked if too rigid an approach is adopted. One must have a high index of suspicion. Better to treat for an ulcer than not. "By treating these cases as ulcer of the stomach we often cure what we cannot diagnose. A triumph of the art over the science of medicine."

Brinton used his postmortem data to look at the epidemiology of gastric ulcer. (Hitherto what was known came from anecdotal evidence.) Some of his findings are of particular interest. For example he noted that ulcers could linger for years or heal spontaneously within months (as half did). The most frightening complication was perforation (fifteen per cent), which was invariably fatal and (as we have seen) seemed to single out young women. On the other hand haemorrhage was common but rarely fatal (three to five per cent) but fatal bleeding was four times more frequent in men. Haematemesis in young women with amenorrhoea was frequently ascribed to vicarious menstruation, which carried a good prognosis, and was often linked to chlorosis.

Knowing that half of all gastric ulcers healed spontaneously Brinton's treatment was largely supportive. Complete rest and a nourishing bland diet (e.g. milk) were important perhaps for several weeks or even months. Opium was the most effective agent for severe pain. He favoured bismuth as particularly beneficial for the relief of pain and vomiting, though he could not explain why. He spoke out against bleeding his patients though it was still popular in his day. Bleeding was based on the notion that it relieved inflammation by reducing vascular congestion in the affected part. Brinton rightly suggested that any theoretical benefit was more than offset by the loss of blood in someone who was often poor, ill fed, old and probably bleeding anyway. But he supported the use of blisters as a local counter-irritant for pain, recommending that turpentine and mustard be applied to the epigastrium. Other suggestions were dry cupping to draw blood away from the ulcer to relieve inflammation or the local application of ice. Nothing really helped vomiting, but dehydration could be corrected by the administration of enemas, or liquids could be applied by wrapping a limb in wet bandages. Iron was a useful tonic.

The risk of perforation might be reduced by avoiding pressure on the stomach, a hazard, for example, in women wearing tight stays or certain occupations such as shoemakers using a last. A contemporary, Thomas Chambers (1817–89), at St. Mary's Hospital blamed perforation on "the habits of half civilised life which females, voluntarily or involuntarily persist in; such as wearing ill fitting stays with rigid beams in front pressing upon the viscera, leaning forward to work immediately after eating, swallowing their meals half masticated, keeping decayed teeth in their heads, allowing mental emotion to check digestion and a variety of other similar causes of the difficulties into which their stomachs fall".[5] But despite this somewhat chauvinistic language Chambers was one of the earliest advocates of medicine as a career for women.

Brinton also wondered why people developed ulcers. He did not know the reason but his conclusions were as good as any put forward over the next century or so. He knew ulcers were more common in old age and more likely to occur in the poor and intemperate. Young women were not unduly prone to have ulcers but among those who did have them, perforation was the awful risk. Gastric juice, especially acid, might prevent healing or even enlarge an ulcer but did not explain why ulceration happened in the first place. And how did so many ulcers manage to heal spontaneously? What would he have given to watch the development of an ulcer in life. But he had to rely on autopsies and he knew the stomach was prone to decomposition after death. One of the questions that intrigued everyone was how the stomach itself escaped digestion while digestion was proceeding within it. The first person to address this point was John Hunter (1728–93) the celebrated anatomist and surgeon.

In 1772 Hunter remarked that occasionally, especially in persons who have died of sudden and violent deaths, much of the stomach is found so dissolved that its contents have escaped into the abdominal cavity. As these people had been in perfect health, Hunter inferred that the phenomenon could not have arisen from disease during life, but must have been due to the action of digestive fluid after death.[6] He ascribed the protection of the stomach in life to a "living principle". By way of illustration, he suggested that were it possible to put a man's hand into the stomach of a living animal such as a lion for a considerable time, no harm would come to it, but if the same hand were separated from the body, the stomach would immediately act upon it. Hunter was convinced that the stomach secreted acid, but not a strong one. Many did not agree with him, for instance the official view in France was that gastric juice was not acid but similar to saliva. Others who agreed that gastric juice was acidic thought it was acetic, phosphoric or even lactic acid. Eventually the composition of gastric secretion was resolved by William Prout (1785–1850) when he presented his paper on "The nature of the acid and saline matters usually existing in the stomachs of animals" to the Royal Society on 1st December 1823.[7] His success can be attributed to his skill as a chemist and biochemist. He confirmed the presence of free hydrochloric acid in the gastric juice of both animals and humans. More important, he made quantitative measurements of the concentration of free and total hydrochloric acid by exact neutralisation with a solution of potash of known strength as well as titrating with silver nitrate to measure the chlorides. Though Prout's work was confirmed by others in Germany, there were some, including Robert Graves (1796–1853), the distinguished professor of medicine in Dublin, who continued to believe that the acid found in the stomach was lactic.[8] Prout also made the first clinical studies of gastric secretion by analysis of the gastric juice ejected from the stomach by three patients with severe dyspepsia. One of these samples was supplied by Sir Astley Cooper, the distinguished surgeon at Guy's Hospital.

Meanwhile Hunter's theory of "The Living Principle" had aroused great curiosity and in due course was put to the test. A young clinician called Frederick Pavy (1829–1911) repeated an experiment by Claude Bernard to show that the living principle did not afford protection from the solvent influence of the stomach.[9] Through an opening into the stomach of a dog, he introduced the hind legs of a living frog and showed that they were digested and dissolved away while the frog was alive. As it could be argued that the wretched frog, a cold-blooded reptilian animal, was not a fair test against the powerful stomach of a warm-blooded animal, he substituted the frog's legs with the ear of a vigorous rabbit. He actually held it in the stomach of the dog for four and a half hours burning his fingers in the process. Again the ear was corroded thus refuting Hunter's "living principle". Bernard had suggested the stomach protected itself by constantly renewing the epithelial layer that with mucus acted as a kind of varnish. Pavy refuted this idea by removing a patch of mucous membrane from the stomach of a living animal and showing that ulceration and perforation did not occur as one might have expected. Indeed repair by cicatrisation took place. So Pavy put forward his theory that the wall of the stomach is protected from acid attack by the neutralising influence of blood permeating it. Furthermore as the acid was secreted, so the local capillary blood became correspondingly alkaline.[†] To support this, he tied the vessels

---

†Prout had postulated that chloride was secreted from blood to lumen by the power of electricity.

of a portion of the stomach in a rabbit and in due course the mucosa was digested and perforated. Pavy was an outstanding exponent of the scientific approach to medicine, though most of his future research lay in the field of diabetes. His work impressed Brinton who concluded that "the ulcer" in short seems to be in its outset a lesion of the vasomotor system, "an accident, so to speak, of extreme gastric congestion".

Brinton acknowledged the work of many distinguished doctors when collecting his cases. One was Matthew Baillie, nephew of William Hunter who ran a famous anatomy school with his brother John. He became engrossed in their work, soon gaining a reputation as a brilliant teacher himself. In 1793 he published his *Morbid Anatomy of Some of the Most Important Parts of the Human Body*, which was based on the specimens in his uncles' museum together with many of his own dissections.[10] In it, he gave the first clear description of the appearance and symptoms of gastric ulcer.

"Opportunities occasionally offer themselves," he wrote, "of observing ulcers of the stomach. These sometimes resemble common ulcers, in any other part of the body, but frequently they have a peculiar appearance. Many of them are scarcely surrounded with any inflammation, have not irregular eroded edges as ulcers have generally, and are not attended with any particular diseased alteration in the structure of the stomach in the neighbourhood. They appear very much as if, some time before, a part had been cut out from the stomach with a knife, and the edges had healed, so as to present an uniform smooth boundary round the excavation which has been made.

"These ulcers sometimes destroy only a portion of the inner coat of the stomach at some one part, but occasionally they destroy a portion of all the coats, forming a hole in the stomach. When a portion of all the coats is destroyed, there is sometimes a thin appearance of the stomach surrounding the hole, which has a smooth surface, and depends on the progress of the ulceration.

"At other times, the stomach is a little thickened round the hole; and at other times still it seems to have the common natural structure.

Interestingly, he published a series of engravings six years later of pathological specimens, among which was one showing a large ulcer of the duodenum, but he makes no mention of acid in the gastric juice even in the eighth edition of his book published in 1833.

Baillie was a pillar of the establishment in contrast to another clinician Edwards Crisp[†] who published a series of 51 cases of perforation of the stomach from simple ulceration. He concluded "the symptoms of a perforated ulcer are so typical I can hardly believe anyone can fail to make the diagnosis. But treatment is hopeless."[11] He thought chlorosis was a very frequent predisposing cause of ulcer.

There was one man whose writings probably influenced Brinton more than any other. John Abercrombie (1780–1844) was born in Aberdeen and qualified in Edinburgh where he became a very successful general practitioner. He visited his patients three or four times a day, a practice unheard of then (and now for that matter). He was connected with the Public Dispensary, an institution for free medical care of the poor, and soon had a large practice that he divided into five districts under the care of senior students apprenticed to

---

[†]   Dr. Edwards Crisp (1806–82) was born in Suffolk and educated at St. Thomas's and Guy's Hospitals. After qualifying with "College and Hall" (MRCS & LSA) he spent two years in Paris before settling in South London where he built up a large and successful practice. He lived to the age of 82 and, over the years, won several prizes and published no fewer than 328 papers on an extraordinary array of subjects from intestinal obstruction to malformation of the heart and from the anatomy of the cuckoo to the oesophagus of the crocodile. Yet he was shunned by the establishment, earned rather grudging obituary notices and is unknown today. Sadly "policy was not a word in his vocabulary". At the age of 42 he presented himself as a candidate for the license of the Royal College of Physicians and was failed "for want of experience". Shocked and furious he spent years vilifying the college examiners even to the extent of founding a journal, *The London Medical Examiner,* through which as editor he hoped to expose the abuses of the examination system and to reform them. Now a bitter critic of the examining bodies and of the nepotism and corruption in hospital appointments, it is hardly surprising that he became unacceptable to his contemporaries. But he was an outstanding figure whose contributions to scientific knowledge deserve greater acknowledgement. Dobson, Jessie. 1952 Dr. Edwards Crisp: A forgotten medical scientist. *J. Hist. Med.* Autumn 384–399

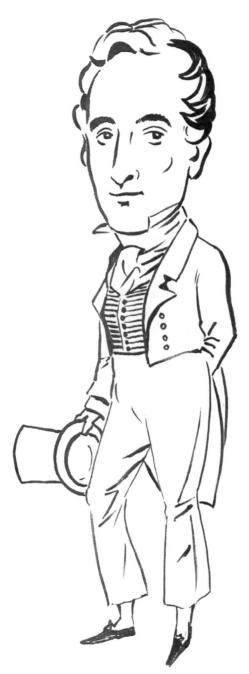

10 *Abercrombie – Successful and married well.*

him. In effect he ran a kind of medical school of his own. In the early nineteenth century there was no systematic teaching of pathology in Scotland and such was Abercrombie's interest in research that he carried out his own autopsies.

His many publications culminated in his book *Pathological and Practical Researches on Disease of the Stomach, the Intestinal Canal, the Liver and Other Viscera of the Abdomen*. This ran to several editions and was popular in America. In it he described several patients with gastric ulcer who had died from perforation, haemorrhage or emaciation. He went on to discuss the vexed problem of attempting the diagnosis before death and distinguishing ulcers from dyspepsia or functional disorders. The microscopic technique was yet to be perfected so Abercrombie was limited to simple morbid anatomy. Furthermore, the nature of gastric juice remained obscure and for him the vagus was still the eighth cranial nerve. Despite this his clinical description of gastric ulcer pre-empted Brinton to a remarkable degree. When it came to treatment he favoured topical bleeding and blistering, a light farinaceous diet and rest. Among internal remedies he recommended oxide of bismuth, lime water and nitric acid among many others. Unlike Brinton he added an appendix on diseases of the duodenum.

> Facts are wanting on this interesting subject, but it is probable the duodenum is the seat of several affections, which are apt to be mistaken for affections of the stomach or the liver. The leading peculiarity of disease of the duodenum, as far as we are at present acquainted with it, seems to be, that the food is taken with relish, and the first stage of digestion is not impeded; but that pain begins about the time when the food is passing out of the stomach, or from two to four hours after a meal. The pain then continues, often with great severity, sometimes for several hours, and generally extends obliquely backwards in the direction of the right kidney. In some cases it gradually subsides after several hours, and, in others, is relieved by vomiting.[12]

He does not describe a case of his own but explains how duodenal ulcer can cause death by bleeding or perforation.

Unfortunately Abercrombie failed to gain the chair of Physic at

Edinburgh University and rather lost interest in medicine. This may partly explain why his work has been almost forgotten.[†] Was duodenal ulcer a rare disease during the nineteenth century? Yes, according to the huge survey of Guy's Hospital post mortems published by Sir Edwin Cooper Perry (1856–1938) and Lauriston Shaw (1859–1923) in 1893. In the preceding 60 years they only managed to find 70 examples of duodenal ulcer, that is 0.4 per cent of all cases.[13] Perhaps a lesion in the duodenum was regarded as so unlikely that the duodenum was not examined with the same thoroughness in every post mortem as the stomach. On the other hand Hugh Baron (born 1931), honorary professorial lecturer at Mount Sinai School of Medicine New York, has recently identified every report of every patient in the USA and Britain with a gastric or duodenal ulcer from 1800 onwards. With the help of Amnon Sonnenberg in Albuquerque, he has found a steady growth from the beginning of the nineteenth century. Both countries show the same rise with duodenal ulcer lagging about ten to twenty years behind gastric ulcer.[14] The same applies in France and Germany, though the Germans were slow to recognise the existence of duodenal ulcer. So if duodenal ulcer was not uncommon it was certainly overlooked because people were unaware of it and missed the significance of it at post mortem. William Osler, the foremost clinician of his day, wrote in 1901 that ulcers were uncommon.[15] He had only diagnosed 25 peptic ulcers in 9 years. Duodenal ulcer was rare (he had seen nine), but even as Osler was writing, a young surgeon in Leeds called Berkeley Moynihan was about to show the world that duodenal ulcer was a common condition, even more common than gastric ulcer.

[†]   In 1808 Dr. Abercrombie married a woman of considerable fortune, which enabled him to keep his carriage. His exceptional qualities were recognised by the award of Fellow of Edinburgh College and his appointment as Physician to George IV in Scotland. It was James Gregory, the Professor of Medicine, who once remarked "that wee fellow will someday be Edinburgh's most sought after consultant", and so he proved to be. Without a hospital appointment, through sheer high quality practice and inspired teaching he achieved the standing foretold by Gregory.

CHAPTER FIVE

EARLY SURGERY FOR PEPTIC ULCER

Abdominal surgery was practically unknown before 1870, except for a few pioneer belly rippers as the ovariotomists were contemptuously called. It was even rare in the 1880s though some of the first ovariotomists had done large numbers of cases by then. Lister's first paper on antiseptic surgery was published in 1867[16] but it was not for some years that surgeons, even the most progressive, had sufficient confidence in it or knowledge of it to encroach on hitherto forbidden territory. Indeed one of the most eminent surgeons of the time, Sir John Eric Erichsen (1818–96) at University College Hospital, prophesised in 1873 that "the abdomen, the chest and the brain would be forever shut from the intrusion of the wise and humane surgeon".[17] Lister himself hardly ever operated on the abdomen.

In Vienna, Theodor Billroth (1829–94) was working out the technique of gastrectomy for cancer of the stomach practising on dogs. His school established a great reputation and some of his students such as Mikulicz-Radecki (1850–1905) and Polya (1876–1944) are still familiar names. Having shown that such operations were feasible in cancer patients it was not long before surgeons turned to the benign but invariably fatal problem of a perforated gastric ulcer. The first successful case was carried out by a relatively obscure surgeon in Wiesbaden in 1892. In this country Hastings Gilford (1861–1941)[18] at Reading repaired a perforated gastric ulcer in June 1893. The patient survived after a stormy convalescence. Gilford did not report this case immediately so credit for the first successful published account in this country goes to Thomas Morse (1859–1921) at Norwich who operated on a girl of twenty in her home in 1894.[19]

Gastro-jejunostomy was introduced for the palliative treatment of pyloric obstruction by Billroth's assistant, Anton Woelfler. Logically it was then applied for the management of benign pyloric stenosis due to gastroduodenal ulceration, but then by some strange step to the treatment of chronic uncomplicated gastric and duodenal ulcer. This was probably because the risk of an abdominal operation at the turn of the century was still considerable. Approximately two thirds of all patients died after abdominal section had been performed on them. "The work was not then a chapter of great surgical achievements, it was a martyrology," wrote Moynihan later.[20] "This was in part due to the large proportion of desperate or 'too late' cases of obstruction and the like that were tackled and in part that the hand of the beginner was heavy."

In 1900 one of the surgical pioneers, Arthur Mayo-Robson (1853–1933) of Leeds (later Sir Arthur) delivered the Hunterian Lectures on the surgery of the stomach. He was able to collect 184 operations performed for gastric ulcer excluding those done for perforation or haemorrhage. The mortality was sixteen per cent. Within eighteen months the same author had a mortality of five per cent and with his colleague Berkeley Moynihan, he was recommending gastroenterostomy for those patients whose ulcer was unresponsive to medical treatment.

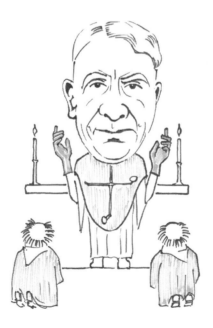

11   Moynihan – Surgeon is the high priest; registrars are his acolytes.

In 1901 Moynhihan (1865–1936) wrote his first paper about duodenal ulcer, describing seven cases on which he had operated.[21] In the next 5 years he operated on a further 100 cases and was soon operating on at least 2 cases a week. He was a master craftsman who revolutionised the technique of the operating theatre with his concept of strict discipline and team work. He lay enormous importance upon the appearance of living tissues seen at operation – what he called "the pathology of the living".[22] The abnormalities seen then, he said, were what gave rise to the patient's pain. Post mortem was well enough but it only told of the end results of illness, it did not reveal what was wrong at the onset of ill health, at a time when cure was most desirable. "The final ruin of an Abbey tells us nothing of the domestic habits of the monks who found shelter within its once unbroken walls." [23]

How did Moynihan diagnose duodenal ulcer without the help of X-rays, acid studies or even the experience of others? At the end of each operation he would draw an exact picture of the abnormalities he had seen and these little sketches were bound in the volume of his case records. Within a decade he was able to pool a group of cases in which the characteristic feature was severe abdominal pain after food. The pain did not come on until at least an hour after the meal had been taken, the patients discovered for themselves that they could relieve their pain by taking more food, drinking a glass of milk, or taking a dose of alkali. These cases differed from the classical symptoms of gastric ulcer, and, by referring to his drawings, Moynihan found that they all had duodenal ulcers. Then he applied the reverse investigation to another group of cases, a group in which his drawings all showed a duodenal ulcer at operation. What were their symptoms? If they had pain relievable by food, the so called "hunger pain" coming on some time after food, then he could claim that the symptoms of a duodenal ulcer differed from those of a gastric ulcer. His enquiry bore him out, the cases did have pain, which was delayed, and was relieved by food.

Moynihan published his views in 1910 in a book entitled simply *Duodenal Ulcer* and he lectured widely on the subject.[24] His fluency as an orator was equalled by his lucid prose. Truly, as Osler wrote soon afterwards, "physicians have been napping, and what the modern gastroenterologist needs is a prolonged course of study at such surgical clinics as Leeds or Rochester, Minnesota (where the Mayo brothers were operating).

Like doubting Thomas, a startled Arthur Hurst visited Leeds to see for himself. He was impressed and one of the first physicians to appreciate Moynihan's work. But he was not overcome. "According to Mr. Moynihan and his followers" (in the provinces and in Scotland) "there is only one treatment of duodenal ulcer, and that is by surgery. I am convinced that this teaching is erroneous, because it is quite common for people with the symptoms, which we now believe to indicate the presence of a duodenal ulcer or a pre-ulceration condition, to get well with fairly simple treatment."[25]

They both agreed that treatment with alkalis was worthwhile. However, though Moynihan was convinced that acid was the key factor in duodenal ulcer, he was less impressed by the benefit of alkalis. They both also believed that removal of chronic sepsis was important. Moynihan claimed that definite appendicular disease was present in 66 per cent of cases of duodenal ulcer. Hurst agreed with this. "The association of chronic appendicitis with acute ulcer is too common to be explained by coincidence," he wrote, "and the causal connection is made still more probable by the frequency with which repeated haematemesis from recurrent acute ulcers" (erosions) "ceases after the removal of an inflamed appendix. As chronic ulcers probably always originate as acute ulcers, the well recognised connection between chronic appendicitis and chronic ulcer, especially of the duodenum, is doubtless of the same nature."[26] Hurst also believed that chronic tonsillar infection and infected teeth (pyorrhoea alveolaris) were important causes of chronic ulcer and recommended that these should be extracted (not to mention problems with nasal sinuses, prostate and gall bladder).

What upset Hurst was that the usual "medical treatment" was quite inadequate. Even when the greatest care was taken with the diet and administration of drugs, often no effort was made to eradicate septic foci from the mouth, nose and throat, and the patient was rarely given sufficiently precise instructions as to his diet and way of life in the future (i.e. no smoking, minimal alcohol, avoid excessive fatigue, eat meals punctually and slowly).

CHAPTER SIX

EARLY RADIOLOGY

As the comparative frequency of chronic duodenal ulcer became accepted, post mortem statistics confirmed the increase. Pathologists were now investigating the duodenum in every case with special care. In Leeds, a chronic ulcer or its scar was found in the duodenum in about six per cent of post mortems as compared with four per cent in the stomach.[27] Clinicians began to diagnose ulcers with more confidence but with treatment now involving several weeks of rest and the possibility of surgery, the need for as certain a diagnosis as possible became paramount. The assistance of X-rays could not have arrived at a more opportune time.

Roentgen (1845–1923) discovered X-rays in 1895 and by the turn of the century bismuth compounds were being swallowed to outline the upper GI tract. To make it more palatable the bismuth was mixed with bread and milk or porridge. The films obtained could only demonstrate gross abnormalities such as a large growth in the stomach, an hourglass deformity or tight pyloric stenosis. They were useful for assessing the motor activity of the stomach, especially spasm, which might suggest an ulcer was present. However, only the craters of large penetrating gastric ulcers could be recognised with any confidence.

Barium was introduced in 1912 by Martin Haudek (1880–1931), a German physician, and soon replaced bismuth because it was more opaque, just as safe and infinitely cheaper. For some years barium meals were done in two stages; the first meal ("the motor meal") was given in the evening and the second the following day to outline the anatomy of the stomach. Great care, skill and patience was required by the radiologist if he was to obtain films of diagnostic quality. With experience it became possible to see most gastric ulcers, but the duodenum was a challenge.

The crater of an ulcer, contraction by scar tissue and spasm gave rise to a most confusing picture, and it was quite impossible to say which of these factors was deforming the bulb. Despite the limitations of early radiography the X-ray became invaluable as a means of diagnosis.

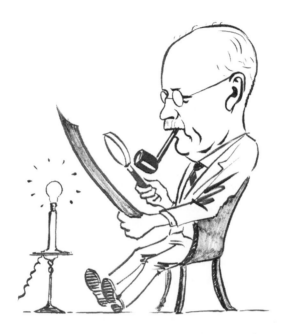

12 Barclay – Pioneer radiologist.

One of the first radiologists to study the stomach was Alfred Barclay (1876–1949) at Manchester. He contributed much to the early art of diagnosis but also to a misconception that Arthur Hurst perpetuated for several years. Barclay thought that a short stomach with active peristalsis and rapid evacuation was characteristic of duodenal ulcer.[28] Hurst and others found that people with these stomachs were prone to hyperchlohydria and called the condition the hypersthenic gastric constitution. "This condition though compatible with perfect digestion is, I believe, the essential predisposing factor in the production of duodenal ulcer."[29] His views seemed to be supported by the work of John Campbell (1891–1973) and John Coneybeare (1888–1967), who studied 54 students at Guy's Hospital in 1924. They found that the six with the highest stomachs had relatively short wide chests and four of these had hyperacidity and stomachs that emptied rapidly.[30] For a decade many believed that body shape provided a clue to the likelihood of a peptic ulcer. However, later evidence did not support these views and people realised that stomach shape was not a biological entity. The shape of a bismuth- or barium-filled stomach was decided by gravity acting on a substance of specific gravity greater than one, contained in an organ of variable tone. A short or steer-horn stomach was a radiological artefact, rarely found by a surgeon at laparotomy. Incidentally Campbell went on to become the first cardiologist at Guy's Hospital. Coneybeare was also a Guy's man through and through, and wrote a popular textbook of medicine that ran to thirteen editions. He was a founder member of the British gastro-enterological club in 1937 and was knighted after attaining the rank of Air-Vice Marshall during the Second World War.

CHAPTER SEVEN

GASTRIC SECRETION

The story of peptic ulcer is inextricably linked with that of hydrochloric acid. From the time of Prout's discovery that gastric acid was hydrochloric, doctors and physiologists have assumed that an understanding of its secretion would be the key to the cause, diagnosis and treatment of peptic ulcer disease. At times they seemed right because after years of study the suppression of acid by refined surgical techniques (highly selective vagotomy) and acid-blocking drugs appeared to heal ulcers. Ironically we now know that acid is only a part of the cause of peptic ulcer disease, the diagnosis no longer relies on the study of acid secretion, and acid suppression plays only a small role in the treatment of the condition.

For years investigators of gastric acidity had different intentions. On the one hand physiologists wanted to unravel the nervous and hormonal mechanisms that control the response of the stomach to feeding, and worked almost entirely on dogs and cats. On the other, clinicians and clinical scientists were interested in the actual amount of acid in the human stomach in so far as it would help them to diagnose and treat ulcers. They worked in isolation for a long time until eventually their discoveries made them indispensable to one another.

The physiologists studied the stomach by a series of painstaking experiments involving innervated gastric pouches (Pavlov type) and denervated pouches (Heidenheim). This type of work required enormous dedication and skill and must have been extremely frustrating. The first important British contribution came from John Edkins[†] who was the

---

[†]   John Edkins (1863–1941) was lecturer in physiology at St. Bartholomew's Hospital and later Professor of Physiology at Bedford College. His main research interest was the stomach and in 1940 he described spirochaetes in the gastric mucous membrane. Sadly he died shortly before the gastrin/histamine controversy was finally settled. He was a superb lecturer and a formidable croquet player.

first to enunciate the gastrin theory. His preliminary communication was given to the Royal Society in May 1905. It occupied a single paper of the proceedings and was entitled "On the chemical mechanism of gastric secretion".

> It has long been known that the introduction of certain substances into the stomach promotes a secretion of gastric juice.... On the analogy of what has been held to be the mechanism at work in the secretion of pancreatic juice by Bayliss and Starling, it is probable that, in the process of absorption of digested food in the stomach, a substance may be separated from the cells of the mucous membrane which, passing into the blood or lymph, later stimulates the secretion cells of the stomach to functional activity. The following observations support this view:

> If an extract in 5 per cent dextrin of the fundus mucous membrane be injected into the jugular veins of an anaesthetised cat, there is no evidence of secretion of gastric juice. If the extract be made with the pyloric mucous membrane, there is evidence of a small quantity of secretion. With dextrin itself there is no secretion.

> Extracts of fundus mucous membrane in dextrose or maltose give no secretion; extracts of pyloric mucous membrane give marked secretion; dextros or maltose alone bring about no secretion.

> If the extracts be made by boiling the mucous membrane in the different media, the effect is just the same, that is to say, the active principle, which may be called "gastrin", is not destroyed by boiling.[31]

Unfortunately Edkins work was followed by a long and unrewarding search for evidence that his antral hormone existed.

For years people thought that gastrin was nothing more than histamine. This was isolated by Henry Dale (1875–1968) in 1907, was found in almost all the tissues in the body, and was shown to be a powerful stimulant of gastric acid a few years later.[32] In fact it took more than 40 years of effort before Mort Grossman (1919–81), working in Andrew Ivy's Laboratory in Chicago, finally confirmed that there was a hormone in the antrum that stimulated acid secretion.[33] One of those working with Ivy was a young English physiologist called Rod Gregory (1913–90) whose name was later to become synonymous with gastrin.

Meanwhile clinicians were trying to study gastric secretion in man. The Germans were the first to devise a simple test meal, notably Carl Ewald (1845–1915) in Berlin in 1885. He gave his patients a "test breakfast" of bread and water and emptied the stomach one hour later using an ordinary stomach tube. The single specimen test gradually developed into the fractional test meal whereby repeated sampling of the gastric contents could be made every fifteen minutes and curves of acidity plotted.

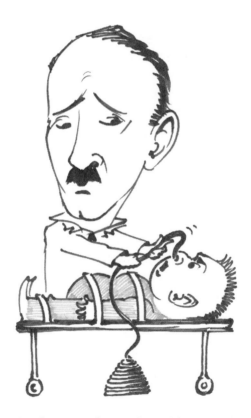

*13 Ryle – **Studies must be conducted humanistically.***

At the end of the First World War two English physicians collaborated in some work that made them household names for decades. After demobilisation Izod Bennett (1887–1946) returned to Guy's Hospital where he became a medical assistant and held a demonstratorship in Professor Pembury's department of physiology. He was very interested in the study of gastric secretion and the method of fractional gastric analysis, but as Pembury pointed out, unless one had knowledge of the normal range it was impossible to interpret the test meal charts.

Bennett joined forces with John Ryle (1889–1950), then a medical registrar at Guy's who invented a thin weighted rubber gastric tube for the collection of gastric samples, remembered to this day as Ryle's tube. Together they set out to perform a hundred gastric analyses on normal people. Swallowing a tube was never a pleasant undertaking and in those days it was more or less unheard of. It required all Bennett's personality to collect his share of the hundred. The volunteers were obtained from anybody that he met and a great many were students. Their results were reported in a classical paper; the subjects had widely differing acid levels ranging from hyperchlorhydria to achlorhydria but most were isochlorhydric.[34] Their "normal range" was used as the reference for decades but there was disagreement as to the degree of reproducibility of the test meal response. Bennett and Ryle claimed that "in several instances identical curves have been obtained on different occasions"; on the other hand James Bell (1896–1969) and William MacAdam (1885–1976) in Leeds did fractional test meals on twenty consecutive days on one normal subject (a cooperative individual) and found large variations from day to day.[35] There were many problems inherent in the test such as the emptying rate of the stomach, the regurgitation of duodenal juice or even dilution by saliva, let alone the meal itself. A single estimate of acidity was attempting to measure several variables, so it was hardly surprising that this ritual, so assiduously practised for half a century (especially in private clinics on the continent) yielded such meagre results. MacAdam later became Professor of Medicine at Leeds and was a founder member of the British Gastroenterological Club.

Not long after histamine had been shown to stimulate gastric acid, it was introduced as a stimulus for test meals instead of food. Though many of the disadvantages of the fractional test meal remained, it was at least feasible to aspirate all the gastric juice without the problem of food contamination and possible, after multiplying volume by acidity, to obtain the total quantity of acid present at a given time. In this country Frank Lee Lander (1906–81) and Noel Maclagan (1904–87), working in Charles Dodds' department of biochemistry at the Middlesex Hospital, eastablished a normal range of acid output in response to histamine, again on a hundred medical students.[36] Maclagan later became the first medically qualified professor of chemical pathology in Britain (at the Westminster Hospital).

Jack Hunt (1917–86), a mercurial clinical physiologist at Guy's Hospital, criticised a common fault in the interpretation of the test meals. Because many workers had failed to recognise that the acidity was the resultant of the interplay between gastric emptying and gastric secretion, he devised the serial test meal in which the whole of the gastric contents was withdrawn on successive days for progressively longer periods each time.[37] He also included a non-absorbable dye so that the volume of gastric contents passing into the duodenum could be calculated. Knowing the amount of acid in the stomach and the amount lost through the pylorus, the total acid secreted could be calculated. Unsurprisingly, the serial test meal did not catch on in clinical practice. Hunt also calculated that the quality of parietal cell secretion is the same in normal and ulcer subjects.

Anthony James (1921–2010), working at St. Mary's Hospital, Paddington at the time, stressed that it was important to know the position of the gastric tube in the stomach by checking with X-rays and he showed that samples of gastric juice from the body, and from the antrum might differ in their acidities.[38] With George Pickering (1904–80), later Sir George of hypertension fame, he measured the pH profile over 24 hours by leaving a thin tube in the stomach and sampling hourly day and night.[39] During the day the most noticeable feature in normal subjects was a drop in acidity on the ingestion of each meal, followed by a gradual acidification until the next meal. During the night, when the stomach was empty, the resting juice was quite acid. Patients with gastric ulcers frequently had neutral gastric contents during the night, unlike patients with duodenal ulcers. Geoffrey Watkinson (1921–96) in Leeds, who repeated these experiments, showed that gastric juice became neutral during the second half of the night. He attributed this to reflux of bile through the pylorus.[40] However, James thought that a fall in acid secretion was the more likely explanation.

In 1952 Wilfrid Card (1908–85) and his colleagues at the Western

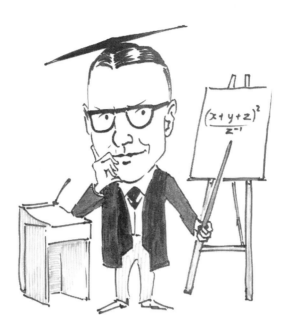

$$\frac{(x+y+z)^2}{z^{-1}}$$

14 Card – Decision-making is mathematical.

General Hospital, Edinburgh emphasised the importance of maximal acid secretion.[41] Card assumed that each parietal cell could make so much acid and no more. If so, the total acid output of the stomach would be related to the total parietal cell mass. Initially he was unable to stimulate the human stomach maximally owing to the unpleasant side effects of histamine, but by giving constant intravenous doses of histamine and measuring the corresponding acid output, he constructed a dose response curve. He concluded that patients with duodenal ulcers did indeed have a large secretory cell mass.

Once it was realised that antihistamines did not affect the stimulant action of histamine on gastric secretion but did counteract the other actions of histamine, it was only a matter of time before Andrew Kay (born 1916), later Sir Andrew, in Glasgow, was able to show that after a dose of the antihistamine mepyramine maleate 30 minutes beforehand, he could give huge doses of histamine.[42] Using his so called augmented histamine test, Kay showed that, with increasing doses of histamine, acid output increased to a maximum, after which further increases in dose led to no change in acid output. Using this technique, Wilfrid Card was able to support his theory of a larger parietal cell mass in many patients with a duodenal ulcer.[43] Subsequently Hugh Baron (born 1931), at the Middlesex Hospital, advocated the measurement of peak acid output as an equally useful but much simpler method of measuring maximal secretion.[44] (See p94.)

The histamine test meal was widely used by surgeons anxious to decide which patients with duodenal ulcers were most likely to benefit from surgery. It was also used to measure the success of their vagotomies.

Meanwhile Rod Gregory who had worked in Ivy's laboratory during the Second World War was now George Holt Professor of Physiology in Liverpool. During his work in America he had become interested in a hormone known as enterogastrone that inhibits gastric secretion after it has been released by the presence of fat in the duodenum. Perhaps isolation of this hormone would lead to a useful treatment for peptic ulcer? Unfortunately most investigators found that whereas their extracts of enterogastrone appeared to inhibit gastric secretion when injected into dogs, instillation of fat into the duodenum had no effect. Gregory realised that in their experiments histamine was used as the stimulus to gastric secretion and that their enterogastrone extracts were crude and contaminated by histamine inhibitors. In a series of meticulous experiments in dogs he showed that fat in the duodenum did indeed liberate enterogastrone even though gastric secretion (stimulated by histamine) was not inhibited.[45] He postulated that enterogastrone might work by inhibiting gastrin released from the antrum and proved this later when he showed that fat in the duodenum did inhibit acid secretion when it was stimulated by gastrin.

These tests for the study of enterogastrone required a stable "background" level of acid secretion that could be reliably inhibited by the enterogastrone extracts, and clearly gastrin was required rather than histamine. At the time the methods of preparing gastrin were still crude. In this country only Alfred Harper (1907–96) in Manchester had an extract.[46] It was of protein character, free of histamine and when injected intravenously into animals caused secretion of a highly acid juice. Once it was recognised that gastrin was a peptide, it was no longer confused with histamine. Gregory realised a purer product was required and with his experience in protein and peptide chemistry found a new method of preparing a potent and highly purified product of gastrin. Working with Hilda Tracy, a biochemist, he isolated a product from Hog's stomachs, obtained from the local abattoir, using ion exchange chromatography resins, which had just become available.[47] His substance was free from histamine and very effective in stimulating acid secretion in dogs and men by subcutaneous, intramuscular and intravenous injection.

Gregory and Tracy submitted their work for publication only to have it bounced back as irrelevant. But Hilda Tracy seized her opportunity when she guessed that the recently described Zollinger-Ellison syndrome was probably due to excessive gastrin secretion from the non-insulin-producing tumours of the islets of the pancreas. It so happened that a physician in Edinburgh called Wilfred Sircus (born 1919) knew of a patient with such a tumour. Sircus knew Gregory well, having worked with him on duodenal mechanisms that inhibit acid secretion. Accordingly a portion of the tumour was brought to Liverpool and its extract tested on a conscious gastric fistula dog. Acid simply poured out. After publication in the *Lancet*,[48] Gregory and Tracy received tumours from all over the world and were able to isolate the active principle, which was identical with gastrin.[†] They worked closely with the peptide chemists in Liverpool who were a rare breed in those days. One was George Kenner (1922–78), Professor of Organic Chemistry, who had little problem establishing the structure of gastrin and synthesising it (very quickly too, much to Gregory's delight).

In his laboratory at the time there was a young chemist from ICI called Jack Morley. With the team, he looked at the structure-function relationships of gastrin, hoping perhaps to find a gastrin antagonist. Though unsuccessful they did discover where the active part of the gastrin peptide lay and before long they had several synthetic gastrins.[49] Gregory came up with pentagastrin, which was shown to be every bit as potent as histamine as an acid stimulant but safer and more comfortable for the patient. So in the end, Gregory, who had started by looking for an acid inhibitor, found he had a potent stimulator, pentagastrin, which soon replaced the augmented histamine test in most laboratories.[50]

---

1   Mort Grossman brought a massive tumour over from the States. It was in a large and conspicuous box that attracted the attention of the customs officer in Liverpool. Asked what was in the box Grossman said, "Well, it's a very, very big tumour and I don't think you want to look inside the box." The customs officer waved him through hurriedly. Grossman visited Liverpool quite frequently and Raymond (Gerry) Kirk, a surgeon at the Royal Free Hospital once said to him, "Isn't Liverpool a marvellous gutsy city?" Grossman replied, "Yes, it's very gutsy, but it's also very ugly. If God ever decides to give the world an enema, that's where he will put the nozzle."

CHAPTER EIGHT

THE RISE IN INCIDENCE OF PEPTIC ULCER

Remarkable changes have occurred in the behaviour of peptic ulcer during the last 200 years. Before 1830, ulceration seems to have been a rare cause of sudden death. The clinical picture of perforation is easy to recognise: sudden agonising pain, board-like rigidity of the abdomen and in most cases collapse and death within 24–48 hours and would hardly have escaped the notice of the fine eighteenth-century physicians. Several cases were in fact reported but they are difficult to verify. These were post mortem accounts of holes in the stomach with food in the peritoneal cavity but were unconvincing because the authors were unsure of the distinction between ante-mortem and postmortem events and gave few clinical details. The most notable English case was that of James Skidmore, reported to the Royal Society by Christopher Rawlinson, a surgeon, in 1727. (Appendix.)

Even early in the nineteenth century perforation was rare. For example Benjamin Travers (1783–1858) Surgeon to St. Thomas's Hospital and one of the original 300 Fellows of the College of Surgeons had only seen two cases of perforated ulcer with a third described to him.[51] His clinical description was brilliant, and we cannot disregard his opinion when he calls the condition rare and unmistakable. However, within the next few years accounts of perforation became common. Many happened in young women in their teens and twenties. They seem to have been acute gastric ulcers near the cardia perforating out of the blue. Practitioners dealing with this illness, which "swept away beautiful and healthy creatures within a few hours", found it one of the most tragic experiences of their lives. In 1857 Brinton reviewed 160 perforations in

women and 74 in men; more than two thirds of the women were under
34 years of age, whereas the men were equally affected throughout life.

Thereafter references in the literature to perforated ulcer became
almost apologetic. There was nothing new to say; Wilhelm Leube
(1842–1912), a German physician, summed up the prevalent attitude in
1876 by describing "euthanasia as the only treatment".[52] However, at the
turn of the century the condition in young women began to decline. We
do not know exactly when this happened but it was probably between
1905 and 1920. In 1905 the registrar general was still able to write,
"Gastric ulcer does not appear frequently as a cause of death until the
attainment of the reproductive period, when the female rate greatly
exceeds the male, while at later ages the male is in excess."[53]

About 1890, when it was realised that surgery gave a chance of
recovery, hospital admissions began to increase. By 1895 recoveries
were becoming common, especially in England, where the importance
of early operation was quickly learnt. After 1900 the diagnosis of ulcer
improved and this coupled with better transport increased the number
of cases going to hospital. Deaths from gastric ulcer were added to the
registrar general's mortality figures in 1901 and deaths from duodenal
ulcer were added in 1911. However, the medical reports of the 1914–18
War do not mention duodenal ulcer as a reason for medical discharge.

After the First World War the incidence of peptic ulcer continued
to rise, especially during the Second World War, reaching a peak in the
1950s. Thereafter the number of ulcers began to decline, a trend that
has continued. Men were more susceptible to the disease than women;
they were three times more likely to have a gastric ulcer and six times
more likely to have a duodenal ulcer. Indeed it was the dramatic rise
in duodenal ulcer that fuelled the numbers during the first half of the
twentieth century and many of these men were young or middle aged.
Clinicians were soon busy and a surgical registrar would feel cheated if
he did not admit "a perforation" during his night on call. These clinical
impressions were supported by several surveys documenting the rise and
subsequent fall of the disease. Apart from highlighting its importance
epidemiologists hoped that they would find some clues that would reveal
the cause of peptic ulcer.

The problem confronting everyone before the arrival of modern
endoscopy in about 1970 was accurate diagnosis. Even by X-rays the
diagnosis of ulcer, especially duodenal ulcer, was imprecise to say the

least. For example the registrar general's mortality statistics were based on death certificates issued in the normal routine of medical practice, and these can be depressingly inaccurate. Death certificates are also unsatisfactory for a disease such as peptic ulcer, which is rarely fatal because changes in prevalence are confused with changes in fatality. An improvement in treatment will clearly improve the mortality rate. In fact the low death rate of peptic ulcer was offset by the sheer number of residents in the United Kingdom with the disease, and data collected over five to ten consecutive years were averaged. The figures confirmed a steady and impressive rise in the number of deaths during the first half of the century followed by an equally impressive fall.

The uncertainties of diagnosis led people to look at autopsy series. These have the great merit that the diagnosis is precise, but unless the pathologist is prepared to examine the stomach and duodenum carefully many ulcer scars may be missed. One of the best series was undertaken in Leeds. Thanks to Moynihan's influence Leeds had become a leading centre for the treatment of peptic ulcer when in 1918 Matthew Stewart (1885–1956) was appointed to the chair of pathology at the age of 33. He had already learned the value of statistical methods and was a keen observer with a remarkable visual memory. Arthur Hurst quickly recognised his talent and by the time they had collaborated on their joint monograph *Gastric and Duodenal Ulcer* in 1929, Stewart had personally supervised nearly 6,000 autopsies. He sought ulcers with almost fanatical care and correlated them with the clinical findings. Continuing to keep meticulous records for another twenty years he inspired his staff to do the same. (His hobby was philately so I can imagine him, catalogue in hand, seeking rare watermarks or misprints.) He retired in 1950 but his work was later analysed by Geoffrey Watkinson, then a senior lecturer at Leeds.[54] Because he had such good material to work with, Watkinson (1921–96) was able to count the number of active and inactive ulcers (scars) in practically every post mortem done by Stewart and his team from 1930–49. He thought that the best estimate of ulcer frequency in the general population was obtained by recording the number of ulcers found incidentally in people dying in hospital, so he deliberately excluded all those who had died as a result of their ulcer. The Leeds figures showed a steady rise in peptic ulcer from ten per cent in 1918 to twenty per cent in 1949, which is probably an overestimate.

Watkinson compared the Leeds figures with a national survey of autopsies he organised in eighteen hospitals in the UK in 1956. By this time the frequency of ulcer had almost halved, suggesting the tide was turning, though Watkinson thought that many inactive ulcers had been missed by the general pathologists (others would argue that the Leeds pathologists saw scars that weren't there). The survey showed that ulcers were more common in Northern England and Scotland because of the high prevalence of duodenal ulcer in young men, especially in Scotland.

Unfortunately many autopsy series were not so scrupulously carried out and the fallacies inherent in this type of analysis discouraged pathologists. The *Lancet* suggested that the time and money spent on this type of examination could well be utilised in more profitable pastimes. Watkinson once admitted "necropsy statistics can be likened to corsets as undesirable, uncomfortable, frequently giving a fallacious impression of truth yet in special selected circumstances forming a basis for deduction and at all times much sought after".[55]

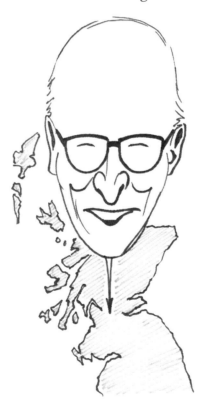

15 Illingworth – Glory of Glasgow medical school.

The admission rate for perforated ulcer was a reliable index of ulcer frequency simply because admission was obligatory. For some reason peptic ulcer was very common in Scotland and especially Glasgow, where Charles Illingworth (1899–1991), later Sir Charles, was appointed Regius Professor of Surgery in 1939. The department was at a low ebb at the time but under his guidance it soon eclipsed all others. Academically the majority of university surgical departments specialised in upper abdominal surgery at the time. The study of gastric secretion in artificial pouches in dogs was popular and for years meetings of the Surgical Research Society were notable for people presenting their work in a Scottish accent.

Illingworth's unit recorded the frequency and incidence of perforated ulcer in the West of Scotland for no fewer than 50 years in a remarkable study from 1924–73.[56] They saw the number of perforations rise steadily, doubling between 1924 and 1934, and this was entirely due to the increase in juxta-pyloric (duodenal) ulcers in men. The trend continued with a spike occuring during the wartime bombing of Glasgow in 1940–41, to reach a peak in the early 1950s.[57] Since then the number of perforated duodenal ulcers has fallen steadily, though they are still by far the most common cause of perforation.[58/59] In contrast, perforated ulcers in women were always a fraction of the number in men, though the number of older women with gastric ulcers has risen recently.

The frequency of peptic ulcer and its implications for both the victim and his employer led others to examine the hospital records of their patients with ulcers, whether perforated or not. Epidemiologically this was fraught with pitfalls. Clearly hospital figures are inappropriate for calculating the incidence of a disease in the population at large. Diagnosis before the arrival of endoscopy was sufficiently uncertain to invalidate the results and the patients were highly selective. Frequently inpatients only were studied, again misleading because patients with a gastric ulcer were more likely to be admitted than those with a duodenal ulcer. This was because patients with a gastric ulcer often looked ill, and radiologically a large lesser curve ulcer was more impressive than a deformed duodenal cap. The pressure on beds before the war (nothing changes) meant that the majority of duodenal ulcer patients were returned to their GP after the X-ray diagnosis had been made.

It was against such a background that in 1940 Francis Avery Jones (1910–2000), later Sir Francis, opened Britain's first specialised gastroenterology unit at the Central Middlesex Hospital. Just 30 years old, he had already made his mark working for Professor Leslie Witts (1898–1982) at St. Bartholomew's Hospital, and was one of the few experts with the semi-flexible gastroscope. During the war, kept at his civilian post by the central medical war committee, Avery Jones kept detailed records of his ulcer patients, and significantly he included outpatients in his study. In common with Illingworth's Scottish study, Avery found that ulcer was largely a male disease and that duodenal ulcer was particularly common in young men.

The ideal way to measure ulcer frequency is by a planned survey of the whole population of a town or locality or a random sample drawn from it. Such studies are difficult to organise and are few and far between; one of the first was undertaken by Avery Jones after the war. By this time he had recruited an exceptional young research assistant, Richard Doll (1912–2005), from the Medical Research Council. Their survey of 6,000 Londoners was particularly interesting as it was done when peptic ulcer was at its height.[60] Some of the cases were diagnosed on symptoms only so we need to be cautious about the results. Once again they confirmed that ulcers were the prerogative of men who comprised 80 per cent of the cases; indeed 10 per cent of middle-aged men had an ulcer at any one time, an extraordinarily high figure. Duodenal ulcer outnumbered gastric ulcer by four to one in younger men but was still twice as common later in life. It was a major scourge of the time.

Another notable population survey was conducted by Norman Pulvertaft (1911–90) in the city and surrounding rural district of York.[61] "Plug" Pulvertaft, as he was known throughout his career, was a radiologist who managed to obtain prevalence rates of ulcers whether perforated or not. He confirmed that duodenal ulcer was more common than gastric ulcer in all age groups, and he also noted that city dwellers were more likely to suffer than country folk, and that people from the lower social classes were especially prone to the disease.

CHAPTER NINE

THE FALL IN INCIDENCE OF PEPTIC ULCER

At a time when this remorseless rise in ulcers was becoming a serious threat to the health and economic welfare of the workforce in the 1950s, a remarkable change occurred. The number of people with gastric ulcer began to fall, closely followed by those with duodenal ulcer. It took a while for the penny to drop. Doll was the first to note a change in mortality from gastric ulcer, which he thought was due to better treatment. But fewer people were being certified as unable to work because of their duodenal ulcer. For example Jerry Morris (1910–2009) from the MRCS social medicine research unit found a falling incidence of duodenal ulcers in doctors as judged by mortality, by hospital admission rates for perforation and by certified incapacity for work.[62] The trend continued and by 1999 there were only 3,500 ulcer deaths compared with 5,000 deaths in 1947, according to the registrar general's mortality figures for England and Wales, during which time the population rose by twenty per cent. The majority of deaths today are in people over the age of 75.

Fewer patients were being admitted to hospital with perforated ulcers. The great study started by Illingworth in the 1930s was continued by Colin Mackay in Glasgow, who completed 50 years of the study in 1973. As we have seen he found that perforated ulcers were becoming relatively less common in men and relatively more common in women, especially older women. Pulvertaft found the same; the incidence of perforated ulcers was falling dramatically in the City of York, especially duodenal ulcers in men.

Perhaps the best evidence came from the Hospital Inpatient Enquiry.

This was established in 1949 by the Office for National Statistics and recorded a sample of discharges and death in hospital from which total admission rates for a given disease could be calculated. Michael Langman, Professor of Therapeutics in Nottingham, analysed the data for peptic ulcer having cut his teeth earlier with Doll at the Medical Research Council's statistical and gastroenterological unit at University College Hospital. He found a steady fall in gastric and duodenal ulcer in men from 1957 to 1977, whether perforated or not.[63] Uncomplicated ulcers also fell in women, unlike perforated ones, which increased slightly. Nevertheless ulcers, especially duodenal ulcers were still much more common in men, though it was now old people who were suffering.[64]

CHAPTER TEN

AETIOLOGY OF PEPTIC ULCER

1) Stress

These (remarkable) changes in the pattern of peptic ulcer during the last 200 years inevitably posed the question – why? Surely, people argued, once they knew this, the cause of ulcers would be obvious. In fact when the answer came, it was dramatic and unexpected and still did not explain all the facts. The sharp rise in morbidity and mortality from peptic ulcer, particularly of the duodenum, during the first half of the twentieth century earned it a place as one of the "diseases of civilisation". However, during the 1950s the incidence of peptic ulcer began to fall. So ulcers could not be just diseases of civilisation in the sense that they were caused by the stresses common to industrial society. If they were, one would have expected them to have increased as society grew more complex and caught up in urban modes of life. The best explanation for the rise and fall in both gastric and duodenal ulcers was put forward by Mervyn Susser, an epidemiologist from South Africa working in the department of social and preventive medicine, Manchester, in 1962.[65] Together with his wife, Zena Stein, he showed that there was a steady rise in peptic ulcer mortality in successive generations born between 1840 and 1880 followed by a fall in all subsequent generations. He suggested that each "cohort" of births must have been exposed to something early in life that affected their future chances of getting an ulcer. Thus each generation carried its own particular risk of bearing ulcers throughout adult life. He could only speculate on what could be responsible, but wondered if ulcers arose from the effect of "early urbanisation", that is before the stress of city life was offset by the benefits of industrialisation such as greater social security and the abolition of extreme poverty. Perhaps too, people learnt to adapt to the demands of industrial society.

Susser was not alone in thinking stress played a part in the life history of patients with peptic ulcer. From the late Victorian period, everyone thought that stress (or mental anxiety as it was then called) was important. "Don't worry or you will get an ulcer," ran the old music hall joke. Brinton wrote that the pain of gastric ulcer was often affected by sudden mental changes. He alluded especially to the "depressing passions of fear, anxiety, or anger, as capable of providing a paroxysm which, in severity and duration, far exceeds the pain excited in the stomach by food".[66] John Ryle, in his Hunterian lecture of 1932 said, "A restless stomach accompanies a restless mind. In many cases (of duodenal ulcer) anxiety and mental conflict seem to play a part in the aggravation of symptoms. In a minority of cases (though it be beyond proof) it is tempting to wonder whether the disease would have developed in the absence of psychological turmoil."[67] Arthur Hurst agreed about the importance of the worry factor in duodenal ulcer, adding that it did not apply to gastric ulcer. The typical duodenal ulcer patient was described as "common in our cities and in the young and vigorous...and in those who drive themselves, drive vehicles and drive other people".

Another who was impressed with the frequency with which some personal tragedy preceded the symptoms of peptic ulcer was Daniel Davies (1899–1966), physician at the Royal Free Hospital and an astute clinician. He was Bradshaw Lecturer at the college in 1935 and entitled his talk "Some observations on peptic ulcer".[68] He showed that the great majority of his ulcer patients had suffered some misfortune shortly before their first attack of dyspepsia. Financial difficulties or a change of job, often a more responsible post, were the most common events. But he stressed that emotional disturbance alone was not enough. The seed must be implanted in the soil. Davies was convinced that his patients were compulsive workers and if they were not at work they were worrying about it. "The sharpness of the ulcer patient depends on a constant tension which is a valuable trait in its minor form but a penalty when it becomes more severe."

Later Richard Doll in his survey with Avery Jones after the Second World War found a high incidence of duodenal ulcer among men holding managerial posts in industry and among foremen rather than workers, which he tentatively suggested may have been the result of anxiety at work. Doctors often suggest a psychological cause for unexplained chronic diseases with a tendency to relapse. One day Richard Asher (1912–69) who, like MacNeice's cat, "lurked and fizzed" in the same hospital, gave Doll an article to read about duodenal ulcer and its cause by psychological stress. Asher wanted to know if it was a fair account of what people thought. Doll said the language was a bit stilted but otherwise he agreed that it was a fair reflection. In fact the article had been written in 1850 about general paralysis of the insane. Asher had merely substituted duodenal ulcer for GPI.[69]

Internal bleeding from an ulcer was also thought to be brought on by stress, so Doll drew up a list of life's disasters (as Davies had done) such as loss of job, family bereavement, divorce, bankruptcy etc., and enquired whether anyone coming into hospital with a bleed had recently experienced such a catastrophe. He found, in fact, that such events were no more likely in these patients than in a control group. Nonetheless, despite the lack of hard evidence, the profession continued to believe that emotional factors were important. After all, counselling was a useful approach to the treatment of ulcers at a time when the medicine cupboard was bare.

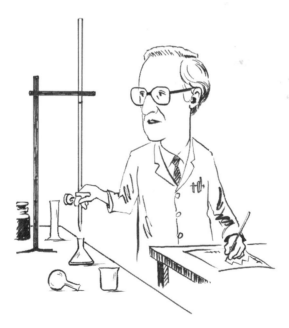

16 Baron – Dedicated follower of acid.

2) Acid

While the epidemiologists were highlighting the social and cultural trends in peptic ulcer, clinicians continued their search for the elusive cause of the disease. The chief of these as we have seen centred on the well known connection between acid and ulcers. The correlation between over and undersecretion of acid and ulcers was finally delineated by Hugh Baron when he formulated his concept of peak acid output. This was a measure of acid output after an intravenous injection of pentagastrin and it was simple to use. The two consecutive highest collection periods (usually fifteen minutes each) were measured, which correlated well with the maximal capacity of the stomach to secrete acid. Baron showed that there was a precise range of acid secretion above which duodenal ulcers were very likely to occur, and below which they were almost impossible. Unfortunately for diagnostic purposes the majority of patients fell within the "normal" range, which begged the question. Baron was among the greatest advocates of gastric function tests in the 1960s, but he was the first to acknowledge that their use in clinical practice became obsolete after the arrival of the easy-to-use fibreoptic gastroscope in the early 1970s.

3) Acute to chronic

If most people with ulcers had normal acid secretion there had to be another factor. We have seen how Arthur Hurst and Matthew Stewart thought that under certain conditions chronic peptic ulcer might develop from an acute ulcer, though they admitted that most acute ulcers healed spontaneously. This was an attractive idea at the time because at least two causes of acute ulcer were known that might be treatable. One was infection elsewhere in the body, notably appendicitis as mentioned earlier. The other was severe burns to the body. It was in 1842 that Thomas Blizard Curling (1811–88), assistant surgeon at the London Hospital and a founder member of the Royal College of Surgeons, presented a paper to the Royal Medical and Chirurgical Society "on acute ulceration of the duodenum in cases of burns".[70] Speaking when Brinton was a medical student, Curling remarked, "In no part of the alimentary canal are the diseases to which it is liable, so obscure, both in their origin and diagnosis, as in the duodenum; and as the following cases of ulceration of this portion of the small intestines in connection with burns may be interesting, as tending to throw some light on its pathology and to awaken some attention to a source of danger in these accidents not generally suspected, I have much pleasure complying with the wishes of the president in submitting them to the consideration of this Society." Curling thought that Brunner's glands in the duodenum oversecreted to compensate for the damaged sweat glands in the skin, and became inflamed and ulcerated in consequence. He recommended the application of leeches to the skin on the corresponding part of the abdomen (provided it was not burnt), opium for pain and bland fluids. In fact all five of Curling's patients were children and all died from bleeding or perforation.

4) Smoking

Another influence on ulcers was smoking. Since the turn of the twentieth century, evidence had accumulated that smoking was strongly associated with peptic ulcer. Prince Albert, later George VI, was a heavy cigarette smoker and developed severe dyspepsia aged twenty. Two years later, in 1917, he had to be taken from active duty by hospital ship from Scapa Flow to Aberdeen. A bland diet and rest provided no relief and in 1917 he was operated upon for a peptic ulcer by Sir Hugh Mallinson Rigby (1870–1944) who was Sergeant Surgeon to King George V. It is likely that a gastro-jejunostomy was done. The advent of cheap cigarettes during the First World War made smoking almost universal, particularly among the unemployed and lower social classes. The most popular padre in the trenches was "Woodbine Willie", the Rev G. A. Studdert-Kennedy who gave the men cigarettes. Arthur Hurst was struck by the connection between excessive smoking and duodenal ulcer. In 1929 he wrote that it was "difficult to say exactly what constituted excessive smoking but in most cases the patient knew that he smoked considerably more than the majority of his friends".[71] He thought smoking could be one of the reasons why duodenal ulcer was so much commoner in men than women. Writing with his usual conviction he said that nicotine blocked the sympathetic synapses thus partially paralysing those fibres that inhibit gastric juice. So the vagus could operate unopposed leading to hyperchlorrhydria, hypertonus and hyperperistalsis. He also thought that one reason why worry aggravates an ulcer was that it was so often an excuse for over-indulgence in tobacco. In contrast, John Ryle, while agreeing that smoking was important, found it "difficult to obtain concise proofs with regard to the part that this habit plays in determining the arrival or perpetuation of symptoms or the different incidence of duodenal ulcer between the two sexes".[72] And that was it. The impression was there, but proof was lacking and doubt persisted.

After the Second World War, while Richard Doll was working with Avery Jones at the Central Middlesex, he met Austin Bradford Hill (1897–1991), who invited him to work on the aetiology of lung cancer with him. Doll accepted and went on to make his name by proving that smoking caused lung cancer, while at the same time continuing his clinical research with Avery Jones who arranged for him to oversee six beds in his department to study factors that might promote peptic ulcer healing. Thus came the first randomised controlled trials in gastroenterology in this country, and they were immaculately carried out. Doll showed that only bed rest in hospital, stopping smoking and the drug carbenoloxone were of any value in the healing of a gastric ulcer. (He did not look at duodenal ulcer because at that time he had to rely on barium meal X-rays to demonstrate healing. Serial films showed the reduction or disappearance of an ulcer crater in the stomach but could not distinguish an active ulcer in the duodenum from an inactive one.) Doll also followed the fortunes of three quarters of the medical profession from 1951 to 1971, comparing smokers with non-smokers.[73] This was a tour de force in which he showed that smokers were more likely to die from a peptic ulcer than their non-smoking colleagues. But the epidemiological evidence connecting smoking and duodenal ulcer remained weak because most of the large surveys were based on questionnaires and symptoms, and without endoscopic proof of ulcers the results were difficult to interpret. Many thought that if there was a correlation between smoking and duodenal ulcer it probably meant they had a common cause rather than that one caused the other. It required many trials of the new ulcer-healing drugs to convince the sceptics. These showed that healing of endoscopically proven ulcers was delayed in smokers and that recurrence of ulceration was more likely.

When it came to explaining how smoking might cause ulcers, nobody knew. One surgeon who spent years of his life trying to find out was Professor Michael Hobsley (born 1929) at the Middlesex Hospital, who was particularly interested in acid secretion. Exactly as Hugh Baron had done, Hobsley showed that the greater the maximal secretion of acid the more likely a person was to get an ulcer, and he went on to show that there was a positive correlation between the total number of cigarettes smoked over a period of years and maximal gastric secretion. He concluded that smoking in so far as it might cause ulcers was working through acid.[74]

Others believed that smoking reduced the protective effect of prostaglandins in the gastric mucosa or that it had a detrimental effect on the blood supply to the stomach lining. It is probable that the question will remain unanswered because we now know the cause of the majority of ulcers, and that any contribution from smoking is trivial compared to its devastating effects elsewhere in the body. However, smoking probably played a part in the rise of ulcers early in the twentieth century and contributed to the fall later as the habit became less prevalent.

5) Anti-inflammatory drugs

The nature of the second factor besides acid, which everyone agreed was necessary for the production of a chronic ulcer, remained elusive. People invoked a "locus minoris resistentiae" (an area of reduced mucosal resistance) as the additional factor but this evaded the real difficulty because the diminished local resistance could only be the result of some active process.[†] Only when this is removed can an ulcer heal. So there had to be an initiating substance. The most likely candidate, for some ulcers at least, appeared to be anti-inflammatory drugs.

Aspirin was introduced into clinical practice in 1899 and soon became a best seller, widely used for all types of pain and inflammation, especially in rheumatic conditions. Before long it was known to cause indigestion, usually as heartburn, occasionally as epigastric pain. In the 1930s the textbooks taught that sodium salicylate irritated the stomach when salicylic acid was released by the hydrochloric acid of the gastric juice. Aspirin, however, was thought to have little effect because hydrochloric acid is very slow to liberate salicylic acid from it.

---

†   According to Virgil Moon (1879–1965), an American pathologist, locus minoris resistentiae was an erudite term under which our predecessors recorded this observation and concealed their ignorance of the essential mechanism involved. Moon V. H. 1938 *Shock and Related Capillary Phenomena*. London and New York. Oxford University Press

Yet it was known that multiple gastric submucous haemorrhages and even haematemesis occurred in aspirin poisoning. This discrepancy between the pharmacological teaching and clinical experience intrigued Arthur Douthwaite (1896–1974), a physician at Guy's Hospital and a founder member of the British Gastroenterological Club. His interest was further aroused by a doctor, who on account of headaches kept himself going in his practice by taking aspirin. "After ten days the doctor awoke one morning in more pain and took two aspirin tablets without water or milk as was his custom. A quarter of an hour later he felt a slight epigastric pain; the same day, four or five hours later, he felt faint and had colic, and soon passed a large tarry stool. As it happened this doctor had had his alimentary tract examined by X-rays and a fractional test meal and a blood count done four or five days before, and apart from hyperchlorrhydria he was shown to be normal. The investigations had been purely precautionary as he had reached middle life (41 years). After the melaena, which lasted for three days, his haemoglobin was 58 per cent. In spite of this he carried on at work, and made a complete recovery. When radiographed twelve days later, again no abnormality was found."[75]

Douthwaite was convinced that aspirin had caused the bleeding so he decided to look at the effect aspirin had on the mucosa of the stomach endoscopically. He had been one of the first physicians to take up gastroscopy using the semi-flexible Schindler gastroscope. With his colleague Gordon Lintott (1908–40) he studied sixteen patients after they had swallowed crushed aspirin.[76] The endoscopies were performed under local anaesthetic and lasted up to ten minutes, which says a lot for his technique and commanding presence. A "positive reaction" i.e. hyperaemia or submucous haemorrhage was found in thirteen cases and they concluded that acetyl salicylic acid was a gastric irritant in itself, irrespective of the acidity of the stomach. They reported their findings to the second meeting of the British Gastoenterological Club (later the BSG) when it met at Cambridge on 9 July 1938. Incidentally when Douthwaite's own duodenal ulcer perforated he diagnosed it himself, drove to hospital and requested an immediate laparotomy.

The following year Hurst and Lintott described a patient who had had a haematemesis caused by aspirin.[77] After excluding other causes, as far as possible, especially the presence of an ulcer, they performed a gastroscopy immediately after the patient had swallowed two aspirin tablets. "Two large fragments of aspirin which had dropped on to the greater curvature, could be seen gripped in the mucous membrane by contraction of the muscularis mucosae. Within a few minutes the mucosa became intensely hyperaemic and actual extravasation of blood occurred." Hurst believed that his patient was unusually sensitive to aspirin and warned that the widespread use and abuse of aspirin should be considered in all cases where the cause of bleeding was not apparent. Indeed he emphasised that he expected to find a history of aspirin in at least half the patients with haemorrhage in whom ulcer, carcinoma and cirrhosis had been excluded. He wrote "the association is never recognised by the patient himself and is discovered only after a careful cross-examination".[78] Lintott was a founder member of the British Gastroenterological Club and visited Germany in order to familiarise himself with the technique of gastroscopy. Appointed Assistant Physician to Guy's Hospital shortly before the Second World War he joined the Army and was posted to Egypt. Almost immediately he contracted dysentery in its most severe form and the hospital learnt that it had lost one for whom a great future had been confidently predicted.

Curiously Avery Jones did not mention aspirin in his Goulstonian lecture on haematemesis and melaena in 1947, though he had described several cases of acute ulceration and erosions seen endoscopically.[79] Later he admitted that some cases of bleeding could possibly be due to aspirin sensitivity. When Bill Summerskill became his senior registrar at the Central Middlesex in 1957, Avery encouraged him to investigate the matter further, particularly as about 4,000 million salicylate tablets were said to be consumed annually in Great Britain alone.

Summerskill (1926–77) was a man of gilded sophistication, head boy of Harrow School, an Oxford scholar and rugby blue, a great clinician and dedicated research worker. Once while a registrar at the Hammersmith he appeared at work in black coat and striped trousers on the day of the Eton and Harrow game at Lord's. To appear for work in such attire at that nest of liberal democracy required a certain panache. With typical enthusiasm he co-opted his house physician to look at 103 consecutive admissions with severe upper gastrointestinal bleeding in just six months.[80] They compared these with a similar number of dyspeptic patients and found that half of the bleeding patients had taken salicylates in the preceding 24 hours, compared with a tiny fraction of their controls. Half of those taking salicylates had chronic ulcers and the rest were thought to have bled from an "acute lesion" seen endoscopically, at laparotomy or necropsy but not identifiable on barium meal. They could not define a "salicylate lesion" and thought that activation of a pre-existing ulcer was common.

As well as looking at "massive gastrointestinal haemorrhage" (patients needing five pints of blood) Summerskill also gave salicylates and paracetamol to a group of 35 people and tested their stools for occult bleeding. Half of the salicylate group bled but none of the paracetamol group. Soon afterwards Summerskill moved to the United States, which was a great blow for British gastroenterology. Severe bleeding due to aspirin was still considered an uncommon event. In 1965 Sidney Truelove wrote "Drugs are an occasional cause (of bleeding) and the chief culprits

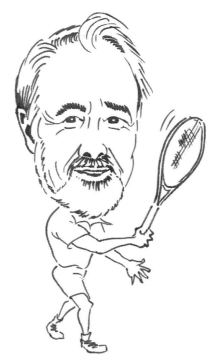

17 Langman – Forty love.

appear to be salicylates, corticosteroids and phenylbutazone (introduced in 1949)."[81]

Summerskill was succeeded as Avery Jones' senior registrar by the young Michael Langman (born 1935). While at the Central Middlesex

Hospital, Langman met Richard Doll (born 1912) from whom he acquired a lifelong interest in epidemiology, particularly in relation to peptic ulcer. He subsequently pursued these studies after moving to Nottingham. Blessed with a healthy degree of scepticism, he reviewed the evidence for the association of aspirin with acute gastro-intestinal bleeding.[82] He found that there were several case control studies showing that patients with bleeding, especially those with no radiological abnormality, were more than likely to have been taking analgesics containing aspirin. But in his view the studies were flawed; often the selection of controls was unsuitable or it was unclear whether aspirin had been taken before the bleeding or afterwards. So he concluded that their evidence was insufficient to incriminate salicylates as a major cause of serious bleeding.

However, Langman was intrigued. He knew from his analysis of the Hospital Inpatient Enquiry that uncomplicated ulcers were becoming uncommon, whereas the incidence of perforated and bleeding gastric ulcers among older people, far from falling, was actually rising. Could this be due to analgesics after all?

During the 1960s and 1970s several new drugs were discovered that shared some of the actions of aspirin, including indomethacin (1963), ibuprofen (1974) and naproxen. These were "aspirin like" and clearly distinct from the glucocorticoids (the other major group of agents used to treat inflammation) so they became known as the non-steroidal anti-inflammatory drugs (NSAIDs). Their popularity was stunning. They soon became the mainstay in the treatment of rheumatic disorders and were widely used as a general purpose painkiller. Their use in the elderly reflected the enormous burden of joint disease in old age. In 1983 for example, 22 million prescriptions were dispensed in Britain alone, quite apart from over-the-counter sales.[83] Rheumatologists and general practitioners found them a valuable and safe treatment and to begin with they were thought to have few serious side effects.

The increasing number of ulcers complicated by perforation or haemorrhage in old people, coupled with the widespread use of NSAIDs, strengthened the suspicion that these drugs might not only cause bleeding from the stomach but actual ulcers themselves. The first reports came from Australia and were followed by studies in the United States. In Britain it was a collective effort. No single study proved that NSAIDs caused ulcers but the weight of evidence was eventually sufficient to convince most people. Nottingham under Langman's influence led the way but reports emerged from several district hospitals. These were usually retrospective case control studies of patients taking NSAIDs using various end points, either simple ulceration or the complications thereof. One of the first came from Exeter where Michael Thompson (born 1965), a surgical registrar, highlighted the link between gastric ulcer and NSAIDs.[84] He simply noted that more patients admitted to hospital with a gastric ulcer had been taking indomethacin than would be expected. He moved to Bristol where he reviewed a further 200 patients with gastric ulcer admitted to the Royal Infirmary and found that most of the patients with NSAID-related ulcers were old ladies.[85] The ulcers were chronic, had often bled and had not caused much dyspepsia. Not long after a report appeared from the department of elderly care in Bolton General Hospital.[86] This analysed a group of 100 patients with benign ulceration, many of whom had bled and reported a significant association with a variety of anti-inflammatory drugs. A neat case control study came from David St. J Collier (born 1954) and James Pain (born 1955), surgeons at the Ipswich Hospital, who found that perforated ulcers in old people were more common if they were taking NSAIDs.[87] Another pair of surgeons in Crewe, Christopher Armstrong (born 1955) and Anthony Blower (born 1956), produced details of all their patients who needed emergency surgery or had died from ulcers.[88] Almost 80 per cent of the patients who died had taken NSAIDs. A similar picture emerged from surgeons working at the Royal Naval Hospital, Haslar.[89]

In Nottingham Langman was now convinced that NSAIDs were responsible for ulcers, bleeding and perforation. He had shown that aspirin was not just coincidental with bleeding but had conducted careful trials confirming the strong association between both aspirin and NSAIDs and ulcers, bleeding and perforation.[90]

Naturally the reason why NSAIDs should cause ulcers was the subject of intense study and the British contribution was impressive. During the 1960s Harry Collier, a distinguished pharmacologist, dubbed aspirin an "antidefensive drug" because it prevented the physiological defence mechanisms of pain, fever and inflammation from functioning normally. Collier suggested that it acted 'by inhibiting some underlying cellular mechanism that takes part to different extents in different responses and mediated by different endogenous substances".[91] While wrestling with the problem, Collier encouraged a young scientist called John Vane (1926–2004) at the Institute of Basic Medical Sciences, Royal College of Surgeons, Lincoln's Inn Fields.[†]

Vane (later Sir John) was interested in the nature of the substances released during anaphylaxis, notably prostaglandins. He noted how a substance released from guinea pig lungs during anaphylaxis, which contracted a rabbit's aorta, could be blocked by aspirin. So he incubated a homogenate from guinea pig lung with arachidonic acid (a precursor of prostaglandins) and different concentrations of aspirin and indomethacin and showed that the drugs could inhibit the formation of prostaglandin. Vane published his classic experiment in *Nature* in 1971 and in the same issue also demonstrated that aspirin could inhibit the prostaglandin, which makes platelets adhere to one another, thus making them less "sticky".[92] For his work Vane was awarded a Nobel Prize in 1982.

A key step in the formation of prostaglandin involves a glycoprotein enzyme known as cyclo oxygenase (Cox), isolated in 1976, which exists in at least two isomeric forms, COX-1 and COX-2. Activation of COX-1 produces prostacyclin, which, if released in the gastric mucosa is cytoprotective, whereas COX-2 is induced by inflammatory stimuli and cytokines. So it was attractive to suggest that the anti-inflammatory actions of NSAIDs are due to inhibition of COX-2, whereas the unwanted side effects (irritation of the stomach lining and reduced platelet stickiness) are due to inhibition of COX-1.

By this time Langman had been joined in Nottingham by Christopher Hawkey, who had been working with prostaglandins in Oxford. Hawkey (born 1948) was a man of persuasive charm and considerable skill who conducted a series of experiments to confirm Vane's work. Over a decade he and his co-workers performed hundreds of endoscopies on unsedated volunteers, taking biopsies, counting erosions and measuring blood loss.[93] Some experiments lasted several days, with their subjects cheerfully swallowing a gastroscope or an orogastric tube many times. He was able to confirm that aspirin caused gastric erosions and that for bleeding to occur, erosions and the anti-haemostatic effects of

---

[†] Once there was a famous exchange between the two at a scientific meeting. Collier presented data on the pharmacology of snails when they were given Chlorpromazine. How, Vane wanted to know, did snails behave when taking Chlorpromazine? "Sluggishly," came the reply.

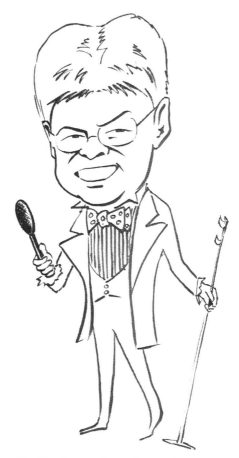

18 Hawkey – I say, I say, I say.

aspirin were necessary. Both effects were caused by the inhibition of prostaglandins and the synthetic prostaglandin, misoprostol, prevented erosions from developing.

6) *Helicobacter pylori*

The damaging effect of aspirin and NSAIDs certainly focussed attention on defects in the mucosal lining of the stomach but the discovery by a young Australian, Barry Marshall (born 1952), that a bacterium in the stomach could cause ulcers was a revelation. Though an Australian discovery, I am including it because some of the key players were British, and a history of peptic ulcer without it would be incomplete.

At the Royal Perth Hospital in Western Australia in 1981, Robin Warren, a histopathologist, observed the presence of "small curved bacilli" in biopsies taken from the stomachs of patients with acute gastritis. "The extraordinary features of these bacteria are that they are almost unknown to clinicians and pathologists alike," he reported, "even though they are present in about half our gastric biopsy specimens in numbers large enough to see on routine histology."[94] By chance at the time Marshall was in the middle of a three-year training programme in internal medicine, which included six months in gastroenterology. Marshall was looking around for a research project, so Warren suggested he might take a close look at the patients with bacilli in their stomachs. Warren may not have appreciated the full significance of his observations, and Marshall had no experience in medical research. Marshall's moment of revelation came by accident when one of the patients with bacilli reported that following a course of tetracycline given for a chest infection, his dyspepsia improved.[95] Marshall promptly had the endoscopy repeated, obtained biopsies and found that the gastritis and bacilli had vanished. The conclusion seemed obvious, the bacteria must have been the cause of his symptoms.

Marshall was fortunate in that by then John Armstrong had arrived from Mill Hill to head the electron microscopy unit at the Royal Perth Hospital. Asked to help, Armstrong and his assistant Wee obtained highly magnified pictures of the spiral bacteria. Later in the same year, 1981, Marshall enrolled the help of Stewart Goodwin (born 1932), an English bacteriologist, who was then head of the department of microbiology in Perth. Together they agreed on a protocol: gastric biopsies would be taken from 100 consecutive patients who were having a routine endoscopy, and these would be processed by the histopathology department and by attempts to culture the organism. The project began in March 1982 under the supervision of John Pearman, Goodwin's colleague in the microbiology department. Because of the risk of overgrowth by contaminants, incubation was restricted to 48 hours but, despite every effort, nothing grew from the first 34 specimens. The 35th culture was interrupted by a five-day Easter bank holiday so unintentionally the culture dishes were incubated for an extra three days. When the plates were finally viewed a pure growth of one millimetre transparent colonies was seen. H. pylori had finally been cultured.[96] The date was 14 April 1982. By a further stroke of luck, the specimen was not contaminated by an overgrowth of pseudomonas. Subsequently specimens were incubated for at least four days and a further ten isolations of the new organism were achieved.

The study took twelve weeks and the bacilli were seen in over half of the patients.[97] In almost every case the infection was associated with active chronic gastritis and duodenal or gastric ulcer. Now convinced that "pyloric campylobacter" were responsible for peptic ulcer, Marshall moved to the Fremantle Hospital where he studied the microbiology of the organism. Here with the help of a very co-operative gastroenterologist, Ian Hislop, he devised selective media for isolating H. pylori and discovered that it was particularly sensitive to bismuth and metronidazole.[98] Finally while in Fremantle, Marshall took the brave step to prove Koch's postulates.[99] In the summer of 1984 he swallowed a cocktail containing large numbers of the bacilli. His first effort failed so he tried again and this time felt very unwell. Ian Hislop performed a gastroscopy, found the organism and cultured it.

Marshall's discovery should not be underestimated. Even if "chance favoured his unprepared mind" and others had seen the bacilli and noted the gastritis, it was his energy and zeal that persuaded senior clinicians, pathologists and microbiologists alike to think the unthinkable – that peptic ulcer might be an infectious disease.[100] His conviction, strong personality and evangelical approach were essential.

Many greeted Marshall's discovery with disbelief and derision. It was asking too much to believe that his organism could cause peptic ulcer. If it did, why were so many infected people in perfect health? Even if campylobacter caused gastritis, there was no proof that it caused ulcers, especially in the duodenum where it was seldom found. Doctors were still conditioned to acid as the main factor in ulcer disease and were unprepared to think in terms of infection. Furthermore they already had an effective and safe treatment for ulcers, though admittedly it needed to be continued indefinitely. Naturally the very people who might have promoted Marshall's work, that is the pharmaceutical industry felt the most threatened by it. If a short course of antibiotics could cure ulcers, lifelong treatment with their products would be obsolete, which would have serious financial implications. Surprisingly the officers of the American Gastroenterological Association and the Council of the British Society of Gastroenterology were also unenthusiastic about the new germ and did little to disseminate the news.

Nevertheless Marshall's discovery was not totally ignored and bacteriologists were excited by it. Martin Skirrow (born 1929), a medical microbiologist at the Worcester Royal Infirmary, was interested in campylobacters and had developed a selective culture medium on which to grow them.[101] When Douglas Annear, the microbiologist in Perth, first cultured the pyloric campylobacter in 1983 he sent two samples to Skirrow who confirmed the characteristics of the bacteria, and like Annear thought that the organism was urease negative.[102] Later in the same year Marshall stayed with Skirrow in Worcester, obtained some gastric biopsies from a patient attending the local endoscopy unit and with Skirrow managed to culture his "Australian" campylobacter-like organism (CLO) using Skirrow's formula. Stimulated by this, Cliodna McNulty (born 1958), a registrar in microbiology at the hospital, managed to culture the organism from a series of gastric biopsies taken from patients, all of whom had gastritis.[103] Not long afterwards the organism was found to possess an abundance of urease by workers in the Central Public Health Laboratory in London, and McNulty seized on this to develop a rapid colour-change test for CLO activity in her biopsies.[104/105] Meanwhile Proctor & Gamble approached her to run a trial, which confirmed that campylobacter pyloridis was strongly correlated with gastritis and that this resolved when the organism was eradicated.[106] McNulty's early work on the diagnosis and treatment of campylobacter was significant and I think overlooked.

The connection between C. pylori and duodenal ulcer remained elusive until two groups working independently found a rational explanation. Kenneth McColl (born 1950) had been brought up in the classical school of ulcers in Glasgow and was well aware that acid secretion was stimulated by gastrin and that patients with duodenal ulcers were unable to switch off gastrin in response to acid, leading to over-secretion of acid. McColl had himself studied patients with porphyria, becoming interested in hepatic enzymes, which included urease, an enzyme that releases ammonia, an alkali, from urea. When he first heard about campylobacter in the stomach and the possibility that they might cause duodenal ulcers he was sceptical. Where was the evidence and how could it fit with what he knew about acid secretion? Fortunately instead of dismissing the matter he made himself familiar with the facts about campylobacter pyloridis (CP) and two things struck him. The organism possessed remarkable urease activity, which helped it to survive in the stomach in a bubble of alkaline ammonia, and the gastritis caused by campylobacter mainly affected the antrum of the stomach, exactly where gastrin is produced. Perhaps the infection by making the antrum alkaline stimulated excessive gastrin, which in turn caused hyperacidity and ulceration in the duodenum. A simple experiment in a few patients with campylobacter infection confirmed his prediction that their gastrin levels would be high. Furthermore, after eradicating the infection the gastrin levels returned to normal. At first it was difficult to prove that the extra gastrin was causing excess acid because the usual stimulant used in experiments was the analogue of gastrin, pentagastrin. Fortunately he was able to circumvent this problem by using the gastrin-releasing peptide, which stimulates acid via gastrin itself. With his research fellow, Emad El-Omar (born 1965), he showed that the acid response in duodenal ulcer patients was sixfold and after treatment of the infection it fell to normal. So he had found a unifying hypothesis: infection with campylobacter disrupted the normal physiology of the stomach, in particular by blocking the control of gastrin by acid, resulting in excess gastrin, excess duodenal acid, gastric metaplasia in the duodenum, infection in the metaplastic mucosa and ulceration. Patches of gastric metaplasia occur in the duodenum as a non-specific response to injury, especially from acid.[107/108]

At the same time John Calam (1948–2001), recently appointed senior lecturer to the Hammersmith Hospital, came to the same conclusion but suggested another stimulus to gastrin in duodenal ulcer patients. Gastro-intestinal peptides had been studied at the Hammersmith for some years, notably by Tony Pearse, Julia Polak and Stephen Bloom. One of these, somatostatin, is synthesised by the so called D cells in the antrum and inhibits the release of gastrin from the G cells of the antrum. With Hugh Baron (their acid expert) the team had shown that duodenal ulcer patients had overactive G cells, causing hyperacidity, and they suggested that they were hyperactive because there was a failure by the D Cells for some reason to produce inhibitory somatostatin. John Calam provided the explanation when he showed that colonisation of the antrum by helicobacter pylori inhibited the D cells.[109] He also showed that eradicating helicobacter pylori with antibiotics reversed the effects on gastrin and somastostatin metabolism.[110] Calam, who had an irrepressible sense of humour was awarded a personal chair in 1997 but died only four years later from a brain tumour.

The link between H. pylori and ulcer disease was gradually being unravelled but key questions remained. Why did so few patients with H. pylori have ulcers and what determined whether a patient acquired a gastric rather than a duodenal ulcer? We still do not know but extensive work by epidemiologists and bacteriologists have provided plausible answers.

Susser's original theory describing the birth-cohort phenomenon has been elaborated with particular reference to H. pylori infection by Sonnenberg.[111] Susser had suggested that urbanisation and the crowded living conditions of expanding cities during the second half of the nineteenth century were unusually stressful for a short time but his argument was unconvincing. It was also difficult to understand why the peak mortality of the birth cohort for gastric ulcer occurred between 1870 and 1890 whereas for duodenal ulcer it lay between 1880 and 1900. Nonetheless the occurrence of a birth-cohort phenomenon indicated that environmental factors were important in the aetiology of gastric and duodenal ulcer. Could this be H. pylori? The decline in hygiene in large sections of the population during the nineteenth century provided ideal conditions for the spread of H. pylori. Subsequent improvements in sanitation probably led to a fall in infection rates at the turn of the century. To find out how early in life H. pylori might be relevant, Sonnenberg pooled the mortality rates of peptic ulcer disease from eighteen countries and was able to show that an environmental factor started exerting its influence before the age of five years in patients with gastric ulcer and before the age of fifteen years in patients with duodenal ulcer. This age-related lag between both ulcer types could explain why the incidence of duodenal ulcer rose and fell ten to fifteen years after gastric ulcer. He surmised that very young children who became infected with H. pylori were more likely to develop chronic or atrophic gastritis, with a subsequent decrease of acid secretion that protected them from developing a duodenal ulcer. These children with atrophic gastritis would be more at risk of a gastric ulcer later. On the other hand older children and adults contracting H. pylori were prone to duodenal ulcer. Hugh Baron and Robert Logan (born 1959) suggested that by then H. pylori is less damaging to the parietal cell mass, and that duodenal ulcer patients can achieve critical levels of acidity despite the ongoing inflammation in the body of the stomach.[112]

Apart from the age when patients acquire infection the virulence of the bacteria, the susceptibility of the host and other environmental factors such as smoking probably decide who will get an ulcer. H. pylori strains possess a high degree of genetic homogeneity and some strains are more virulent than others. Focussing on specific genes, in 1988 the vac A. gene (encoding a vacuolating toxin) and the cag A. gene (cytotoxin associated gene) were identified in H. pylori of patients who were more likely to have a duodenal ulcer. Much of this work has been done in America and Europe but Jean Crabtree, a microbiologist at the University Hospital, Leeds, was the first person to find that the cag A. protein produced an antibody in the serum that was easy to measure and potentially a useful marker of patients with duodenal ulcer.[113] However, Crabtree was unable to show a definite relationship between cytotoxicity of H. pylori and peptic ulcer.

About this time, John Atherton (born 1963), a research fellow in Nottingham, was working on treatment strategies for eradicating H. pylori. Becoming intrigued by the work of the bacteriologists, he joined Martin Blaser's group in Nashville whose interest was in the toxicity of H. pylori. There he helped to show that the structure of the vac A. gene varies, exchanging genes with other H. pylori strains, mutating and forming a mosaic.[114] This seemed to explain why though all the strains contained toxin, only some were cytotoxic. Research continues but the occurrence of peptic ulcer disease seems to depend, in part at least, on the properties of the bacterial strain.

The host, that is man himself, is more or less susceptible. Fifty years ago Cyril Clarke (1907–2000), later Professor of Medicine, Liverpool University and President of the Royal College of Physicians, discovered that anti-D immunisation prevented Rhesus haemolytic disease. Continuing his interest in blood groups, he confirmed Ian Aird's earlier report that patients with blood group O were more likely to have a duodenal ulcer.[115] The link was modest and Doll and Langman were unable to confirm it. However, they did find an association in their control group who were blood donors. Realising that these were people who had frequently had a gastro-intestinal bleed themselves, they concluded that patients with complicated ulcers were more likely to belong to blood group O. These observations implied a genetic susceptibility to the development of a duodenal ulcer but the basis of it was unclear. Recently, Emad El-Omar, now Professor of Medicine, Aberdeen University, has shown that there are also polymorphic differences in human genes that control inflammatory mediators, which could explain the raised (gastrin-stimulated) acid output often seen in patients with duodenal ulcer.[116] Genetic changes may also explain why the inflammatory response to H. pylori is so variable.

It is over 30 years since the discovery of H. pylori, which is not a long time in the annals of medicine. Yet there has been intense activity worldwide in order to understand the bacterium with significant contributions from the United Kingdom. The subject is complex and it will be some years before the definitive history of H. pylori can be written.

CHAPTER ELEVEN

EARLY MEDICAL TREATMENT

John Buchan's illness illustrates the difficulties that confronted doctors trying to treat peptic ulcer at the beginning of the twentieth century. Buchan's problems began in his early thirties when what he called "the viper" began to attack him in earnest.[117] His pain would last for several months at a time and he needed long spells in bed. He refused to stop work and went on with business and politics as hard as ever. In this sense he was not a "good patient". His doctors must have told him repeatedly to cut down his commitments, diet, go to bed early and generally relax. But this was not his nature. After three months in bed at the beginning of the First World War he was enjoined to make a long convalescence. This he took as *Times* Correspondent at the Front. In 1916 he was appointed to Haig's staff in France but had to be invalided back to England, and early in 1917 he underwent a gastro-jejunostomy by Berkeley Moynihan. After a brief convalescence he was back in the thick of things again, now Director of Information at the War Office. He was also writing his novels and gave the character Blenkiron a duodenal ulcer in *Greenmantle*. Blenkiron was lucky because Buchan allowed him to be cured of his ulcer in his next novel, *Mr. Standfast*. This appeared in 1918 at a time when Buchan was still able to hope that his own operation might be a success. Sadly it proved a failure. The pain returned at regular intervals and his doctors seemed unable to find a cure for it. He could not put on weight, always looked much too thin and often downright ill. Later all his teeth were removed in the hope of eliminating infection, but this merely added to his discomfort and made his dreary diet yet more boring.

In Buchan's day the medical management of peptic ulcer had changed little since Brinton's time. William Osler in 1901 recommended absolute rest in bed and a bland diet given at regular intervals.[118] If the stomach was very irritable, lavage could be practised every morning with alkaline water, and fluids administered per rectum. This could continue for weeks or even months. Medicines were thought to be ineffective but all sorts of agents were tried including bismuth, nitrate of silver and Carlsbad salts (sulphate of sodium, bicarbonate of sodium and chloride of sodium). The pain if severe warranted opium but milder attacks responded to 20 or 30 drops of chloroform. Counter irritants placed on the abdominal wall such as mustard or cantharides (the dried bodies of the blister beetle or Spanish fly) were useful. If the stomach was intractable, the patient might be tube-fed with beef solution or milk and an unlikely fricassee of cracked ice, chloroform, oxalate of cerium (a metal), bismuth or hydrocyanic acid.

When symptoms abated, recurrences would follow and it was difficult to decide how active an ulcer was or how well it was responding to treatment. So it was not surprising that physicians experienced in the treatment of ulcer disease frequently recommended surgery. Who better could Buchan turn to than Moynihan? He was the foremost surgeon of his day with a unique experience of ulcer surgery. Initially Moynihan recommended surgery for all cases of gastric and duodenal ulcer. "No other treatment than that which the surgeon offers can do more than relieve the patient to some extent of his sufferings when once a chronic ulcer is established in the stomach.... The recognition of duodenal ulcer is most necessary, for it is, I feel sure, a far more serious disease than gastric ulcer, and it is, moreover, one which, in my judgement, should always be treated by operation."[119]

So for a while surgery for ulcers was allowed to monopolise the interest of the medical profession, until Bertram Sippy (1866–1924), a physician in Chicago, re-emphasised the need to control the nocturnal secretion of acid.[120] Though not new, Sippy's attempt to produce complete neutralisation by means of hourly feeds and alkaline powders between feeds restored belief in the possibility of medical treatment.

In this country his views were widely adopted and championed by Arthur Hurst, already the leading advocate for medical treatment of ulcers. He fiercely maintained that if only the principles of treatment were properly followed, the majority of ulcers would heal and remain healed.[121] Recurrence was usually the patient's fault because he had not followed his instructions with sufficient care, but occasionally he conceded it might be the doctor's fault because the precautions laid down had been insufficiently strict. Most of his advice was not new nor was it based on particularly sound evidence but rather on his charisma and conviction.

Rest and warmth were important so it was best to keep the patient in bed. Like Brinton and Sippy, Hurst recommended milk as the basis of the diet. Most patients found it acceptable, it was nourishing, helped to neutralise the acid, and the fat content inhibited the secretion of gastric juice. Ulcer diets were precise and tedious, requiring exact quantities of bland food every two hours of the day. Cream was helpful and his colleague John Ryle had shown by means of the fractional test meal that it inhibited acid secretion.[122] The patient should not smoke nor drink alcohol. Hurst favoured magnesium oxide as an effective antacid. For a time he used bismuth but stopped after his colleague, Professor C. S. Gibson in the biochemistry department at Guy's Hospital, showed that it was a poor antacid.[123] Nonetheless he was intrigued that so many physicians and patients were convinced of its value. He also recommended belladonna and atropine for their inhibitory effect on the vagus nerve, thus reducing the secretion of gastric juice. Izod Bennett (1887–1946) had demonstrated this effect by means of the fractional test meal.[124]

Hurst believed in the infective factor behind ulcers and thought it essential to eradicate as completely as possible all foci of infection. Foremost was pyorrhoea alveolaris (dental caries). The patient must be scrupulous about oral hygiene and the tongue should be frequently scraped with a wooden spatula to remove the fur from it. Teeth with apical infection should be extracted, infected gums incised and the bone scraped. Sinusitis must be drained, the appendix removed if chronic appendicitis was thought to be present (Moynihan strongly supported this) and occasionally cholecystectomy was necessary. The startled patient should even have his urine examined before and after prostatic massage to exclude prostatitis.

It was difficult to decide when an ulcer had healed. As pain and tenderness usually resolved quickly, the doctor had to rely on evidence of occult bleeding in the faeces and X-rays. Unfortunately X-rays were of little help in the case of duodenal ulcers, though useful for gastric ulcer.

Hurst was particularly concerned to prevent recurrence "when the ulcer has healed our duty to the patient is only half done".[125] He admitted that to insist on a lifetime of tedious restrictions to a vigorous working man who was feeling better was not easy. The patient had to be made to understand that he was prone to ulcers and that there was always a danger of recurrence. Hurst blamed recurrence on carelessness with the diet, over-indulgence in alcohol or excessive smoking. He insisted on small regular meals, slowly eaten and thoroughly chewed. Many desirable foods were forbidden including various vegetables, nuts, chutney, meat, new bread, most cheeses, strong tea and coffee and effervescent drinks such as champagne.

Few patients will have been fortunate or wealthy enough to be treated by physicians such as Arthur Hurst. Many probably never visited a doctor at all, preferring to endure recurrent attacks of pain with the help of simple antacids so long as they could remain at work, smoke and enjoy the odd pint of bitter. They would not be found dead in a dentist's chair. A number might visit their general practitioner who would recommend rest, some variant of the "Sippy diet" and alkalis. The symptoms would settle for a while only to recur. An X-ray might confirm the diagnosis. Treatment would be repeated. Sooner or later a complication of the ulcer might arise, requiring immediate admission to hospital. Perforation was nearly always treated by simple closure, pyloric obstruction by gastroenterostomy and haemorrhage by rest, starvation and, occasionally, blood transfusion.

CHAPTER TWELVE

THE RISE OF SURGERY

Eventually after years of torment a patient would be deemed "to have earned his operation". This ascetic attitude came about for two reasons. Firstly Hurst and his followers preached that it was extremely rare for an ulcer not to heal on medical treatment, so an operation was rarely necessary. Secondly the risk and complications of surgery were quite significant, and sometimes disastrous. For many years the standard operation was a gastroenterostomy and the well-to-do patient was referred to a name such as Moynihan or one of his protégés, for example Leonard Braithwaite (1878–1942) in Leeds. Moynihan called Braithwaite "unsurpassed" and Gordon-Taylor spoke of his "artistry and gentleness rivalling those of Moynihan himself" and described a gastroenterostomy by Braithwaite as probably the most accomplished operation he had ever watched.[126] But for most people the surgeon was a man of mixed ability. Mixed in the sense that he was a generalist happy to turn his hand to whatever was required, amputations, thyroidectomies, abdominal emergencies or trauma cases. Mixed also in his ability and training. One might be a general practitioner operating at the local hospital, while another may have learnt his trade before Moynihan "threw open the abdomen to all surgeons"[127] and come to ulcer surgery late in his career. The morbidity and mortality figures of these surgeons are unknown but it is easy to see why gastroenterostomy enjoyed such wide usage and high repute. It seemed to fulfil all the criteria for success, for it relieved pyloric obstruction and put the diseased duodenum at rest, it was simple to perform and relatively free from risk. It was in fact very effective for duodenal ulcer, and initially Moynihan believed that it would also heal gastric ulcers. He reasoned that it helped to empty the stomach quickly, which was conducive to healing, and it also encouraged alkaline juice from the proximal loop of the jejunum to mix with and dilute the acid in the stomach. But most gastric ulcers failed to heal after gastroenterostomy and Moynihan himself described three cases in which a gastric ulcer actually developed after gastroenterostomy had been performed for a duodenal ulcer.[128] Clearly if it was possible for an ulcer to develop in the stomach after gastroenterostomy, it was hardly logical to perform the same operation to cure one that was already present. Moynihan was also aware of the risk of cancer with gastric ulcer and later agreed that gastrectomy and removal of the ulcer was the operation of choice. His mortality for partial gastrectomy was less than two per cent (a remarkably low figure) and he claimed never to have had a recurrence of ulceration.[129] But he stuck to gastroenterostomy for duodenal ulcer throughout his career. "I do not practise resection (gastrectomy), it is an operation which is unnecessary and dangerous and is attended by a risk of secondary ulceration not less than in the short circuiting operation (gastroenterostomy)." Admittedly in his last 1,000 cases of operation for duodenal ulcer he had only one death. But his enthusiasm for the short-circuiting operation slowly brought it into disrepute.

As early as 1908, Herbert Paterson (1867–1940), assistant surgeon at the National Temperance Hospital in London, wrote a classic paper on jejunal and gastrojejunal ulceration after gastroenterostomy.[130] He believed acid was the cause and warned that fear of the condition was casting a faint shadow over the admirable results of the operation. Optimistically he suggested that the incidence was less than two per cent. Moynihan in his great book *Abdominal Operations* agreed but ignored the role of acid. He attributed stomal ulcers to the use of unabsorbable sutures, ischaemia caused by intestinal clamps or the presence of an untreated septic focus. After the First World War, Garnett Wright (1878–1945), senior surgeon at the Royal Infirmary, Salford, published three cases of secondary gastrojejunal ulceration and reviewed 142 cases from the literature.[131] Like Paterson he stressed the importance of gastric acid and the inability of the jejunal mucosa to withstand a digestive action to which it was not accustomed. But he simply excised the new ulcer or fashioned a new gastroenterostomy. Not surprisingly he noted that further surgery had only very moderate success and in some cases failed dismally.

As the surgeon's skill and experience increased, some form of partial gastrectomy became the standard method of treating gastric ulcer. Partial gastrectomies were of two main varieties. The Bilroth I operation involved joining the gastric stump to the duodenum, thus mimicking the normal anatomical arrangements. The Polya variant of the Bilroth II operation involved bringing up a loop of proximal jejunum and joining it to the gastric stump. The object of doing a partial gastrectomy was to remove the actual ulcer and at the same time to take away a substantial proportion of the stomach, so reducing gastric secretion and the risk of recurrent ulceration. As surgeons became more aware of stomal ulceration, many on the continent and in the United States advocated gastrectomy as the primary procedure in duodenal as well as gastric ulcer. Hurst agreed and wrote in 1929 that the only indication for gastrojejunostomy in duodenal ulcer was sufficient pyloric obstruction to cause gastric stasis.[132] But many British surgeons were still unwilling to agree to this big operation for so small a lesion. This was certainly Moynihan's view and he was supported by his friend Charles Mayo (1865–1939) in Rochester, Minnesota. "If any man wanted to cut out half of my good stomach in order to cure a little ulcer of my duodenum I would run faster than he." According to Moynihan gastrectomy for duodenal ulcer was neither safe nor simple, nor did it bring an adequate reward. "…we know the worst of gastroenterostomy, the best is unsurpassable; we have yet to learn the worse of gastrectomy, though what we know is bad enough."[133] What they knew was that a significant number of patients certainly did come back with marginal or stomal ulcers, and the operation itself was much more risky with a mortality in good hands of ten per cent and further complications later. But some rose to the challenge and began doing a much more radical gastrectomy in an attempt to eliminate acid. Notable among those was Arthur Hedley Visick (1897–1949).

Visick was elected surgeon to the York County Hospital in 1928 and soon became particularly interested in gastric surgery. While a Rockefeller scholar in Michigan he had reorganised their methods of clinical record-keeping, which stood in him in good stead when in 1936 he began a careful six-monthly follow-up of a consecutive group of 500 patients whom he had treated by gastrectomy. He was fanatical about the follow-up of his patients and tried to see them all himself. Patients who failed to keep their appointments were written to, and if this failed they were visited in their own homes, usually by Visick himself on a

Sunday afternoon. The study lasted twelve years and he lost track of only 3 patients out of the 500.[134] Initially like most surgeons he removed up to "two thirds to three quarters" of the stomach but found that among the first 150 patients 5 had developed a recurrent ulcer within eighteen months of operation. So he perfected his so-called measured radical gastrectomy, which concentrated on the exact size of the stomach remnant left in place rather than making a vague guess at the proportion of stomach he intended to remove. Early on his mortality figure was high (twelve per cent) but this fell dramatically as the study progressed. None of the later patients had stomal ulcers but up to fifteen per cent had some symptoms particularly the weakness syndrome and "dumping", and a sense of fullness with early satiety. Only a handful had intractable symptoms (two to three per cent) and he felt many of these were just one step nearer to incurable mental and moral breakdown. "These were an insoluble problem who were not so much failures of gastrectomy as failures of selection for gastrectomy."

But even as late as 1944 when a discussion was held at the Royal Society of Medicine, British surgeons for the most part were still worried about partial gastrectomy for duodenal ulcer.[135] It was still a relatively risky operation and no guarantee against recurrent ulceration. Another concern was the problem of anaemia. Removing part or most of the stomach can prevent the absorption in the ileum of vitamin B12, a substance essential in the production of red blood corpuscles by the bone marrow. This was anticipated by the gastric surgeons who knew that idiopathic or progressive pernicious anaemia was associated with atrophy of the stomach lining. Credit for this belonged to one Samuel Fenwick (1821–1902), a Victorian physician working at the London Hospital. In 1877 Fenwick described four cases of anaemia in all of whom "a well-marked lesion of the glandular structure (of the stomach) was discovered after death".[136] He believed that gastric atrophy and the anaemia were related in some way,[137] and later it was shown that such patients were invariably achlorrhydric (using the fractional test meal technique). In 1927 William Castle (1897–1990), in Boston, discovered that the stomach secretes a ferment-like substance that he called intrinsic factor. Intrinsic factor is necessary for the absorption of B12, which is the extrinsic factor. So gastric atrophy and gastrectomy can cause pernicious anaemia, which worried the surgeons. Indeed Hans Finsterer (1877–1955) in Vienna, one of Europe's foremost surgeons, proposed an operation in 1930 called "physiological gastrectomy". The idea was to leave the pyloric antrum in situ to provide the intrinsic factor required by the bone marrow. This was supported by William Heneage Ogilvie (1887–1971), later Sir William, at Guy's Hospital[138] and by Charles Wells (1898–1989), later the first professor of surgery in Liverpool,[139] who performed the operation on a small group of patients in 1937. Both surgeons discovered almost immediately that recurrence of ulceration was speedy and frequent. The reason was pointed out by Eric Pearce Gould (1886–1940), surgeon to the Middlesex Hospital, who himself died of a perforation shortly afterwards, who suggested that the residual antrum must be responsible for the continuing acidity. Inadvertently Ogilvie and Wells had carried out a neat little experiment on the site of origin and importance of the hormone gastrin in the secretion of hydrochloric acid.

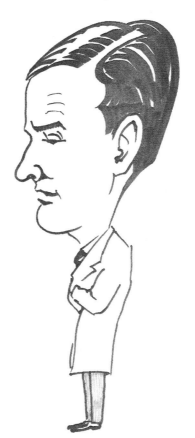

19 Witts – Dr Don of the Lancet 1939.

Iron deficiency, usually as a result of chronic blood loss, is the commonest cause of anaemia. But as early as 1929, Gordon Gordon-Taylor (1878–1960), later Sir Gordon, remarked on the occurrence of superficial glossitis, a sign of iron deficiency, after gastrectomy.[140] Over the next few years, the link between gastrectomy and lack of iron was studied extensively by Leslie Witts (1898–1982), a youthful professor of medicine at St. Bartholemew's Hospital, working closely with the surgical unit directed by Paterson Ross (1895–1980).[141] Witts' early work on chronic microcytic (iron deficiency) anaemia was so comprehensive and influential that for the next decade the condition was often referred to as Witts' anaemia. Apart from recurrent ulcer Witts thought that the poor absorption of iron after gastrectomy was because the duodenum was bypassed and food hurried through the jejunum (the very places were iron is usually absorbed). People also had a poor appetite so their iron intake was often minimal. During his short tenure at St. Bartholomew's Hospital, Witts made another contribution that was to change long established clinical practice.

It had been generally held by Hurst and others that patients who bled from their ulcers should be kept immobile with complete rest of the stomach. This meant not only strict rest in bed and morphia but total starvation until the bleeding had stopped for 48 hours. But in 1932 Edward Cullinan (1901–65) and Roy Price (1905–79), young doctors on the staff at St. Bartholomew's Hospital, analysed 105 cases of severe bleeding from peptic ulcer.[142] They noted that patients who had been starved for 24 or 48 hours were much more likely to bleed again than those patients who were fed immediately. Shortly after a Swedish physician, Einar Meulengracht (1887–1976), treated a large group of patients with bleeding ulcers by encouraging them to eat a bland diet immediately and only one per cent died.[143] Leslie Witts confirmed these results. He realised that far from resting the stomach, to withhold food and drink was to invite the strongest waves of peristalsis. He fed his patients on admission with a nourishing milk-based diet and they did well. He argued that they were better nourished, and he doubted the wisdom of keeping the stomach empty and exposed to gastric juice. He also emphasised the importance of blood transfusion to prevent haemorrhagic shock and discouraged early surgery. Most of the patients submitted to operation for gastroduodenal haemorrhage at the time died. He said, "It is best to wait…" because "…it is impossible by clinical methods to decide whether the patient is bleeding from an acute or chronic ulcer," implying that an operation for an acute ulcer was never justified.[144]

CHAPTER THIRTEEN

LIMITATIONS OF MEDICAL TREATMENT DURING MID-TWENTIETH CENTURY

By 1950 peptic ulcer was a national scourge. A physician on his round could expect to have several ulcer patients in the ward. The diet kitchen served up a variety of milk drinks and puddings and vegetable purees to the new arrivals while those on the road to recovery were promoted to steamed fish, rabbit, tripe and cheese custard, delicacies disliked intensely by the average labourer. The patient might stay in hospital for six to twelve weeks simply for rest and a bland diet though only a few of those prepared to come into hospital could be found a bed. Though it was known by physicians that ulcers often healed without a single dose of alkali or other medicine, most used them. Alkalis and bismuth salts remained popular, sedatives, especially phenobarbitone, were widely used and antispasmodics such as bella donna and poldine were considered valuable.[†]

In fact there was no evidence that any treatment influenced the rate of ulcer healing. Indeed in 1947 Alan Morton Gill (1909–85), a physician at the West London Hospital, cast doubt on the value of any therapy other than that necessary to gain the patient's confidence.[145]

[†] While most agreed with the use of a bland diet, Surgeon Captain T. L. 'Peter' Cleave known in the Navy as '"the bran man" was unimpressed. During the last war, while based at Scapa Flow, Cleave treated the admiral for a duodenal ulcer but before his patient could be admitted for treatment, the German battleship put to sea and the admiral had to go after it. Cleave agreed on condition his patient ate an ulcer diet of steak, roast potatoes and baked apples with wholemeal bread. The admiral happily complied and on his return his ulcer had healed.

With one exception he found that twenty patients with chronic gastric ulcer treated only with daily injections of distilled water lost their pains as quickly as did a control series treated on orthodox lines. He was a pioneer gastroscopist and showed that healing of the ulcer took place in the usual time. Today his personal gastroscope is on display in the London Science Museum. Another to cast doubt on the value of medical treatment was Laurence Martin (1910–81), a physician at Addenbrooke's Hospital, Cambridge. He pointed out that treatment to ease the pain of a relapse was not synonymous with curing an ulcer or any guarantee against further trouble, even if treatment was continued indefinitely. He criticised the publication of short-term results and the vaunting of ephemeral cures. To support his views he looked at the fate of 356 patients who had received treatment for peptic ulcer ten years earlier. At least a quarter of them had died with active ulcers. Among the survivors there was no evidence that medical treatment had influenced the natural course of the disease, and Martin came to the conclusion that anyone who had had an ulcer for ten years merited a gastrectomy.[146]

At the time, the cornerstone of reliable knowledge in medicine was the cumulative wisdom acquired through everyday practice. The notion that the validity of specific treatments might be objectively tested was hardly ever raised. This all changed in 1950 when Austin Bradford Hill (1897–1991) used the randomised controlled trial to prove that tuberculosis could be cured by drugs. This was a brilliant piece of work after which the randomised trial blossomed to become the standard way of evaluating new drugs. As we have seen, Richard Doll had joined Bradford Hill but continued his clinical research with Avery Jones at the Central Middlesex Hospital. Doll was aware of the many, often bizarre treatments in vogue at the time and was intrigued by Morton Gill's observations. So he set up a series of randomised controlled trials and with so many treatments to test he devised a factorial design whereby he could test three at once. He took eight blocks of eight patients, which gave him every possible combination of the three treatments. Only gastric ulcers were studied. Barium meals were repeated monthly for three months and the size of the ulcer crater measured by the radiologist, Frank Pygott (1911–95). In their first study they showed that phenobarbitone and ascorbic acid (then widely recommended) were ineffective and that strict bed rest in hospital helped to heal ulcers.[147] Even then he was worried that the study was flawed because the inpatients were fed a "gastric diet" that may have been more strictly enforced in hospital than at home, raising the possibility that diet rather than rest was the therapeutic factor.

About this time John Lawrence (1908–96), a physician at the Herts and Essex Hospital (later known for his work as Director of the Arthritis and Rheumatism Council Unit at Manchester University), treated alternate patients with either a bland diet or a "full convalescent" diet that included fried foods, cheese and pork pies.[148] 93 per cent of his patients in each group healed. Some of the patients on the full diet "were at first dubious of a regime so much at variance with their earlier instructions but their anxiety was allayed when it was explained to them that such food was required to inactivate their over-potent gastric juice".

Another physician from the Royal Victoria Hospital, Belfast, Sydney Allison (1899–1978), better known for his work on multiple sclerosis, also suggested that a bland diet was unnecessary.[149] Allison had acquired an interest in diseases of the gastro-intestinal tract while working as assistant physician at the Ruthin Castle in North Wales, where he was influenced by Sir Edmund Spriggs (1871–1949), a founder member of the British Society of Gastroenterology.

Subsequently Doll confirmed these findings with further randomised trials and also proved that an intragastric milk drip (six pints per day for three weeks) did not heal ulcers.[150] Like Lawrence he found it difficult to persuade people to have a normal diet, which illustrates just how ingrained the notion of a bland diet was at the time. Indeed Doll felt obliged to advise his patients to avoid something so he suggested fried food simply to reassure them that they were having some dietary advice. Years later Doll said that his most important contribution to gastroenterology was to show that such diets were unnecessary.

Ulcer disease was so common and debilitating that people were prepared to clutch at any straw. Some of the treatments were ingenious, moderately plausible and worth recording. One was cabbage juice, recommended on the grounds that it contained a factor termed "Vitamin V", which was capable of preventing histamine-induced ulcers in guinea pigs. This "anti-peptic ulcer dietary factor" was present in several foodstuffs but especially fresh cabbages. There were claims from America of astonishingly rapid healing in a group of ulcer patients given a quart of cabbage juice daily, obtained from four to five pounds of fresh cabbage. However, Doll was unable to show any benefit in a randomised trial.[151]

Another was a tissue extract known as "robaden", which was popular on the continent. It was a proprietary extract of gastric and intestinal tissue that had been found to protect pylorus-ligated rats against the development of gastric ulcers, and guinea pigs against histamine-induced ulcers. It was chemically distinct from enterogastrone, and could be given intramuscularly or in tablet form. A particular claim for robaden was that it prevented relapses in people going about their daily lives on a normal diet. Many uncontrolled studies suggested it was effective but a small controlled trial in England by Philip Evans (1917–84), physician to the Wrexham group of hospitals did not.[152] Again Doll subjected the drug to a rigorous controlled trial and showed it did not help to heal gastric ulcers.

One might have thought that extract of liquorice would also prove a disappointment when put to the test. Liquorice root was a well known folklore remedy for indigestion, but did not attract attention until a Dutch pharmacist, Mr Revers in Holland during the last war, noticed that patients taking it did surprisingly well. Revers showed that it helped to heal gastric ulcers but his trial did not contain a control series and similar results might have been obtained with an inert preparation. Furthermore many patients became oedematous and it failed to catch on. But it was clearly a pharmacologically active drug causing salt and water retention and was investigated extensively in animals in whom it was found to be anti-inflammatory and to improve wound healing. So Doll decided that it merited a randomised trial and indeed he showed unequivocally that liquorice or "carbenoloxone" promoted the healing of gastric (but not duodenal) ulcers.[153] Soon several trials confirmed Doll's findings and carbenoloxone was widely used for a decade. But the side effects were a problem so a deglycyrrhinised liquorice was produced in which the mineralocorticoid activity causing these effects was removed. Unfortunately the beneficial effects of liquorice were probably eliminated at the same time, and the product, marketed as Caved-S, also contained bismuth, aluminium and magnesium salts and sodium bicarbonate so any benefit of the deglycyrrhinised liquorice itself was never proved. Though carbenoloxone healed gastric ulcers, it was rapidly absorbed and very little reached the duodenum. To get round this the manufacturers devised "Duogastrone" an ingenious preparation of carbenoloxone in a hygroscopic gelatine capsule. This was designed to fragment as it passed through the pylorus, releasing its ingredients directly into the duodenal cap. It was evaluated by Dr. Thomas Hunt (1901–80), a physician at St. Mary's Hospital and a founder member of the British Society of Gastroenterology. Hunt co-ordinated a long-term multi-centre controlled trial in England, which showed a favourable effect on duodenal ulcers, but the results were less convincing than those for gastric ulcer and it is unlikely that the capsule really delivered the goods as claimed.[154]

Desperate diseases require desperate remedies. As we have seen, one of the conspicuous features of duodenal ulcer was its predeliction for the adult male. Women seemed to be protected and if unlucky enough to get an ulcer they often got better during pregnancy. Could female hormones help to heal or prevent ulcers in men? Certainly the idea had occurred to a number of people and a few patients on the continent had apparently responded well to oestrogens. So in 1952 Sidney Truelove (1913–2002), a physician at the Radcliffe Infirmary, Oxford, carried out a randomised trial comparing stilboestrol with a placebo.[155] The trial was identical in design to those run by Richard Doll at the Central Middlesex, except that Truelove looked at duodenal ulcer not gastric ulcer. This was long before the duodenum could be inspected endoscopically and he had to rely on X-ray findings and the expert help of his radiologist, Dr. Kenneth Lumsden (1908–95). Eighty men with a duodenal ulcer were invited to volunteer for inclusion in the trial. They were told that an experiment was being made in treatment and none of those invited refused. Half of the forty men who received stilboestrol healed compared with only one tenth of the placebo group. The obvious snag was the feminising effect with breast enlargement and loss of sexual potency, though both reversed promptly after treatment was stopped. Truelove hoped that a chemical analogue without feminising properties would be found, but nobody followed this up, which was surprising. One would imagine that a cure from the misery of a duodenal ulcer would justify the temporary side effects. After all, anti-androgens are regularly used to mitigate the effects of prostate cancer, admittedly in an older age group.

CHAPTER FOURTEEN

VAGOTOMY

While the physicians were casting around for a cure and systematically refuting one time honoured treatment after another, the surgeons were steadily perfecting their latest weapon, vagotomy. In fact vagotomy was not new, it was first employed at the beginning of the twentieth century. European surgeons hoped that by dividing the nerve supply to the intestine they would relieve the pain and vomiting of their patients, many of whom had tabes dorsalis, a form of neurosyphilis. Thereafter there were flurries of interest in vagotomy but it petered out until Lester Dragstedt (1893–1975), a surgeon working in Chicago, revived the procedure in 1943.[156] He was convinced by experiments in the dog, which showed that the secretions and activity of the stomach could be blocked by cutting the vagus nerve. In fact a cardiothoracic surgeon in Liverpool, Ronald Edwards (1910–83), had already published a paper on the neurogenic origin of duodenal ulcer in which he stated the case for vagotomy.[157] Unfortunately his technique was imperfect, the procedure proved unreliable and he abandoned the project. But Dragstedt's early results were promising. He operated on patients specially selected for their intractable symptoms, who immediately felt better, lost their pain and reduced their acid secretion. Soon many surgeons were emulating him, though in Britain vagotomy was regarded as exciting but unproven and still experimental. The first to adopt vagotomy here were Ian Orr (1906–66) and Harold Johnson (1910–80), both surgeons at the British postgraduate medical school, Hammersmith, who reported fifty cases.[158] Unlike Dragstedt, who favoured a transthoracic operation, Orr and Johnson preferred an abdominal approach, which let them explore the abdomen and exclude the possibility of other lesions. None of their patients died and all of them lost their pain and returned to work.

For a while, vagotomy on its own seemed the answer; it was simple, avoided mutilating surgery and was physiologically appealing. This prompted Harold Burge (1913–81), a surgeon at the West London Hospital and himself an enthusiastic vagotomist, to ask a research fellow at the hospital medical school, Alan Pollock (born 1920), to review the results of vagotomy by several leading surgeons in Britain. The results were disappointing with nearly half the patients classed as unsatisfactory.[159] If the vagotomy was incomplete, recurrent ulceration was likely; if on the other hand vagotomy was complete, severe gastric retention occurred with an uncomfortable fullness and foul eructations. One disgruntled Scotsman complained that he had to give up smoking because the gas he eructed was highly inflammable. Diarrhoea was also common. Soon all vagotomies were combined with a drainage procedure to overcome this gastric atony, and there was little to choose between gastrojejunostomy and pyloroplasty. Even so the naturally conservative British surgeon was wary of vagotomy, particularly when G. F. Henson and Charles Robb (1909–94) reported a hundred cases of vagotomy and gastroenterostomy from St. Mary's Hospital, London, concluding that it was an unsatisfactory operation.[160] A few years later Illingworth added his weight suggesting that vagotomy was obsolete.

Thus in the early 1950s when duodenal ulcer was as its peak surgeons were still undecided between partial gastrectomy and vagotomy with a drainage procedure or even old fashioned gastroenterostomy on its own. So various trials took place, notably in Glasgow and Leeds. In Glasgow Patrick Forrest (born 1923), later Sir Patrick, soon showed that gastroenterostomy alone was unacceptable because of the recurrence of ulceration.[161] But he was unable to distinguish between partial gastrectomy and vagotomy with gastroenterostomy.

The landmark trial was done in Leeds and York under the leadership of John Goligher (1912–98), Professor of Surgery at the General Infirmary, Leeds.[162] Goligher had the advantage of working with Geoffrey Watkinson (1921–96) and Norman Pulvertaft, who helped him to run the trial and could draw on the rich tradition of ulcer surgery in both cities. They also compared partial gastrectomy with vagotomy and gastroenterostomy but added a third arm, vagotomy and antrectomy. Remarkably there was not one death among 634 cases. Recurrent ulceration was negligible but almost ten per cent had problems. The gastrectomy patients were underweight and nearly a quarter of the

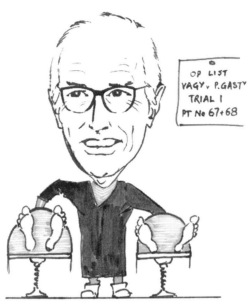

20 Golligher – Prolific triallist.

vagotomy patients developed diarrhoea. Meanwhile Harold Burge in London continued to study vagotomy. He believed that recurrent ulceration was usually due to incomplete vagotomy and with John Vane he invented a little electrode that could tell the surgeon if the vagotomy was complete.[163] Over more than twenty years he accumulated a series of 700 vagotomies becoming a strong advocate of so-called selective vagotomy whereby only the stomach was denervated.[164] His results were good with very few recurrent ulcers and hardly any complaints of diarrhoea. But his dream that a drainage operation might be unnecessary was not realised; gastric retention, bilious vomiting and dumping saw to that.

Vagotomy finally reached its peak after further refinements culminated in the highly selective "vagotomy" or "proximal gastric vagotomy". This operation denervated the parietal cell area of the stomach but preserved the nerve supply to the antrum and pylorus. Gastric stasis was avoided as the distal end of the stomach was able to empty itself through the pylorus in the normal way. In this country David Johnston (born 1937) in Leeds was the prime proponent of this operation.[165] He amassed a huge series of cases reporting excellent results but steadfastly refused to conduct a randomised trial on the grounds that the results were so much better, with almost no diarrhoea afterwards. However, in Belfast, Terence Kennedy (1919–93) a pioneer of prospective randomised controlled surgical trials, filled the gap. He showed conclusively that a highly selective vagotomy was extremely safe and effective.[166] Recurrent ulceration was rare and the side effects that had bedevilled vagotomy for years were eliminated. At last the surgeons had designed an operation that cured ulcers but was not mutilating; a triumph of years of experiment and effort. Admittedly it was a time-consuming and painstaking operation, which appealed to the specialist, and the average surgeon still found simple truncal vagotomy and pyloroplasty the most satisfactory procedure. However, just as David Johnstone was reporting the excellent results of a huge survey of 5,500 patients,[167] the physicians hit back with a hammer blow, the histamine H2 receptor antagonist.

CHAPTER FIFTEEN

HISTAMINE RECEPTOR ANTAGONISTS

From the time he introduced his augmented histamine test in 1953 Andrew Kay had wondered why the anti-histamines did not block the action of histamine on the parietal cells of the stomach. It did seem strange and a review in the *British Medical Journal* suggested that investigation of the anti-histamines should be rewarding.[168] But after the isolation of gastrin by Rod Gregory in 1960, everyone was expecting an effective anti-gastrin would be found to inhibit acid and heal ulcers. Indeed in 1971 Russell Johnstone went so far as to say, "acid secretion, no place for histamine", which effectively summed up interest in histamine as far as acid secretion was concerned.

During the 1950s James (later Sir James) Black (1924–2010), a physiologist and research chemist, was working in the veterinary school in Glasgow. His interest in ventricular fibrillation led him to show that it was possible to block some of the effects of adrenaline on the heart and his discovery of the beta adrenergic receptor-blocking drugs such as propanolol made his name. While Black was in Glasgow he was joined by a young gastroenterologist called Adam Smith, who had found that when anaesthetised cats were treated with five hydroxy-tryptamine, their stomachs were full of mucus. Black and Smith confirmed this and also showed that 5 H-T was a potent inhibitor of histamine-stimulated acid secretion. Black was well aware that conventional anti-histamines had no effect on acid secretion, and it occurred to him that histamine and adrenaline shared something in common. They were quite similar molecules derived from amino acids; adrenaline had several actions, some of which could be blocked by one group of anti-adrenaline drugs but others that could only be blocked by another group. Similarly histamine had several actions, some of which could be blocked by conventional anti-histamines but not others. So he reasoned that as with adrenaline there must be a histamine beta receptor that deserved to have its antagonist.[169]

By this time Black had moved to the Research Institute, Smith, Kline & French Laboratories Ltd., Welwyn Garden City where he began work on his theory in 1974. Shortly after, it so happened that the term H1 receptor was coined to describe the receptors blocked by conventional anti-histamines, so Black had little option but to call his proposed beta receptor an H2 receptor. He used guinea pig ileum (an H1 system) and guinea pig atrium (a non-H1 system) to test his compounds. Clearly histamine itself would stimulate both. At first things did not go well. Both adrenaline and histamine have a hydroxyl group on one end of their molecule. The adrenaline antagonist had been found by changing the hydroxyl group but this did not work for histamine. The chemistry was difficult so in between times he did some simpler things, that included adding a methyl group to every substitutable position on the histamine molecule. One happened to be 4-methyl histamine that selectively stimulated guinea pig atrium (H2) and another was 2-Methyl histamine that selectively stimulated guinea pig ileum (H1). He had proved the existence of two receptors. It was then a long hard slog substituting the side chain of histamine to find a competitive antagonist. Before he came up with burimamide, the first H2 receptor antagonist, 700 compounds were synthesised and tested.[170]

Tests on rats and dogs in vivo confirmed the activity of the drug; burimamide suppressed gastric acid whether this was stimulated by histamine or pentagastrin. Finally Black enrolled the help of John Wyllie (born 1933), a surgeon at the University College Hospital Medical School to test the drug in man.[171] Wyllie and his volunteers underwent standard augmented histamine stimulation tests and sure enough the secretion of gastric acid was almost switched off by burimamide.[†] Acid production fell by 80 per cent, far beyond anything seen before.

James Black's discovery was the result of a brilliant piece of deduction combined with determination to see his idea through. The H2 receptor was waiting to be discovered every time that Kay's augmented histamine

---

†   During the histamine infusion John Wyllie developed a headache, red face and engorged conjunctivae despite a large dose of mepyramine, a conventional anti-histamine. But after the addition of burimamide he became quite pale again which made Black realise that both the H1 and H2 receptors were involved in the cardiovascular response of histamine.

test was performed and it was being done countless times in research and clinical laboratories. No one took the imaginative leap until Black. He was supported throughout by the pharmaceutical industry, though at one stage they threatened to close him down, explaining that there was already a big programme concerned with inhibiting acid secretion in the United States. Fortunately Black convinced the industry that he was not trying to inhibit acid secretion, he was trying to block a new histamine receptor. Later he said with his customary modesty that once he was launched on his project, it was character that mattered more than intellect, the determination to keep going, year after year, when nothing seemed to be happening. His discoveries of the beta-adrenergic blocking compounds and H2–receptor antagonists won him the Nobel Prize and in 2000 he was invited to join the Order of Merit.

Burimamide was a valuable prototype that tested Black's ideas but it was relatively weak when taken orally and was soon replaced by metiamide. Smith, Kline & French were naturally excited by their new discovery but not in their wildest dreams could they have realised how successful it would be. In 1973 they hosted an international symposium in London in order to release details of the pharmacology and toxicology of the compounds. Soon groups of investigators around the United Kingdom were testing metiamide.

George Misiewicz (born 1930) was a senior lecturer at the Central Middlesex Hospital with Avery Jones and was interested in ulcer disease. He was aware of the work by John Lennard Jones (born 1927) at the hospital who had studied the effect of various diets on 24-hour gastric acidity.[172] When he heard Black lecture on the H2 receptor he persuaded Smith Kline French to let him study metiamide for them. Misiewicz adapted Lennard Jones' technique and showed that a single dose of the drug could inhibit gastric secretion overnight.[173] This was a crucial observation as no other drug had succeeded in doing this before. He did this work with David Jenkins, and with John Williams and Godfrey (later Sir Godfrey) Milton Thompson (1930–2012), both physicians in the Royal Navy, whom he had met at St. Marks Hospital and with whom he was to co-operate productively for some years.

Smith, Kline & French also turned to Ken Wormsley (born 1928) in Dundee, a gastroenterologist who was interested in gastric secretion. Wormsley confirmed that metiamide almost abolished acid secretion in

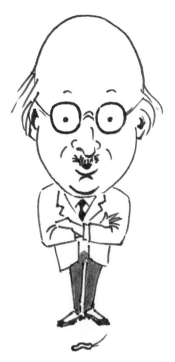

21 Misiewicz – Can a spirochaete really cause an ulcer?

patients with gastric and duodenal ulcer and was highly effective when given by mouth.[174]

At the same time David Shearman's team in Edinburgh showed that metiamide inhibited the stimulating effect of the vagus on gastric secretion.[175] This meant that the H2 antagonists were now known to block all known stimuli to acid secretion; clearly a clinical trial was indicated.

The first was a trial by Misiewicz and Milton Thompson who had now been joined by Roy Pounder (born 1944), a registrar at the Central Middlesex Hospital. Misiewicz persuaded him to forsake the immunology field in favour of his own more practical and well funded project. They compared metiamide with a placebo in patients with symptomatic duodenal ulcers and showed that their symptoms settled.[176] But this trial was inconclusive so far as ulcer healing was concerned because they could not believe that patients would tolerate a second gastroscopy.

The other study did show that metiamide healed ulcers. Roger Celestin (born 1925), a surgeon in Frenchay Hospital, Bristol, had had a duodenal ulcer since childhood but despite his training he had never believed that surgery was the appropriate treatment for ulcers. So he had written to several pharmaceutical companies offering his services should they have a product they wished to try. His chance came when the medical director of Smith, Kline & French sought his help. Soon he was co-ordinating a trial with workers from Bristol, Dundee, Edinburgh, Gloucester, University College Hospital and Newcastle, all of whom were experienced endoscopists.[177] Every patient had an endoscopically proven duodenal ulcer before treatment began and a further endoscopy after the trial to assess healing. After four weeks nearly three quarters of the patients on metiamide had healed compared to only a quarter of those on placebo.

About 600 patients enjoyed the almost magical benefits of metiamide before it had to be withdrawn. Six people had developed agranulocytosis, a potentially lethal condition in which the white blood corpuscles are destroyed exposing the victim to overwhelming infection. The bone marrow is full of histamine and it was unclear whether the agranulocytosis was specific to metiamide or the result of H2 blockade itself on cell maturation. The future of H2 receptor antagonists hung in the balance but was saved by a patient with Zollinger-Ellison syndrome under the care of Duncan Colin-Jones (born 1938) in Portsmouth. The ZE syndrome is characterised by very high acidity and intractable ulcers usually as a result of a gastrinoma. In this case the unfortunate patient had life-threatening haemorrhages despite a vagotomy and pyloroplasty, further undersewing of his duodenal ulcer and finally a partial gastrectomy in the space of three weeks. The situation was transformed by metiamide and he went home. Eight weeks later he returned with a severe staphylococcal infection that had broken down his wound, attacked his nasal septum and given him a nasty conjunctivitis. There were no neutrophils in his blood and metiamide was stopped. Fortunately he responded to antibiotics and his neutropenia began to recover, whereupon he started to bleed heavily from his ulcer again. Permission was given by a senior executive of Smith, Kline & French to try another H2 receptor antagonist, cimetidine. This was still under trial but to everyone's relief the bleeding stopped and significantly the patient's neutrophils returned to normal levels. Colin-Jones had shown that metiamide-induced agranulocytosis could recover during treatment with another H2 receptor antagonist.[178]

Metiamide contained a thiourea moiety on its side chain akin to neomercazole, an antithyroid drug well known to cause agranulocytosis. Cimetidine, which replaced it, has a cyanoguanidine group in place of the thiourea portion. By the time cimetidine was marketed in November 1976 it had undergone several clinical trials in patients with ulcers, which showed that it was effective and safe. By now endoscopy was widely used and all the trials were able to look at duodenal ulcer healing easily and objectively. One of the earliest was by John Wyllie, a small open trial that showed that duodenal ulcers nearly all healed in six weeks but appeared to relapse quite quickly. Even then he warned that treatment might have to be prolonged.[179]

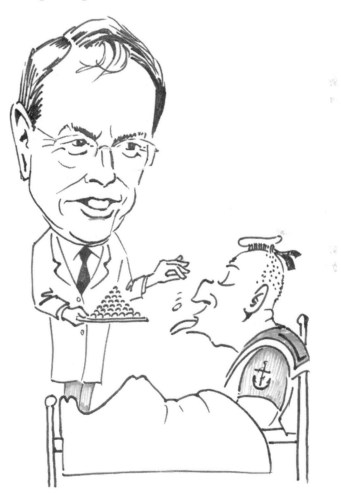

22 Pounder – Cimetidine for naval ratings at Haslar.

A larger trial took place at the Royal Naval Hospital, Haslar run by the Central Middlesex pair, Pounder and Misiewicz and the Royal Navy specialists, John Williams and Milton-Thompson. They confirmed ulcer healing and again measured the effect of cimetidine on 24-hour acid secretion.[180] At first they were horrified to find that the acidity was hardly affected. They had based the dose of cimetidine on earlier fasting experiments, and it was only when they realised that the patients were stimulating their acid with regular meals that they increased the dose, and all was well. Clinical research was not so sophisticated in those days.

Ken Wormsley in Dundee also confirmed the effectiveness of cimetidine but noted the high relapse rate within a few months of stopping treatment.[181] The drug was not curing the ulcer and needed to be continued, perhaps indefinitely. Eliminating acid provided ideal conditions for ulcer healing but was not a cure. So he maintained his patients on H2 receptor antagonists for years and he was one of the first to use ranitidine when it became available in 1979.

But there were fears about the safety of long-term cimetidine. Could the widespread use of a drug that reduces gastric acid predispose to gastric cancer? It was suggested that bacteria might proliferate in the stomach and convert dietary nitrites and nitrates to potentially carcinogenic nitrosamines. Accordingly the medical director of Smith, Kline & French, Bill Burland decided to fund a large study. In 1978 Colin-Jones (Portsmouth), Langman (Nottingham), David Lawson (Glasgow) and Martin P. Vessey (Oxford) began a post-marketing surveillance study to detect any adverse effects.[182] This was a remarkable effort in the days before personal computers and the analysis was done by John Beresford on an IBM main-frame computer at night when it was not in use. Nearly 10,000 patients were recruited and followed up for twenty years. No evidence to suggest an extra risk of cancer was found, which was most reassuring for the patients and their medical advisors.

The fact that patients needed to take H2 receptor antagonists indefinitely to prevent relapses may have worried some but it was sweet music to the ears of the manufacturers. Dr. John Wood (born 1949) of Glaxo-Smith-Kline (as it became in 2000) has estimated that more than 500 million people received this category of drug. Put another way ranitidine, which gradually superseded cimetidine, was worth £2.3 billion in sales annually at its peak.[183] But once again the wheel of fate was to spin in a way that few could have anticipated.

CHAPTER SIXTEEN

HELICOBACTER PYLORI

As we have seen, bismuth was often recommended by the Victorian physicians, and later Hurst himself used it, though he could not understand why it should work because it was a weak antacid. I would have expected Richard Doll to have tested it in one of his controlled trials, but he and Avery Jones were not prepared to co-operate with the manufacturers at the time, who were rather aggressive. However, the maker's persistence prevailed elsewhere, by which time modern endoscopy was available. One of the earliest trials was carried out by Paul Salmon (born 1937) in Alan Read's (1926–93) department in Bristol.[184] He showed that colloidal bismuth (De Nol) undoubtedly healed ulcers and another trial by David Shreeve (born 1937) in North Manchester found the same. Both groups stressed the importance of endoscopy in the assessment of treatment of duodenal ulcer. However, their trials did not attract much attention as the H2 antagonists were launched soon afterwards.

In 1978 Derrick Martin (born 1949), who was lecturer in medicine and gastroenterology in the university department of medicine at Withington

---

1   Shreeve recalls that one weekend in November 1976 the northern circulation manager of *The Times* and *Sunday Times* was admitted with abdominal pain and vomiting with a history of previous indigestion. He was slightly tender in the epigastrium and his liver tests were mildly abnormal, which were attributed to alcohol. Gastroscopy revealed a large duodenal ulcer. The patient was aware from a special report in *The Sunday Times* that a new treatment for duodenal ulcer was about to be launched and requested Shreeve to ring SKF to see if he could get some of this treatment for him. Only on the Monday morning did Shreeve realise that his patient was requesting cimetidine, which had been announced in the press before warning the medical profession. There was quite a furore during the week but intravenous cimetidine was obtained and given to the patient without benefit. Laparotomy revealed a gall stone ileus and the patient recovered.

Hospital, did a further trial with fascinating results.[185] De Nol was popular in the department because Iain Dymock (born 1939), the senior lecturer had been involved in some studies and knew it was effective. After cimetidine was introduced, Martin and Paul Miller (who had replaced Dymock by this time) decided to compare De Nol with cimetidine, which was by then everyone's favourite drug. A double blind study showed an excellent response to both treatments within a few weeks. As an afterthought they prolonged the study and re-endoscoped any patient whose symptoms recurred. They were astonished to find that the patients treated with De Nol were much less likely to have relapsed a year later than the cimetidine group. At first they did not believe their results but the evidence was solid so they decided to publish.[†] Try as they might they were unable to explain why De Nol should confer this long-term benefit. They were probably aware that Howard Steer and Duncan Colin-Jones in Southampton had observed gram negative bacilli in 80 per cent of their patients with gastric ulcer in 1975[186] but naturally had no reason to connect this observation with the benefits of bismuth in their patients.

Soon afterwards, Barry Marshall made his great discovery, which explained how bismuth, by killing H. pylori, cured ulcers once and for all. Few took him seriously at first, though Cliodna McNulty, with the help of Skirrow's experience, confirmed that campylobacter-like organisms caused gastritis and showed that peptobismol (a bismuth preparation from Proctor & Gamble) eradicated the organism and cured the gastritis.[187] This was the first work of its kind in this country and she had difficulty getting it published. The results were greeted by a deafening silence and after publication she received no correspondence at all. A submission of her work was turned down by the American Gastroenterological Association.

[†]   The results of the study might not have been published. Derrick Martin read the paper at a plenary session of the BSG and was harangued from the audience by a very prominent gastroenterologist who had done a great deal of work on cimetidine. However, he was confident that his data were correct and pushed on to publish. He sent the paper to the *Lancet* and received one reviewer's report, which was fairly damning. The reviewer was clearly the gastroenterologist who had attacked Martin at the BSG, as many of the points discussed were reflected in his review. Martin felt that these were spurious so he looked back at the reviewer's own publications and found that these refuted most of the comments which he had made in his report. Martin passed this on to the editor of the *Lancet* who had originally rejected the paper and shortly afterwards it was published.

But other pathologists were intrigued and began to find the organism, including Terence Rollason (born 1952) in Birmingham[188] and Ashley Price (born 1941) at Northwick Park Hospital. Price was supported enthusiastically by Jonathan Levi (1933–99), one of the few clinicians who believed that De Nol was a better drug than cimetidine and treated all duodenal ulcers with it. Gradually Price and Levi became convinced that campylobacter pylori was a pathogen and had to be eliminated if ulcers were to remain healed.[189] One man to be impressed by Levi's opinion was an Irishman, Colm O'Morain (born 1946), his senior medical registrar.[†] When he returned to Dublin O'Morain enlisted the support of the pathologists and microbiologists to compare De Nol with cimetidine.[190] Bismuth was certainly superior to cimetidine in healing ulcers but it was rather a weak antibacterial agent and only eradicated the organism from a third of the patients. Marshall, Warren and Stewart Goodwin found the same in Australia.[191] O'Morain realised that additional antibiotics were needed and carried out further trials showing that a combination of bismuth, metronidazole and amoxicillin were much more effective.

Until then, testing for H. pylori required an endoscopy to obtain biopsies for histological examination and culture. This was not only invasive but biopsies often missed the organism because its distribution within the stomach was patchy. This was clearly a significant drawback especially as it became apparent that large trials to find a suitable combination of antibiotics would be needed. A simple non-invasive test to confirm successful helicobacter eradication would be invaluable and it appeared right on cue.

While he was a senior lecturer in medicine in Nottingham Duncan Bell (born 1945) had developed a breath test to study aspects of liver metabolism.[192] He moved to Ipswich in 1983 where he did some work with Brocades, the makers of De Nol. Consequently he soon became interested in H. pylori and with his colleague John Trowell developed a simple half-gram stain for identifying the organism in gastric biopsies.[193] He knew the bacteria were urease positive and realised that he could

---

†   Levi believed in De Nol and used it routinely to treat duodenal ulcer. One of his patients in Northwick Park Hospital was a brother of the managing director of Smith, Kline & French in Dublin. When O'Morain moved to Dublin he met the managing director who admitted that he had regularly sent free samples of cimetidine to his brother. But after the treatment with De Nol, the demand for cimetidine had mysteriously stopped.

exploit this activity with a new breath test.[194] His patients drank a solution of urea labelled with radioactive carbon 14C and the high urease activity of H. pylori hydrolysed the urea forming ammonia and labelled carbon dioxide. The carbon dioxide in the patient's breath was collected for two hours and if isotope was present it confirmed the presence of H. pylori. Bell initially had difficulty convincing his colleagues that his idea would work but finally submitted a paper for publication in 1987. He was then mortified to learn that the *Lancet* were about to publish an almost identical study using a stable isotope 13C from David Graham in Houston, Texas. Recognising the significance of Bell's work, the editor published it in letter form ahead of Graham's paper.

Now that there was a simple way to measure the effectiveness of treatment, Bell and others were able to run large trials looking at antibiotic combinations. Some used Bell's breath test but others preferred the non-radioactive version of David Graham. This was taken up by Misiewicz's group at the Central Middlesex Hospital and simplified by Robert Logan (born 1959).[195] Logan, Misiewicz's senior registrar, was encouraged to study the breath test by his brother Richard, a physician in Nottingham, who had helped Bell with the statistical side of his work. At first Misiewicz was hesitant. He had spent his life studying acid and found it hard to accept that peptic ulcer could be an infective disease. But after attending the first European campylobacter pylori study group workshop in Bordeaux in 1988 he was converted and joined forces with Hugh Baron at St. Mary's Hospital to form the Parkside Helicobacter Study Group. Logan refined and shortened the 13C urea breath test, which was more suitable than the 14C test for repeated use in the same subject and for children and women of child-bearing age. But it was more expensive and required access to a mass spectrometer. Using the urea breath tests, groups all over the United Kingdom studied various combinations of antibiotics with bismuth and in 1990 an international working party at the World Congress of Gastroenterology in Sydney agreed an effective regimen.[196] This consisted of bismuth, metronidazole and tetracycline (or amoxycillin).

Even so treatment of peptic ulcer with antibiotics was slow to catch on. Clinicians could rely on their trusted H2 receptor antagonists and still found it hard to accept that ulcers were caused by infection. Advertising has a profound effect on prescribing habits and there was no promotion from the pharmaceutical industry. Compliance with treatment that required three drugs to be taken four times a day for two weeks was inevitably poor, and tedious for those who enjoyed a drink because alcohol interacts with metronidazole. Furthermore H. pylori was often resistant to metronidazole so the regimen left a lot to be desired.

Shortly before the Sydney guidelines were produced, Astra launched omeprazole, a new and remarkably effective acid inhibitor, which blocked the proton pump mechanism. Studies in the United Kingdom by Roy Pounder's group at the Royal Free had already confirmed its ability to decrease intragastric acidity.[197] A multicentre study led by Klaus Schiller (1927–2010) at St. Peter's Hospital, Chertsey showed that it healed ulcers even more quickly than the H2 receptor antagonists and they remained healed for longer.[198] Karna Bardhan (born 1941), a gastroenterologist in Rotheram with a seemingly inexhaustible supply of patients with peptic ulcer, also showed that omeprazole could heal ulcers that were refractory to H2 receptor antagonists.[199] Why was a course of omeprazole so much more effective? Using his breath test Bell showed that the drug could suppress the activity of H. pylori, though it was unable to eradicate it.[200] The most likely reason for this was its ability to eliminate gastric acid. H. pylori is adapted to live in an acid environment but Ken McColl had shown that if there was no acid, the ammonia produced by the bacteria was not neutralised and could actually damage the bacteria – 'suicidal destruction' he called it.[201]

These observations stimulated a profusion of trials comparing different combinations and strengths of proton pump inhibitor and antibiotics to treat H. pylori. Glaxo also invested heavily in a product, ranitidine bismuth citrate, which was effective and well received in America.[202] But it could not compete with the all-conquering proton pump inhibitors and never caught on in this country.

Barry Marshall, now in the United States, was becoming increasingly frustrated by the inertia of the medical profession. In 1993 only 25 per cent of gastroenterologists in Britain were using eradication therapy as first-line treatment for duodenal ulcers and 20 per cent per cent did not use it at all. Marshall appeared on television in a programme, *Horizons on Helicobacter,* accusing the pharmaceutical industry of their lack of support.[203] Why, he wanted to know, was the National Health Service spending millions of pounds on treating peptic ulcer when he could cure the disease in two weeks for a pittance?

The same debate was happening in the United States and in 1994 a peculiarly American event took place in Bethesda, Maryland.[204] The National Institute of Health convened a meeting on helicobacter pylori in peptic ulcer disease bringing together specialists in gastroenterology, surgery, infectious diseases, epidemiology, pathology and, significantly, members of the public. Britain was represented by Ken Wormsley (born 1928) from Dundee. After one and a half days of presentations by experts and discussion by the audience, a consensus panel weighed the evidence and prepared their statement. They concluded that ulcer patients with H. pylori infection required treatment with antibiotics in addition to antisecretory drugs. This was the turning point in attitude to peptic ulcer disease and it coincided with the arrival of the most effective and simple regimens to treat H. pylori.

By now duodenal ulcer was becoming a relatively uncommon disease (apart from those caused by non-steroidal anti-inflammatory drugs) so John Misiewicz set up a multicentre study with Karna Bardhan (Rotherham), Sassoon Levi (Wexham Park), Colm O'Morain (Dublin), Brian Cooper (Birmingham), Graeme Kerr (Shrewsbury) and Michael Dixon (Leeds).[205] Gastroenterologists from 55 hospitals in Great Britain and Ireland took part and over 500 patients were treated. The study showed conclusively that a one-week course of a combination of a proton pump inhibitor with two antibiotics effectively eradicated H. pylori in patients with duodenal ulcer or non-ulcer gastritis or both.

The story of peptic ulcer is far from over. The genetics of H. pylori and the response of its host, man, are yet to be unravelled. Should H. pylori be eradicated in everyone and if so will a vaccine become available? Physicians cannot afford to be complacent about ulcers. One authority wrote, "Isn't it therefore really a joy to be an ulcer physician in 1995?"[206] Perhaps, but I think James Penston (born 1952), then consultant medical advisor to Glaxo Wellcome, was nearer the mark when he said, "...whilst it may not be a joy to be an ulcer patient in 1996, it is certainly better than being an ulcer patient in earlier times".[207] John Buchan would have agreed with him.

REFERENCES

SECTION TWO

1   Brinton W. 1858 *Lectures on the diseases of the stomach*. First edition John Churchill & Sons, London

2   Brinton W. 1857 *On the Pathology, Symptoms, and Treatment of Ulcer of the Stomach*. John Churchill, New Burlington Street, London.

3   Price, W. 1956 *Textbook of the Practice of Medicine* 9th edition p577

4   *Plague, Pox & Pestilence* 1997 edited by Kiple K. F. Weidenfeld and Nicolson 160–5

5   Chambers T. 1856 *Digestion and its Derangements* Churchill, London p402

6   Hunter J. 1772 On the stomach itself being digested after death. *Phil. Trans. R. Soc.* 62: 447–454

7   Prout W. 1824 On the nature of acid and saline matters usually existing in the stomach of animals. *Phil. Trans. R. Soc.* 1: 45–49

8   Graves R. J. 1824 An account of the chemical properties of an acid found in the human stomach, together with remarks upon the manner in which it is formed both in disease and in health. *Trans. Assoc. Fell. Licen.* Kings Queens Coll. Phys. Ireland 4 316–331

9   Pavey F. 1869 *A Treatise on the Function of Digestion*. 2nd edition John Churchill & Son

10 Baillie M. 1833 *The Morbid Anatomy of Some of the Most Important Parts of the Human Body*. 8th London pp86–87

11 Crisp E. 1842–43 Cases of perforation of the stomach from simple ulceration. *Lancet* ii 639

12 Abercrombie J. 1830 *Pathological and Practical Researches on Diseases of the Stomach, the Intestinal Canal, the Liver, and Other Viscera of the Abdomen*. Philadelphia, Carey and Lea p119

13 Cooper E. C., Shaw L. E. 1893 On Diseases of the Duodenum. *Guy's Hosp. Reports* 50: 171-308

14 Baron J. H., Sonnenberg A. 2002 Hospital admissions for peptic ulcer and indigestion in London and New York in the 19th and early 20th centuries. *Gut* 50: 568–570

15   Osler W. 1901 *The Principle and Practice of Medicine*. Young J. Pentland 4th edition p478

16   Lister J. 1867 On a new method of treating compound fractures. *Lancet* i 327

17   Erichsen J. E. 1873 *Lancet* Oct 4th quoted by Sir St. Clair Thomson 1938 *Lancet* Oct 15 th: 911

18   Gilford H. 1894 A case of perforated gastric ulcer for which gastrorrhaphy was performed: death on the 31st day. *Brit. Med. J* 1-944

19   Morse T. H. 1894 Ruptured gastric ulcer treated by laparotomy, gastric suture, and washing out of the peritoneum; Recovery. *Med. Chir. Trans.* 77, 187–191

20   Moynihan B. G. 1907 The pathology of the living. *Brit. Med. J.* ii 1381

21   Moynihan B. G. 1901 Duodenal ulcer. *Lancet* ii 1656

22   Moynihan B. G. 1907 The pathology of the living. *Brit. Med. J.* ii 1381

23   Moynihan B. G. 1913 The gifts of surgery to medicine. Annual address to Brit. Med. Assoc.

24   Moyhihan B. G. 1910 *Duodenal Ulcer* London

25   Hurst A. 1909 *Guy's Hosp. Gaz.* 23: 332–335

26   Hurst A., Stewart M.J. 1929 *Gastric and Duodenal Ulcer*. Oxford University Press p48

27   Stewart M.J. 1923 The pathology of gastric ulcer. *Brit. Med. J.* ii 955 & 1021

28   Barclay A. E. 1915 *The Radiology of the Alimentary Tract*. Oxford University Press London

29   Hurst A., Stewart M.J. 1929 *Gastric and Duodenal Ulcer*. p59

30   Campbell J. M.H., Coneybeare J. J. 1924 Comparison of the test meal and X-ray examination of the stomach in health. *Guy's Hosp. Reports*. 74: 354–366

31   Edkins J. S. 1905 On the chemical mechanism of gastric secretion. *Proc. Roy. Soc. B.* 76: 376

32   Dale H. H., Laidlaw P. P. 1910 The physiological action of B-iminazolylethylamine. *J. Physiol*. 41: 318

33   Robertson C. R., Langlois K., Martin C. G., Slezak G., Grossman MI. 1950 *Amer. J. Physiol*. 163: 27

34   Bennett T. I., Ryle J. A. 1921 Studies in gastric secretion. V. A study of normal gastric function based on the investigation of one hundred healthy men by means of the fractional test meal. *Guy's Hosp. Reports*. 71: 268–318

35   Bell J. R., MacAdam W. 1924 *Quart. J. Med*. 17: 215

36   Lander F. P. L., Maclagan N. F. 1934 One hundred histamine test meals on normal students. *Lancet* ii 1210–13

37   Hunt J. N. 1959 Gastric emptying and secretion in man. *Physiol. Rev*. 39: 491–533

38   James A. H. 1951 Duodenal intubation with magnet-tipped tubes. *Lancet* I 209–10

39   James A. H., Pickering G. W. 1949 Role of gastric acidity in pathogenesis of peptic ulcer. *Clin. Sci*. 8: 181–210

40   Watkinson G. W. 1951 A study of the changes in pH of gastric contents in peptic ulcer using the 24–hour test meal. *Gastroenterology* 18 377–390

41   Card W. I. 1952 Peptic ulcer: Aetiology. In Avery Jones. F. (ed) Modern Trends in *Gastroenterology*, Butterworths, London 380–388

42   Kay A. W. 1953 Effect of large doses of histamine on gastric secretion of HCl *Brit. Med. J.* 2: 77–80

43   Card W. I., Marks I. N. 1960 The relationship between the acid output of the stomach following "maximal" histamine stimulation and the parietal cell mass. *Clin. Sci.* 19:147–163

44   Baron J,H., Burrows L., Wildstein W., Kark A. E., Dreiling D. A. 1965 The maximum histamine response of denervated fundic pouches in dogs. *Amer. J. Gastroenterol.* 44: 333–344

45   Gregory R. A., Tracy H. J. 1959 The action of enterogastrone on gastric secretion *J. Physiol.* 149: 58P & 70P

46   Harper A. A. 1946 The effect of extracts of gastric and intestinal mucosa on the secretion of hydrochloric acid by the cat's stomach. *J. Physiol.* 105: 31P

47   Gregory R. A., Tracy H. J. 1961 The preparations and properties of gastrin. *J. Physiol.* 156: 523

48   Gregory R. A., Tracy H. J., French J. M., Sircus W. 1960 Extraction of a gastrin-like substance from a pancreatic tumour in a case of Zollinger-Ellison syndrome. *Lancet* I 1045–48

49   Morley J. S., Tracy H. J., Gregory R. A. 1965 Structure-function relationships in the active C-terminal tetrapeptide sequence of gastrins. *Nature* 207: 1356–59

50   Baron H. J. 1969 Timing of peak acid output after pentagastrin. *Gastroenterology* 56: 641–643

51   Travers B. 1816 Rupture of the stomach and escape of its contents into the cavity of the abdomen. *Medico-Chir Trans.* 8 231–240

52   Leube W. 1876 *Ziemssen's Handbuch der Speziellen Pathologie und Therapie.* Leipzig.

53   Registrar General's Annual Reports (1905–35)

54   Watkinson G. 1960 The incidence of chronic peptic ulcer found at necropsy. *Gut* 1: 14–30

55   Watkinson G 1960 ibid page 15

56   Illingworth C. F. W., Scott L. D. W., Jamieson R. A. 1944 Acute perforated peptic ulcer *Brit. Med. J.* 2: 617–620 & 655–658

57   Jamieson R. A. 1955 Acute perforated peptic ulcer – frequency and incidence in West of Scotland. *Brit. Med. J.* 222–227

58   MacKay C. 1966 Perforated peptic ulcer in the West of Scotland: a survey of 5,343 cases during 1954 – 63. *Brit. Med. J.* 1: 701–705

59   MacKay C., MacKay H. P. 1976 Perforated peptic ulcer in the West of Scotland 1964–73. *Proc. Surgical Research Society* 157–8

60   Doll R., Jones F. A. 1951 Occupational factors in the aetiology of gastric and duodenal ulcer. With an estimate of the incidence in the general population. HMSO, London. MRC Special report series No 276

61   Pulvertaft C. N. 1968 Comments on the incidence and natural history of gastric and duodenal ulcer *Postgrad. Med. J.* 44: 597–602

62   Meade T. W., Arie T. H. D., Brewis M., Bond D. J., Morris J. N. 1968 Recent history of ischaemic heart disease and duodenal ulcer in doctors. *Brit. Med. J.* 3: 701–704

63   Brown R. C., Langman M. J. S., Lambert P. M. 1976 Hospital admissions for peptic ulcer during 1958–72 *Brit. Med. J.* 1: 35–37

64   Coggon D., Lambert P., Langman M.J. S. 1981 20 years of hospital admissions for peptic ulcer in England and Wales. *Lancet* i: 1302–04

65   Susser M., Stein Z. 1962 Civilisation and peptic ulcer. *Lancet* I: 115–9

66   Brinton W. 1864 *Lectures on Diseases of the Stomach*. 2nd edition Churchill & Son. p115

67   Ryle J. A. 1932 *Lancet* i: 327

68   Davies D. T. 1935 Some observations on peptic ulcer. Bradshaw Lecture *Lancet* I 521 & 585

69   Doll R. 2002 Peptic ulcer: Rise and Fall. *Wellcome Witnesses to Twentieth Century Medicine* Vol 14 ed. Christie D. A., Tansey E. M. p9

70   Curling T. B. 1842 On acute ulceration in the duodenum in cases of burn. *Med. Chir. Transact.* London 25 260

71   Hurst A. F., Stewart M. J. 1929 *Gastric and Duodenal Ulcer*. Oxford Med. Pub. Chap 2 69–70

72   Ryle J. A. 1932 Hunterian Lecture *Lancet* i: 339

73   Doll R. Peto R. 1976 Mortality in relation to smoking; 20 years observations on male British doctors. *Brit. Med. J.* 2: 1525–36

74   Whitfild P. F., Hobsley M. 1987 Comparison of maximal gastric secretion in smokers and non-smokers with and without duodenal ulcer. *Gut* 28 557–560

75   Douthwaite A. H. 1938 Some recent advances in medical diagnosis and treatment. *Brit. Med. J.* 1: 1143–46

76   Douthwaite A. H., Lintott G. A. M. 1938 Gastroscopic observation of the effect of aspirin and certain other substances on the stomach. *Lancet* ii 1222–25

77   Hurst A. F., Lintott G. A. M. 1939 Aspirin as a cause of haematemesis: a clinical and gastroscopic study. *Guy's Hosp. Reports.*, 89, 173–6

78   Hurst A. F. 1941 Aspirin and Gastric Haemorrhage. Letter to *Brit. Med. J.* 1: 768

79   Jones F. A. 1947 Haematemesis and mealaena. *Brit. Med. J.* 2: 441 & 477

80   Alvarez A. S., Summerskill W. H. J. 1958 Gastrointestinal haemorrhage and salicylates. *Lancet* ii 920–25

81   Truelove S. C., Reynell P. C. 1965 in *Diseases of the Digestive System*. Blackwell, Oxford 2nd ed p216

82   Langman M. J. S. 1970 Epidemiological evidence for the association of aspirin and acute gastrointestinal bleeding. *Gut* 11: 627–634

83   Walt R., Katchinski B., Logan R., Ashley J., Langman M. J. S. 1986 Rising frequency of ulcer perforation in elderly people in the United Kingdom. *Lancet* I 489–492

84   Thompson M. R. 1980 Indomethacin and perforated duodenal ulcer. *Brit. Med. J.* I 448

85   Thompson M. R. 1981 The unnatural history of drug-associated gastric ulcers. *Gut* 22: A877

86 Clinch D., Banerjee A. K., Ostick G., Levy D. W. 1983 Non-steroidal anti-inflammatory drugs and gastrointestinal adverse effects. *J. R. Coll. Gen. Pract.* 17 228–230

87 Collier D. St. J., Pain J. A. 1985 Non-steroidal anti-inflammatory drugs and peptic ulcer perforation. *Gut* 1985 26 359–363

88 Armstrong C. P., Blower A. L. 1987 Non-steroidal anti-inflammatory drugs and life threatening complications of peptic ulceration. *Gut* 28 527–532

89 Walker A. J., Dewar E. P. 1985 Emergency peptic ulcer surgery – an association with NSAIDs *Gut* 26 A1118

90 Somerville K., Faulkner G., Langman M. J. S. 1986 Non-steroidal anti-inflammatory drugs and bleeding peptic ulcer. *Lancet* i 462–464

91 Collier H. Personal communication

92 Vane J. 1971 Inhibition of prostaglandin synthesis as a mechanism of action for aspirin-like drugs. *Nature (New Biology)* 231–232

93 Hawkey C. J., Hawthorne A. B., Hudson N., Cole A. T., Mahida Y. R., Daneshmend T. K. 1991 Separation of the impairment of haemostasis by aspirin from mucosal injury in the human stomach. *Clin. Sci.* 81 565–573

94 Warren J. R., Marshall B. J. 1983 Unidentified curved bacilli on gastric epithelium in active chronic gastritis. *Lancet* i 1273–75

95 Marshall B. J. 1989 History of the discovery of Campylobacter Pylori. In Blaser M. J. ed *Campylobacter Pylori in Gastritis and Peptic Ulcer Disease* New York. Igakushoin 7–23

96 Marshall B. J., Royce H., Annear D. I., Goodwin C. S., Pearman J. W., Warren J. R., et al 1984 Original isolation of Campylobacter Pyloridis from human gastric mucosa. *Microbios Letters* 25 83–88

97 Marshall B. J., Warren J. R. 1984 Unidentified curved bacilli in the stomach of patients with gastritis and peptic ulceration. *Lancet* I 1311–13

98 Marshall B. J., McGechie D. B., Rogers P. A., Glancy R. J. 1985 Pyloric campylobacter infection and gastroduodenal disease. *Med. J. Aus.* 142 439–444

99 Marshall B. J., Armstrong J. A., McGechie D. B., Glancy R. J. 1985 Attempt to fulfil Koch's postulates for pyloric campylobacter. *Med. J. Aus.* 142 436–439

100 Le Fanu J. 1999 in *The Rise and Fall of Modern Medicine*. Little, Brown & Co., UK. chap 12 p186

101 Skirrow M. B. 1977 Campylobacter enteritis : a "new disease". *Brit. Med. J.* ii 9–11

102 Skirrow M. B. 2001 Personal communication.

103 McNulty C. A. M., Watson D. M. 1984 Spiral bacteria of the gastric antrum. *Lancet* I 1068–69

104 McNulty C. A. M., Wise R. 1985 Rapid diagnosis of Campylobacter-associated gastritis. Letter *Lancet* I 1443–44

105 McNulty C. A. M., Dent J. C., Uff J. S., Gear M. W. L., Wilkinson S. P. Detection of Campylobacter pylori by the biopsy urease test: an assessment in 1445 patients *Gut* 30 1058–62

106 McNulty C. A. M., Gearty J. C., Crump B. et al. 1986 Campylobacter pyloridis and associated gastritis: investigator blind placebo- controlled trial of bismuth salicylate and erythromycin ethylsuccinate. *Brit. Med. J.* 293 645–649

107 McKoll K. E. L., El Omar E. 1994 Effect of H. pylori infection on gastrin and gastric acid secretion. In Hunt R. H., Tytgat G. N. J., eds. *Helicobacter Pylori: Basic Mechanisms to Clinical Cure.* Boston; Kluwer Academic 245–256

108 McKoll K. E. L., El Omar E. 1995 Review article: gastrin releasing peptide and its value in assessing gastric secretory function. *Aliment. Phar.and Ther.* 9: 341–347

109 Levi A., Beardshall K., Haddad G., Playford R., Ghosh P., Calam J. 1989 Campylobacter pylori and duodenal ulcer: The gastrin link. *Lancet* i 1167–68

110 Moss S. F., Calam J. 1993 Acid secretion and sensitivity to gastrin in patients with duodenal ulcer: effect of eradication of Helicobacter pylori. *Gut* 34 888–892

111 Sonnenberg A. 1995 Temporal trends and geographical variations of peptic ulcer disease. *Alimentary Pharmacology and Therapeutics* 9 (Suppl.) 3–12

112 Baron J. H., Logan R. P. H. 1994 Infection by Helicobacter pylori is the major cause of duodenal ulcer. *Proc. R. Coll. Physicians Edinb.* 24: 21–36

113 Crabtree J. E., Taylor J. D.,Wyatt J. I., Heatley R. V. et al. 1991 Mucosal IgA recognition of Helicobacter pylori 120 KDa protein, peptic ulceration, and gastric pathology. *Lancet* 338 332–335

114 Atherton J. C., Peek R. M., Tham K. T., Cover T. L., Blaser M. J. 1997 Clinical and pathological importance of heterogeneity in vacA, the vacuolating cytotoxin gene of Helicobacter pylori. *Gastroenterology* 112 92–99

115 Clarke C. A., Edwards J. W., Haddock D. R. W., Howel Evans A. W., McConnell R. B., Sheppard P. M. 1956 ABO blood groups and secretor character in duodenal ulcer. *Brit. Med. J.* ii 725–731

116 El-Omar E. M., Carrington M., Chow W. H., McKoll K. E., Bream J. H. et al. 2000 The role of interleukin-1 polymorphisms in the pathogenesis of gastric cancer. *Nature* 404: 398–402

117 Tweedsmuir 1982 *John Buchan a Memoir.* Iola

118 Osler W. 1901 *The Principle and Practice of Medicine* Y. J. Pentland Lon. & Edin. 4th ed. 485–486

119 Moynihan B. 1907 The pathology of the living. *Brit. Med. J.* ii 1381–84

120 Sippy B. W. 1915 Gastric and duodenal ulcer: Medical cure by an efficient removal of gastric juice corrosion. *Trans. Assoc. Am. Physicians* 30: 129–148

121 Hurst A. F., Stewart M. J. 1929 *Gastric and Duodenal Ulcer* Ox. Univ. Press Part VIII 387

122 Ryle J. A. 1921 Inhibition of gastric secretion by butter and cream *Guy's Hosp. Reports.* lxxi 54

123 Freezer C. R. E., Gibson C. S., Matthews E. 1928 Neutralisation of HCl by various alkalies. *Guy's Hosp. Reports* lxxviii 191–

124 Bennett T. I. 1921 Action of atropine and belladonna on gastric secretion. *Guy's Hosp. Reports.* lxxi 54–57

125 Hurst A. F., Stewart M. J. 1929 *Gastric and Duodenal Ulcer* p438

126   Gordon-Taylor G. 1943 obit. *Brit. Med. J.* i 24

127   Finch E. 1960 *The Moynihan Chirurgical Club* (1909–59)

128   Moynihan B. G. A. 1928 development of gastric ulcer after gastrojejunostomy *Brit. Med. J.* ii 1021

129   Moynihan B. G. A. 1932 The prognosis of gastric and duodenal ulcer *Brit. Med. J.* i 1–3

130   Paterson H. J. 1909 Jejunal and gastrojejunal ulcer following gastroenterostomy. *Annals of Surgery* 50: 367–440

131   Wright G. 1919 Secondary jejunal and gastro-jejunal ulceration. *Brit. J. Surg.* 6: 390–401

132   Hurst A. F., Stewart M. J. *Gastric and Duodenal Ulcer* p438

133   Hurst A. F., Stewart M. J. 1929 quoted in *Gastric and Duodenal Ulcer* p440

134   Visick A. H. 1948 A study of the failures after gastrectomy. Hunterian Lecture. *Ann. Roy. Coll. Surg. (Eng.)* 3: 266–284

135   Walton A. J. et al. 1944 Discussion on treatment of duodenal ulcer. *Proceedings of the Royal Society of Medicine* 38: 91

136   Fenwick S. 1877 Lecture on atrophy of the stomach *Lancet* ii 1–4, 39–41, 77–78

137   Fenwick S. 1880 *On the Atrophy of the Stomach and on the Nervous Affections of the Digestive Organs.* Churchill, London

138   Ogilvie W. H. 1938 The approach to gastric surgery. II -Ulcer of the stomach. *Lancet* ii 295–299

139   Wells C. A. 1957 Duodenal ulcer: a study in the development of method. *Irish J. Med. Sci.* 7 32–41

140   Gordon-Taylor G. 1929 mentioned by Wells in Welbourn Hughes & Wells 1951 vit B defic. *Lancet* I 939

141   Witts L. J. 1966 *The Stomach and Anaemia.* Athlone Press, London

142   Cullinan E. R., Price R. K. 1932 Haematemesis following peptic ulceration: prognosis and treatment. *St. Barts. Hosp. Rep.* 65: 185

143   Meulengract E. 1935 Treatment of haematemesis and melaena with food: the mortality. *Lancet* ii 1220–2

144   Witts L. J. 1937 Haematemesis and melaena. *Brit. Med. J.* I 847–852

145   Gill A. M. 1947 Pain and the healing of peptic ulcers. *Lancet* i: 291

146   Martin L. C., Lewis N. 1949 Peptic ulcer cases reviewed after ten years. Effect of medical treatment and indications for gastrectomy. *Lancet* ii: 1115–20

147   Doll R., Pygott F. 1952 Factors influencing the rate of healing of gastric ulcers. *Lancet* i: 171–5

148   Lawrence J. S. 1952 Dietetic and other methods in the treatment of peptic ulcer. *Lancet* i: 482–485

149   Rae J. W., Allison R. S. 1953 The effect of diet and regular living conditions on the natural history of peptic ulcer. *Quart. J. Med.* 22: 439–455

150   Doll R., Friedlander P. H., Pygott F. 1956 Dietetic treatment of peptic ulcer. *Lancet* i: 5–9

151   Doll R., Pygott F. 1954 Clinical trial of Robaden and of cabbage juice in the treatment of gastric ulcer. *Lancet* ii: 1200–04

152   Evans P. R. C. 1954 The value of strict dieting, drugs and Robaden in peptic ulceration. *Brit. Med. J.* I 612

153   Doll R., Hill I. D., Hutton C., Underwood D. J. 1962 Clinical trial of a triterpenoid liquorice compound in gastric and duodenal ulcer. *Lancet* ii: 793–796

154   Hunt T. C. 1972 Symposium on carbenoloxone. *Br. Med. Week.* Tokyo

155   Truelove S. C. 1960 Stilboestrol, phenobarbitone and diet in chronic duodenal ulcer. *Brit. Med. J.* ii: 559–566

156   Dragstedt L. R., Owens F. M. 1943 Supradiaphragmatic section of the vagus nerves in treatment of duodenal ulcer. *Proc. Soc. Exp. Biol.*, N. Y. 53: 152 also 1945 Vagotomy for gastroduodenal ulcer. *Annals of Surgery* 122: 973 -989

157   Edwards F. R. 1939 On the neurogenic origin of duodenal ulcer. *Brit. J. Surg.* 181–198

158   Orr I. M., Johnson H. D. 1947 Vagal resection in the treatment of duodenal ulcer. *Lancet* ii: 84–89

159   Pollock A. V. 1952 Vagotomy in the treatment of peptic ulceration: review of 1524 cases. *Lancet* ii: 795–802

160   Henson G. F., Rob C. G. 1955 Duodenal ulcer treated by vagotomy and gastro-enterostomy. Results of 100 consecutive cases. *Brit. Med. J.* ii: 588–589

161   Forrest A. P. M. 1958 The treatment of duodenal ulcer by gastroenterostomy, gastroenterostomy and vagotomy, and partial gastrectomy. *Gastroenterology* 89: 307–311

162   Goligher J. C., Pulvertaft C. N., de Dombal F. T., Conyers J. H., Duthie H. L., Feather D. B., Latchmore A. J. C., Harrop Shoesmith J., Smiddy F. G., Willson-Pepper J. 1968 Five- to Eight-year results of Leeds/York controlled trial of elective surgery for duodenal ulcer. *Brit. Med. J.* i: 781–789

163   Burge H., Vane J. R. 1958 Method of testing for complete nerve section during vagotomy. *Brit. Med. J.* i: 615–618

164   Burge H., Stedeford R. D., Hollanders D. 1970 Recurrent ulceration after vagotomy and drainage with electrical stimulation test, 1957–69. *Brit. Med. J.* ii: 372–375

165   Johnston D., Goligher J. C., Pulvertaft C. N., Walker B. E., Amdrup E., Jensen H. E. 1972 The two- to four-year clinical results of highly selective vagotomy (parietal-cell vagotomy) without a drainage procedure for duodenal ulcer. *Gut* 13: 842

166   Kennedy T., Johnston G. W., Macrae J. D., Anne Soencer E. F. 1975 Proximal gastric vagotomy: interim results of a randomised controlled trial. *Brit. Med. J.* ii 301–303

167   Johnston D. 1975 Operative mortality and postoperative morbidity of highly selective vagotomy. *Brit. Med. J.* 4 545–547

168   Anonymous. 1948 Antihistamine drugs and gastric secretion. *Brit. Med. J.* ii: 1028

169   Black J. W. 2002 in Peptic Ulcer: Rise and Fall. *Wellcome Witnesses to Twentieth Century Medicine* vol 14. eds. Christie D. A., Tansey E. M. 63–67

170 Black J. W., Duncan W. A. M., Durant C. J., Ganellin C. R., Parsons E. M. 1972 Definition and Antagonism of Histamine H2–receptors. *Nature* 236 385–390

171 Wyllie J. H., Hesselbro T., Black J. W. 1972 Effects in man of histamine H2–receptor blockade by burimamide. *Lancet* ii: 1117–20

172 Lennard-Jones J. E., Fletcher J., Shaw D. G. 1968 Effect of different foods on the acidity of the gastric contents in patients with duodenal ulcer. *Gut* 9: 177–182

173 Milton-Thompson G. J., Williams J. G., Jenkins D. J. A., Misiewicz J. J. 1974 Inhibition of nocturnal acid secretion in duodenal ulcer by one oral dose of metiamide. *Lancet* i: 693–694

174 Thjodleifsson B., Wormsley K. G. 1974 Gastric response to metiamide *Brit. Med. J.* ii: 304–306

175 Carter D. C., Forrest J. A. H., Werner M., Heading R. C., Park J., Shearman D. J. C. 1974 Effect of histamine H2–receptor blockade on vagally induced gastric secretion in man. *Brit. Med. J.* iii: 554–556

176 Pounder R. E., Williams J. G., Milton-Thompson G. J. 1975 Effect of metiamide on duodenal ulcer: a controlled trial *Brit. Med. J.* ii 307–309

177 Celestin L. R., Harvey V., Saunders J. H. B., Wormsley K. G., Forrest J. A. H., Logan R. F. A., Shearman D. J. C., Fermont D., Haggie S. J., Wyllie J. H., Albinus M., Thompson M. H., Venables C. W., Burland W. L. 1975 Treatment of duodenal ulcer by metiamide. A multicentre trial. *Lancet* ii: 779–781

178 Burland W. L., Sharpe P. C., Colin-Jones D. G., Turnbull P. R. G., Bowskill P. 1975 Reversal of metiamide-induced agranulocytosis during treatment with cimetidine. *Lancet* ii: 1085

179 Burland W. L., Duncan W. A. M., Hesselbro T., Mills J. G., Sharpe P. C., Haggie S. J., Wyllie J. H. 1975 Pharmacological evaluation of cimetidine, a new histamine H2–receptor antagonist in healthy man. *Br. J. Clin. Phar.* 2 481–486

180 Pounder R. E., Williams J. G., Milton-Thompson G. J., Misiewicz J. J. 1975 24–hour control of intragastric acidity by cimetidine in duodenal ulcer patients. *Lancet* ii: 1069–72

181 Boyd E., Johnston D., Penston J. G., Wormsley K. G. 1988 Does maintenance therapy keep duodenal ulcer healed? *Lancet* i: 1324–28

182 Colin-Jones D. G., Langman M. J. S., Lawson D. H., Logan R. F. A., Paterson K. R., Vessey M. P. 1992 Postmarketing surveillance of the safety of cimetidine: 10 years mortality report. *Gut* 33: 1280–84

183 Wood J. 2002 in Peptic Ulcer: Rise and Fall. *Wellcome Witnesses to Twentieth Century Medicine* vol 14 eds. Christie D. A., Tansey E. M. 73–76

184 Salmon P. R., Brown P., Williams R., Read A. E. 1974 Evaluation of colloidal bismuth (De-Nol) in the treatment of duodenal ulcer employing endoscopic selection and follow up. *Gut* 15: 189–193

185 Martin D. F., May S. J., Tweedle D. E., Hollander D., Ravenscroft M. M., Miller J. P. 1981 Difference in relapse rates of duodenal ulcer after healing with cimetidine or tripotassium dicitrato bismuthate. *Lancet* i: 7–10

186 Steer H. W., Colin-Jones D. G. 1975 Mucosal changes in gastric ulceration and their response to carbenoloxone sodium. *Gut* 16: 590–597

187   McNulty C. A. M., Gearty J. C., Crump B., et al. 1986 Campylobacter pyloridis and associated gastritis: investigator blind, placebo controlled trial of bismuth salicylate and erythromycin ethylsuccinate. *Brit. Med. J.* 17 309–314

188   Rollason T. P., Stone J., Rhodes J. M. 1984 Spiral organisms in endoscopic biopsies of the human stomach. *J. Clin. Pathol.* 37: 23–26

189   Smith A. C., Price A. B., Borriello P., Levi A. J. 1988 A comparison of ranitidine and tripotassium dicitratobismuth (TDB) in relapse rates of duodenal ulcer. The role of campylobacter pylori (CP) *Gut* 29: A 711

190   Humphries H., Bourke S., Dooley C., McKenna D., Power B., Keane C. T., Sweeney E. C., O'Morain C. 1988 Effect of treatment on Campylobacter pylori in peptic ulcer disease: a randomised prospective trial. *Gut* 29: 279–283

191   Marshall B. J., Goodwin C. S., Warren J. R., et al. 1988 Prospective double-blind trial of duodenal ulcer relapse after eradication of Campylobacter pylori. *Lancet* ii: 1437–42

192   Henry D. A., Sharpe G., Chaplain S., Cartwright S., Kitchingman G., Bell G. D., Langman M. J. S. 1979 The (14C) – aminopyrine breath test. A comparison of different forms of analysis. *Br. J. Clin. Phar.* 8: 539–545

193   Trowell J. E., Yoong A. K. H., Saul K. J., Gant P. W., Bell G. D. 1987 A simple half-gram stain for demonstrating Campylobacter pyloridis in sections. *J. Clin. Pathol.* 40: 702

194   Bell G. D. et al. 1987 14C-urea breath analysis, a non-invasive test for campylobacter pylori in the stomach. *Lancet* i: 1367–68 Letter

195   Logan R. P. H., Polson R. J., Misiewicz J. J., Rao G., Karim N. Q., Newell D., Johnson P., Wadsworth J., Walker M. M., Baron J. H. 1991 Simplified single sample 13 Carbon urea breath test for Helicobacter pylori: comparison with histology, culture, and ELISA serology. *Gut* 32: 1461–64

196   Anonymous. 1990 Gastroenterologists in Sydney. *Lancet* 336: 779–780

197   Sharma B. K., Walt R. P., Pounder R. E., Gomes M de F. A., Wood E. C., Logan L. H. 1984 Optimal dose of oral omeprazole for maximal 24 hour decrease of gastric acidity. *Gut* 25: 957–964

198   Schiller K. F. R., Axon A. T. R., Carr-Locke D. L., Cockel R., Donovan I. A., Edmondstone W. M., Ellis A., Gilmore I. T., Harvey R. F., Linaker B. D., Morris A. I., Wastell C., Williams J. G., Gillon K. R. W. 1989 Duodenal ulcer recurrence after healing with omeprazole or cimetidine treatment: a multicentre study in the U. K. *Gut* 30: A1490

199   Bardhan K. D., Naesdal J., Bianchi Porro G., Petrillo M., Lazzaroni M., Hinchliffe R. F. C., Thompson M., Morris P., Daly M. J., Carroll N. J. H., Walan A., Rikner L. 1991 Treatment of refractory peptic ulcer with omeprazole or continued H2–receptor antagonists: a controlled clinical trial. *Gut* 32: 435–438

200   Weil J., Bell G. D., Powell K., Morden A., Harrison G., Gant P. W., Jones P. H., Trowell J, E. 1991 Omeprazole and Helicobacter pylori: temporary suppression rather than true eradication. *Alimentary Pharmacology and Therapeutics* 5: 309–313

201 Greig M. A., Neithercut W. D., Hossack M., MacDonald A. M. I., El Nujumi A. M., McColl K. E. L. 1990 Suicidal destruction of H. pylori mediated by its urease activity. *Gut* 31: A600

202 Dixon J. S., Pipkin G. A., Mills J. G., Wood J. R. 1997 Ranitidine bismuth citrate plus clarithromycin for the eradication of H. pylori. *J. Physiol. Pharmacol.* 48: 47–58

203 Ulcer Wars. Broadcast on 16 May 1994. *Horizon*, BBC2.

204 NIH Consensus Conference. 1994 Helicobacter pylori in peptic ulcer disease. *J.A.M.A.* 272: 65–69

205 Misiewicz J. J., Harris A. W., Bardhan K. D., Levi S., O'Morain C., Cooper B. T., Kerr G. D., Dixon M. F., Langworthy H., Piper D. Lansoprazole Study Group. 1997 One week triple therapy for Helicobacter pylori: a multicentre comparative study. *Gut* 41: 735–739

206 Labenz J., Borsch G. 1995 Towards an optimal treatment of Helicobacter pylori-positive peptic ulcers. *Amer. J. Gastroenterol.* 90: 692–694

207 Penston J. G. 1996 Review article: clinical aspects of Helicobacter pylori eradication therapy in peptic ulcer disease. *Alimentary Pharmacology and Therapeutics* 10: 469–486

APPENDIX

A preternatural Perforation found in the upper Part of the STOMACH, with the SYMPTOMS it produc'd,

by Mr. CHRISTOPHER RAWLINSON, surgeon.

JAMES SKIDMORE had complain'd for Three or Four Years last past, of a violent Pain in his Stomach and Bowels, never being able to rest in his Bed at Night, 'till he had vomited up the greatest Part of what he had eat or drank the Day before. He would often compare his Pain to some great Weight laying upon the Region of the Stomach, which he in some Measure alleviated, by pressing hard with his Hand upon that Part. When he turn'd himself in Bed from one Side to the other, he told me, he could plainly perceive that some Fluid or other fell down with Noise to the depending Side; which Fluid he believ'd to be the Occasion of all his Misery: For which Reason he often said, he would willingly consent, nay, often earnestly press'd that the Surgeons would cut him open (as he expressed it) and let it out.

He had no apparent TUMOUR upon the Part, nor was his Belly more EXTENDED than usual. He had had the Advice of several able Physicians before he came into the Hospital, but all without the least Amendment to his Disease. When he died we were desired to open him, and try if we could find out the Cause of his Complaints. As soon as we had penetrated the PERITONEUM, there flow'd out a whitish LIQUOR, not much unlike to WHEY, only a little more thick and faeculent; nor did it emit so noisome a Smell as might be expected from its long Residence in that Place. We computed there were above Four Quarts of this Liquor contain'd in the CAVITY of the ABDOMEN.

When we came at the STOMACH we found it PERFORATED in its UPPER Part, about the middle Space betwixt the Two Orifices, wide enough to contain the End of one's Finger. We cut it open Length-ways, and found it pretty full of a thick glutinous Matter, inclining to be yellow; and to its inner Coat, on the lower Side,there firmly adher'd the Stone of a PRUNE, or some other Fruit resembling it. On its Inside, near the Preternatural Perforation, twas gangreen'd for two or three Inches; and on the other Side of the Perforation there was an ULCER near the same Bigness. The whole Stomach was agreat deal thicker than usual; but that Part next the Pylorus was above Four Times thicker than in a natural State. It ADHER'D closely to all the Parts about it; and to the PANCREAS 'twas so firmly ty'd down, that it could not be separated without tearing. The Spleen did not exceed a Quarter of an Ounce in Weight. The PANCREAS was SCHIRROUS, tho' pretty near its natural Size. In the LIVER and KIDNEYS there was no apparent Defect, nor had the Parts of the THORAX receiv'd any visible Alteration, except that the LUNGS adher'd more than firmly to the Pleura than usual. The INTESTINES and the VISCERA contain'd in the ABDOMEN were of a whiter Colour than usual, by being so long sodden in the Liquor they floated in.

Philosophical Trans. Roy. Soc., London, 35: No 400, p361–2 1727–28

SECTION THREE

THE SMALL INTESTINE: COELIAC DISEASE

CHAPTER SEVENTEEN

GEE'S DISEASE

The Victorians died young. A typical family with five children could expect two of them to be dead by the age of fifteen and as recently as 1871 four out of five Englishmen were under the age of 45. Death from smallpox had virtually disappeared but had been replaced by epidemics of dysentery and gastroenteritis and various respiratory infections. To some extent breast feeding protected infants from gastrointestinal infection but this was little help to sick and undernourished mothers unable to provide sufficient milk. If their children managed to survive infancy they were weaned on bread, margarine and jam and 50 per cent of them had rickets. It was hardly surprising that twelve-year-old boys at private schools were on average five inches taller than their less fortunate compatriots in council schools. Wealthy Victorians were lucky. For the first time well-to-do mothers had a measure of control over their children's survival. Earlier, when smallpox was rife, rich and poor alike succumbed. Now effective breast feeding, good sanitation and fresh air meant the rich could avoid life-threatening dysentery and respiratory disease. The "sanitary idea" also led to a decline in tuberculosis. Pulmonary TB was the commonest form of the disease but there was a type, peculiar to children, caused by intestinal infection from drinking infected milk. The child became puny, wasted and anaemic, with a large belly and offensive diarrhoea, and usually died.

Occasionally this "consumption of the bowels" as it was known would pick out a child regardless of social class when everyone else in the family was healthy. The child either died or survived as a rickety dwarf and an invalid. Attributed to tuberculosis these cases were easily overlooked as a distinct entity by physicians preoccupied by infectious disease and malnutrition. Perhaps it was the very fact that this mysterious and debilitating disease singled out the well-to-do as often as the poor that eventually brought it to somebody's notice, though it needed somebody with considerable experience to recognise it. Such a person was Dr. Samuel Jones Gee.

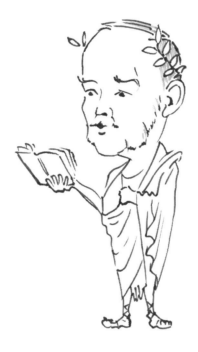

23 Gee – A classicist.

Gee (1839–1911) was a physician at St. Bartholomew's Hospital and Great Ormond Street. He was a shy man with few social graces and had certain mannerisms that his students liked to mimic, but he was an astute clinician and his writings reveal a classical education and a deep sense of history. He first drew attention to coeliac disease in a lecture at Great Ormond Street on 5 October 1887 and the following year published his account in St. Bartholomew's Hospital reports.[1] He had a motto "thrift in words", and his paper is a classic of concise presentation. It has been much admired and is reproduced in Appendix 1, Section 3 in full.[1]

---

1 Curiously Norman Moore (1847–1922) who knew Gee well does not mention Gee's account of coeliac disease in his history of St. Bartholomew's Hospital. To Gee perhaps the description of coeliac disease was unremarkable by comparison with the rest of his work.

Some years ago two paediatricians, Bryan Dowd and John Walker-Smith (born 1936) analysed Gee's paper.[2] They suggested that Gee's literary style was deliberately archaic. It may have seemed bookish, even to his contemporaries, but reflected his familiarity with seventeenth-century literature, his respect for the ancient writers, and his delight in teasing his readers. In the opening paragraph he expected them to recognise a couplet he quotes and assumed they would understand the significance of the "half sod meat". A clue to the source of the couplet comes in a lecture he gave five years later, when he spoke of "old books, such for instance as the writings of those learned anatomists Robert Burton and Phineas Fletcher, contemporaries of Harvey". Fletcher (1582–1650) was hardly an anatomist but a poet who fascinated Gee. He had written an allegory of the human body and mind *The Purple Island or the Isle of Man*.[3] In the preface to this poem there is a short appreciation written by his friend Francis Quarles (1592–1644).

> Mans *Bodie's* like a house: his greater *bones*
> Are the main *timber*; and the lesser ones
> Are smaller *splints*; his ribs are *laths*, daub'd o're,
> Plaister'd with *flesh*, and *bloud*: his mouth's the *doore*,
> His *throat's* the narrow *entrie*, and his heart
> Is the *great chamber*, full of curious art:
> His midriffe is a large partition-wall
> Twixt the great chamber, and the spacious *hall*:
> His *stomack* is the *kitchin*, where the meat
> Is often but half sod, for want of heat:

Gee seized on this couplet to take his reader back to the writings of Aretaeus whose vivid clinical description of coeliac disease he admired. Aretaeus was a Cappadocian from Asia Minor who lived in the first century AD. The Cappadocians were regarded as "dull and submissive and prone to vice"[4] so clearly Aretaeus was an exception. He believed that digestion (pepsis) and absorption of food depended on 'natural or indwelling heat'. Pepsis in its non-medical sense implied a softening or change under the influence of heat, like the ripening of fruit by the sun or the cooking of food. It was natural to apply this idea to the "cooking" or the coction of food in the stomach. Indeed the word concoction used by Gee is a fair rendering of pepsis.

Aretaeus thought the coeliac state only occurred in adults. He stressed that it was a chronic illness causing general debility and starvation. The stool looked white, lacked bile and was offensive. There were foul smelling eructations and rumblings in the gut with emission of flatulent material which was thick and looked like clay. The patient was emaciated, pallid and feeble.

It was probably Gee's paediatric experience that enabled him to recognise coeliac disease in infants. He was on the staff of Great Ormond Street and jealous of his broad medical experience. He once declared "there is a name I hate, yea there are two names that my soul abhoreth, the name of a Specialist and the name of a Consultant".[5] He considered the disease to be rare in adults unless they had been living in India.

Gee was not in fact the first Englishman to draw attention to malabsorption. Thirty years earlier Sir William Gull (1816–90), doyen of physicians of his time at Guy's Hospital, described fatty diarrhoea and emphasised the difference between steatorrhoea due to pancreatic insufficiency and that resulting from disease of the small intestine. He too acknowledged the older writers: "Diarrhoea chylosa or fluxus coeliacus was recognised by them, and attributed to some impediment in the absorbent system." Writing in Guy's Hospital reports in 1855 Gull said, "The normal absorption of fatty matters is prevented from two causes; either from a defect in the digestive or emulsifying process, or from disease of the absorbent system. The instances of fatty stools from disease of the pancreas and the duodenum, as described by Dr. Bright and others, belong to the former, and are characterised by the fat passing from the intestines, more or less separate from the general mass of the faeces, and concreting upon them; but in the latter case, where the disease is in the absorbent system, the fat, being emulsified, becomes incorporated with the evacuation, and is consequently not so easily recognised. If, however, there be, with defective absorption, an inflammatory condition of the mucous membrane and diarrhoea, the oily matters rise to the surface of the evacuation as a creamy film, and produce the pale, chalky, and soapy appearance so characteristic of chronic muco-enteritis and mesenteric disease."[6] Post mortem examination on Gull's patients revealed tuberculosis of the intestine (tabes mesenterica) causing obstruction of the lacteals.

Gee's crucial observation was his inability to find anything "unnatural" in the intestines of the children who died. He does not say how many he examined, but he is thought to have performed over 600 necropsies in his lifetime so he was an experienced morbid anatomist and unlikely to have overlooked mesenteric tuberculosis. He was describing a new disease even though he chose to acknowledge the older writers in his report. Aretaeus' patients were adult or even elderly and almost certainly had TB; Gee's patients were children and were not tuberculous.

Gee's decision to call the condition coeliac disease or belly affection, from koilia (belly), was wise. It alluded to the flaccid distended abdomen and implicated the abdominal viscera without attempting to explain the cause or pathogenesis of the disease. The works of Aretaeus had recently been translated by the scholar Francis Adams (1796–1861)† and published by the Sydenham Society in 1856.[7] Gee may have adopted the title "on the coeliac affection" from Adams' English version, but he was quite capable of reading Greek so he may have chosen the title partly as a compliment to the ancients.

Despite his experience and clinical acumen, Gee was a sceptic with little time for the new biochemistry. Laboratory data are conspicuously absent from his report. The possibility that coeliac disease could be caused by some as yet undetected pathological process in the lining of the intestine would have appealed to him, which was the reverse of the opinion put forward by Robert Gibbons (1854–1934) after Gee had shown him examples of the disease. Gibbons was Resident Medical Officer at Great Ormond Street when he described four children with coeliac disease, though he implies that he had seen several more. Only one came to post mortem and no abnormality was found in the intestinal tract. On this basis he concluded that there must be "a functional disturbance of the nervous supply of the liver, pancreas, glands of Brunner and follicles of Lieberkuhn, possibly also of those of the stomach and salivary glands".[8] Gee would not have agreed with this. He demanded precision and fact. "Anatomy not physiology," he used to say, "in anatomy you have facts; in physiology more or less theory."[9]

---

†   Adams was a GP in Banchory, a remote town in Scotland, who had a remarkable gift for translating classical Greek. He was a good doctor though a paradox; he obstinately refused to believe that the sounds of the foetal heart could be heard at auscultation.

CHAPTER EIGHTEEN

TROPICAL SPRUE

Both Gee and Gibbons had noticed the resemblance between children with coeliac disease in England and malabsorption in the tropics, which was the scourge of Europeans living in India and the Far East. To understand the relationship between the two diseases a brief digression on the subject of tropical sprue is necessary.

Towards the end of the Victorian era large numbers of Europeans were hastening to colonise the Eastern Tropics. With their arrival came a "new" disease consisting of mouth ulceration and severe malabsorption which was frequently fatal. The troops who first occupied Saigon and Annam were devastated by the disease, and civilian settlers paid a heavy toll to its ravages. Many names were used to describe it, notably psilosis (loss of hair or epithelium), white chronic tropical diarrhoea, diarrhoea alba, Ceylon sore mouth, tropical apthae and stomatitis intertropica. With more consistency the Dutch physicians in the East adhered to the local term current in Java – Indische Spruw (thrush or stomatitis) – and this word, anglicised into Sprue, was adopted by Sir Patrick Manson in China in 1880. Manson[†] (1844–1922) was at the time medical officer in the service of the Chinese Imperial Maritime Customs, and it was in their report for the half-year ended 31 March 1880 that he wrote his *Notes on Sprue*. He pointed out that the condition had received little attention from medical writers and went on to describe it in detail. He stressed the importance of mouth ulceration and described the insidious onset,

---

[†]   Manson retired in 1889 but lost all his money when the Chinese dollar crashed, so he had to come out of retirement. In the event this was fortunate for tropical medicine as he founded the London Hospital for Tropical Disease and Hygiene and became the father of tropical medicine.

the slow progress and the tendency to relapse. Manson insisted that the affection was a disease "sui generis", entirely apart and distinct from all other intestinal affections. He must have been pleased the catchy word sprue caught on. "Much good may be done by associating this deadly disease with a specific name"; by doing so it should be possible to persuade the victim of an "absolute necessity for leaving the country".[10]

In the Lettsomian lectures delivered in 1881, which contain a reference to Manson's work, Sir Joseph Fayrer (1824–1907) described "chronic white tropical diarrhoea", a disorder that he said was one of the most tedious and intractable affections to which Europeans in India were liable. He was undoubtedly describing sprue though all his cases were seen in England. Clinical investigation in tropical countries was not easy in his day. Patients with sprue were sent home and usually recovered, so opportunities for post mortem studies were few. Nonetheless he was impressed by the pathology. If death occurred early, the intestine was contracted and the mucous membrane congested or ulcerated. If death occurred later, the membrane was atrophied and the seat of fatty or lardaceous degeneration. Frequently there was ulceration in both ileum and colon with atrophy of the mesenteric glands.[11]

Gibbons was aware of Fayrer's work and felt sure that coeliac disease and tropical sprue were not the same condition. It was inconceivable that Gee could have overlooked such obvious pathology in his patients.

CHAPTER NINETEEN

STEATORRHOEA

Apart from a brief paragraph in Osler's text book of medicine (1892), Gee's publication excited little comment for several years until Walter Cheadle (1835–1910) gave a lecture at St. Mary's Hospital Medical School in 1903. Cheadle was on the staff of the Hospital for Sick Children, Great Ormond Street, and enjoyed a considerable reputation as a consultant on children's diseases. He was 67 when he drew attention once more to coeliac disease.

He called it acholia because he was convinced that the white stool indicated a complete absence of bile. He described five children with typical symptoms and compared them with an adult whom he thought had sprue. His problem was to explain the acholia in the absence of jaundice or biliary obstruction. The best he could propose was an "arrest of the chologenetic function of the liver" from nervous inhibition "perhaps linked to teething". His treatment included bismuth and opium for troublesome diarrhoea, and brandy as a hepatic stimulant together with the chlorides of arsenic, mercury and iron.[12] Cheadle's paper is important because he was the first person to draw attention to the excess of fat in the stool which was analysed "by his friend Dr. W. H. Willcox", lecturer on chemistry and chemical pathology at St. Mary's Hospital. (Sir William Willcox, 1870–1941)

Coeliac disease was rediscovered in 1908 by an American, Christian Herter (1865–1910), who was apparently unaware of Gee's account. Herter published a short book *Infantilism From Chronic Intestinal Infection*, recording the cases of ten children. None of the children died so he was unable to study the morbid anatomy, but he emphasised, as the title implies, that infection must be the cause. By this time the science of bacteriology was well established and the organisms responsible for most bacterial diseases had been isolated. Herter thought that an overgrowth of gut flora caused an inflammation of the intestine but his evidence was weak. However, he was a good biochemist and carried out some fine metabolic studies showing that his children were losing calcium. He also noted that the fat in the stool was in the form of fatty acids. "These losses cannot of course be attributed to any failure of fat splitting in the intestine, but are clearly referable to a diminished power of absorption."[13] The next year an eminent and influential paediatrician in Berlin, Otto Heubner (1843–1926), was inspired by Herter's book to publish his own account which attracted sufficient attention in Germany for it to be referred to as his disease.[14] By now the names for the disease were many and various with coeliac disease known as Gee's disease, Gee-Herter's disease, Herter-Heubner's disease, acholia and intestinal infantilism.

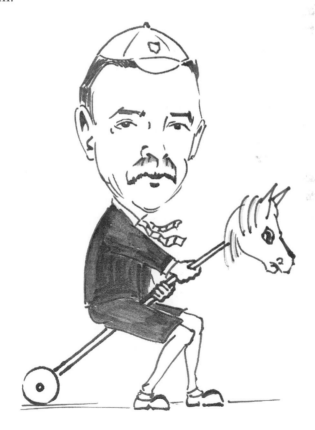

24 Still – First professor at Gt. Ormond St.

Twenty years after Gee's original description, Sir Frederic Still (1868–1941), the first professor of paediatrics at Great Ormond Street Hospital, rectified matters when he delivered the Lumleian lectures to the College of Physicians on coeliac disease.[15] He could add little to what was known but his observations were sharp and beautifully written. "The most striking feature is the surprising inconsistence of the child's size with its age. What appears to be an infant little more than twelve months old, startles one by unexpectedly talking and so reveals the fact that it is at least a year or two older, perhaps three or four years older, than its appearance would suggest." Still drew attention to the similarity between coeliac disease and sprue and speculated about its cause, but he was hampered by a lack of post mortem evidence. Aware of only two autopsies he described an inflammation of the whole intestinal tract, which was obvious to the naked eye as well as under the microscope. He said "the marked thickening of the wall of the bowel was something quite unusual". But he could not explain it. "The bacteriological findings, it must be admitted, are far from conclusive of any specific infective cause." The best he could suggest was that "in coeliac disease there is a primary infective catarrhal condition of the mucosa in the small intestine where in health the absorption of fat occurs chiefly or entirely". This worried him because other causes of catarrh of the upper intestine, for example, common summer diarrhoea, did not affect fat absorption. On treatment, he agreed with Gee that the diet was crucial. "The element in the food which requires most consideration is the fat, and the form of fat which seems most obnoxious to children is the fat of cow's milk." He also noted some difficulty dealing with starches, though much less than with fats. "Unfortunately, one form of starch which seems particularly liable to aggravate the symptoms is bread." He concluded his lectures with a note of resignation: "I have raised many questions, I have answered few, and if any apology is needed, I should say, in the words of Heraclitus: *"Those who seek for gold dig much earth and find little."*

Unfortunately with respect to coeliac disease this aphorism was true for the next 25 years. There were minor improvements in its management but the cause remained elusive. Though the mortality was approximately 30 per cent post mortems were seldom done. Reginald Miller (1879–1948) physician to St. Mary's Hospital and Paddington Green Children's Hospital, reported one autopsy he did himself on a child aged five. A provisional diagnosis of abdominal tuberculosis had been made but the post mortem was normal. He too wondered about the cause of coeliac disease and concluded that it "was independent of organic changes and this must be due to a digestive fault – probably a defective action of bile on fat absorption".[16]

A little later, John Ryle (1889–1950), now physician at Guy's Hospital with an international reputation for his work on gastric function, put forward his ideas on the cause of the disease at a meeting of the Association of Physicians in 1923. He dismissed Miller's hypothesis that the production of bile was inadequate because there was no evidence of liver dysfunction. Ryle himself described two cases of typical coeliac disease in young adults who underwent laparotomy. In each case the intestinal lymphatics were grossly distended with fat and obstructed by caseous tuberculous glands in the mesentery. Realising his mistake, Ryle suggested that healthy lymphatics were necessary for normal absorption and wrote "the inability to absorb fats in coeliac disease and the attendant complications such as infantilism and tetany, can best be accounted for by an obstructive lesion of some part of the lacteal tree". He urged that fat should be restricted, and added two interesting comments. One was that pancreatic disease was not, as generally thought, a common but a rare cause of steatorrhoea. Secondly tropical sprue and idiopathic steatorrhoea in adults "might be similarly explained", implying that people who had never been to the tropics could acquire steatorrhoea or so-called non-tropical sprue.[17]

CHAPTER TWENTY

CALCIUM DEFICIENCY

Ryle highlighted two of the most distressing features of coeliac disease: infantilism and tetany thought to be due to excessive calcium loss in the faeces. Tetany was first described in 1815,[18] and almost 50 years later Armand Trousseau (1801–67) described his famous sign.[19] He also recognised that tetany could be a complication of diarrhoea "especially when abundant and chronic".[20] But until it was possible to measure blood calcium the cause of tetany remained baffling. For example, in 1911, Frederick Langmead (1879–1969), one of the first full-time professors of medicine in England and physician-in-charge of the children's department at St. Mary's Hospital, recorded fourteen cases of 'colonic tetany' with distension of the colon, pultaceous, pale offensive stools and stunted growth. He attributed the tetany to toxic absorption from the putrefying contents of the colon.[21]

Even Frederic Still, who described three cases in his Lumleian lectures, was puzzled by tetany, though he was aware that hypocalcaemia was probably responsible. At the time investigators had to rely on balance studies to decide if a patient was calcium deficient. Measurement of blood calcium only became feasible in the 1920s when simpler titration methods were introduced but these were laborious and unavailable in most laboratories.

Tetany was also a recognised, if somewhat rare, complication of tropical sprue, being first reported by James Cantlie (1851–1926) in 1913, who observed six cases.[22] It was rediscovered in 1919 by Percy Bassett Smith (1861–1927) who recorded a case of very severe tetany occurring shortly before the patient's death.[23] Though tetany was rare, this fact did not prevent the promotion of an extraordinary theory for the aetiology of tropical sprue implicating the parathyroids. The disease was now a major problem in the East, incapacitating Europeans who had to be sent home for treatment, usually to the Hospital for Tropical Disease in London. In 1923 extract of parathyroid hormone became available for the first time, which coincided with a brief vogue for its use in sprue.

This was championed by Harold Scott (1874–1956), a man of conviction and strong personality, who wrote prolifically and rose to become Director of the Bureau of Hygiene and Tropical Disease, an authority responsible for the publication of regular bulletins on tropical matters. Scott argued that in the East people ate an excess of protein and fat, which stimulated overproduction of acid. Excess acid in the duodenum stimulated the production of secretin, which led to overstimulation of the pancreas and an upset in the balance of the endocrine glands, among them the parathyroids. He also believed that alimentary toxaemia exhausted the parathyroids, causing a disturbance of calcium metabolism and a decrease in tissue resistance. The fact that the blood calcium was usually normal in his patients did not deter him; he argued that the ionic calcium was deficient, though he did not measure it. Scott was the first to obtain parathyroid extract and gave it by mouth with calcium lactate, claiming excellent clinical results.[24]

Others including Philip Manson-Bahr (1881–1966), son-in-law of Sir Patrick Manson, followed suit and for five years parathyroid extract was widely recommended until the credibility of the theory was questioned and it was abandoned. This episode illustrates just how anxious doctors were to help patients with sprue, a debilitating and often fatal disease. Another physician at the Hospital for Tropical Disease, Carmichael Low (1872–1952), treated his patients empirically, relying on months of strict bed rest and a bland diet, mainly milk; a miserable time for the patient apart from a liberal intake of strawberries, which he thought were beneficial.[25] In fact what really helped was repatriation from the tropics as Manson originally insisted.

It was the discovery of vitamin D that transformed the treatment of the spasms and deformities of coeliac disease. Cod liver oil was first used in medicine at the Manchester Infirmary in 1772 for patients with rheumatism. At first it was applied as an inunction to the skin, until "an accidental circumstance", wrote Dr. Robert Darbey to Dr. Thomas Percival (1789), "discovered to us a remedy...the cod or ling liver oil, taken by mouth".[†/26] John Hughes Bennett (1812–75) revived interest in its use in 1841 and no less than 811 gallons at five shillings a gallon were bought by St. Bartholomew's Hospital in 1877.[27] Gee himself wrote (1868) "in cod liver oil we possess a pharmaceutical agent worthy of a place beside iron, Peruvian Bark and mercury" (used for green sickness, quartan agues and the pox respectively).[28] He was writing about its use in rickets but cannot have known how it worked.[§]

The breakthrough came in 1906 when the father of British biochemistry, Frederick Gowland Hopkins (1861–1947), later Sir Frederick, President of the Royal Society and Nobel Prize winner, postulated the existence of accessory food factors, which prevent some diseases such as scurvy and rickets.[29] The term vitamine was coined in 1912 by Casimir Funk (1884–1967), a Polish-born chemist working at the Lister Institute in London, to describe "special substances which are the nature of organic bases which we call vitamines".[30] It was later realised that the amine groups were not essential, and in 1920, J. C. Drummond, later Sir Jack Drummond (1891–1952) at the Ministry of Food, proposed the omission of the 'e' and vitamin passed into universal use.[‡/31]

Just before the First World War, an American physiologist, Elmer McCollum (1879–1967), showed that certain fats contained an essential ingredient for growth. Shortly afterwards the Medical Research Committee (later Council) decided to promote research into the nature and cause of rickets, and Hopkins recommended his protégé Edward Mellanby (1884–1955), a precocious professor of physiology in the University of London to carry out this work. By the end of the war, in a series of laborious experiments done in Cambridge, Mellanby was able to produce the clinical, radiological and histological bone changes of rickets in dogs by depriving them of the fat-soluble vitamin that had been discovered by McCollum. He showed too that adding cod liver oil but not vegetable oils prevented the disease.[32] Two years later, McCollum

---

†   The healthcare company, Smith and Nephew, was founded in 1879 in order to market cod liver oil. Smith started it and brought in his nephew.

§   Sir John Bland Sutton (1855–1936), a cockney who became President of the RCS, cured rickets that frequently killed lion cubs born in the London Zoo with a mixture of cod liver oil and crushed bones (1889), but did not follow up his discovery.

‡   Drummond was murdered in mysterious circumstances in Provence while on holiday in 1952 in what became known as the Medici affair.

identified this as vitamin D,[33] and workers in Germany found that ultraviolet light helped rickets by activating a provitamin into vitamin D, and in 1927 the provitamin was identified as ergosterol. Within a few years Mellanby's work led to the rational treatment of rickets in infants.

Once it was possible to measure blood calcium, several people began to report the occurrence of hypocalcaemia in coeliac disease, notably Leonard Parsons[†] (1879–1950). As far back as 1913 Parsons had shown a case of coeliac disease before the Midland Medical Society, suggesting that rickets was not an uncommon complication of the disease.[34] In due course he became one of the early professors of medicine with his appointment to the chair of diseases of children in the University of Birmingham. Parsons carried out extensive studies of the biochemical changes in coeliac disease over several years and was one of the first to measure ionised calcium in the blood. He concluded: "the bone deformities of coeliac infantilism are rachitic in nature…. The rickets is of the low calcium type which is the explanation of the frequent occurrence of tetany. The cause is to be found in deficient absorption of fat and therefore of vitamin D, calcium and phosphorus."[35]

Any doubt that tetany in chronic diarrhoea might result from deficiency of the parathyroids was finally dispelled by the work of two doctors at St. Bartholomew's Hospital. Geoffrey Linder (1892–1981) had been assistant physician at the Rockefeller Institute for Medical Research in New York. While there he came under the influence of D. D. van Slyke (1883–1971) with whom he did research of the biochemistry of patients with nephritis. Returning to England he met Charles Harris (1900–74) who had also been in the States with a Rockefeller fellowship at Johns Hopkins University Medical School. Supported by their professor, the legendary Francis Fraser (1885–1964), who was about to become the inspiration behind the new Postgraduate Medical School at Hammersmith, Linder and Harris studied three young women with steatorrhoea and tetany. The patients were in hospital for several months, during which calcium and phosphorous balances studies were carried out. One patient was studied continuously for five months and required re-admission the following year for further studies lasting four

---

†   Parsons' influence on paediatrics was founded on a solid experience of original research and his enthusiasm and pertinacity helped to give the subject appropriate status in Great Britain. He received a knighthood in 1946 and was elected FRS in 1948.

months. Their research showed unequivocally that tetany was due to hypocalcaemia resulting from malabsorption. The blood phosphorus was low and intramuscular parathormone was useless in relieving tetany. Fat restriction improved the steatorrhoea and calcium supplements raised the blood calcium slightly. Linder and Harris agreed with Parsons that fat-soluble vitamin D was being lost in the stool and found that water-soluble irradiated ergosterol had a dramatic effect on tetany and blood calcium. Their patients were studied consecutively from 1926 to 1928 and began a new era in metabolic medicine in this country.[36]

Afterwards, Linder's and Harris' paths diverged. Harris became the first physician to be in charge of a separate children's department at St. Bartholomew's and later Dean of the Medical School. His administrative skills led to his appointment as Vice-Chancellor of London University and a knighthood. Linder emigrated to South Africa where he started a diabetic clinic and continued his research. He was appointed first professor of chemical pathology at the university of Cape Town.

CHAPTER TWENTY-ONE

ANAEMIA

The anaemia of coeliac disease began to attract attention. In his Lumleian lectures, Still had noted that anaemia was common but usually mild. Only 3 of his 41 children were severely anaemic with a low colour index, suggesting iron deficiency.

As blood films began to be examined for the first time, hypochromic anaemia was found to be common in malnourished infants, an impression that was confirmed by a remarkable paediatrician Helen Mackay (1891–1965). Mackay became interested in the dietetic deficiencies of children while working with Clemens Pirquet (1874–1929) in Vienna where every child had rickets by the age of fifteen.[37] Pirquet thought the cause was infective akin to childhood tuberculosis. However, Mackay was able to prove that cod liver oil could prevent rickets by carrying out a clinical trial, "with the accuracy of a laboratory experiment" as Pirquet put it. Her success not only helped the children but was an excellent response to those who taunted Mellanby that "vitamins were the latest dietetic stunt". Returning home, she applied her skills to the study of anaemia and showed that nutritional deficiency was extremely common. Her work, carried out with meticulous attention to detail, was published by the Medical Research Council as a special report in 1931.[38] Mackay's contribution was recognised by the Royal College of Physicians when she was elected Fellow – the first woman to receive this honour.

Though iron deficiency was common in coeliac disease, people were also describing a megalocytic anaemia seemingly identical to Addisonian or pernicious anaemia. One of the first examples was presented by Sir Henry Tidy (1877–1960) to the Royal Society of Medicine in 1920 in a child thought to have renal dwarfism.[39] At the age of thirteen the boy was sent home from a public school said to be suffering from "pernicious anaemia". His haemoglobin was 45 per cent and many megalobasts were found in the blood, but he did not have proteinuria, so he may well have had coeliac disease rather than renal disease.

Another case of megalocytic anaemia was described by two medical students at Guy's Hospital, Arthur Hampson (1894–1972) and J. W. Shackle. The patient, a girl of sixteen, was also thought to have renal dwarfism but her blood urea was normal and albumin was not found in her urine. Hampson (1894–1972) while still a medical student, albeit a mature one with the Military Cross to his credit, went on to study the anaemia of sprue with Shackle. Together they published Price Jones curves, an index of red cell size popular at the time, from a number of patients with megalocytic anaemia, and highlighted just how difficult it was to distinguish Addisonian anaemia from the anaemia of idiopathic steatorrhoea or non-tropical sprue. To illustrate the point they quoted a case thought to have Addison's anaemia by Arthur Hurst and sprue by Carmichael Low. She was a lady aged 65 who had lived for many years in Barbados and gave a two-year history of fatty diarrhoea, buccal ulcers, weakness and weight loss. Investigations showed complete achlorrhydria, haemoglobin 62 per cent and many megalocytes in her blood film. Diplomatically the students did not take sides and her progress is not recorded.[40]

Pernicious anaemia was a universally fatal disease until the 1920s, when George Minot (1885–1950) in Boston decided to investigate the value of a diet rich in liver in patients with the condition. By 1926 he was able to report with his colleague William Murphy (1892–1936) that liver produced a striking remission in 45 patients, work which was to earn them the Nobel Prize.[41] Liver had to be given in huge amounts if swallowed, but extract of liver could be prepared for intramuscular injection.

At about this time a doctor working in the department of chemical pathology at the Royal Free Hospital, Lucy Wills (1888–1964), was invited to investigate "pernicious anaemia of pregnancy" prevalent among the poor in Bombay. She soon realised that this "tropical macrocytic anaemia" as she preferred to call it, was a distinct disease frequently associated with pregnancy and often complicated by malaria, hook worm disease or sprue. Liver injections were effective but she was working under difficult conditions. Her patients were uneducated, very frightened and suspicious. They were unwilling to stay in hospital; "if a woman could crawl", Wills wrote, "she must attend to her home duties". So they would not stay in hospital and treatment with liver, even if acceptable, was too expensive. Wills examined their diets and noted that the women did not eat vegetables. At first she thought they might be lacking vitamin A or C but treatment was a failure. In a series of experiments she found that rats fed on the women's diet became anaemic. If this was nutritional could it be due to a deficiency of vitamin B? She gave the rats a yeast extract, a potent source of vitamin B, and they recovered.[42]

Experiments with patients followed and Wills chose Marmite, a yeast extract, as the most suitable preparation. The extract was supplied by the Marmite Food Extract Company and a sample was tested by Dr. Harriet Chick of the Lister Institute who found it was rich in vitamin B_1 and B_2. The response to Marmite was "amazing" and Wills recommended its use routinely to prevent the macrocytic anaemia of pregnancy. She realised that it was not B_1 or B_2 that was curative and the "Wills factor" became a household name in medicine until the discovery of folic acid in 1945. The anaemia was known as "Wills anaemia" for a time, and shortly after her discovery, Stanley Davidson in Aberdeen published two cases of true pernicious anaemia confirming that liver, and only liver as opposed to Marmite, was beneficial in this disease.[43]

Haematology was still in its infancy in this country when one of the pioneers in the use of liver extracts, Janet Vaughan (1899–1993), was working with Minot in his laboratory in Boston. The recipient of a Rockefeller fellowship, she was inspired by the exciting discoveries of Minot and Murphy and their assistant William Castle (1897–1990), who discovered intrinsic factor, and she often prepared extracts of liver at home by herself.

On her return to England she was one of the first people to examine the morphology of the red cell in detail, carefully measuring the size and shape of cells in anaemia. Now the holder of a Beit Memorial Fellowship, she met Donald Hunter (1898–1978), physician to the London Hospital who later became well know for his work on occupational disease. At the time Hunter was interested in disorders of calcium metabolism and the parathyroid glands. He had several patients with steatorrhoea and was collaborating in a study of the condition with Izod Bennett at the Middlesex Hospital, who also had some cases. Bennett (1887–1946) was a distinguished gastroenterologist, the author of numerous books and papers, notably *The Stomach and Upper Alimentary Canal in Health and Disease*, and a future founder member of the British Society of Gastroenterology.

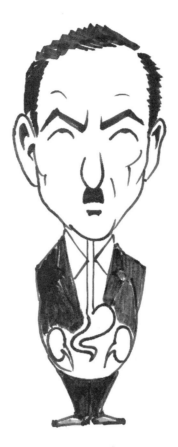

25 Bennett – Mordant wit.

Hunter and Bennett asked Janet Vaughan to classify the anaemia in their group of fifteen patients. Several were iron deficient and responded to massive doses of iron, and two patients had a megalocytic anaemia. Both had free hydrochloric acid in their stomachs and Vaughan realised that they were similar to the cases of nutritional anaemia described by Lucy Wills. As they were not starving they must for some reason be unable to absorb vitamin B. Vaughan gave them Marmite, which she knew contained all the constituents of the vitamin B complex, and they responded immediately.[44] This was good news for them and even better news for the manufacturers of marmite.† It is easy to see why coeliac disease was once thought to be a deficiency disease. Apart from the severe cases who died from starvation, many patients only had a selective deficiency of iron, vitamin B or vitamin D. It was this that brought them to the attention of the nutritionists, Helen Mackay and Lucy Wills, and the haematologist Janet Vaughan, who probably regarded their contribution to the understanding of coeliac disease as trivial in comparison with their other achievements. These women were outstanding examples of the small band of women doctors in a world dominated by men.

All were born into privileged families; Helen and Lucy were both educated at Cheltenham College for Young Ladies while Janet Vaughan, whose father was headmaster of Rugby School, received her education at home. They were exceptionally intelligent and this combination of brains and private means was essential for a girl wishing to pursue a career in medicine. They were also highly motivated; Lucy Wills obtained a double first honours degree in botany and geology at Cambridge after which she became deeply interested in the work of Freud and enrolled as a student at the London School of Medicine for Women, with a view to a career in psychiatry. Helen Mackay also qualified at the London School for Women (later the Royal Free Hospital Medical School), which was the only medical school available to women in England at the time. Within three years of qualification in 1914 she had written her MD and passed the MRCP. Janet Vaughan, after a struggle, managed to get admitted to Somerville College, Oxford, where she obtained a first class degree in physiology. She had a keen interest in politics so she turned to medicine in the belief that a career in medicine would best enable her to fight social injustice and poverty. Lucy Wills, who gave her name to a vitamin and a disease, was a legend in her own lifetime. Her only qualification was MBBS, and apart from several trips to India in the 1920s, she stayed in the Pathology Department at the Royal Free Hospital all her life. Naturally aristocratic, she was anti-establishment and

---

†   Marmite was introduced in 1902 and was originally sold in small earthenware pots – hence the name which comes from the French. It should be pronounced marmeet which the makers hoped would give the impression that it contained meat but this never caught on with the English who are not celebrated for their French pronunciation. The discovery that it was a rich source of vitamin B did wonders for its sales a few years later.

critical of the conservative scientific and medical committees on which she served. This may explain why greater honours did not come her way. Helen Mackay became a paediatrician in the East End of London where her clinical work and her research were always complementary. Her clinics were full of infants and children with nutritional disorders, which stimulated her to conduct surveys of the problems and how to prevent them. Her special MRC reports brought her worldwide recognition and many honours and changed the whole pattern of infant feeding. However, neither Lucy nor Helen achieved as much in their lives as Janet Vaughan. After a successful early career in haematology at the Post Graduate Medical School, Hammersmith, she organised the blood transfusion service in London during the war. Afterwards she left London and haematology to become Principal of her old college, Somerville, Oxford. She became interested in the problems of nuclear energy, for both civil and military purposes, directing an MRC unit for research on bone-seeking isotopes. Eventually she was regarded as a world authority on plutonium. At Oxford she promoted the cause of Science in the university and worked indefatigably on behalf of her college. She had the ability to get things done, which earned her the title of "the Active Principal (or Principle?)". Honoured as a Dame of the British Empire in 1957, she was one of six women who were featured in the BBC series *Women of Our Century*. She was married with two children and died aged 93.

CHAPTER TWENTY-TWO

A CONTINUING ENIGMA, TROPICAL AND NON-TROPICAL SPRUE AND COELIAC DISEASE

Apart from anaemia, Bennett and Hunter looked at the clinical aspects of their patients in detail, especially the tetany and deformities of osteomalacia caused by calcium deficiency, and concluded that the catastrophic effects of idiopathic steatorrhoea were simply due to malabsorption of essential nutrients. "Starvation in the midst of plenty" as they called it.[45] They showed that a low fat intake controlled the steatorrhoea, that calcium supplements and ergosterol relieved tetany and to some extent the pain of osteomalacia, and that iron and Marmite as we have seen could alleviate the anaemia. But one can sense their feeling of frustration that they could not pinpoint the underlying pathology. A careful history often traced the illness back to infancy or childhood, so they believed that idiopathic steatorrhoea or non-tropical sprue was the adult form of coeliac disease. In contrast, tropical sprue, despite the similarities, was a different disease, which almost invariably began in adults while living abroad. Their view was vigorously opposed by many at the time, notably a Danish authority Hess Thaysen (1883–1944) from Copenhagen, who was convinced that the three conditions were all one and the same disease, which he preferred to call idiopathic steatorrhoea.[46] In this he was supported by Arthur Hurst (1879–1944) who as late as 1942 wrote "tropical sprue, non tropical sprue and coeliac disease are varients of the same disorder – the sprue syndrome – which differs only in the part of the world in which the disorder originated and in the age of the patient".[47] To illustrate his point he described a severe case of sprue syndrome.

Christoper R, aged eight (not the Christopher Robin who was born three years later) was sent to him as a case of coeliac disease in 1925. He was born in Penang and became ill with offensive diarrhoea on board ship on his way home aged two. Within two years he was emaciated and unable to stand. His father, who was living in Malaya and was not a doctor, read Still's *Diseases of Children* and came to the conclusion that the boy had coeliac disease. This was confirmed by Sir Frederic Still in 1924, by which time he was having severe attacks of tetany about twice a week. One attack lasted eighteen hours, during which he suffered agony and his hands became oedematous. When Hurst first met him he weighed two stone, five and three-quarter pounds and his height was only three foot four inches. His abdomen was greatly distended and he had frequent attacks of abdominal pain. He passed three or four bulky unformed stools a day. The dried faeces contained a great excess of fat, almost entirely in the form of fatty acids and soaps (i.e. digested fat). He was anaemic (haemoglobin 50 per cent) and X-rays showed that both small and large intestines contained excess of gas. He was given a fat-free diet, iron and calcium. From this moment he improved "at an amazing pace". Three months after admission he was able to walk upstairs. The haemoglobin percentage was 90, and there had been no further attacks of tetany. A year later his mother wrote that he had been able to enjoy a life of full activity, but he had to continue his strict fat free diet for another eight years. In 1940, at the age of 23, he passed A1 for a commission in the Royal Air Force. Hurst comments, "This case shows very well the advantage of the designation 'sprue syndrome' over sprue, non tropical sprue and coeliac disease, as it might have been diagnosed as 'tropical sprue occurring in a child' and coeliac disease originating in the tropics with equal propriety."[48] Personally I think he had coeliac disease and was lucky to respond so well to treatment. I like to think he lived long enough to enjoy the benefits of a gluten-free diet in his later years.

The inability to explain coeliac disease gave rise to some curious notions. No sooner had Scott's theory of the exhausted parathyroids been discredited than adrenal insufficiency was fancied. Thaysen in Copenhagen suggested that a failure to absorb the vitamin B complex depressed suprarenal function causing intestinal asthenia. This rather nebulous concept reflected Thaysen's problem; he was convinced that the intestinal wall of sprue patients was histologically normal. Unfortunately his problem became everyone else's because his writings, notably his monograph, *Non-tropical Sprue: a Study of Idiopathic Steatorrhoea* (1932) dominated medical thought at the time.[49]

Vitamin B was certainly helpful in the treatment of coeliac disease but his theory did not explain how deficiency of the B vitamins occurred in the first place, quite apart from their supposed effect on the adrenal glands. Nonetheless many people still thought of steatorrhoea as a deficiency disease.

More convincing was the work of Frigyes Verzar, a physiologist in Switzerland who had spent many decades studying absorption in dogs. In 1936 he published a book *Absorption From the Intestine* in which he described experiments showing that adrenalectomy depressed absorption of triglycerides.[50] From this he concluded that coeliac disease was caused by adrenal insufficiency. In fact there was no clinical support for his suggestion; patients with Addison's disease do not have steatorrhoea.

Verzar thought that intestinal absorption could be explained simply on the basis of osmosis and diffusion and that it was not an active process. His book was influential and shaped the thinking of physiologists for the next decade. Arthur Hurst was impressed by it. Verzar had shown that the movement of intestinal villi depended upon stimulation of Meissner's (submucosal) nerve plexus. In his view fat droplets in the villi were propelled by a pumping action into the lymphatic channels. Hurst seized on this theory to propose that paralysis of the mucous membrane, in the villi would prevent the absorption of fat. He was aware of the recent X-ray changes described in steatorrhoea in which the normal markings of the valvulae conniventes were often absent. Paralysis of the main layer of the mucous membrane, he surmised, would prevent the pumping action of the villi and would explain the flattening or disappearance of the valvulae conniventes. Conveniently such a paralysis would not alter the microscopic appearances of the mucous membrane, which Hurst assumed was normal. Hurst's difficulty was that he could not explain why Meissner's plexus should fail to function in the first place. "Could it be an absence of the unknown constituent of the chyme which stimulates the plexus," he wondered, "or the effect of vitamin deficiency or some specific of non specific toxaemia on the plexus itself?"

Everyone was struggling to explain the cause of coeliac disease, and I have sympathy for Izod Bennett who adopted a rather pragmatic approach to the problem. With disarming candour he suggested that until the cause was known the syndrome should be called chronic jejuno-ileal insufficiency. This would indicate the gross disturbance of function without attempting to explain it, rather in the way that terms such as pancreatic insufficiency or renal insufficiency were used.[51]

CHAPTER TWENTY-THREE

FAT ABSORPTION

In this country after the Second World War probably no one knew more about fat transport than Alastair Frazer (1909–69). "Fats" Frazer as he was known was a big man with tremendous energy and an all-embracing geniality. He was appointed Professor in Pharmacology and Medical Biochemistry at Birmingham in 1942 where he built up a large department and became particularly interested in the mechanisms of fat absorption. He put forward the partition hypothesis to explain the two ways in which fat was absorbed; first and most importantly as triglyceride particles into the lymphatic system, but also as fatty acids via the portal venous system. In his view the sprue syndrome was essentially a defect of fat absorption, which he realised was due to a block in the absorption of triglycerides by the mucosa. Absorption of fatty acids took over, resulting in a switch from the particulate absorption of triglycerides to the less efficient molecular absorption of fatty acids. Believing like everyone else that the mucosa was anatomically normal Frazer pondered long and hard about the basic fault and gradually came to the conclusion that it was mechanical due to the excessive secretion of mucus by the intestine.[52]

His evidence was based on radiological studies and in this he was assisted by Jim French (1911–90). French had been fascinated by the aetiology of sprue while serving with the Indian Medical Service during the war and joined Frazer as a research fellow in 1947. A likeable and modest man with a ready sense of humour French was a hands-on research worker and was often to be seen carrying cans of faeces about the hospital corridors.

For several years patients with nutritional deficiencies including many with steatorrhoea had been observed to have an abnormal X-ray

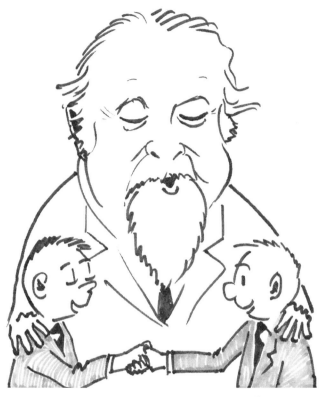

26 Frazer – all-embracing geniality.

appearance of the small intestine on barium follow-through examination. Instead of showing the normal feathery appearance, the barium became clumped and the valvulae conniventes smooth, an appearance known as the "deficiency pattern". As this was also seen in normal infants and occasionally in normal adults it was thought to have little diagnostic value, but Frazer was intrigued and decided to reinvestigate the phenomenon. With French he persuaded student volunteers to swallow gastric and duodenal tubes simultaneously, poured in barium and as expected obtained pictures of the normal feathery pattern. Next various substances including hydrolysed fats and even faecal fat recovered from cases of sprue were added. Clumping and segmentation of the barium occurred proving that the so-called deficiency pattern was simply a response to fat and not caused by nutritional deficiencies as had been thought.[53]

Frazer and French went on to show that the main reason for segmentation and clumping was flocculation of the barium by mucus secretion, and that fatty acids seemed to aggravate this secretion. When they used a complex gelo-colloid preparation of barium that did not flocculate they were able to show an apparently normal but dilated and rather sluggish intestine in infants with coeliac disease.[54] So they concluded that malabsorption might be due to excessive mucus secretion or a lack of intestinal motility or to both. But why should mucus block fat absorption and what was it doing there in the first place?

CHAPTER TWENTY-FOUR

CHRONIC JEJUNITIS

One man who thought he knew was a physician in Ipswich, Dr. John Paulley (1918–2007). For some time Paulley had been convinced that the small intestine was inflamed in patients with coeliac disease but he had difficulty in persuading anyone to agree with him. For years people had accepted Thaysen's opinion that all morbid changes in the jejunum of these patients were due to post mortem autolysis. In their view the small bowel was histologically normal in coeliac disease. Another problem for Paulley was his belief that idiopathic steatorrhoea was usually, if not always, a psychosomatic disorder. Most people found this impossible to accept and regarded Paulley as an eccentric provincial. But Paulley was his own man, a giant of six-foot-seven inches, sporting a monocle, who drew strength from his own convictions and would not be deterred no matter how unconventional his ideas might seem to others.

These ideas originated during the Second World War when he was looking after patients with sprue who had been evacuated from India and Burma. He wrote in 1945, "The sprue patient's intestine (prior to his disease) appears to react more violently in the face of infection than that of his more placid companion".[55] Encouraged by how often he could anticipate the development of post-dysenteric bowel looseness in introspective and asthenic individuals, Paulley undertook a large survey of patients with ulcerative colitis after the war and found that all of them had morbid personalities.[56] Next he looked at patients with Crohn's Disease of the ileum and found that they too had the same personality traits.[57] He then argued that if the duodenum (peptic ulcer), colon and ileum were all sites of psychosomatic disease, surely it was illogical to exclude the jejunum. "Was not the gut," he asked, "embryologically and physiologically a tube with much of its blood and nerve supply in

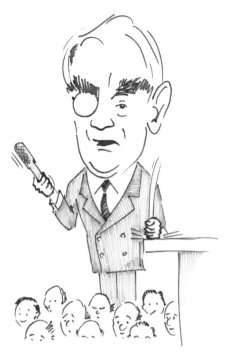

27 Paulley – Speaking at a meeting to ensure publication.

common? Would not the same changes in vascularity, secretion and motility observed in the colon and stomach in response to emotion, also affect the small intestine?" Sure enough a study of ten patients with steatorrhoea revealed the same immaturity and dependence that he had noted in ulcerative colitis.[58] Admittedly it was difficult to explain the disease when it began in infancy but older patients could always be traced back to childhood restriction and parental possessiveness. In support of his theory he later recalled the remarkable case of a boy of fifteen months with coeliac disease who remitted without a gluten-free diet following psychological intervention in 1950.[59] (Appendix 2.)

So with colitis and ileitis in mind, Paulley came to the conclusion that some form of chronic jejunitis could be causing idiopathic steatorrhoea and coeliac disease. He drew support from the radiographic changes recently described in the small bowel and was particularly interested by French's discovery that "clumping" was due to flocculation of the barium by mucus. This was consistent with his theory of a low-grade chronic inflammation or irritation of the small intestine.

He was also aware of the early reports, notably by Manson-Bahr describing villous atrophy and round-cell infiltration of the mucosa in patients with sprue,[60] and sceptical of Thaysens monograph (1932) in which these findings were dismissed as the result of post mortem autolysis. Thaysen reported only two post mortems of his own (one of sprue and one non-tropical sprue) and Paulley thought his conclusions were unsound. "Mucosal changes in the steatorrhoeas may well be more apparent in life than after death," he prophesied.[61]

The next step was to test his jejunitis hypothesis by obtaining biopsy material from a living patient. This would not be easy as he would have to persuade a surgeon to take a jejunal biopsy during a laparotomy – a rare procedure in patients with idiopathic steatorrhoea.

The first patient was a man aged 56 under the care of Dr. Marriott (1900–83)[†] at the Middlesex Hospital where Paulley was first assistant. He clearly had steatorrhoea but malignancy was suspected and a laparotomy performed. Paulley was present and saw the dilated and thickened jejunum. The surgeon was unwilling to take a biopsy from it but did agree to remove one of the enlarged lymph nodes from the jejunal mesentery. Histological examination showed chronic inflammatory changes with much destruction by fibrosis.

Paulley had to wait over two years before his next opportunity arose, by which time he had taken up his appointment as Consultant Physician at Ipswich. The patient was a man aged 39 with severe steatorrhoea who needed a laparotomy for suspected intestinal obstruction. In fact obstruction was not found but the whole of the gut appeared "wet" and glistening with an oedematous mesentery and many enlarged lymph nodes. A wedge biopsy of the jejunum showed broad villi packed with plasma cells and eosinophils. The histologist called it "an extreme form of sinus catarrh".

Paulley felt he had proved his point but the journals disagreed. Both the *Lancet* and *Gastroenterology* rejected his findings though he was told that Chester Jones, editor of the *New England Journal of Medicine*, wanted to publish but his assessors disagreed. Undaunted Paulley presented his cases to the British Society of Gastroenterology meeting in Leeds in 1951 during a discussion of Frazer's work on the cause of the Sprue

---

[†]   Hugh Marriott was the only British physician, other than McCance, to work on salt and water metabolism during the 1940s and 1950s, and wrote some splendid articles in the *Brit. Med. J.* and *Lancet.*

syndrome. His comments attracted little attention but the transactions were at least published.[62] This was a decade before the publication of the journal *Gut* when proceedings of the British Society of Gastroenterology appeared in *Gastroenterologia*.

The following year he obtained biopsies from two more cases, which he compared with biopsies from normal jejunum taken from a patient having a partial gastrectomy. This time he spoke at a meeting of the Royal Society of Tropical Medicine and Hygiene, the transactions of which he knew would be published.[63] He emphasised how few pathologists had had the opportunity to study normal human jejunum, and how they should take every opportunity to do so. He also suggested that the excess of mucus seen by Frazer and French in the jejunum was a response to the inflammation he had described akin to that seen in colitis.

Paulley now had four cases of jejunitis from patients with steatorrhoea and, crucially, photomicrographs from two of them, which could be compared to a normal subject. This was enough finally to persuade the *Brit. Med. J.* to publish his work. His paper "Observations on the aetiology of idiopathic steatorrhoea" was a seminal work and a triumph for Paulley himself, whose self-belief was thoroughly vindicated.[64] Though his theory on the cause of coeliac disease may have been misconceived his ability to think for himself and to act on his conviction completely changed medical opinion about malabsorption. In his publication reference to the psychosomatic nature of idiopathic steatorrhoea was restrained, perhaps because Paulley knew his views were controversial but also because by this time dramatic advances in the treatment of coeliac disease had occurred.

CHAPTER TWENTY-FIVE

GLUTEN

For decades speculation about the cause of coeliac disease was matched only by ideas on how to treat it. Confusion reigned as virtually every form of diet was tried. Early on Fanconi in Italy recommended a fruit and vegetable diet, others favoured an exclusive milk diet and yet others preferred the "beef steak cure". Many believed that the disease was a deficiency disorder requiring vitamin supplements alone. Most agreed that fat intake should be limited to reduce the severity of the steatorrhoea. From the start carbohydrates were thought to be poorly absorbed and gradually starches became the focus of attention. During the 1920s and 30s an American, Sidney Haas, believed that all starches except bananas were harmful and should be avoided. He claimed that his "banana diet" was a specific cure that would prevent the notorious and often fatal relapses of coeliac disease.[65] During the Second World War coeliac children in the UK were permitted a special allowance of bananas at a time when supplies were exceedingly difficult to obtain. Though over-optimistic, his diet was moderately successful because starches include cereals such as bread. His ideas were later supported by Dorothy Andersen (1901–63), a paediatrician in New York, who had made her name by distinguishing fibrocystic disease of the pancreas from the coeliac syndrome in 1942. Andersen agreed that starch intolerance was the key feature in coeliac disease after she found that amylase was usually absent from the duodenal juice.[66]

In this country the starch hypothesis was championed by one of our leading paediatricians, Sir Wilfrid Sheldon (1901–83). Sheldon qualified at King's College Hospital and was appointed Assistant Physician to the children's department when he was only 26 years old. There he worked with Frederic Still, who probably inspired his interest in coeliac disease.

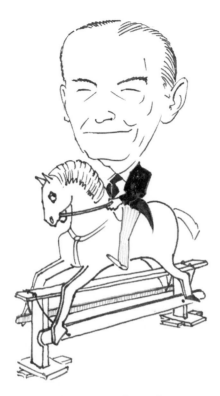

28 Sheldon – Royal paediatrician.

Sheldon's views about starch intolerance were based on astute clinical observation: (1) coeliac disease usually begins between six months and two or three years of age, whereas before this, at a time when their diet consists of milk, the children who eventually develop the disorder show no indication of what is to come. (2) The principal dietetic change coinciding with coeliac symptoms consists of a steadily increasing intake of starches. (3) Abdominal distension is due to fermentation of carbohydrates. Sheldon confirmed this impression by experiments on fifteen coeliac children showing that fat absorption improved when starch was removed from the diet. The children managed to tolerate a virtually normal fat intake, gained weight and felt and behaved better.[67] Sheldon must have felt he was close to solving the riddle of coeliac disease and indeed he was. At the very time of these experiments, a Dutch paediatrician in the Hague began work on his doctoral thesis, which was to prove that wheat flour was the toxic agent, not starch.

The story of how Karel Dicke (1905–62) discovered the beneficial effect of a wheat-free diet is well known but it was such an achievement that no chapter on coeliac disease would be complete without it. According to G. P. Van Bere-Henegouwen and C. J. J. Mulder, "Dicke's attention was caught by a case report presented in 1932 by two paediatricians, Dusseldorp and Stheeman, concerning relapses of diarrhoea that had been preceded by consumption of bread or rusks."[68] However, Sir Christopher Booth who met Dicke later wrote "He was quite clear in his conversation with me that it was a young mother's statement that her coeliac child's rash improved if she removed bread from the diet that first alerted his interest."[69] That was in 1936, and the same year Dicke began a meticulous study lasting two years at the Juliana Children's Hospital in a boy with coeliac disease. A wheat-free diet had a favourable effect on his clinical symptoms, weight and growth.

In 1941 Dicke wrote, "In recent literature it is stated that the diets of Haas (bananas) and Fanconi (fruit and vegetables) give the best results in the treatment of patients with this syndrome. At present (World War II) these items are not available therefore I give a simple diet, which is helping these children at this time of rationing. The diet should not contain any bread or rusks. A hot meal twice a day is also well tolerated. The third meal can be sweet or sour porridge (without any wheat flour)."[70]

So Dicke was convinced by the beginning of the war that the staple food of Western man, wheat, was toxic. He preached this to every physician who was willing to listen to him, but nobody believed him. Laboratory proof was needed. His opportunity came in 1948 when his colleague, Professor Ten Bokkel Hunink, introduced him to Dr. van Eekelen, then Director of the Central Institute for Nutritional and Food Research in Utrecht. "Van Eekelen, this is my colleague Dicke, the man who is convinced that your good old wheat is deleterious to our little coeliacs. But two young chaps here, one working at your institute, the other in my department, both are extremely good at determining fat in faeces. I feel sure that these two boys will be able to prove within some months, Dicke, that your fantastic ideas are wrong."[71]

The two "boys" were a biochemist J. H. van de Kamer and a paediatrician H. A. Weijers who had developed an accurate and easy way to measure fat in the faeces. The next day they began to investigate Dicke's idea. The meticulous experiments were done with standardised diets over several months in just five children. Each was challenged with different cereals in turn under an exact protocol during which faecal fats were measured and the so-called fat absorption coefficient was calculated. To van de Kamer's surprise they showed that wheat did indeed have an adverse effect on the children, just as Dicke had forecast. Wheat flour but not wheat starch cause anorexia, diarrhoea and steatorrhoea. Potatoes, maize and rice were absolutely harmless, and they had indisputable data to convince the sceptics.[72]

Unfortunately Dicke[73] and Weijers[74] both published the results in Dutch as the subject of their doctoral theses – not easy to obtain, let alone translate. However, about this time James Smellie (1893–1961), Professor of Paediatrics in Birmingham, was about to collaborate with Frazer and French in a study of children with coeliac disease to see if they had the same alteration in gastrointestinal function as adults with idiopathic steatorrhoea. This was of course before jejunal biopsy was available when the diagnosis was made clinically, aided by extensive biochemical tests and small bowel radiography. By this time Frazer had adopted the simpler Dutch method of measuring faecal fat and knew van de Kamer well.[75] In the light of Dicke's work and with his blessing, the study was extended to look at the effect of wheat on these children. The work was co-ordinated by Charlotte Anderson (1915–2002), a young research fellow from Melbourne who was later to succeed Douglas Hubble to the Chair of Paediatrics. As anticipated they showed that coeliac children had a generalised absorption defect similar to that seen in adults. Exclusion of wheat reversed all the defects, confirming Dicke's work and showing that coeliac disease was at last curable.[76]

CHAPTER TWENTY-SIX

"ADULT COELIAC DISEASE"

Izod Bennett's belief that idiopathic steatorrhoea was the adult form of coeliac disease was slow to catch on because most people thought that coeliac disease cleared up at about the age of twelve. For example just before the Second World War Christopher Hardwick (1911–2008), Outpatient Registrar at Great Ormond Street, looked at the progress of 73 children with coeliac disease. This was well before the gluten-free era and 30 per cent of the children died in hospital. The survivors did well and appeared to recover completely, though they were in hospital for months or even years. Four did relapse and Hardwick found that they still had steatorrhoea, so he suggested that coeliac disease could lie dormant and occasionally resurface in adult life as idiopathic steatorrhoea.[77]

Later Wilfrid Sheldon wrote that "by 7 or 8 years of age most cases... have recovered, a few drag on to puberty, and there have been instances recorded in adult life".[78] In fact most clinicians were only vaguely aware of idiopathic steatorrhoea; the patients had non-specific symptoms and the diagnosis was usually overlooked. An attempt to estimate the incidence of "sprue syndrome" by Stanley Davidson (1894–1981) in 1950 illustrates this. He made use of the fact that during the Second World War all people with steatorrhoea were entitled to priority rations. The diagnosis had to be ratified by a special diets advisory committee who reported to the Ministry of Food if a grant of extra rations was justified. The data were carefully recorded and Davidson obtained the figures and calculated that the average incidence was 44 cases per year in England and Wales or 1 per 700,000 of the population over fifteen years of age. He believed his estimate was a true reflection of the incidence even though he only managed to collect 1,614 cases in six years. He also sent a questionnaire to the doctors of 100 of these patients and from their replies deduced that 34 per cent had probably had coeliac disease in childhood.[79]

The diagnosis of patients with chronic diarrhoea was imprecise. Patients with inflammatory bowel disease, spastic colon and steatorrhoea were easily confused as indeed they are today. Rigid sigmoidoscopy was done by surgeons looking for cancer, single contrast barium enemas were inaccurate and performed by general radiologists, and faecal fat estimation was never popular with the laboratory.

It was only in centres such as Birmingham where Alastair Frazer was well known for his work on fat absorption that a sizeable number of patients with steatorrhoea could be found; so when two young physicians, Trevor Cooke (1911–87) and Clifford Hawkins (1915–91), who had worked with Frazer, emphasised that idiopathic steatorrhoea was not rare and could be easily recognised if one was alert to it, they were able to select 100 patients from a series of more than 300 with some form of steatorrhoea.[80]

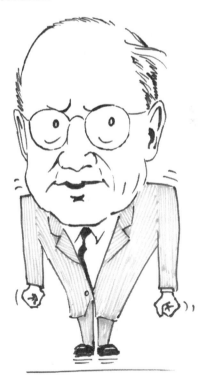

29 Cooke – Fiery temper.

Though steatorrhoea was the *sine qua non* for the diagnosis, over half of their patients did not complain of diarrhoea unless carefully questioned. Indeed up to twenty per cent regarded themselves as constipated. So what led them to suspect the diagnosis in patients without diarrhoea? First a high index of suspicion in any patient complaining of constitutional disturbances such as lassitude, weight loss, glossitis and symptoms of anaemia. Next the general appearance of a rather short, pale, fair haired, sometimes oedematous patient with a desquamating rash was helpful. Then a blood count nearly always showed macrocytosis or anaemia of some kind. Indeed a persistently normal blood picture was strong evidence against the diagnosis. Finally an abnormal X-ray of the small bowel showing a "deficiency" pattern was always found. If this collection of symptoms and signs was present, fat balance tests were essential whatever the errors in collection or estimation of stool fat. During this study Cooke and Hawkins noted that 43 per cent of their patients had a history of severe diarrhoea, anaemia, "tuberculous peritonitis" or "consumptive bowels" in childhood, which was enough to convince them that coeliac disease and idiopathic steatorrhoea were one and the same condition, and Cooke later introduced the term adult coeliac disease.

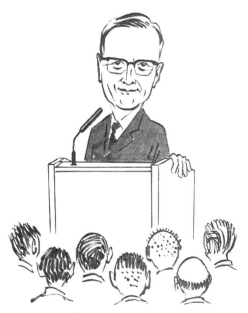

30 Hawkins – Born communicator.

Despite their common interests and research together, Cooke and Hawkins were no more alike than chalk and cheese. Clifford Hawkins was an urbane and sociable man who excelled at speaking and writing in medicine; indeed he wrote a book on the subject. Beneath the veneer, however, lay remarkable drive and energy and later he worked closely with his friend and colleague Jim French (1911–90), who became Reader in Medicine when Cooke resigned in 1955.

Trevor Cooke was a dedicated gastroenterolgoist who later became President of the BSG. But he was a shy and sensitive man who seemed to cultivate anger and impatience to overcome what he thought were the shortsighted views of others. When he failed to get the Chair of Medicine he resigned as Reader and moved to the General Hospital in Birmingham. Many predicted the end of his career but they were wrong. Over the next twenty years he built up a gastroenterology unit of international repute.

After Cooke left Queen Elizabeth Hospital, French and Hawkins decided that if coeliac disease and idiopathic steatorrhoea were the same disease, surely adults, especially those with a childhood history, should respond to a gluten-free diet like the children? At the time a few cases had been treated rather briefly with disappointing results. So drawing once more on the resources available in Birmingham they looked at 22 patients with idiopathic steatorrhoea who were carefully selected according to the usual strict criteria. Each patient was persuaded to avoid gluten and their response was monitored by daily faecal fat measurement, in some cases for six months. Nearly all of them responded satisfactorily though some took several months to achieve normal fat absorption. A few relapsed when challenged with wheat only to improve when gluten was again withdrawn. This painstaking study convinced them that gluten caused idiopathic steatorrhoea, analogous to coeliac disease. French and Hawkins also noticed a dramatic improvement in those patients who were underweight and worn out but who had minimal steatorrhoea. It seemed that steatorrhoea could be a late sign of malabsorption, occurring long after the small intestine had been damaged. This could explain why adults took much longer to respond to treatment than children, reflecting years of damage to the intestine.[81]

CHAPTER TWENTY-SEVEN

SMALL BOWEL BIOPSY

Despite Paulley's discovery that idiopathic steatorrhoea was associated with inflammation of the jejunum, laparotomy was scarcely feasible in every adult suspected of the disease, let alone children. Yet the diagnosis and response to treatment was inexact and relied on time-consuming and tedious tests – difficult enough in adults let alone a miserable infant or a fractious child. A simpler way to obtain tissue was needed, and it came with the timely arrival of the tube biopsy technique pioneered by Margot Shiner (1923–98).

Shiner was born in Berlin in 1923. The family were Jewish and fled to London in 1938. She qualified in Leeds and was Senior House Officer at Great Ormond Street, after which she decided to pursue a career in research. She managed to obtain an honorary appointment at the Royal Postgraduate Medical School, Hammersmith Hospital, working in Sheila Sherlock's (1920–2001) department. At the time Selwyn Baker, an Australian postgraduate, was working with David Mollin (1917–89), a dynamic haematologist with a particular interest in the megaloblastic anaemias. Mollin knew of a patient with pernicious anaemia who had normal gastric acidity and Baker suggested that a gastric biopsy might help to elucidate the problem. Baker was aware that Sir Ian Wood (1903–86), Head of Clinical Research in Melbourne, had pioneered a suction biopsy technique with a guillotine cutting device, which provided a full thickness specimen of gastric mucosa.[82] Baker encouraged Shiner to learn the technique, which clearly had research potential. Shiner soon became familiar with the instrument and before long had obtained more than 100 gastric biopsies. It was then that she took the innovative step to extend the technique beyond the pylorus to sample duodenal and even jejunal mucosa. Initially she thought this would be helpful in the diagnosis of conditions such as steatorrhoea, Crohn's Disease, duodenitis or X-ray negative dyspepsia. But not in her wildest dreams did she foresee the impact it would have on coeliac disease and research into the small intestine.

Enlisting the help of a technician from the genito-urinary manufacturing company, she constructed a longer version of Wood's tube and eschewing animal experiments managed to obtain duodenal biopsies from twelve patients with dyspepsia or peptic ulcer.[83] She had several failures initially because it was difficult to manoeuvre the tube into the duodenum[†] and frequently the suction device failed to obtain a specimen. Nonetheless, she was sufficiently encouraged by her results to modify the tube by adding a balloon to the headpiece, which encouraged peristalsis to guide it into the jejunum.[84] This worked well and she soon had biopsies from the jejunum of fifteen patients.[85] Recognising the potential of her technique Francis Avery Jones (1910–98) invited her to join his new department at the Central Middlesex Hospital, where she became a full-time member of the MRC unit. Her success was beginning to attract attention, particularly from those interested in steatorrhoea. Within eighteen months of joining Avery Jones, she had taken biopsies from 65 patients with steatorrhoea of all sorts sent to her from physicians at the Central Middlesex and Hammersmith Hospitals and from Trevor Cooke in Birmingham. Only 22 of these original 65 patients had classical idiopathic steatorrhoea, which indicates how uncommon the diagnosis was in the late 1950s.[86]

From the start Margot Shiner worked closely with her friend and colleague, Israel Doniach (1911–2001), a pathologist at the Postgraduate Medical School, Hammersmith and later Professor of Pathology at the London Hospital. "Sonny" Doniach as he was known examined all Shiner's biopsies in meticulous detail, including dozens of control cases, and described the morphological changes of idiopathic steatorrhoea that are used today.[87] With the zeal of a stamp collector chasing a philatelic rarity he measured the height and width of the villi with a calibrated micrometer, observed the degree of cellular infiltration and thickness of the submucosa and counted the number of mitoses in the young

---

†   Here she was helped by a remarkable lady called Miss Winnie Wernli, who was employed to keep the place clean and tidy but also provided technical help when necessary. She had a remarkable knack of persuading the tube to pass through the pylorus, using appropriate pressure on the patients' abdomen.

epithelial cells in the crypts. Most of the patients had what he described as subtotal villous atrophy with stumpy villi too small to measure. The submucosa was thickened by glandular hyperplasia and invaded by lymphocytes. He thought that the epithelial cells on the surface of the villi originated from the crypts of Lieberkuhn and ascended like the steps of a moving staircase to be cast off from the villous tips – a process that took about two days. Cell production had to keep up with cell loss and as he found an increased mitotic rate in the crypts, he assumed this was an attempt to compensate for the reduced lifespan or viability of the mature enterocytes. He likened the situation to that seen in haemolytic anaemia.

He thought the changes were irreversible because some of the patients had been on a gluten-free diet for as long as three and a half years, though he acknowledged that French had proved the clinical benefit of gluten withdrawal.

The significance of Shiner and Doniach's work cannot be over-emphasised. For the first time samples of the jejunum could be obtained without the need for a laparotomy, something that was to transform the study of the small intestine in the years to come. At first few doctors were in a position to take advantage of the technique. Gastroenterology was undertaken by general physicians and though the BSG was then twenty years old it was still a cosy little club restricted to 65 members. With the exception of Trevor Cooke in Birmingham and some paediatricians, only a few clinicians who were studying anaemia showed any interest.

Trevor Cooke was particularly anxious to examine the pathology of his cases. This was hardly surprising for a man who had spent years of his professional life concerned with the classification and treatment of coeliac disease. However, Cooke and his colleagues found Shiner's instrument difficult to use and frequently failed to obtain a biopsy. Fortunately they were rescued by an alternative device invented by a brilliant American, Lt Col William Crosby (1914–2005) and his engineer colleague, Heinz Kugler. Bill Crosby was working with the US Army's sprue team in Puerto Rico and found Shiner's tube was unsatisfactory. The cable was too rigid to activate the knife reliably so he devised an instrument consisting of a capsule containing a knife that was spring-activated and triggered by suction.[88] Its great advantage was that the capsule was attached to a thin polyurethane tube rather than a cable which made it much easier to use – in particular it slipped through the pylorus more readily.

Cooke used Crosby's capsule with considerable success. Within two years he had biopsies from no fewer than 58 patients with adult coeliac disease.[89] He wanted to prove that coeliac disease in children and adults was one and the same condition and to find out whether coeliac disease was a single entity or a syndrome with several causes.

Of the 58 patients, 4 had normal biopsies, so he reviewed their histories carefully and concluded that the original diagnosis was wrong. The rest had abnormal biopsies, of whom half had villous atrophy identical to that seen in children. This group with "flat" biopsies had been ill in childhood and clearly had coeliac disease, though most were eating normally, felt well and thought they were cured.

Cooke found it difficult to categorise the rest of his patients who had partial villous atrophy, an appearance Doniach had described in two of Shiner's patients. The villi were stunted and contained a heavy infiltrate of inflammatory cells. Many of these patients had also responded clinically to a gluten-free diet and felt fine, but some were profoundly anaemic.

He wondered if the "flat" mucosa was the end result of a process that began with partial atrophy and conversely whether partial villous atrophy indicated regeneration of a flat mucosa. He was unable to commit himself and decided that only those people with a "flat" biopsy could be labelled coeliac. The second group with abnormal villi probably had another cause for their disease.

Soon after Margot Shiner joined Avery Jones at the Central Middlesex Hospital, she was approached by the paediatrician Jack Sakula (1908–82), who had just admitted a boy aged seven with typical coeliac disease. Would she attempt to obtain a duodenal biopsy on this little fellow who was three and a half feet tall and weighed four stone he wondered? Indeed she would, using her adult biopsy tube, which was a brave step at a time when the risks of haemorrhage and perforation were still unknown. Using local anaesthetic she managed to obtain four specimens from the duodenum, all showing villous atrophy similar to her adult cases.[90] It did seem as Cooke thought that coeliac disease and idiopathic steatorrhoea were the same disease.

Her success quickly caught the attention of several paediatricians who were keen to learn her technique. But intestinal biopsy proved to be more difficult in children than adults and when Shiner published her first small series in the first edition of *Gut* in 1960 she had only managed to obtain biopsies from ten out of eighteen children. Nonetheless all the eight children with coeliac disease had villous atrophy. One of these, in fact the boy referred by Jack Sakula, was given a gluten-free diet and underwent repeat biopsies without sedation on three occasions over the next two years. By this time he was clinically better but Shiner had difficulty convincing herself that his biopsies had improved with treatment.[91]

With practice Shiner's success rate improved but others found her technique difficult. In their hands the child needed heavy sedation or a general anaesthetic, the biopsy tube was difficult to position and required prolonged screening, and if the jejunum was reached, the biopsies were frequently fragmented. There was considerable relief when Bill Crosby introduced his capsule, particularly a smaller one for use in infants. Paediatricians found this much easier to manage and it was widely adopted. Success rates soared, screening time was halved and good samples of mucosa were obtained.

Meanwhile Charlotte Anderson had left Birmingham to continue her research into coeliac disease in Melbourne, and James Smellie had retired, but his chair was more than adequately filled by Douglas Hubble (1900–81). A youthful 58 years old, urbane and compassionate, yet abounding in energy, he soon capitalised on the department's rich experience of coeliac disease to organise a large study of children by jejunal biopsy. Hubble's arrival coincided with Shiner's biopsy technique but after a brief flirtation with her tube, his team changed to the Crosby capsule. In a little over two years they had obtained duodenal/jejunal biopsies from 51 children and were able to show unequivocally that the mucosal changes reverted to normal in response to gluten withdrawal.[92] They also confirmed that many older children, who seemed well on a normal diet, still had villous atrophy. This began a debate about whether such children, or rather adolescents, should be kept on a gluten-free diet. Should, Hubble mused, the doctor, pace W. H. Auden, be:

"an endomorph with gentle hands
who will not make absurd demands
that I abandon all my vices"

or should he be a perfectionist who pursues the way of complete rectitude for himself and his patients? Wisely at the time, he thought parents and children should be given the facts and encouraged to choose for themselves but be strict until the age of ten years and preferably till after puberty.[93]

Simultaneously another large study of children with coeliac disease was undertaken by Sir Wilfrid Sheldon at Great Ormond Street. This study too began with the help of Margot Shiner, though Sheldon insisted that the biopsies should be obtained under general anaesthetic. Like everyone else his team found her technique too difficult and changed to the Crosby capsule. Sheldon agreed with Hubble's findings and was equally unsure about long-term treatment. While acknowledging that gluten sensitivity seemed to be permanent he agreed that if a child was completely well the diet could be relaxed.[94] But four years later he reviewed his older children, now young adults off diet, and found that only 25 per cent were healthy. So he revised his policy and recommended that gluten should be withheld indefinitely.[95]

When folic acid and vitamin B12 were first isolated after the Second World War clinical haematology as a speciality did not exist. For a further twenty years patients with anaemia were managed entirely by the physicians.

Leslie Witts was well known for his work bridging haematology and the gut and was now the Nuffield Professor of Clinical Medicine at the Radcliffe Infirmary, Oxford. In 1949 he took on a graduate student, John Badenoch (1920–96), to study the absorption of iron in patients with steatorrhoea. Within a few years Badenoch had accumulated a personal series of more than 100 patients. In his Goulstonian Lectures in 1960, he emphasised how few of these people had bowel symptoms and how many were simply tired or underweight.[96] Most were iron or folate deficient and indeed he came to suspect malabsorption in anyone with hypochromia and immature red blood cells. Badenoch found intestinal biopsy helpful to distinguish the various causes of steatorrhoea but unfortunately did not take matters further, forsaking research for an NHS appointment.

Similarly Stanley Davidson, Professor of Medicine in Edinburgh, had long been interested in pernicious anaemia and after the war he encouraged his lecturer, Ronald Girdwood (1917–2006), to study the absorption and excretion of folic acid.[97] Girdwood's real interest was anaemia and he claimed that he saw very few cases of coeliac disease. Nonetheless when jejunal biopsy became available he was one of the first to use the technique and obtained biopsies from 24 patients with malabsorption, which confirmed Trevor Cooke's findings. Clinically the patients with "flat" biopsies were inseparable from those with stunted villi so Girdwood argued that they probably had the same disease. Three of his patients happened to have a malignant stricture in the ileum but he thought this was a coincidence.[98]

However, it was the haematology department at the Hammersmith Hospital in London that provided the catalyst that was to influence research into coeliac disease for the next two decades. By now most people knew that the macrocytic anaemia of idiopathic steatorrhoea was caused by poor absorption of folic acid and iron; nevertheless pernicious anaemia due to vitamin B12 deficiency was often confused with it until it became possible to measure vitamin B12 directly in blood. David Mollin managed this with a new assay when he was working in Professor John Dacie's department. Later, with the help of Lester Smith from the research division of Glaxo Laboratories, he obtained some highly radioactive B12 intending to study its clearance from the body. This was in 1954 at which time he took on Christopher Booth (1924–2012) as a research fellow.

Booth thought that it would be more interesting to study vitamin B12 absorption from the gut and compare patients with pernicious anaemia with controls. However, when he fed the vitamin to normal subjects he found that it took much longer than he expected for the B12 to appear in the blood. Either it was held up by the jejunal mucosa or it was being absorbed lower down in the ileum. Experiments in rats indicated the latter[99] so Booth gave B12 to patients having a laparotomy and, using a hand-held Geiger counter, found the isotope concentrated in the ileum. This was highly significant because it showed for the first time that a particular part of the gut could actively absorb a substance.[100] Furthermore Booth saw that this could be used as a test for ileal function.

Many substances including most water-soluble vitamins and glucose are readily absorbed high in the jejunum. Protein and fat are also absorbed in the jejunum but the process is slower because they have to be digested first, so some protein and fat reaches the lower jejunum or even the ileum before absorption takes place. Absorption of B12 by the ileum is unique. So when surgeons resected a segment of small bowel, Booth was able to predict the pattern of malabsorption that might occur and recommend appropriate supplements. He also drew attention to the remarkable reserve capacity of the intestine, stressing the ability of the ileum to take over the function of the jejunum if necessary.[101]

CHAPTER TWENTY-EIGHT

VILLOUS ATROPHY

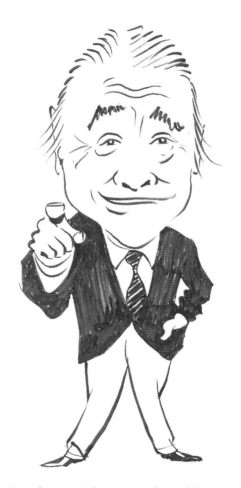

31 Booth – And that's not for publication.

Booth was now fascinated by the small intestine and working next door to Margot Shiner he was quick to recognise the potential of her technique. He must have looked down the microscope when Sonny Doniach was first describing the histology of coeliac disease. When Sheila Sherlock left in 1959 to take the Chair of Medicine at the Royal Free Hospital, Professor Sir John McMichael (1904–93) recognised and rewarded Booth for his enthusiasm and work on the small intestine by appointing him to succeed her. At the time clinical science at the Hammersmith was carried out in a prefabricated hut known as the lower medical corridor, an unattractive building sandwiched between the medical wards. Booth surrounded himself with clinicians and scientists, embraced new techniques as they came along and opened up the small intestine. He always said he was not a gastroenterologist: "I start at the pylorus and I finish at the ileo-caecal valve."

Already the Americans were building on Shiner's results, especially Cyrus Rubin and his group in Seattle. They insisted that biopsy of the proximal small bowel was essential for the diagnosis of coeliac disease and pointed out that as the jejunum bore the brunt of undigested gluten it naturally suffered the greatest damage. Some of their patients with a flat mucosa were well but these had a normal ileum, confirming Booth's prediction that the degree of malabsorption depended on the extent of the lesion down the gut.

One of the first tasks Booth set himself was to clarify the relationship between sub-total villous atrophy and partial villous atrophy. Rubin had suggested that examination of fresh biopsies under the dissecting microscope might be helpful and Booth decided to follow this up. With the help of his senior house officer, Raymond (Ted) Holmes (1927–2009) and a registrar in pathology, Dermot Hourihane, he obtained three-dimensional pictures of the mucosa. Healthy people had beautiful long slender finger-like villi but in coeliacs with villous atrophy the villi were completely flattened.[102] A few patients showed a curious whorled or ridged appearance, which he called convoluted. Histologically these patients had partial villous atrophy.

With his new registrar, Jimmy Stewart (born 1929), and the haematologists Booth went on to compare the structure and function of the jejunum and ileum in patients with coeliac disease. Almost every patient had a flat proximal intestinal mucosa but the appearance improved further down the gut where it became convoluted or normal.

Furthermore the flat lesions changed to a convoluted pattern after treatment with a gluten-free diet. Though seldom used today, the dissecting microscope technique was invaluable at the time proving that the two forms of villous atrophy simply reflect the severity of the coeliac lesion. This important study also confirmed that the degree of steatorrhoea depended upon the reserve capacity of the ileum rather than the severity of the jejunal lesion.[103]

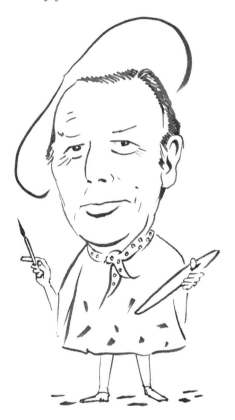

32 Creamer – Painter.

The re-modelling of the intestinal villi in response to treatment was remarkably rapid and intrigued several workers, notably Brian Creamer (1926–2005), senior lecturer at St. Thomas's Hospital, who had recently worked with Charles Code, Professor of Physiology at the Mayo Clinic, on oesophageal motility. On his return to St. Thomas's Hospital he persuaded the governors to build him a wooden clinical research unit affectionately known as the gut hut. He learnt to use Shiner's tube and began to study the dynamics of cell turnover in the intestine. Research was unusual among the physicians at the hospital (apart from the professorial unit) but what Creamer lacked in research fellows was well compensated by a series of registrars anxious to enlarge their CVs.

Whereas Doniach and others thought that the crypts of Lieberkuhn were hyperplastic to compensate for the loss of surface enterocytes, Creamer championed the alternative view that some factor was preventing the young enterocytes from maturing. He began by comparing the number of adult enterocytes on the surface mucosa with the number of immature cells in the crypts, a painstaking task that meant counting the mitotic activity of thousands of cells. Unlike normal cells the crypt cell population in coeliacs far outnumbered the adult cells but failed to mature and died in situ before they could migrate from the pits.[104] There were no villi because there were not enough adult cells to cover them. Using the dissecting microscope he went on to show that the shape of the villi, whether finger-like or convoluted, correlated nicely with the population of adult cells.[105]

Creamer extended the concept of cell turnover when Desmond Croft (born 1932) joined him as Senior Registrar. Croft was one of the first to use radionucleotides in clinical medicine. He had developed a technique for measuring desquamation from the gastric mucosa, using DNA, at the West Middlesex Hospital with Nelson Coghill (1912–2002). All cells have the same amount of DNA so he could calculate the number of cells being shed by measuring the DNA in the washings. Croft and his colleague at St. Thomas's Hospital, Christian Loehry (born 1936), devised a technique for isolating and perfusing a five-centimetre segment of the jejunum[106] and showed that the cell turnover was much more rapid in coeliacs than normal. Patients with a flat mucosa had a turnover time of under six hours compared to the normal four days.[107] They called this condition an exudative enteropathy and showed with the electron microscope that the cells were indeed enterocytes, not merely inflammatory cells.[108] So it seemed that Doniach's original suggestion that the crypts were hyperplastic to compensate for the increased cell turnover was correct after all. Creamer gave a masterly account of his work in the second Arthur Hurst Lecture to the British Society of Gastroenterology in 1968

One would have thought that the diagnosis of coeliac disease was now relatively straightforward. A flat biopsy invariably pointed to the disease, especially in children, but for several years Brian Creamer argued that villous atrophy was a non-specific appearance with several causes.[109] Even a response to gluten withdrawal, he argued, did not necessarily imply a patient had coeliac disease, any more than someone with a megaloblastic anaemia responding to B12 had pernicious anaemia. Some patients with villous atrophy did not respond to gluten withdrawal anyway.[110] Furthermore the coeliac syndrome, as he called it, was often found in association with other diseases, notably malignancy.

CHAPTER TWENTY-NINE

COELIAC DISEASE AND MALIGNANCY

Malignancy associated with steatorrhoea was recognised before the Second World War by Fairley and Mackie at the Hospital for Tropical Disease, London. Sir Neil Hamilton Fairley (1891–1966), an Australian, had served in Egypt and Palestine during the First World War, where he was noted for his work on schistosomiasis. Later in Bombay he became interested in the treatment of tropical sprue and was finally appointed to the Hospital for Tropical Disease, London in 1929. There he was joined by Frederick Percival Mackie (1875–1944) who had worked with him on sprue in Bombay. Mackie had recently retired after a distinguished career with the Indian Medical Service and was now a pathologist at the hospital. They described three patients who had lymphoma of the mesenteric glands, thought to be blocking the lymphatics, and compared the situation to that described by Ryle of a patient with tabes mesenterica and steatorrhoea.[111]

After this there were several more reports but in every case it was assumed that the reticulosis was the cause of the steatorrhoea. Certainly diffuse involvement of the gut could be responsible but in many of the cases there was no tumour in the gut itself or at most a single discreet deposit, which was hardly enough to cause steatorrhoea. A typical example was described by C. N. Best and Peter Cook (1926–2000), two registrars working with Reginald Nassim (1908–75), physician to the Royal National Orthopaedic Hospital, Stanmore, who was interested in metabolic bone disease. Their patient had typical idiopathic steatorrhoea and responded well to a gluten-free diet. Three years later he relapsed with fever and weight loss and laparotomy revealed reticulosarcoma of the mesentery, though the gut was normal. Best and Cook thought the sarcoma was the cause of the steatorrhoea which just happened to be gluten sensitive. In some way the tumour was assumed to have produced coeliac-like changes in the intestine.[112]

If steatorrhoea was an unlikely complication of lymphoma could the reverse be true? Could lymphomas arise as a complication of coeliac disease? This was the inspired suggestion of a senior house officer, Kenneth Gough (born 1931), at the Bristol Royal Infirmary. Gough was working on the professorial unit in Bristol and regularly attended the surgical teaching round of the Professor of Surgery, R Milnes-Walker (1903–85), whom he greatly admired. One Saturday morning the surgical registrar presented the case of a 59-year-old woman with a reticulosarcoma of the ileum, who had suffered from steatorrhoea for four years before her death. Gough was struck by the length of her history and his interest quickened when a few months later a 54-year-old-man was admitted to the medical unit with a 25-year history of steatorrhoea. For a time he had done well on a gluten-free diet but had stopped it and relapsed. His small bowel meal was typical of malabsorption and jejunal biopsies showed villous atrophy. He did not improve and laparotomy six months later revealed a reticulosarcoma obstructing the ileum. Sections of small bowel distant from the tumour showed villous atrophy.

About the same time another physician in Bristol, John Naish (1915–2009), at Frenchay Hospital, admitted a 48-year-old woman who had had steatorrhoea for two years. X-ray studies and jejunal biopsy were consistent with adult coeliac disease. She improved briefly but relapsed after four months when laparotomy revealed an extensive reticulosarcoma of the jejunum. Encouraged by Alan Read (1926–93), who had recently arrived from the Hammersmith to be Lecturer in Medicine in Bristol, Gough and Naish reviewed the literature and found 16 cases of intestinal reticulosis including the case described by Best and Cook. Several had a long history of steatorrhoea and many, like Best and Cook's case, had minimal involvement by tumour of the gut itself.[113]

It seemed obvious to Gough and his friends in Bristol that lymphoma was occurring as a complication of coeliac disease, though they could not prove it. Reaction to their ideas was mixed. Brian Creamer was sceptical and believed that malignancy was more likely to be the cause of villous atrophy rather than the reverse.[114] But Alan Read, now Reader in Medicine, enthusiastically promoted Gough's original observation. The Bristol team suggested that patients with steatorrhoea and villous atrophy were also at risk of cancers as well as lymphoma. [115] However, the numbers were small and the argument might have continued for years had not Trevor Cooke been able to draw upon his huge experience in Birmingham.

Cooke reviewed 202 patients who had had coeliac disease for at least 25 years, a remarkable series by any standards, especially in 1965. Most had been under surveillance for ten years, several for much longer and he confirmed that malignancy was much more common than expected. Thirteen patients eventually succumbed to carcinoma, usually of the oesophagus or stomach but only after they had had coeliac disease for nearly 40 years. Similarly fourteen patients developed an intra-abdominal lymphoma after twenty years. The sheer length of time that Cooke's patients had had coeliac disease was tantamount to proof that malignancy was indeed a complication. [116]

CHAPTER THIRTY

DEFINING COELIAC DISEASE

Interest in coeliac disease was now widespread but many questions remained. How common was it and were coeliac disease and adult coeliac disease the same illness? How did gluten damage the mucosa and would a gluten-free diet prevent malignant change? These questions proved extremely difficult to answer and have preoccupied research workers to this day. Many still disagreed about its management, especially the paediatricians.

If further evidence was needed that childhood and adult coeliac disease were the same condition it had come from a remarkable study by Archibald Norman (born 1912) and Christopher Booth, who managed to track down some of the children originally seen by Christopher Hardwick before the war. In fact, Norman, who was a paediatrician, had already traced 28 of Hardwick's cases in 1954.[117] That was before the days of jejunal biopsy and Norman concluded that the "majority would have passed any routine examination" though four were clearly unwell with malabsorption. Ten years later Norman joined forces with Booth to examine biopsies from eight of these children who were now in their thirties.[118] They all had subtotal villous atrophy with one exception, a man who probably never had coeliac disease in the first place. Yet they were all comparatively well and enjoying a normal diet in spite of a flat mucosa. This was consistent with Booth's opinion that the ileum often compensated for the jejunum. In fact most of the patients were deficient in folic acid and they felt that treatment with a gluten-free diet seemed more rational than the use of dietary supplements.

Insisting that someone who feels well should restrict himself to a gluten-free diet has never been easy, and certainly not in the early days of uncertainty when gluten-free products were not so available and the co-operation of education authorities was poor. Even those patients who were underweight or small in stature were often unimpressed by such advice. John Badenoch in Oxford, which is close to good galloping country, recalls that steatorrhoea was known locally as the jockey's disease. More than once he was accused of spoiling a promising future by making a young man grow again with gluten restriction.

The merit of a lifelong gluten-free diet was strongly supported by two paediatricians, Winifred Young (1909–69) and Elizabeth Pringle (1905–91), at the Queen Elizabeth Hospital for children, Hackney, London. They undertook a Herculean study of 110 children with coeliac disease over a period of nineteen years.[119] Sadly Winifred Young died in 1969 before the work was published. All the children were treated with a gluten-free diet and responded well as expected. Forty-four children were followed up for periods as long as nineteen years. Twenty who remained on the diet gained weight, grew normally and had no complications. The rest, who did not, developed sub-optimal growth and chronic ill health and were prone to diarrhoeal attacks, iron deficiency and megaloblastic anaemia. One who claimed she was symptom-free had a crisis in pregnancy.

Though villous atrophy was the gold standard for diagnosis, subjecting a child to a jejunal biopsy was not a procedure to be undertaken lightly, and as late as 1966 Sheldon sounded a note of caution. Even with the Crosby capsule his failure rate was 35 per cent and he had three major complications – one perforation, one severe bleed and a child in whom the capsule remained stuck to the wall of the jejunum. Not surprisingly, he felt that intestinal biopsy was unjustified as a routine procedure.[120] Young and Pringle agreed with him and felt that biopsy "should be done by persons who are in a situation to gain experience and to continue that experience". This was sound advice in those days of "see one, do one, teach one".

Despite these warnings, Sandy McNeish (born 1938) a registrar in paediatrics in Glasgow was obtaining satisfactory biopsies from nine out of ten children at the Royal Hospital for Sick Children.[121] McNeish used a paediatric Crosby capsule attached to a softer tube that slipped through the pylorus easily, and he had no complications from 100 consecutive biopsy procedures. Moreover three quarters of his children were under the age of five years. As soon as jejunal biopsy was shown to be practical and safe, the door was opened for its widespread use by clinicians, especially paediatricians, throughout the country.

In 1968 two enterprising people, Elizabeth Segall and Peter Benenson[†] (1921–2005) founded the Coeliac Society, a lay organisation run by coeliacs for the welfare of their members in Great Britain. The society provides advice on diet and management of the disease and has grown steadily; by the year 2000 there were 40,000 members. Allied to the Society, the Coeliac Trust supervises its financial assets and in 1969 supported the first international conference on coeliac disease. The meeting was the brainchild of Christopher Booth, who wanted to bring together the paediatricians and gastroenterologists and remove the unnecessary barriers between the two. The meeting was highly successful and concluded with a vigorous debate on the precise definition of the disease.[122]

Everyone agreed that a characteristic flat mucosal biopsy was essential for the diagnosis together with an unequivocal response to a gluten-free diet. Difficulties arose over the meaning of the word unequivocal because patients often felt better with treatment, though the mucosa remained flat. So it was agreed that a second biopsy was essential to prove that the mucosa had recovered. Even then some paediatricians wanted proof that children were definitely gluten-sensitive by a further biopsy after a gluten challenge. One in ten children, they argued, had a transient enteropathy which was not coeliac disease. If it was put to a family that a lifelong diet may be unnecessary they would gladly agree to a gluten challenge to find out. This was safe and jejunal biopsy should be repeated after three months and if still normal at intervals of two years thereafter.[123]

Despite this advice, a survey of members of the European Society of Paediatric Gastroenterologists later revealed that few paediatricians were so rigorous in practice.[124] The simple fact that 95 per cent of children were known to relapse when exposed to gluten was enough to satisfy them that a challenge was unnecessary. [†]

---

† The founder of Amnesty International and a coeliac himself.

CHAPTER THIRTY-ONE

EPIDEMIOLOGY OF COELIAC DISEASE

Once it was possible to make a firm diagnosis of coeliac disease, doctors naturally wondered about its prevalence and looked to epidemiologists for clues.

For years people had noted that more than one case was not unusual in a family. This impression was confirmed by Cedric Carter (1917–84), a medical geneticist at Great Ormond Street, who showed that children attending Wilfrid Sheldon's clinic were more likely to have relatives with the disease, though the mode of inheritance was far from obvious.[125]

The first person to study this was Morrice McCrae (born 1932), a paediatrican in Glasgow. He took 100 children with biopsy proven coeliac disease and managed to interview nearly 3,000 relatives, only 6 of whom had clear evidence of coeliac disease though none had biopsies taken. This indicated a family incidence of 1 in 465 which was slightly more common than in the general population, which he estimated was 1 in 1850. He went on to calculate the average number of cases in hospital from 1948 to 1960 and related the number to the size of the population served by the hospital. From this he concluded that the small increase in the disease among relatives meant that it was not inherited as the result of a single major gene effect. The genetic component of coeliac disease made people prone to damage by a number of environmental factors and this susceptibility was inherited as a polygeric variation. In effect, genetic factors determined the degree to which an individual was susceptible.[126]

McCrae was the first to agree that he was probably under-estimating the frequency of coeliac disease. He knew that many cases went undetected and were able to eat wheat with impunity despite their villous atrophy. Less than a quarter had the classical signs of steatorrhoea, osteomalacia or anaemia. Often an unexplained macrocytosis was the only clue to the diagnosis. The figures depended entirely on the enthusiasm with which the clinicians sought the disease. For example ,some community health services referred all small but otherwise healthy schoolchildren many of whom were coeliacs. Surveys also showed that coeliac disease was common in old people with over a quarter of cases presenting in the seventh decade, tagged "very adult coeliac disease".[127]

McCrae also acknowledged that there was a much higher incidence of villous atrophy among relatives compared to the small number of cases he had found. Doctors in Seattle had managed to obtain biopsies from relatives who seemed to be in perfect health and found they were a hundred times more likely to have villous atrophy than expected. Similarly in London, Patricia Mortimer (born 1930), a paediatrician, carried out a study with Christopher Booth, selecting relatives with folate deficiency for biopsy.[128] No fewer than eight per cent of these people had a flat mucosa. This discrepancy between the mucosal lesion and the clinical syndrome led McCrae to conclude that environmental factors were more important than the inherited predisposition itself.

He discovered that when wheat imports to Scotland stopped during World War Two, coeliac disease fell dramatically. Homegrown wheat was relatively harmless. What, he wondered, were the factors causing the mucosal damage and what caused the difference between silent and overt clinical cases?[129]

One clue lay in the west coast of Ireland where coeliac disease seemed to be particularly common. Paediatricians in the regional hospital in Galway led by Brian McNicholl estimated that the disease was about ten times more frequent than in England.[130] No one knew why but Edmund Moynahan (1908–99), a dermatologist at Guy's Hospital, suggested that the high incidence could have arisen because wheat was not eaten by the Irish until after the potato blight in 1847. Susceptible genes causing wheat intolerance, which would have been eliminated over the centuries in, say, wheat-eating Englishmen, would have persisted in Ireland. Once Irishmen began to eat wheat, coeliac disease flourished.[131]

But only when a simple test to diagnose coeliac disease became available would the real incidence reveal itself. Even so it seemed unlikely that epidemiology alone would explain the disease.

CHAPTER THIRTY-TWO

PATHOGENESIS OF COELIAC DISEASE

Exactly how wheat damaged the mucosa had puzzled doctors since Dicke's original discovery that bread caused coeliac disease. Indeed this became the Holy Grail of research and only now are we close to the solution. The work has been frustrated by the extreme complexity of wheat proteins and by the fact that for years the precise site of attack on the mucosa was far from clear.

(a) Missing peptidase hypothesis

At first the biochemists hoped they would find the answer when Dicke and his colleagues showed that the toxic fraction in wheat was gluten. In a series of laborious experiments in Birmingham, Alastair Frazer showed that the harmful properties of gluten were unaffected by gastric or pancreatic digestion but further digestion by pig intestine rendered it harmless. In other words partial digestion of gluten to polypeptides leaves the harmful effect intact but complete proteolysis to amino acids makes it harmless. Frazer was working before the days of jejunal biopsy and had to rely on careful feeding studies and faecal fat measurements. He called his peptic/tryptic digest of gluten "fraction III" and Frazer's fraction III became the standard starting point for gluten challenge studies thereafter.[132] He thought coeliac disease was due to a missing mucosal enzyme and put forward his missing peptidase hypothesis.[133] This held that in coeliac disease there was a genetically determined deficiency of an intra-cellular peptidase allowing toxic peptides to accumulate and damage the enterocyte.[†]

[†]   He actually wondered for a time if his fraction III was acting as an antigen but couldn't prove it.

As soon as jejunal biopsy became available, Christopher Booth decided to test this hypothesis. Now senior lecturer at the Hammersmith, Booth needed a new registrar. John McMichael introduced him to Jimmy Stewart (born 1929) and they clicked immediately: "I'm Doctor, call me Chris, Booth." To support Stewart during his research Booth managed to obtain an obscure fellowship from the Royal College of Physicians.[†] Stewart was at the Hammersmith for five years and recalls that one of the most enjoyable things about working with Booth was the loyalty and mutual support he inspired within the unit.

Histochemistry was expanding rapidly and at the Hammersmith Tony Pearse (1916–2001), a pathologist, was a leader in the field.[‡] In his department he had a brilliant biochemist, Ernst Riecken from Germany. They were the ideal people to help Booth, who had little experience in biochemistry but whose enthusiasm was infectious. They examined the brush border of the enterocyte as well as the other intracellular structures and Pearse was able to locate a variety of enzymes and peptidases in different parts of the cell.[134] The flat biopsies of coeliac patients were mirrored by a corresponding decrease in enzyme activity, but this always recovered after treatment. In other words the enzyme changes were a secondary phenomenon and there did not seem to be a specific enzyme deficiency to explain coeliac disease. However, the study of peptide digestion by the enterocyte was now underway.

In 1966 Booth was appointed Professor and Director of Medicine at the Royal Post Graduate Medical School and the following year opened his intestinal research unit funded by the Medical Research Council. At last the small intestine was on level terms with the heart, lungs and kidney. Several new research fellows arrived including Adrian Douglas from Newcastle and Tim Peters (born 1941) from Dundee.[§] These two developed Booth's ideas and helped to unravel how peptides were absorbed by the mucosa.[3]

If the coeliac enterocyte was lacking a crucial peptidase it would be

---

[†] T K Stubbins.

[‡] He was later to define the hormone peptides showing that the gut is the largest endocrine organ in the body.

[§] Peters was a registrar in Dundee. One of the medical secretaries was suspected of coeliac disease and was advised to go to the Hammersmith (500 miles away) for a biopsy. This stimulated Peters to visit the Hammersmith with an introduction from Ken Lowe who had worked at the Hammersmith on the first artificial kidney.

unable to digest the peptides of gluten and release the corresponding amino acids. To find out Douglas incubated homogenates of coeliac mucosa with Frazer's Fraction III and found that the amount of amino acid released was indeed less than normal. However, after treatment the levels returned to normal showing that treated coeliacs and normal subjects behaved the same.[135] This should have laid the peptidase theory to rest but curiously both Douglas and Peters were loathe to let it go.

Douglas went on to postulate the lectin hypothesis suggesting that abnormal brush border glycoproteins bind to gluten because of its lectin properties.[136] Cell damage ensues and the villi are destroyed. It was an ingenious theory but was never substantiated. He later embraced the immune theory and returned to Newcastle before emigrating to America.

Peters did much to bring cell biology into gastroenterology. He carried out exhaustive studies of the enzymes in the enterocyte and showed how protein digestion was a multi-step process with progressive luminal, brush border and intracellular hydrolysis of peptides. For some years he championed the theory that coeliac disease might be due to a primary increase in mucosal permeability allowing the absorption of toxic peptides. Ultimately this theory was not substantiated. However, he did show that transglutaminase activity was increased in biopsies from coeliac patients both in remission and relapse and wondered if this had a role in gluten-cell membrane interactions.[137] The crucial role of tissue transglutaminase was to become apparent some years later.

(b) Immunological theory

As support for an enzyme theory waned people began to think some form of allergy to gluten could be causing coeliac disease. Frazer himself had considered the possibility after noting that his peptide fraction III caused tachyphylaxis in sensitised guinea pigs but he was put off because FF IIIa (autoclaved FF III) had no such effect.

Immunology was still in its infancy in the 1950s. Philip Gell (1941–2001) in Birmingham and Robin Coombs (1921–2006) in Cambridge had recently classified the four types of hypersensitivity reaction, distinguishing antibody or humoral responses from lymphoctye mediated or delayed hypersensitivity. Though John Humphrey (1915–81) had founded the division of immunology at the National Institute for Medical Research, Mill Hill in 1957, clinical immunologists were almost unknown.

The early work on coeliac disease was done by gastroenterologists feeling their way in this new field and it is remarkable how much they achieved. Even so there was considerable doubt at first and it was several years before the immune theory was finally accepted.

The earliest evidence came from Sidney Truelove (1913–2002) in Oxford who had recently made his reputation by proving that cortisone was effective in ulcerative colitis, which was thought to be an immune-related disease. Aware that steroids were also helpful in coeliac disease he thought an immunological type of response was more likely than an enzyme deficiency. He had already found circulating antibodies to milk proteins in colitis patients and next discovered there were antibodies to gluten peptides in coeliac disease.[138] He was assisted by Ralph Wright (1930–90), a South African who had recently emigrated to Britain.[†] Truelove also found antibodies to milk and egg proteins in his patients so he was unsure if his gluten antibodies were significant.[139] Perhaps they were simply a response to abnormal absorption of these proteins and nothing to do with the cause of coeliac disease. By this time antibodies, i.e. immunoglobulins, had been subdivided according to their function into immune classes including IgG, IgA and IgM, and intestinal plasma cells were known to secrete IgA in response to bacterial and other antigens. In 1965 Cyrus Rubin, a coeliac pioneer in America, showed that plasma cells in the mucosa of coeliac patients produced antibody to gliadin (a fraction of gluten).

At the Hammersmith Jack Hobbs (1929–2008), a haematologist interested in immunoglobulins, worked closely with Adrian Douglas on Booth's unit. At first they were highly sceptical that an immune process was involved but the effect of prednisolone in untreated disease helped to change their minds.[140] They found raised levels of IgA in the serum of patients with coeliac disease indicative of an antibody response and confirmed the American discovery that there were an increased number of plasma cells in the jejunal mucosa which secreted the immunoglobulin IgM.[141] They also agreed that patients with selective deficiency of IgA were more likely to have coeliac disease, which had recently been described by Heremans in Leiden, though quite why this should be was the subject of much speculation.[142]

[†]   Wright was to become one of the founders of modern hepatology and to share the discovery that hepatitis B infection can progress to chronic hepatitis and cirrhosis.

Meanwhile Margot Shiner at the Central Middlesex took the opportunity to study coeliac children who were having a second jejunal biopsy after a gluten rechallenge to confirm the diagnosis. She found an infiltration of plasma cells and lymphocytes in the lamina propria (not the epithelium) and immuno-fluorescent staining showed IgA (not IgM) immune complexes in the region of the basement membrane, which she thought might indicate an Arthus reaction (tissue damage due to complexes of antigen, antibody and complement).[143]

Shiner's findings were confirmed by Bill Doe (born 1941) a young Australian who like others had attended the Hammersmith Postgraduate Course and joined the Department of Medicine.

Doe was struck by the impressive nature of the coeliac mucosa. Despite the loss of villi, the mucosa was angry and swollen, indeed anything but atrophic. He met Joseph Heremans (1927–75) on a visit to Leiden who showed him his immuno-fluorescent antibody technique. Doe challenged treated coeliacs with gluten and demonstrated deposits of IgM and complement in the gut wall as Shiner had done. He too wondered if this reaction (Arthus) was damaging the gut but was unable to find anti-gluten antibody in the mucosa and no one could see immune complexes under the electron microscope.[144] Doe went on to have a distinguished career in Australia before returning to take a chair of medicine at Birmingham University.

In 1976 Christopher Booth left the Hammersmith to become Director of the MRC Clinical Research Centre at Northwick Park, London. His departure coincided with the growth of gastroenterology units throughout the country. Several, especially Birmingham, Bristol, St. Bartholomew's Hospital, Leeds, Manchester, Newcastle, Edinburgh and Glasgow were already actively engaged in research including the pathogenesis of coeliac disease. The humoral theory was beginning to lose favour and in 1981 David Webster (born 1940), an immunologist at Northwick Park Hospital, described a patient with coeliac disease who was known to have severe hypogammaglobulinaemia.[145] In his view this effectively ruled out an antigen/antibody reaction as the cause of coeliac disease.

(c) Cell mediated immunity

If not humoral, could coeliac disease be caused by a cell mediated immune response? This was the view of Peter Asquith (born 1937) who was Trevor Cooke's senior registrar in Birmingham. He had come under the influence of Philip Gell FRS, the celebrated geneticist who introduced him to immunology and as a result he learnt how to culture lymphocytes, obtaining his MD on coeliac disease and the role of lymphocytes. He resigned from his senior registrar post to become an honorary research fellow and won a Wellcome fellowship in the States for his work on lymphocyte transformation.[†] At the time tissue typing was done by mixing lymphocytes from the donor and the recipient. If the lymphocytes transformed, the patients were incompatible. He happened to notice that when he performed the mixed lymphocyte reaction on patients with coeliac disease, the lymphocytes did not transform. In other words coeliacs must have a similar set of antigens on the surface of their lymphocytes. These he realised could only be the HLA antigens that had been described a few years earlier.

(d) HLA Histo-compatibility antigens

The HLA antigens, which are glycoproteins, had been discovered about ten years earlier. They coat the surface of most cells and are encoded by genes found in the short arm of chromosone 6. The antigens govern the fate of transplanted tissue, hence the name histocompatibility antigens, and the group of genes encoding them is known as the major histocompatibility complex (MHC). They are inherited on Mendelian principles and individual antigens had already been found in association with various diseases.

In collaboration with Pauline Mackintosh at the Regional Blood Transfusion Centre, Asquith decided that given its familial nature coeliac disease was an obvious choice for HLA typing, especially if it was caused by an immunological reaction and could be complicated by lymphoma.

They began with 49 patients using sera that recognised twelve HLA antigens from the region on chromosone 6, later defined as class I. To their delight they found a four-fold increase in one of the antigens (HLA-1-B8).[146] Encouraged by this they extended the study and included children. Several clinicians co-operated in the work; the adult patients were under

---

[†]   Asquith worked on Joseph Kirsner's unit in Chicago and recalls that at the Billings Hospital there were no fewer than twenty gastroenterologists on the staff – this was in 1971.

the care of Trevor Cooke and were traced by Peter Stokes, a research fellow from New Zealand and Geoffrey Holmes (born 1943), his senior registrar; the children came from Charlotte Anderson's clinic and were traced by Sandy McNeish (recently moved from Glasgow) and Chris Rolles (born 1942) – all to become familiar names in the coeliac world. Pauline Mackintosh did the HLA typing and confirmed the original findings.[147]

Soon other groups with access to tissue typing found the same, by which time another part of chromosone 6, defined as class II, was noted to have a much closer association with coeliac disease than the class I marker. This was the HLA-DR-3 marker. Results from family studies by several groups in Birmingham, Liverpool and Galway suggested that there was a genetic inheritance linked to HLA, but how this increased susceptibility to coeliac disease remained a puzzle. Asquith himself speculated that HLA antigens might allow epithelial cells to bind specifically with gluten or that there might be an immune response gene influenced by HLA, which controlled the ability of the host to react to gluten.[148]

The problem was that though distinct HLA antigens were commonly found in association with coeliac disease, over 99 per cent of the population with these same antigens were perfectly healthy. The situation was quite different from that, say, in ankylosing spondylitis, where there is a very close association (90 per cent) with an otherwise infrequent antigen, HLA-B27. So early hopes that HLA typing might be useful in spotting people at risk were dashed. Indeed no less an authority than Sir Cyril Clarke (1907–2000), doyen of clinical genetics, once said that if he were young again he would not want to be involved in studying further associations of HLA types and disease. It was unlikely to be of clinical benefit though he acknowledged that it had great academic interest.[149] In a sense he was right, HLA status has not been helpful clinically yet but it has given us considerable insight into the molecular basis of the disease. Coeliac disease is rather special because the cause, gluten, can be removed, making it an excellent model for dissecting immunological disease.

(e) Animal studies

Patients with steatorrhoea sometimes have a small spleen. This was well known but was reinvestigated by Alan Read in Bristol after his discovery that lymphoma can complicate coeliac disease.[150] He assumed there must be some dysfunction in the reticulo endothelial system, a view that was echoed by Jimmy Stewart at the Hammersmith[151] and by Anne Ferguson (1941–98), a trainee gastroenterologist in Glasgow.[152] Ferguson thought the atrophic spleen was not caused by cachexia or starvation but represented part of a widespread immunological disturbance.

Anne Ferguson made a significant contribution to our understanding of coeliac disease.[†] She was a brilliant student and after several years as Senior Lecturer in Edinburgh she belatedly received a personal Chair. She worked closely with the paediatricians and built up an impressive research programme with a succession of PhD students passing through

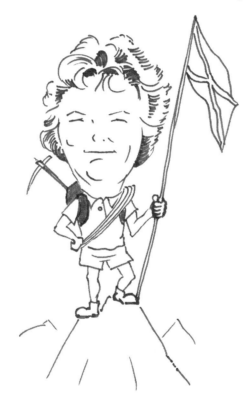

33 Ferguson – Bonny Scot.

[†]   Anne Ferguson was proud of her Scottish ancestry. Given the chance she would have repealed the Act of Union and happily stood as Anne, Queen of Scots.

her Unit. Her first paper as a registrar was a post mortem study of the intestinal villous pattern in stillborn infants.[153] This work combined with her interest in splenic atrophy led her to join one of the first departments of immunology in the country, set up by the eminent but difficult Bob White at the Western Infirmary, Glasgow.[†]

Ferguson was in the right place at the right time. A few years earlier would have seen her investigating humoral mechanisms in disease rather than cell-mediated immunity but she was aware of Shiner's recent demonstration of lymphocytes and plasma cells in the mucosa of children with coeliac disease.[154] Furthermore lymphocytes had now been divided into T (thymus dependent) and B (bursa) or bone-marrow-derived lymphocytes, and plasma cells were recognised to be mature lymphocytes. What, she wondered, was the role of these lymphocytes in the epithelium?

Ferguson's mentor was Delphine Parrott, a notable bacteriologist who helped her with the first detailed study of intra-epithelial lymphocytes using the electron microscope. She began by confirming that lymphocytes did indeed infiltrate the epithelium of people with coeliac disease and that they dispersed after treatment.[155]

Next she showed that in mice at least, most of the lymphocytes were T cells.[156] She suspected that a cell-mediated process was at work but the usual method of demonstrating this with a skin test failed. To get round this she grafted foetal intestine from mice under the kidney capsule of adult mice. As expected the grafts grew for a few days, became infiltrated with lymphocytes and were rejected, all typical of a local delayed hypersensitivity reaction.[157] The exciting discovery came when Ferguson, with her training in gastroenterology, noticed that the morphology of rejection was identical to that seen in coeliac disease, a fortuitous observation that could easily have been overlooked by those unfamiliar with coeliac disease.[158] Bearing in mind that the implanted foetal intestine carried no antigens such as food or micro-organisms, Ferguson knew that the pathological changes could only be caused by the rejection process itself, i.e. T lymphocytes. Moreover the mucosal damage preceded the appearance of antibody by several days emphasising the cellular nature of the reaction.

This was the first evidence that villous change was caused by the

---

†   Humphrey (in Mill Hill, p37) and White's (in Glasgow) book on immunology was the standard work for many years.

action of stimulated lymphocytes and Ferguson went on to examine how the villi were damaged. Her first PhD student was Tom MacDonald, an unemployed zoology graduate working in Tennants Brewery at the time, where he happened to meet Anne's husband. An informal interview took place while she was collecting her first adopted child and soon afterwards MacDonald found himself implanting foetal grafts into mice kidneys.

Ferguson and MacDonald noticed that during the process of villous atrophy the epithelial cells were shed into the lumen relatively unscathed. On the other hand there was an intense infiltration of lymphocytes in the lamina propria implying that villous atrophy was not caused by damage to the enterocytes but by inflammation of the underlying tissue. The crypts of Lieberkuhn were hyperplastic and it seemed that hyperplasia was not a compensatory response to damaged enterocytes as generally thought.[159]

Finally they took jejunal biopsies from patients with coeliac disease and cultured them in the presence of the peptide, alpha gliadin. After incubation the culture medium contained a substance that inhibited the migration of normal human leucocytes in a chamber. They thought this migration inhibition factor (MIF) was a lymphokine – i.e. a mediator of cellular immunity secreted by sensitised lymphocytes in response to an antigen, in this case gliadin.[160]

(f) Dermatitis herpetiformis

Further evidence of a cell-mediated response came from another unexpected quarter. In 1967 Sam Shuster (born 1926), a dermatologist at the Royal Victoria Infirmary, Newcastle, gave a lecture at the Royal College of Physicians entitled "Dermatogenic Enteropathy", in which he described a group of patients with dermatitis herpetiformis who had villous atrophy.[161] He thought the bowel lesion was due to the skin disease or possibly that patients with villous atrophy were unable to absorb dapsone, the usual treatment for dermatitis herpetiformis. In the audience was Lionel Fry (born 1934), an MRC research fellow in dermatology at the London Hospital, who during questions disagreed with Shuster's conclusions, arguing that these patients probably had coeliac disease. Behind him a voice he didn't recognise agreed. This was Victor Hoffbrand (born 1935), then Professor Dacie's registrar in haematology at the Hammersmith Hospital. They were well qualified to comment because Fry had learnt the technique of jejunal biopsy with Badenoch and written his MD on coeliac disease, while Hoffbrand was familiar with the condition through his interest in folic acid deficiency and his association with Chris Booth. They got together and showed that all patients with dermatitis herpetiformis had gluten-sensitive enteropathy and that both the mucosal lesion and the skin disease responded to the diet.[162] This took several years to gain general acceptance. Many of these patients were symptomless and it was only the dermatitis that alerted them to the diagnosis. They were therefore in the privileged position of examining biopsies showing the earliest changes of gluten enteropathy rather than the typical advanced lesions seen in the full-blown disease. Their pathologist, Robert McMinn (born 1924), Professor of Anatomy at King's College, was the first to describe the classical intestinal lesion of dermatitis herpetiformis comprising normal mucosal architecture in which the villous epithelium is heavily infiltrated with plasma cells and lymphocytes, a key observation.[†] This was exactly what Shiner was seeing in her children and what Ann Ferguson was describing in her experiments.

(g) Studies of intestinal lymphoid tissue I–XV

"For more than 30 years, mucosal abnormalities have been qualitatively described in terms of varying degrees of villous atrophy, a system of terminology that is not only inappropriate but also seems to have paralysed any new intellectual activity that might elucidate afresh the immuno-pathological basis of the mucosal response." M. N. Marsh, 1992, Manchester University School of Medicine.[163]

I suspect that few gastroenterologists knew Michael Marsh (born 1939) yet he had a large and busy practice and contributed much to our understanding of coeliac disease. His studies of intestinal lymphoid tissue, published over two decades, revealed a man with a mission and his writing was scholarly. He was a fierce critic who did not endear

---

[†] They may not have recognised the significance of their findings at the time as they agreed with the current hypothesis that immune complexes and an arthus-type reaction involving complement was probably the cause.

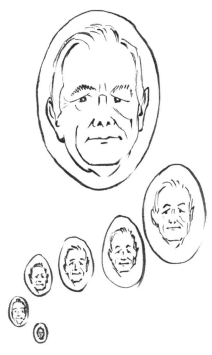

34 Marsh – Sequential – lymphocytes.

himself to those whose work he felt was substandard and furthermore he did not seek office within the BSG.

Marsh believed that it was essential to follow the evolution of the mucosal lesion of coeliac disease under the microscope; only then would the immunopathology be understood. He loved the microscope and measuring things. He gained a first class degree in anatomy and cell biology in Oxford and later became medical registrar to Booth at the Hammersmith where he linked with scientists at Unilever to produce some beautiful scanning EM pictures of the villi to complement Booth's dissecting microscope studies.[164] With the help of an MRC travelling fellowship he spent a year in Boston with Jerry Trier, where he learned to cut ultra-thin sections of mucosa for examination under oil emersion. Returning to Southampton he predicted that if the intraepithelial lymphocytes were being activated by antigens crossing the epithelium they would be actively mitotic and blastoid. But it was essential to use small doses of gluten to see the early changes; hitherto large doses had been used. Indeed when he added tiny doses of gluten to biopsies (approximately one gram instead of the usual 25 to 40, the lymphocytes reacted as he anticipated, returning to normal afterwards.[165]

He counted the intraepithelial lymphocytes very carefully and found that though the absolute number was decreased in coeliac disease they did rise in response to gluten.

Marsh took an appointment at the Hope Hospital, Salford, Greater Manchester where he continued his research using mini-challenges of gluten. He took serial biopsies from well treated patients and showed the evolution of a flat mucosa. At first there was lymphocytic infiltration, next crypt hypertrophy and finally mucosal destruction with flat villi.[166] This sequence fitted nicely with Ferguson's original graft versus host lesions in mice but in addition he had shown that gluten was the antigen responsible. Later he suggested that the mere infiltration of the epithelium with lymphocytes was apparently harmless because they were found in many patients with dermatitis herpetiformis and close relatives of coeliac patients.[167] Only when the dose of gluten was critically increased did the mucosal lesion progress. His picture strongly supported the growing immunological evidence that the mucosal damage began in the lamina propria of the villi and not in the enterocyte.

Marsh became Reader in Medicine in Manchester but failed to obtain a personal chair. Still buzzing with ideas he was promised a grant for a five-year project by the Coeliac Society, which was subsequently withdrawn after a change in policy. Embittered by this lack of support and recognition for years of dedicated work, he resigned from his position and retired to read theology in Oxford.

h) T-Lymphocytes

While Marsh was looking at lymphocytes, the immunologists were making great strides. In 1978 it became possible using monoclonal antibodies to sub-divide T-lymphocytes according to their function as either CD4 (helper) cells or CD8 (cytotoxic) cells. George Janossy (born 1940), a Hungarian doctor, had emigrated to Britain in 1970 to work with Melvyn Greaves (born 1941), a biologist at Mill Hill and later Professor of Cell Biology at the Institute of Cancer Research. Janossy was recruited by Victor Hoffbrand to the Royal Free Hospital to work on leukaemia and shortly afterwards noticed that the T-lymphocytes were seeking different environments (as he put it). The CD4 T cells tended to seek the company of HLA Class II antigen presenting cells (macrophages and dendritic cells) and CD8 T cells favoured HLA Class I rich sites such as epithelium. This was a brilliant observation, which he recorded in *Nature* with other distinguished immunologists and a young research fellow, Warwick Selby (born 1948), from Australia.[168]

Also at the Royal Free Hospital at the time was Derek Jewell (born 1941), Senior Lecturer with Professor Sheila Sherlock, who liked to have a gastroenterologist to look after the luminal side of gastroenterology while she ran the hepatology (the gut was a poor second to the liver at the Royal Free). Jewell had looked at IgE antibodies to milk proteins in colitis with Sidney Truelove at Oxford and was interested in the immunology of gut disease. Now that monoclonal antibodies were available, he was keen to characterise the intra-epithelial lymphocytes in the GI tract, as the proportion of T cells to B cells was still the subject of debate. So he joined forces with Janossy and Selby and they duly proved that nearly all the intraepithelial lymphocytes were T cells as they had suspected. What was more interesting, the great majority of these T cells were CD8 (cytotoxic-suppressor) T cells whereas the T cells in the lamina propria were mostly CD4 (helper/inducer) cells.[169] Bearing in mind that coeliac disease was strongly associated with HLA Class II antigens, which were now known to present antigen only to CD4 lymphocytes, their finding was highly significant and opened up a new field of research in coeliac disease.

Derek Jewell was appointed Consultant Physician in Oxford and left the Royal Free, taking Selby with him. They went on to show that the CD8 cells in the epithelium were not activated in coeliac disease suggesting that the main role of CD8 cells was likely to be suppressor rather than cytotoxic, acting as the first line of defence against foreign antigens in the gut.[170]

Warwick Selby was supported by various fellowships during this research and his future was insecure. There were few openings in this country and coeliac disease does not attract much support from the pharmaceutical companies. After some agonising Selby returned to Australia later becoming Clinical Associate Professor of Medicine at the Royal Prince Albert Hospital, Sydney. He was a loss to academic medicine in Britain and Derek Jewell was sad to see him go.

About this time, Ludwik Trejdosiewicz (born 1945), known as "Les", a Polish biologist and colleague of Janossy, left the Royal Free and moved to Leeds. Leeds was an attractive option because Monty Losowsky (born 1932) had built a fine department at the university hospital. Losowsky's early interest was in haematology and he had worked with William Castle in Harvard. On his return he came across several cases of coeliac disease

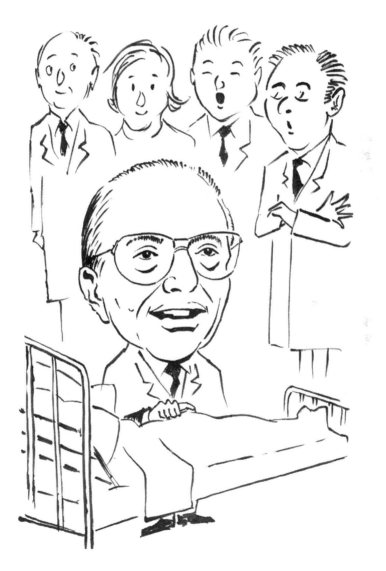

35 Losowsky – Teacher.

which prompted him in 1972 to write a book *Malabsorption in Clinical Practice*. The book sold out and established his name in the coeliac world. With his appointment to the chair of medicine, Losowsky headed the only professorial unit outside London wholly devoted to coeliac disease. The department was productive and successive registrars prospered there. HLA Associations, hypersplenism, dermatitis herpetiformis, humoral and cellular immune mechanisms all came under their scrutiny.

Trejdosiewicz and Janossy co-operated with Losowsky and his lecturer Peter Howdle (born 1948), who had set up a successful in-vitro organ culture of the intestine.[171] They took Jewell's work further and showed that unlike the CD8 cells in the epithelium the CD4 T helper cells in the lamina propria were indeed stimulated in coeliac disease and began to accumulate in the epithelium or close by in the lamina propria.[172] Even so the cells did not necessarily activate a full-blown inflammatory response, which was presumably dose related. CD4 T helper cells help B lymphocytes (plasma cells) to secrete immunoglobulin and Brian Scott, a physician in Lincoln from the Leeds stable, had recently demonstrated an increased number of plasma cells in untreated coeliac disease.[173] This amplified the original observation by Douglas that immunoglobulin levels are raised in coeliac disease but left open the question whether they actually contributed to the mucosal damage.[174]

Why and how the inflammatory response sometimes led to crypt hypertrophy and villous flattening was unclear, particularly as a similar cascade of inflammatory mediators might, for example, cause a lesion such as Crohn's Disease. But an ingenious experiment by Tom MacDonald, now in the Department of Paediatric Gastroenterology at St. Bartholomew's Hospital shed some light on this problem.

After his work with Anne Ferguson in 1976 MacDonald went to the States for two years "to learn all about T lymphocytes", later becoming Associate Professor in Microbiology at Thomas Jefferson University, studying mucosal immunology in mice. He then worked briefly and unhappily in Merck, Sharp and Dohme's laboratories and in 1985 visited England to attend a meeting where he met an old friend, John Walker-Smith (born 1936), Professor of Paediatric Gastroenterology at St. Bartholemew's Hospital, who offered him a research fellowship.[†]

---

†   Funded by CICRA (Chron's in Childhood Research Appeal).

At the same meeting MacDonald met his future wife, Jo Spencer from University College, London, a fellow immunologist.

A new centre for clinical research had recently opened at St. Bartholemew's Hospital where a medical research council fellow, Robert Dourmashkin, had managed to establish a very successful foetal organ culture system.[†] Spencer had used this to show that the foetal human small intestine contained T and B lymphocytes from about fourteen weeks of gestation. On his arrival at St. Bartholomew's Hospital MacDonald decided to see what would happen if he stimulated the foetal lymphocytes with a mitogen. He chose the pokeweed mitogen and to his delight reproduced all the changes of coeliac disease exactly as he had with Anne Ferguson in mice fifteen years earlier.[175] He and Spencer showed that this response was due to stimulation of lamina propria CD4 T helper cells, some of which crossed into the epithelium to activate B lymphocytes. Somehow or other activation of T lymphocytes by whatever means (mitogen or gluten) caused crypt hypertrophy, though the process itself was unexplained.[176]

i) Molecular mimicry

Though coeliac disease is caused by gluten in genetically predisposed patients, only a small proportion of susceptible people who eat wheat actually have the disease. Furthermore several monozygotic twins and HLA-identical siblings have been reported where only one partner has coeliac disease. Could there be another factor that triggers the response to gluten? For a time there was considerable excitement when Martin Kagnoff (born 1942), a gastroenterologist in California and David Kasarda, a cereal chemist, noticed a remarkable similarity between a peptide of A gliadin and a peptide in the adenovirus 12, a common gut virus. Perhaps infection with the virus could predispose genetically susceptible patients to coeliac disease. Kagnoff and Kasarda collaborated with Parveen Kumar (born 1942) at St. Bartholomew's Hospital and Joe Unsworth (born 1956), a PhD student studying antibodies in coeliac disease.[177] They found that patients with coeliac disease were more likely to have antibodies to the coat proteins of adenovirus 12, indicating past

---

[†]   Though critically correct at the time, subsequent amendments to the Abortion Act prevented further use of foetal implants after 1994

infection. Their theory gained further support when Derek Jewell in Oxford found that T cells of patients with coeliac disease recognised and reacted to synthetic gliadin and synthetic viral peptides identically.[178]

The crucial step was to show an immune response to the viral protein itself and it so happened that in Leeds, Eric Blair (born 1960), a biochemist, was particularly interested in the adeno virus. Working with Peter Howdle and other members of Losowsky's unit he was unable to show specific antibodies to the viral protein.[179] He went on to isolate DNA from jejunal biopsies and using the polymerase chain reaction he found that patients with coeliac disease were no more likely to be infected with adeno virus than normal.[180] This dampened enthusiasm for the hypothesis, particularly when two groups from Newcastle and Dublin also failed to find evidence of infection even in infancy.[181]

j) Gluten

In 1974 Paul Ciclitira (born 1948), a research fellow at Cambridge, set himself the task of finding a new cereal capable of making "normal" flour. Almost forty years and several millions of pounds later, he has achieved a great deal. He is single-minded and believes he should succeed.

Ten years after Dicke and his colleagues showed that wheat proteins caused coeliac disease, gluten was subdivided into soluble proteins called gliadins and insoluble glutenins. The gliadins were subdivided into alpha, beta, gamma and omega by electrophoresis. Frazer's fraction III obtained by peptic/tryptic digestion of gluten contains glutenins and gliadins and has been used for years as the starting point for gluten challenge experiments. A decade later Sidney Truelove and Robin Offord, a molecular biophysicist in Oxford, managed to filtrate smaller peptides from Frazer's fraction III, which were still toxic when fed to coeliac patients and served to show how extraordinarily complex the peptides were.[182]

Ciclitira's interest in wheat began when he worked with Professor E. S. Lennox at the Laboratory of Molecular Biology in Cambridge on plant proteins and the pathogenesis of coeliac disease.[183] He joined Hermon Dowling's (born 1936) unit at Guy's and showed that all forms of gliadin could exacerbate coeliac disease and that there was considerable immunological cross reactivity between them.[184] In 1983 he moved to St. Thomas's Hospital where he succeeded Brian Creamer and continued his research at the Rayne Institute.[†] By this time monoclonal antibodies were widely used and the complete sequencing of the gliadins had been achieved. It was now possible to produce synthetic analogues of these peptides. Ciclitira began to dissect the antigenic structure of these cereal peptides using monoclonal antibodies. It was costly, tedious and painstaking work, as other European workers, notably in Oslo, Holland and Italy would agree. However, over the years he managed to clone T cells from biopsies of patients with coeliac disease and show that they react to re-stimulation with individual synthetic peptides releasing various cytokines in the process.[185] He could block this reaction with antibody to HLA antigens confirming the importance of HLA in the binding of T cells to gluten antigens. So at last, like others on the continent, he had pinpointed some of the actual peptides causing coeliac disease. Recently he has managed to alter one of the peptides by substituting a single amino acid in the peptide chain, which prevents its recognition by T cells. Ciclitira's goal is to manufacture a safe and acceptable form of wheat. There are many peptides to be altered and the response of the T cell to them is diverse, so he has a job on his hands before the safe but cumbersome gluten-free diet is replaced.

---

†   Lord Rayne (1918–2003), property developer and philanthropist, was a governor of St. Thomas's Hospital and a member of the council of its medical school for 30 years.

CHAPTER THIRTY-THREE

SCREENING…TO TREAT OR NOT TO TREAT?

a) *Endoscopic biopsy*

Meanwhile clinicians continued to recommend a gluten-free diet confident of success. In theory diagnosis of coeliac disease was now accurate and treatment effective. However, the Crosby capsule technique was tedious and time-consuming and X-ray screening was needed to ensure that the device had reached the jejunum. The capsule could take only one piece of tissue at a time and frequently failed to obtain a biopsy. Brian Scott (born 1945) in Leeds had shown that the coeliac lesion was patchy so a single biopsy could be misleading.[186] He did this by using a hydraulic biopsy device capable of taking of dozens of biopsies in quick succession, which had been developed by Quinton and Rubin in America. Unfortunately the instrument was quite a mouthful and though useful as a research tool, was unsuitable for general use.[187]

By now fibreoptic endoscopy was widely practised and it occurred to Brian Prout (1933–85), physician to the new Royal Cornwall Hospital (Treliske), that a Crosby capsule could be muzzle-loaded through a gastroscope and fed into the jejunum.[188] The technique was quick and avoided the need for X-rays but failed to catch on because it still relied on the Crosby capsule obtaining a specimen.

Greg Holdstock (born 1950), Senior Registrar in Bournemouth and Southampton, used this technique for a time but decided to go one better by taking biopsies with forceps directly from the descending duodenum.[189] Hitherto the duodenal bulb had been considered unsuitable for the diagnosis of coeliac disease because acid-related duodenitis and villous blunting commonly confused the picture, but Fiona Stevens and Ciaron McCarthy in Galway had shown that villous atrophy could be demonstrated in duodenal cap biopsies.[190] Holdstock enlisted the help of Peter Isaacson (born 1937), a pathologist in Southampton with a particular interest in coeliac disease, who later was to define the T-cell lymphoma that occasionally complicates the disease. He showed that biopsies obtained with endoscopic forceps were adequate for histological evaluation.[191] Others confirmed this, notably Brian Scott with the help of his pathologist David Jenkins in Lincoln.[192] The seal of approval came from Peter Cotton (born 1939) and his group at the Middlesex Hospital who showed unequivocally that obtaining multiple biopsies from the descending duodenum was the most reliable method for diagnosis.[193]

This was a great advance on the Crosby capsule technique and changed practice overnight. Obtaining biopsies was now simple and quick and the detection of coeliac disease doubled. Many patients with, for example, obscure iron-deficiency anaemia were found to have coeliac disease.

A gluten-free diet was effective but not every patient was prepared to accept the restrictions of a diet day in and day out. No harm seemed to accrue from the occasional or even regular dietary indiscretion. Why ruin a good dinner with friends or a holiday abroad?

When Morrice McCrae and Bill Sircus in Edinburgh bewailed how frequently their young patients were lost to follow-up and "neglected", the reason was simple. The patients thought they were cured and no longer needed a special diet. Among more than 100 patients only two felt ill enough to seek medical advice.[194]

A survey by Christine Swinson (born 1949), honorary senior registrar to Jonathan Levi (1933–99) at Northwick Park Hospital, indirectly made the same point when bemoaning the fact that coeliac disease was being overlooked in many parts of the country.[195] Her point was that many coeliacs had trivial symptoms but felt vastly better after treatment. But how many patients would adhere to a diet if their symptoms were so trivial? Was there a case for a low-gluten diet as opposed to a gluten-free diet? Parveen Kumar thought there was.

Parveen Kumar was born in Lahore and the family fled to England during partition in 1947. She qualified at St. Bartholomew's Hospital and began her career in bacteriology, where she taught herself the rudiments of immunology. In her MD thesis she compared the mucosal changes

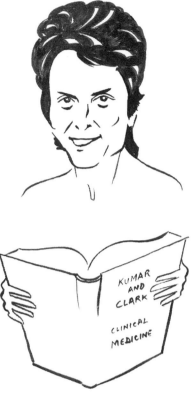

36 Kumar – Popular textbook.

of coeliac disease with dermatitis herpetiformis stimulating her lifelong interest in malabsorption. She joined the gastroenterology unit at Bartholomew's Hospital headed by Anthony (later Sir Anthony) Dawson (1928–97), a distinguished physician who ran a fine research department. Kumar's colleagues included Michael Clark (born 1935), with whom she wrote her well-known textbook of general medicine, Michael Lancaster-Smith (born 1939), who had developed immunofluorescent antibody techniques with John Holborow at Taplow,[196] and Michael Farthing (born 1949), whose interest lay in nutrition. Dawson had forged close links with John Harries (1934–83) at Great Ormond Street and with his successor Peter Milla (born 1944), after Harries' death at the early age of 49. He also collaborated closely with John Walker-Smith, Professor of Paediatric Gastroenterology at St. Bartholomews Hospital and the Queen Elizabeth Hospital for Children, taking over the coeliac patients as they became adolescent.

Kumar soon realised that very few of the teenage patients were bothering with a strict diet so Tony Dawson suggested that they should find out if it was really necessary. The next thirteen patients were allowed one 2.5 gram item of gluten each day and monitored closely. They did well and serum IgA antibody levels fell to normal, as expected. Folate deficiency was corrected and the intestinal mucosa recovered, apart from a mild infiltration of lymphocytes in the epithelium. Though the study was short and the long-term significance of the lymphocytosis uncertain, Kumar and her colleagues concluded that a small amount of gluten was harmless and a reasonable compromise if it improved compliance.[197]

At about the same time in March 1989 Geoffrey Holmes (born 1943) published his long-term follow up of the late Trevor Cooke's patients which showed for the first time that a strict gluten-free diet reduced the chances of malignancy in coeliac disease. Malignancy was uncommon so some years earlier Chris Booth, by then at the Clinical Research Centre, Northwick Park Hospital, had set up a national collaborative study to look at the size and nature of the problem.[198] A register of approximately 400 patients from all over the country with coeliac disease and malignancy was collated by Christine Swinson and the details verified by a panel of histologists chaired by Gordon Slavin (born 1933). Lymphoma was twice as common as expected. Adenocarcinoma of the small intestine was almost a hundred times more common than usual but even this meant an incidence of only 50 per 100,000 per annum, about the same as colon cancer in the ordinary population. Clearly to establish that a gluten-free diet prevented these rare cancers would take a long time.

Holmes' study was remarkable and his paper in *Gut* attracted considerable attention, becoming one of the most cited papers of the decade.[199] It was a masterpiece of epidemiology, typical of the Birmingham group, which extended over 25 years, beginning with Cooke's original study, which had shown that malignancy could complicate coeliac disease. At the time (1967) Cook summarised that a gluten-free diet might protect patients from malignant complications but he felt that his evidence was inconclusive.[200] Ten years later Holmes, who had joined Cooke's team, reviewed the progress of the original patients and included several more so that he now had over 200 patients with biopsy-proven coeliac disease.[201] He was still unable to say that a strict diet prevented malignant complications. "The evidence that coeliac disease harboured malignant potential was very strong" but he believed it would be several years before he could show that a gluten-free diet reduced the risk. He thought this would need an analysis of a huge group of patients treated from childhood.

Nonetheless twelve years later Holmes returned with his final report. Once again non-Hodgkin's lymphoma was the commonest form of malignancy and oddly he had no examples of carcinoma of the small intestine, which was easily the commonest cancer on Swinson's national register. Holmes showed that the 108 patients who had been on a strict gluten-free diet for more than five years were no more likely to get cancer than normal. In contrast 102 patients who had been slack about their diet remained at risk. Even so two patients on the strict diet developed lymphoma indicating that even five years treatment was insufficient to reverse the effect of an oncogenic stimulus present since infancy (unless of course they were not on as strict a diet as he thought). After this most clinicians insisted on a strict diet for life, though the relative risk of developing cancer for an individual coeliac patient was small.

Thanks to small-intestinal biopsy, coeliac disease was much more common than previously thought. In Nottingham, Michael Langman collaborated with Leonard Arthur (1926–83), a paediatrician in Derby. They reviewed all the children with villous atrophy born between 1965 and 1972 and calculated that the prevalence was 1 in 900, which roughly agreed with the figures from Anne Ferguson in Edinburgh.[202] This was twice as common as McCrae had found in the West of Scotland before the days of biopsy. Then curiously several paediatricians noticed that the clinical disease seemed to be disappearing.

James Littlewood (born 1933) in Leeds realised that no one was making use of his jejunal biopsy service[203] and David Challacombe (born 1937) in Taunton reported that he did not have a single case of coeliac disease in 1980.[204] It was the same in Glasgow where Sandy McNeish saw a dramatic fall in numbers.[205] Membership of the Coeliac Society even fell for a time.[206]

In fact coeliac disease was not disappearing at all, it was being postponed.

In 1974 the Department of Health and Social Security encouraged a return to breast feeding and a bi-product of this advice was delayed exposure to gluten. John Walker-Smith looked at children born between

1960 and 1985 and found that the disease was indeed presenting later, which he thought reflected the changes in feeding practice.[207]

The rising number of people with the disease reflected the ability of doctors to recognise it, though it could still be overlooked by both clinicians and pathologists.[208] Many patients had trivial symptoms and symptomless cases were common, for example, among healthy relatives. Pathologists argued about so-called latent coeliac disease. What would be reported as normal mucosa by most pathologists might have subtle changes only apparent to specialists in the field. The true prevalence of coeliac disease would only become apparent when it was possible to make the diagnosis with a simple blood test.

b) Antibody tests

Intestinal biopsy was invasive so for years doctors had looked for a simple antibody test. They began in earnest when the possibility of an immune basis to the disease became apparent. Early on immunoglobulin abnormalities were recognised, notably by Jack Hobbs and Gershon Hepner (born 1938) at the Hammersmith[209] but also by John Walker-Smith, then in Sydney, who found elevated serum IgA levels in coeliac children, which returned to normal on a gluten-free diet.[210] Falchuk and Strober, two pioneers in coeliac disease in America, showed that much of the immunoglobulin produced by the jejunum was an antibody to gliadin. People disagreed about the significance of these antibodies, which were often undetectable yet frequently found in patients without coeliac disease. One view promoted by Christopher Booth and William Doe at the Hammersmith[211] and supported for several years by Sidney Truelove in Oxford,[212] suggested these antibodies reflected an underlying Arthus phenomenon.[†] Indeed Truelove thought he had found a skin test using a gluten extract specific for coeliac disease but no one else could make it work.[213]

As support for the lymphocyte-mediated response grew, people began to realise that circulating antibody to gliadin could be simply an epiphenomenon and its inconsistency frustrated early hopes of its use in diagnosis. But a chance observation in 1971 was eventually to prove highly significant. This was the discovery of an auto antibody by John Holborow (1918 -2009).

[†]   Tissue damage due to an antigen antibody and complement reaction.

Holborow had served in the Middle East where he became interested in rheumatic fever and streptococcal disease. His colonel, John Dacie, helped him to obtain an appointment in bacteriology at the Hammersmith Hospital, where he met Eric Bywaters (1911–2002), a pioneer rheumatologist. When Bywaters moved to the Canadian Red Cross War Memorial Hospital in Taplow to set up the new MRC Rheumatism Unit, he took Holborow with him. Like other bacteriologists, Holborow became interested in the new science of immunology (against Bywaters' advice) and was one of the first people in England to find auto-antibodies using the new staining technique of immuno-fluorescence.[214] He added patients' serum to various organs in the rat and examined the sections with conjugates of fluorescein-labelled immunogloublin, usually IgG. Antibodies if present could be seen fluorescing under a filtered microscope.

It was to Holborow that Lionel Fry at St. Mary's Hospital turned when he hoped to find an immunological abnormality linking dermatitis herpetiformis with an enteropathy. Holborow duly obliged and found a new antibody directed against connective tissue, which he had not seen before. He thought this was an auto-antibody reacting with connective tissue or reticulin and called it anti-reticulin antibody.[215] Many coeliacs had it, especially children, and it also occurred in some patients with Crohn's Disease, but it was rarely found in normal people.[216] It usually faded in response to a gluten-free diet so he thought it was probably specific for coeliac disease.[217]

Others, notably Ralph Wright in Southampton,[218] Trevor Cooke in Birmingham[219] and the Galway group[220] all confirmed Holborow's discovery and showed that the anti-reticulin antibody was even more sensitive and specific for coeliac disease if IgA-class antibody was used rather than IgG. Even so the test still missed too many patients with coeliac disease to be useful as a screening procedure.

In 1975 Holborow moved to the London Hospital to head the MRC Immunology Group, Bone and Joint Research Unit. Here he took on a PhD student, Joe Unsworth[†] to study antibody responses in coeliac children in collaboration with John Walker-Smith at the Queen Elizabeth Hospital for Children in Hackney. Unsworth's task was to see if he could

---

†   Unsworth heard of Holborow through his ABC series on immunology in the *Brit. Med. J.* By the time he applied for the PhD, the job had been filled. Fortunately there was money for another project in coeliac immunology.

block the anti-reticulin antibody with a surfeit of gliadin by adding it to the sera of coeliac patients with the antibody. He did not succeed but in the process inadvertently added gliadin to patients without anti-reticulin antibody and to his surprise they appeared to become positive. Intrigued the team realised that gliadin antigen/antibody complexes must be adhering to the reticulin and went on to show that gliadin itself was capable of binding selectively to reticulin fibres.[221]

They capitalised on this discovery by introducing a new immuno-fluorescent test for gluten sensitivity, which detected antibodies to gliadin in blood of coeliacs.[222] (The beauty of the test was that it was very similar to the anti-reticulin antibody test.) The test was very good at detecting gluten sensitivity but unfortunately many children without coeliac disease tested positive. It still seemed that antibody tests would never replace a biopsy as the definitive diagnostic tool.

The breakthrough came, as so often, rather unexpectedly. A group of dermatologists in America were studying the immunology of bullous skin lesions. Skin is a poor substrate for antibody testing because it is so rich in immunoglublin G. Consequently a skin substitute was used, in this case the oesophageal lining from a marmoset monkey. Furthermore dermatologists use IgA antisera rather than IgG antisera. Therefore when Chorzelski and his colleagues in Buffalo, USA, decided to look at anti-reticulin factor in patients with dermatitis herpetiformis they naturally used the monkey (a primate) oesophagus rather than rat kidney, and IgA antisera rather than IgG, and found an antibody that they called endomysial antibody (EMA).[223] This was virtually identical to the reticulin antibody but proved to be far more sensitive and specific in the detection of dermatitis herpetiformis and coeliac disease. It was invariably present in untreated coeliac disease but never found in patients with other bowel diseases. The combination of an anti-gliaden antibody test and the EMA test could now be safely used to screen for coeliac disease. Indeed these tests proved even more reliable than biopsy evidence of coeliac disease.

The exact nature of the endomysial antibody remained elusive until 1997 when immuno-chemists in Germany led by Ernst Riecken[†] identified it using human umbilical cord (an alternative to monkey oesophagus). They exposed the antibody to a soup of antigens and

---

†   Riecken had worked with Chris Booth at the Hammersmith Hospital during the 1960s on lysosomal damage in the coeliac enterocyte and its recovery with steroid treatment.

using sequenced proteins and computers whittled away the possibilities until they had a glutamin-rich peptide that turned out to be the enzyme tissue transglutaminase.[224] This was a painstaking and brilliant example of immuno-chemistry with far-reaching consequences. The test for endomysial antibody could now be done using an immuno-assay technique (ELISA) rather than the immuno-fluorescent technique. This allowed the detection of lower titres of endomysial antibody than was possible with immuno-fluorescence and could be automated saving a great deal of staff time.

Identification of tissue transglutaminase (TTG) as the auto-antigen provided a further clue to the pathogenesis of coeliac disease. It transpired that TTG influences the cellular immune response to gluten. Scientists in Oslo and the Netherlands have recently identified several gluten peptides that can cause coeliac disease and much of the research over 40 years is falling into place. Only patients with certain HLA class II molecules get coeliac disease. These molecules, which are found on the surface of antigen-presenting cells, bind gluten peptides and present them to CD4 T lymphocytes. But they can only do this with the help of tissue transglutaminase so TTG is an essential element in the pathogenesis of coeliac disease as well as providing a valuable diagnostic test through its antibody, EMA.[225]

The discovery of a reliable blood test transformed the diagnosis of coeliac disease. It was now feasible to pick out people at risk, such as relatives of patients with the disease. People with conditions known to be associated with coeliac disease such as diabetes mellitus or Down's syndrome can be screened and patients with unexplained osteomalacia or anaemia can have coeliac disease excluded without the need for an intestinal biopsy.

Such simple case-finding has inevitably increased awareness of coeliac disease and the incidence in the population has risen dramatically. Old estimates based on clinical and biopsy diagnosis of 1 in 500 or more increased to 1 in 200.[226] Recently a large survey of the adult population from the Cambridge area found that 1 in 100 of perfectly healthy people had coeliac disease.[227] The coeliac iceburg, first described by Carlo Catassi and his colleagues from Ancona in 1994, was reaching Titanic proportions.[228]

This provoked a debate over the merits of mass screening for coeliac disease. The protagonists argue that coeliac disease is common and easily overlooked. Effective treatment is available and prevents complications such as chronic ill health, stunted growth, skeletal disorders and malignancy. The case seems compelling but, as Parveen Kumar argues, is it?

If only a minority of these patients have symptoms the benefit of detecting "occult" disease has yet to be shown. There is a world of difference between case-finding and mass screening. Whether screening will reduce mortality is highly debatable and there is as yet no evidence to suggest that a gluten-free diet prevents malignancy or metabolic bone disease in occult cases. The recent survey in Cambridge by Kay-Tee Khaw (born 1950) in collaboration with Geoff Holmes in Derby and Richard Logan (born 1947) in Nottingham, failed to show any harm among those discovered to have coeliac disease. Indeed there was some evidence that the coeliacs were less at risk from cardiovascular disease. Even if treatment was justified, compliance has always been a problem, even among symptomatic patients. "We should not," wrote Kumar in 2003, "be the harbingers of yet another source of anxiety for the general population (often helped by the media), making us an even more neurotic population. Pragmatism must win over misguided purism."[229]

Coeliac disease has fascinated doctors for over a century. We are now close to understanding how gluten damages the villi of the small intestine and many hope an alternative to the safe but tedious gluten-free diet is not far away. Whether the likes of Paul Ciclitira can fool the T lymphocytes by substituting amino acids in the offending gliadin peptides, or whether inhibitors of tissue transglutaminase or other compounds that can prevent T cell activation will be developed remains to be seen.

REFERENCES

SECTION THREE

1   Gee S. 1888 On the coeliac affection. *St. Bart. Hosp. Rep.* 24 17–20

2   Dowd B., Walker-Smith J. A. 1974 Samuel Gee, Aretaeus, and the coeliac affection. *Brit. Med. J.* i 45–47

3   Fletcher P. 1633 *The Purple Islands or The Isle of Man: Together with Piscatorie Eclogs and Other Poeticall Miscellanies.* Cambridge, Universitie of Cambridge.

4   Lempriere J. 1788 *A Classical Dictionary.* Reading T. Cadell, London

5   Moore N. 1918 *The History of St. Bartholemew's Hospital.* C. Arthur Pearson Ltd. London vol 2 733

6   Gull W. 1855 Fatty stools from disease of the mesenteric glands. *Guy's Hosp. Reports.* i: 369

7   Adams F. 1856 *The Extant Works of Aretaeus, the Cappadocian.* Printed for the Sydenham Society

8   Gibbons R. A. 1889 The coeliac affection in children. *Edin. Med. J.* 35: 321–330 and 420–428

9   Bodley Scott R. 1974 *The Royal Hospital of St. Bartholemew 1123–1973.* ed. by Medvei V. C., Thornton J. L. London p188

10 Manson P. 1880 China. *Imperial Maritime Customs. Medical Reports for the half-year ended 31st March 1880.* 19th Issue. Published by order of the Inspector General of Customs. Shanghai 33–37

11 Fayrer J. 1881 *Tropical Dysentery and Chronic Diarrhoea.* J & A Churchill, London 121–171

12 Cheadle W. B. 1903 A clinical lecture on Acholia. *Lancet* i: 1497–1500

13 Herter C. A. 1908 *Infantilism From Chronic Intestinal Infection.* Macmillan New York

14 Heubner J. O L. 1909 *Jahrb. f. Kinderheilk* Berlin 70 667

15 Still G. F. 1918 The Lumleian lectures on coeliac disease. *Lancet* ii: 163, 193, 227

16 Miller R. 1921 A fatal case of coeliac infantilism. *Lancet* i: 743–746

17 Ryle J. A. 1924 Fatty stools from obstruction of the lacteals. *Guy's Hosp. Reports* 74: 1–8

18 Clarke J. 1815 *Commentaries on Some of the Most Important Diseases of Children.* Longman, Herst, Rees, Orme & Brown, London p86–90

19   Trousseau A. 1862 Clinique medicale de l'Hotel Dieu de Paris, 2, 112–4

20   Trousseau A. 1867 *Lectures on Clinical Medicine*. New Sydenham Soc., London. 35: 370

21   Langmead, F. 1913 Discussion on Alimentary Toxaemia; its Sources, Consequences and Treatment. *Proceedings of the Royal Society of Medicine* 6: (Gen. Rep.) 319–320

22   Cantlie J. 1913 Some recent observations on sprue. *Brit. Med. J.* ii 1296–97

23   Bassett-Smith P. 1919 A case of sprue with associated tetany. *Lancet* I 178

24   Scott H. H. 1923 The nature and treatment of sprue. *Brit. Med. J.* ii 1135–37

25   Low G. C. 1928 Sprue. An analytical study of 150 cases. *Quart. J. Med.* 21 523–534

26   Percival T. 1789 *Essays Medical, Philosophical and Experimental*, 4th ed., vol 2

27   Franklin A. W. 1954 Rickets, in *The History and Conquest of Common Diseases*. ed. By W. R. Bett, University of Oklahoma Press.

28   Gee S. 1868 Rickets. *St. Bart. Hosp. Rep.* 4, 69

29   Baldwin E. 1961 Gowland Hopkins The discovery of vitamins. Van Den Bergh

30   Funk C. 1914 *Die Vitamine*. Wiesbaden

31   Jones F. A. 1992 New concepts in human nutrition in the twentieth century: the special role of micronutrients. The Caroline Walker Lecture, 1992

32   Mellanby E. 1919–20 Discussion on the importance of accessory food factors (vitamines) in the feeding of infants. *Proceedings of the Royal Society of Medicine. Sect. Dis. Child.* 13 52

33   McCollum E. V. et al. 1922 An experimental demonstration of the existence of a vitamin which promotes calcium absorption. *J. Biol. Chem.* 53 293

34   Parsons L. G 1913 Intestinal infantilism – discussion. *Birmingham Med. Review.* 74: 33

35   Parsons L. G. 1927 The bone changes occurring in renal and coeliac infantilism and their relationship to rickets. *Arch. Dis. Child.* ii 1 & 98

36   Linder G. C., Harris C. F. 1930 Calcium and phosphorus metabolism in chronic diarrhoea with tetany. *Quart. J. Med.* 23: 195–211

37   Mackay H. M. M. 1923 Studies of rickets in Vienna 1919–22. MRC Special Report series No 77

38   Mackay H. M. M. 1931 Nutritional anaemia in infancy. MRC Special Report series No 157

39   Tidy H. L. 1920 in discussion of paper by Fletcher H. M. A case of renal infantilism. *Proceedings of the Royal Society of Medicine* (Sect. Child Dis.) xiii, 123

40   Hampson A. C., Shackle J. W. 1924 Megalocytic and non-mgalocytic anaemias. *Guy's Hosp. Reports* 74: 193–216

41   Minot G. R., Murphy W. P. 1926 Treatment of pernicious anaemia by a special diet. *J.A.M.A.* 87: 470–476

42   Wills L 1931 Treatment of "pernicious anaemia of pregnancy" and "tropical anaemia". *Brit. Med. J.* i: 1059–64

43   Davidson S. 1931 Vitamin B in anaemia. *Lancet* ii 1395–98

44   Vaughan J. M., Hunter D. 1932 The treatment by Marmite of megalocytic hyperchromic anaemia occurring in idiopathic steatorrhoea. *Lancet* i 829–834

45   Bennett T. I., Hunter D., Vaughan J. M. 1932 Idiopathic steatorrhoea (Gee's disease). A nutritional disturbance associated with tetany, osteomalacia and anaemia. *Quart. J. Med. n.s.* 4: 603–6677

46   Thaysen T. E. H. 1929 The "Coeliac Affection" – idiopathic steatorrhoeas. *Lancet* i 1086–89

47   Hurst A. F. 1942 The pathogenesis of the sprue syndrome as seen in tropical sprue, non-tropical sprue and coeliac disease. *Guy's Hosp. Reports.* 91: 1–21

48   Hurst A. F. 1942 Severe case of the sprue syndrome. *Guy's Hosp. Reports* 91: 22–24

49   Thaysen T. E. H. 1932 *Non-tropcal Sprue: a Study of Idiopathic Steatorrhoea.* Oxford University Press

50   Verzar F., McDougall E. J. 1936 *Absorption From the Intestine.* Longmans, Green & Co, London

51   Bennett T. I., Hardwick C. 1940 Chronic jejuno-ileal insufficiency. *Lancet* ii 381–384

52   Frazer A. C. 1951 *Fat Absorption* chapter 21 Steatorrhoea 528–546

53   Frazer A. C., French J. M., Thompson M. D. 1949 Radiographic studies showing the induction of a segmentation pattern in the small intestine in normal human subjects. *Brit. J. Radiol.* 22 123–136

54   Astley R., French J. M. 1951 The small intestine pattern in normal children and in coeliac disease: its relationship to the nature of the opaque medium. *Brit. J. Radiol.* 24: 321–330

55   Paulley J. W. 1959 quoted in Emotion and Personality in the etiology of steatorrhoea. *Amer. J. Dig. Dis. n.s.* 4 352

56   Paulley J. W. 1950 Ulcerative colitis – a study of 173 patients. *Gastroenterology* 16 566

57   Paulley J. W. 1948 Regional ileitis. *Lancet* i 923

58   Paulley J. W. 1949 Chronic diarrhoea symposium *Proceedings of the Royal Society of Medicine* 42: 241–244

59   Paulley J. W. 1959 Emotion and personality in the aetiology of steatorrhoea. *Amer. J. Dig. Dis.* 4 352–360

60   Manson-Bahr P. 1924 Sprue histology *Lancet* I 1148

61   Paulley J. W. 1949 op. cit. 243

62   Paulley J. W. 1951 Discussion on the aetiology of the sprue syndrome *Gastroenterologia* 78 Fasc 6 361

63   Paulley J. W. 1952 *Transactions of the Roy. Soc. Trop. Med. & Hyg.* 46: 594–595

64   Paulley J. W. 1954 Observations on the aetiology of idiopathic steatorrhoea; Jejunal and lymph node biopsies. *Brit. Med. J.* ii 1318–29

65   Haas S. V. 1924 The value of the banana in the treatment of celiac disease, *Amer J. Dis. Child* 24: 421–437

66   Andersen D. H. 1947 Celiac syndrome VI The relationship of celiac disease. starch intolerance, and steatorrhea. *J. Paed.* 30: 564–582

67   Sheldon W. 1949 Coeliac disease: a relation between dietary starch and fat absorption. *Arch. Dis. Child.* 24: 81–87

68   Van Berge-Henegouwen G. P., Mulder C. J. J. 1993 History of Dicke's discovery of the gluten-free diet for coeliac sprue. In *Gastro-intestinal Disease* Ed M.H. Sleisenger and J. S. Fordtran W. B. Saunders 5th ed chap 50 1072–77

69   Booth C. C. 1989 History of coeliac disease. *Brit. Med. J.* I 527

70   Dicke W. K. 1941 Simple dietary treatment for the syndrome of Gee-Herter. *Ned. Tijdschr. Geneeskd.* 85 1715 (in Dutch)

71   Van de Kamer J. H. 1974 Coeliac disease: a Historical Review. *J. Irish Med. Assoc.* 67 405–406

72   Dicke W. K., Van de Kamer J. H., Weijers H. A. 1953 Coeliac disease II The presence in wheat of a factor having a deleterious effect in cases of coeliac disease. *Acta. Paediatr.* 42: 34

73   Dicke W. K. 1950 Coeliac disease. Investigation of the harmful effects of certain types of cereal on patients with coeliac disease. Thesis. Univ. of Utrecht, The Netherlands (in Dutch).

74   Weijers H. A. 1950 Fat absorption in normal and diseased neonates and children, especially in patients with coeliac disease. Thesis. Univ. of Utrecht. The Netherlands (in Dutch).

75   Van de Kamer J. H., Ten Bokkel Huinink H., Weijers H. A. 1949 Rapid method for the determination of fat in faeces. *J. Biol. Chem.* 177: 347

76   Anderson C. M., Frazer A. C., French J. M., Gerrard J. W., Sammons H. G., Smellie J. M. 1952 Coeliac disease: gastro-intestinal studies and the effect of dietary wheat flour. *Lancet* I 836–842

77   Hardwicke C. 1939 Prognosis in coeliac disease: a review of seventy-three cases. *Arch. Dis. Child* 14: 279–294

78   Sheldon W. 1955 *Diseases of Infancy and Childhood.* p217 Churchill, London

79   Davidson L. S. P., Fountain J. R. 1950 Incidence of sprue syndrome with some observations on the natural history. *Brit. Med. J.* i: 1157–61

80   Cooke W. T., Peeney A. L. P., Hawkins C. F. 1953 Symptoms, signs, and diagnostic features of idiopathic steatorrhoea. *Quart. J. Med. n.s.* 22: 59–77

81   French J. M., Hawkins C. F., Smith N. 1957 The effect of a wheat-gluten-free diet in adult idiopathic steatorrhoea. A study of 22 cases. *Quart. J. Med. n.s.* 26 481–499

82   Wood I. J., Doig R. K., Motteram R., Hughes A. 1949 Gastric biopsy *Lancet* i 18–21

83   Shiner M. 1956 Duodenal biopsy. *Lancet* i: 17–19

84   Shiner M. 1956 Jejunal-biopsy tube *Lancet* i: 85

85   Shiner M. 1957 Duodenal and jejunal biopsies. I. A discussion of the method, its difficulties and applications. *Gastroenterology* 33: 64–70

86   Shiner M., Doniach I. 1960 Histopathologic studies in steatorrhoea. *Gastroenterology* 38: 419–440

87   Doniach I., Shiner M. 1957 Duodenal and jejunal biopsies II Histology. *Gastroenterology* 33: 71–76

88   Crosby W. H., Kugler H. W. 1957 Intraluminal biopsy of the small intestine. The intestinal biopsy capsule. *Amer. J. Dig. Dis. n.s.* 2 236–241

89   Fone D. J., Cooke W. T., Meynell M. J., Brewer D. B., Harris E. L., Cox E. V. 1960 Jejunal biopsy in adult celiac disease and allied disorders. *Lancet* i: 933–938

90   Sakula J., Shiner M. 1957 Coeliac disease with atrophy of the small-intestine mucosa. *Lancet* i: 876–877

91   Shiner M. 1960 Coeliac disease: Histopathological findings in the small intestinal mucosa studied by a peroral biopsy technique. *Gut* 1 48–54

92   Cameron A. H., Astley R., Hallowell M., Rawson A. B., Miller C. G., French J. M., Hubble D. V. 1962 Duodenal-jejunal biopsy in the investigation of children with coeliac disease. *Quart. J. Med.* n s 31: 125–140

93   Hubble D. V. 1963 Diagnosis and management of coeliac disease in childhood. *Brit. Med. J.* ii: 701–6

94   Sheldon W., Tempany E. 1966 Small intestine peroral biopsy in coeliac children. *Gut* 7: 481–489

95   Sheldon W. 1969 Prognosis in Early Adult Life of Coeliac Children Treated with a Gluten-free Diet. *Brit. Med. J.* i; 401–404

96   Badenoch J. 1960 Steatorrhoea in the adult. *Brit. Med. J.* ii: 879 & 963

97   Davidson L. S. P., Girdwood R. H., Innes E. M. 1947 *Folic Acid in the Treatment of the Sprue Syndrome.*

98   Girdwood R. H., Delamore I. W., Williams A. W. 1961 Jejunal biopsy in malabsorptive disorders of the adult. *Brit. Med. J.* i; 319–323

99   Booth C. C., Chanarin I., Anderson B. B., Mollin D. L. 1957 The site of absorption and tissue distribution of orally administered 56Co – labelled vitamin B12 in the rat. *Brit. J. Haematol.* 3: 253–261

100   Booth C. C., Mollin D. L. 1959 The site of absorption of vitamin B12 in man. *Lancet* i: 18

101   Booth C. C. 1961 The metabolic effects of intestinal resection in man. *Postgrad. Med. J.* 37: 725–739

102   Holmes R., Hourihane D. O'B., Booth C. C. 1961 Dissecting microscope appearance of jejunal biopsy specimens from patients with idiopathic steatorrhoea. *Lancet* i: 81–83

103   Stewart J. S., Pollock D. J., Hoffbrand A. V., Mollin D. L., Booth C. C. 1967 A study of proximal and distal intestinal structure and absorptive function in idiopathic steatorrhoea. *Quart. J. Med.* n s 36: 425–444

104   Creamer B. 1962 Dynamics of the mucosa of the small intestine in idiopathic steatorrhoea. *Gut* 3: 295–300

105   Creamer B. 1964 Variations in small-intestinal villous shape and mucosal dynamics. *Brit. Med. J.* ii: 1371–73

106   Croft D. N., Loehry C. A., Taylor J. F. N., Cole J. 1968 DNA and cell loss from normal small-intestinal mucosa. *Lancet* ii: 70–73

107   Croft D. N., Loehry C. A., Creamer B. 1968 Small bowel cell-loss and weight-loss in the coeliac syndrome. *Lancet* ii: 68–70

108   Pink I. J., Croft D. N., Creamer B. 1970 Cell loss from the small intestinal mucosa: a morphological study. *Gut* 11 217–222

109   Creamer B. 1966 Coeliac thoughts. *Gut* 7 569–571

110   Pink I. J., Creamer B. 1967 Response to a gluten-free diet of patients with the coeliac syndrome. *Lancet* i: 300–304

111   Fairley N. H., Mackie F. P. 1937 The clinical and biochemical syndrome in lymphadenoma and allied diseases involving the mesenteric lymph glands. *Brit. Med. J.* i: 375–380

112   Best C. N., Cook P. B. 1961 Case of Mesenteric Reticulosarcoma Associated with Gluten-sensitive Steatorrhoea. *Brit. Med. J.* ii: 496–498

113   Gough K. R., Read A. E., Naish J. M. 1962 Intestinal reticulosis as a complication of idiopathic steatorrhoea. *Gut* 3: 232–239

114   Creamer B. 1964 Malignancy and the small intestinal mucosa. *Brit. Med. J.* ii: 1435–36

115   Austad W. I., Cornes J. S., Gough K. R., McCarthy C. F., Read A. E. 1967 Steatorrhoea and malignant lymphoma. *Amer. J. Dig. Dis.* n s 12: 475–490

116   Harris O. D., Cooke W. T., Thompson H., Waterhouse J. A. H. 1967 Malignancy in Adult Coeliac Disease and Idiopathic Steatorrhoea. *Amer. J. Med.* 42: 899–912

117   Lindsay M. K. M., Nordin B. E. C., Norman A. P. 1956 Late prognosis in coeliac disease. *Brit. Med. J.* i: 14–18

118   Mortimer P. E., Stewart J. S., Norman A. P., Booth C. C. 1968 Follow-up Study of Coeliac Disease. *Brit. Med. J.* ii: 7–9

119   Young W. F., Pringle E. M. 1971 110 Children with Coeliac Disease, 1950–69 *Arch. Dis. Child.* 46: 421–436

120   Sheldon W., Tempany E. 1966 op. cit. p488

121   McNeish A. S. 1967 Jejunal biopsy in infants and underweight children. *Arch. Dis. Child* 42 623–625

122   Booth C. C., Dowling R. H. 1970 *Coeliac Disease* Churchill Livingstone, Edinburgh

123   Meeuwisse G. 1970 Diagnostic criteria in coeliac disease. *Acta. Paed. Scand.* 59:461–464

124   McNeish A. S., Harms H. K., Rey J., Shmerling D. H., Visacorpi J. K., Walker-Smith J. A. 1979 The diagnosis of coeliac disease. *Arch. Dis. Child.* 54: 783–786

125   Carter C., Sheldon W., Walker C. 1959 The inheritance of coeliac disease. *Ann. Hum. Genet.* 23 266–278

126   McCrae W. M. 1969 The inheritance of coeliac disease. *J. Med. Genet.* 6: 129–131

127   Kirby J., Fielding J. F. 1984 Very adult coeliac disease! The need for jejunal biopsy in the middle aged and elderly. *Irish Med. J.* . 77: 263–267

128   Mortimer P. 1970 quoted by Booth C. C. in *Coeliac Disease*. Ed. Booth C. C., Dowling R. H. Churchill Livingstone, Edinburgh & London p62

129   McCrae W. M. 1970 The inheritance of coeliac disease. In *Coeliac Disease*, ed. Booth C. C., Dowling R. H. Churchill Livingstone, Edinburgh & London, 55–63

130   Mylotte M., Egan-Mitchell B., McCarthy C. F., McNicholl B. 1973 Incidence of coeliac disease in the West of Ireland. *Brit. Med. J.* i: 703–706

131   Moynahan E. J. 1973 Coeliac disease in the West of Ireland. *Brit. Med. J.* i: 484

132 Frazer A. C., Fletcher R. F., Ross C. A. C., Shaw B., Sammons H. G., Schneider R. 1959 Gluten-induced enteropathy: the effect of partially digested gluten. *Lancet* ii: 252–255

133 Frazer A. C. 1960 Pathogenetic concepts of the malabsorption syndrome. *Gastroenterology* 38: 389–398

134 Riecken E. O., Stewart J. S., Booth C. C., Pearse A. G. E. A histochemical study on the role of lysosymes in idiopathic steatorrhoea before and during a gluten-free diet. *Gut* 7 317–332

135 Douglas A. P., Booth C. C. 1970 Digestion of gluten peptides by normal human jejunal mucosa and by mucosa from patients with adult coeliac disease. *Clin. Sci.* 38: 11–25

136 Weiser M.M., Douglas A. P. 1976 An alternative mechanism for gluten toxicity in coeliac disease. *Lancet* i: 567–569

137 Peters T. J., Bjarnason I. 1984 Coeliac syndrome: biochemical mechanisms and the missing peptidase hypothesis revisited. *Gut* 25: 913–918

138 Taylor K. B., Thompson D. L., Truelove S. C., Wright R. 1961 1961 An immunological study of coeliac disease and idiopathic steatorrhoea. *Brit. Med. J.* ii 1727–31

139 Taylor K. B., Truelove S. C., Wright R. 1964 Serological reaction to gluten and cow's milk proteins in gastrointestinal disease. *Gastroenterology* 46: 99–108

140 Wall A. J., Douglas A. P., Booth C. C., Pearse A. G. F. 1970 Response of the jejunal mucosa in adult coeliac disease to oral prednisolone.*Gut* 11 7–14

141 Hobbs J. R., Hepner G. W., Douglas A. P., Crabbe P. A., Johansson S. G. O. 1969 Immunological mystery of coeliac disease. *Lancet* ii: 649–650

142 Crabbe P. A., Heremans J. F. 1966 Distribution of immunoglobulin – containing cellsalong the gastrointestinal tract. *Gastroenterology* 51: 305

143 Shiner M., Ballard J. 1972 Antigen-antibody reactions in jejunal mucosa in childhood coeliac disease after gluten challenge. *Lancet* i: 1202–05

144 Doe W. F., Henry K., Booth C. C. 1975 Complement in coeliac disease. In *Coeliac Disease*. Ed. W. Th. J. M. Thekkens and A. S. Pena, pp189–194, Stenfert Kroese, Leiden

145 Webster A. D. B., Slavin G., Shiner. M., Platts-Mills T. A. E., Asherson G. L. 1981 Coeliac disease with severe hypogammaglobulinaemia. *Gut* 22: 153–7

146 Stokes P. L., Asquith P., Holmes G. K. T., Mackintosh P., Cooke W. T. 1972 Histocompatibility antigens associated with adult coeliac disease *Lancet* ii: 162–4

147 Mackintosh P., 1981 A critical analysis of HLA in coeliac family studies in Birmingham. In *The Genetics of Coeliac Disease*. Ed. R. B. McConnell MTP Press Ltd. Lancaster pp201–206

148 Mackintosh P., Asquith P. 1978 HLA and Coeliac Disease. *British Medical Bulletin* 34: 291–294

149 Clarke C. A. 1981 Clinical genetics: the wider horizon. In *The Genetics of Coeliac Disease*. Ed R. B. McConnell MTP Press Ltd. Lancaster pxxiii

150 McCarthy C. F., Frazer I. D., Evans K. T., Read A. E. 1966 Lymphoreticular dysfunction in idiopathic steatorrhoea. *Gut* 7: 140

151 Marsh G, W., Stewart J. S. Splenic function in adult coeliac disease. *Brit. J. Haematol.* 19: 445–57

152 Ferguson A., Hutton M.M., Maxwell J. D. 1970 Adult coeliac disease in hyposplenic patients. *Lancet* i: 163–4

153 Ferguson A., Maxwell J. D., Carr K. E. 1969 Progressive changes in small intestinal villous pattern with increasing gestation. *J. Pathology* 99: 87–91

154 Shiner M. 1973 Ultrastructural changes suggestive of immune reactions in the jejunal mucosa of coeliac children following gluten challenge. *Gut* 14: 1–12

155 Ferguson A., Murray D. 1971 Quantitation of intraepithelial lymphocytes in human jejunum. *Gut* 12: 988–994

156 Ferguson A., Parrott D. M. V. 1972 The effect of antigen deprivation on thymus-dependent and thymus-independent lymphocytes in the small intestine of the mouse. *Clin. & Exp. Immunol.* 12 477–488

157 Ferguson A., Parrott D. M. V. 1973 Histopathology and time course of rejection of allografts of foetal mouse intestine. *Transplantation* 15: 546–554

158 Ferguson A., MacDonald T. T. 1977 Effects of local delayed hypersensitivity on the small intestine. In *Immunology of the Gut*. Ciba Foundation Symposium No 46 p322

159 MacDonald T. T., Ferguson A. 1976 Hypersensitivity reactions in the small intestine – 2 –- effects of allograft rejection on mucosal architecture and lymphoid cell infiltrate. *Gut* 17 81–91

160 Ferguson A., MacDonald T. T., McClure J. P., Holden R. J. 1975 Cell-mediated immunity to gliadin within the small-intestinal mucosa in coeliac disease. *Lancet* i: 895–897

161 Shuster S., Marks J. 1965 Dermatogenic enteropathy. *Lancet* i 1361–63

162 Fry L., Seah P. P., McMinn R. M. H., Hoffbrand A. V. 1972 Lymphocytic infiltration of epithelium in diagnosis of gluten-sensitive enteropathy. *Brit. Med. J.* iii: 371–374

163 Marsh M. N. 1992 Gluten, Major Histocompatibility Complex, and the Small Intestine. A Molecular and Immunobiologic Approach to the Spectrum of Gluten Sensitivity ("Celiac Sprue") *Gastroenterology* 102 p337

164 Marsh M. N., Swift J. A., Williams E. D. 1968 Studies of Small-intestinal Mucosa with the Scanning Electron Microscope. *Brit. Med. J.* iv 95–96

165 Leigh R. J., Marsh M. M., Crowe P. J., Garner V., Gordon D. B. 1985 Studies of intestinal lymphoid tissue IX – Dose-dependent gluten-induced lymphoid infiltration of coeliac jejunal epithelium. *Scand. J. Gastroenterol.* 20 715–719

166 Marsh M. N. 1990 Grains of truth: evolutionary changes in small intestinal mucosa in response to environmental antigen challenge. *Gut* 31 111–4

167 Marsh M. N., Bjarnason I., Shaw J., Ellis A., Baker R., Peters T. J. 1990 Studies of intestinal lymphoid tissue XIV-HLA status, mucosal morphology, permeability and epithelial lymphocyte populations in first degree relatives of patients with coeliac disease. *Gut* 31 32–36

168   Janossy G., Tidman N., Selby W. S., Thomas J. A., Granger S., Kung P. C., Goldstein G. 1980 Human T lymphocytes of inducer and suppressor type occupy different microenvironments. *Nature* 288: 81–84

169   Selby W. S., Janossy G., Jewell D. P. 1981 Immunohistological characterisation of intraepithelial lymphocytes of the human gastrointestinal tract. *Gut* 22 169–176

170   Selby W. S., Janossy G., Bofill M., Jewell D. P. 1983 Lymphocyte subpopulations in the human small intestine. The findings in normal mucosa and in the mucosa of patients with coeliac disease. *Clin. Exp. Immunol.* 52: 219

171   Howdle P. D., Corazza G. R., Bullen A. W., Losowsky M. S. 1981 In-vitro diagnosis of celiac disease: an assessment. *Gut* 22 939–947

172   Malizia G., Trejdosiewicz L. K., Wood G. M., Howdle P. D., Janossy G. Losowsky M. S. 1985 The microenvironment of celiac disease: T cell phenocytes and expression of the T2 "T Blast" antigen by small bowel lymphocytes. *Clin. Exp. Immunol.* 60 437

173   Scott B. B., Goodall A., Stephenson P., Jenkins D. 1984 Small intestinal plasma cells in coeliac disease. *Gut* 25 41–46

174   Wood G. M., Shires S., Howdle P. D., Losowsky M. S. 1986 Immunoglobulin production by celiac biopsies in organ culture. *Gut* 27 1151–60

175   MacDonald T. T., Spencer J. M. 1988 Evidence that activated T cells play a role in the development of enteropathy in human small intestine. *J. Exp. Med.* 167: 1341–49

176   Spencer J. M., MacDonald T. T., Diss T. C., Walker-Smith J. A., Ciclitira P. J., Isaacson P. G. 1989 Changes in intraepithelial lymphocyte subpopulations in coeliac disease and enteropathy associated T cell lymphoma (malignant histiocytosis of the intestine). *Gut* 30 339–346

177   Kagnoff M. F., Paterson Y. J., Kumar P. J., Kasarda D. D., Carbone F. R., Unsworth D. J., Austin R. K. 1987 Evidence for a role of a human intestinal adenovirus in the pathogenesis of coeliac disease. *Gut* 28 995–1001

178   Mantzaris G. J., Karagiannis J. A., Priddle J. D., Jewell D. P. 1990 Cellular hypersensitivity to a synthetic dodecapeptide derived from human adenovirus 12 which resembles a sequence of A-gliadin in patients with coeliac disease. *Gut* 31 668–673

179   Howdle P. D., Zajdel M. E., Smart C. J., Trejdosiewicz L. K., Blair G. E., Losowsky M. S. 1989 Lack of a serologic response to an EIB protein of adenovirus 12 in celiac disease. *Scand. J. Gastroenterol.* 24: 282–6

180   Mahon J., Blair G. E., Wood G. M., Scott B. B., Losowsky M. S., Howdle P. D. 1991 Is persistent adenovirus 12 infection involved in coeliac disease? A search for viral DNA using the polymerase chain reaction. *Gut* 32 1114–16

181   Carter M. J., Willcocks M. M., Mitchison H. C., Record C. O., Madely C. R. 1989 Is a persistent adenovirus infection involved in celiac disease? *Gut* 30: 1563–67

182   Dissanayake A. S., Jerrome D. W., Offord R. E., Truelove S. C., Whitehead R. 1974 Identifying toxic fractions of wheat gluten and their effect on the jejuna mucosa in celiac disease. *Gut* 15: 931–946

183 Ciclitera P. J., Hunter, J. O. and Lennox E. S. 1980 Clinical testing of bread made from millisonic 6A wheats in coeliac patients. *Lancet*, ii 234–236

184 Howdle P. D., Ciclitira P. J., Simpson F. G., Losowsky M. S. 1981 Are all gliadins toxic in coeliac disease? *Gut* 22: A 874

185 Ellis H. J., Pollock E. L., Engel W., Fraser J. S., Rosen-Bronson S., Wieser H., Ciclitira P. J. 2003 Investigation of the putative immunodominant T cell epitopes in coeliac disease. *Gut* 52 212–217

186 Scoott B. B., Losowsky M. S. 1976 Patchiness and duodenal-jejunal variation of the mucosal abnormality in coeliac disease and dermatitis herpetiformis. *Gut* 17: 984–992

187 Scott B. B., Losowsky M. S. 1976 Peroral small-intestinal biopsy: experience with the hydraulic multiple biopsy instrument in routine clinical practice. *Gut* 17: 740–743

188 Prout B. J. 1974 A rapid method of obtaining a jejunal biopsy using a Crosby capsule and gastrointestinal fibrescope. *Gut* 15: 571–572

189 Holdstock G. 1978 Jejunal biopsy without the need for screening. *Lancet* i: 1236–37

190 Stevens F. M., McCarthy C. F. 1976 The endoscopic demonstration of celiac disease. *Endoscopy* 8 177–180

191 Holdstock G., Eade O. E., Isaacson P., Smith C. L. 1979 Endoscopic duodenal biopsies in coeliac disease and duodenitis. *Scand. J. Gastroenterol.* 14: 717–720

192 Scott B. B., Jenkins D. 1981 Endoscopic small-intestinal biopsy. *Gastrointestinal Endoscopy* 27 162–7

193 Mee A. S., Burke M., Vallon A. G., Newman J., Cotton P. B. 1985 Small bowel biopsy for malabsorption: comparison of the diagnostic adequacy of endoscopic forceps and capsule biopsy specimens. *Brit. Med. J.* iii: 769–772

194 McCrae W. M., Eastwood M. A., Martin M. R., Sircus W. 1975 Neglected celiac disease. *Lancet* i: 187–190

195 Swinson C. M., Levi A. J. 1980 Is coeliac disease underdiagnosed? *Brit. Med. J.* iv 1258–60

196 Lancaster-Smith, M. J., Parveen Kumar, Marks, R., Clark, M. L. and Dawson, A. M. 1974 Jejunal mucosal immunoglobulin-containing cells and jejuna fluid immunoglobulins in adult celiac disease and dermatitis herpetiformis. *Gut*, 15, 371–376

197 Montgomery A. M. P., Goka A. K. J., Kumar P. J., Farthing M. J. G., Clark M. L. 1988 Low gluten diet in the treatment of adult coeliac disease: effect on jejunal morphology and serum anti-gluten antibodies. *Gut* 29 1564–68

198 Swinson C. M., Slavin G., Coles E. C., Booth C. C. 1983 Coeliac disease and malignancy *Lancet* i: 111–5

199 Holmes G. K. T., Prior P., Lane M. R., Pope D., Allan R. N. 1989 Malignancy in coeliac disease: effect of a gluten-free diet. *Gut* 30 333–338

200 Harris O. D., Cooke W. T., Thompson H., Waterhouse J. A. H. 1967 Malignancy in adult celiac disease and idiopathic steatorrhoea. *Amer. J. Med.* 42: 899–912

201 Holmes G. K. T., Stokes P. L., Sorahan T. M., Prior P., Waterhouse J. A. H., Cooke W. T. 1976 Coeliac disease, gluten-free diet, and malignancy. *Gut* 17: 612–619

202   Arthur L. J. H., Langman M. J. S. 1981 Prevalence of celiac disease in Derby. In *The Genetics of Coeliac Disease,* ed. R. B. McConnell, M.T. P. Press 15–17

203   Littlewood J. M., Crollick A. J., Richards I. D. G. 1980 Childhood celiac disease is disappearing. *Lancet* ii: 1359–60

204   Challacombe D. N., Bayliss J. M. 1980 Childhood coeliac disease is disappearing. *Lancet* ii 1360–61

205   Dossetor J. F. B., Gibson A. A. M., McNeish A. S. 1981 Childhood celiac disease is disappearing. *Lancet* i: 322–3

206   Langman M. J. S., McConwell T. H., Sigelhalter D. J., McConwell R. B. 1985 Changing patterns of coeliac disease frequency: an analysis of celiac society membership records. *Gut* 26: 275–278

207   Kelly D. A., Phillips A. D., Elliott E. J., Dias J. A., Walker-Smith J. A. 1989 Rise and fall of coeliac disease 1960–85. *Arch. Dis. Child* 64 1157–60

208   Logan R. F. A., Tucker G., Rifkind E. A., Heading R. C., Ferguson A. 1983 Changes in clinical features of celiac disease in adults in Edinburgh and the Lothians 1960–79. *Brit. Med. J.* i: 95–97

209   Hobbs J. R., Hepner G. W. 1968 Deficiency of M-globulin in coeliac disease. *Lancet* i: 217–220

210   Kenrick K. G., Walker-Smith J. A. 1970 Immunoglobulins and dietary protein antibodies in childhood coeliac disease. *Gut* 11: 635–640

211   Doe W. F., Henry K., Booth C. C. 1974 Complement in celiac disease In *Coeliac Disease: Proceedings of the 2nd Internat. Coeliac Symposium, Leyden* Ed. W. Th. J. M. Hekkens, A. S. Pena Stenfert Kroese, Leyden

212   Anand B. S., Piris J., Jerrome D. W., Offord R. E., Truelove S. C. 1981 The timing of histological damage following a single challenge with gluten in treated coeliac disease. *Quart. J. Med. n.s.* 197 83–94

213   Anand B. S., Truelove S. C., Offord R. E. 1977 Skin test for celiac disease using a subfraction of gluten. *Lancet* i: 118–120

214   Holborow E. J., Weir D. M., Johnson G. D. 1957 A serum factor in Lupus Erythematosus with affinity for tissue nuclei. *Brit. Med. J.* ii: 732–734

215   Seah P. P., Fry Lionel, Hoffbrand A. V., Holborow E. J. 1971 Tissue antibodies in dermatitis herpetiformis and adult coeliac disease. *Lancet* i: 834–836

216   Seah P. P., Fry Lionel, Rossiter M. A., Hoffbrand A. V., Holborow E. J. 1971 Antireticulin antibodies in childhood celiac disease. *Lancet* ii: 681–682

217   Seah P. P., Fry Lionel, Holborow E. J., Rossiter M. A., Doe W. F., Magalhaes A. F., Hoffbrand A. V. !973 Antireticulin antibody: Incidence and diagnostic significance. *Gut* 14: 311–315

218   Eade O. E., Lloyd R. S., Lang Celia, Wright R. 1977 IgA and IgG reticulin antibodies in coeliac and non-coeliac patients. *Gut* 18: 991–993

219   Mallas E. G., Williamson N., Cooper B. T., Cooke W. T. 1977 IgA class reticulin antibodies in relatives of patients with celiac disease. *Gut* 18: 647–650

220   Stevens F. M., Lloyd R. S., Egan-Mitchell B., Mylotte M. J., Fottrell P. F., Wright R., McNicholl B., McCarthy C. F. 1975 Reticulin antibodies in patients with celiac disease and their relatives. *Gut* 16: 598–602

221 Unsworth D. J., Johnson G. D., Haffenden G., Fry L., Holborow E. J. 1981 Binding of wheat gliadin in vitro to reticulin in normal and dermatitis herpetiformis skin. *J. Invest. Dermatol.* 76: 88–93

222 Unsworth D. J., Manuel P. D., Walker-Smith J. A., Campbell C. A., Johnson D. G., Holborow E. D. 1981 New immunofluorescent blood test for gluten sensitivity. *Arch. Dis. Child* 56: 864–868

223 Chorzelski T. P., Beutner E. H., Sulej J., Chorzewska H., Jablonska S., Kumar V. et al. 1984 IgA anti-endomysium antibody. A new immunological marker of dermatitis herpetiformis and coeliac disease. *Brit. J. Dermatol.* 111 395–402

224 Dieterich W., Elmis T., Bauer M., Donner P., Volta U., Riecken E. O. 1997 Identification of tissue transglutaminase as the auto-antigen of celiac disease. Nat Med. 3 797–801

225 Molberg O., McAdam S. N., Korner R., Sollid L. M., Lundin K. E. A. 1998 Tissue transglutaminase selectivity modifies gliadin peptides that are recognised by gut derived T cells. Nat Med 4 713–717

226 Hin H., Bird G., Fisher P., Jewell D. P. 1999 Coeliac disease in primary care: a case finding study. *Brit. Med. J.* 318 164–7

227 West J., Logan R. F. A., Hill P. G., Lloyd A., Lewis S., Hubbard R., Reader R., Holmes G. K. T., Khaw K-T. 2003 Seroprevalence, correlates,and characteristics of undetected celiac disease in England. *Gut* 52: 960–965

228 Catassi C., Ratsch I. M., Fabiani E., Rossini M., Bordicchia F., Candela et al. 1994 Coeliac disease in the year 2000: exploring the iceberg. *Lancet* 343: 200–203

229 Kumar P. J. 2003 Debate. European and North American populations should be screened for coeliac disease – Antagonist *Gut* 52: 170–1

APPENDIX ONE

ON THE COELIAC AFFECTION

by SAMUEL JONES GEE

There is a kind of chronic indigestion which is met with in persons of all ages, yet is especially apt to affect children between one and five years old. Signs of the disease are yielded by the faeces; being loose, not formed, but not watery; more bulky than the food taken would seem to account for; pale in colour, as if devoid of bile; yeasty, frothy, an appearance probably due to fermentation; stinking, stench often very great, the food having undergone putrefaction rather than concoction.

> "His *stomack* is the *kitchin*, where the meat
> Is often but half sod, for want of heat."

The pale loose stool looks very much like oatmeal porridge or gruel. The hue is somewhile more yellow, otherwhile more drab. The paleness is commonly supposed to signify lack of bile; but the colour of faeces is a very rough measure of the quantity of bile poured into the duodenum; nay, more, the colour of faeces is a very rough measure of the quantity of bile which they contain. Whitish stools are not always so wanting in bile as they seem to be; in particular, opaque white food, such as milk-curd, undigested, will hide the colour of much bile.

Diarrhoea alba is a name employed in India to denote the coeliac affection; not that it is always a coeliac flux, a diarrhoea strictly speaking. True the dejections are faecal, more liquid and larger than natural, but they are not always more frequent than natural; it may be that the patient voids daily but one large, loose, whitish stinking stool. Diarrhoea chylosa is another name used formerly, and which seems to mean that the faeces consist of chyle unabsorbed. Aretaeus and Aurelian speak of the coeliac diathesis, ventriculosa passio (as who should say in English, wambecothe or belly sickness), names which are to be preferred, inasmuch as they connote nothing relative to the precise seat or nature of the disorder. It is one of a few diseases called by the common people consumption of the bowels, a phrase similar to that of pulmonary consumption; the term consumption referring to the wasting of the whole body, and the qualifying words, bowels or lungs, signifying the parts affected first and foremost.

The coeliac disease is commonest in patients between one and five years old: it often begins during the second year of life. Sometimes from India Englishmen return sick with the coeliac affection: seldom is it met with in adults who have never left our island.

The causes of the disease are obscure. Children who suffer from it are not all weak in constitution. Errors in diet may perhaps be a cause, but what error? Why, out of a family of children all brought up in much the same way, should one alone suffer? This often happens. Nor can we deem the coeliac passion always a consequence of accidental diarrhoea, for costiveness is sometimes a forerunner of the disorder. Nor need we call upon teething and worms to explain this, more than every other disease of childhood.

Naked-eye examination of dead bodies throws no light upon the nature of the coeliac affection; nothing unnatural can be seen in the stomach; intestines, or other digestive organs. Whether atrophy of the glandular crypts of the intestines be ever or always present, I cannot tell.

The onset is usually gradual, so that its time is hard to fix: sometimes the complaint sets in suddenly, like an accidental diarrhoea; but even when this is so, the nature of the disease soon shows itself.

The patient wastes more in the limbs than in the face, which often remains plump until death is nigh. In the limbs, emaciation is at first more apparent to hand than to eye, the flesh feeling soft and flabby. Muscular weakness great: muscular tenderness often present.

Cachexia, a fault of sanguification, betokened by pallor and tendency to dropsy, is a constant symptom: the patients become white and puffy; the loss of colour sometimes such as to resemble the cachectic hue of ague or splenic disease: the spleen sometimes enlarged. Examination of the blood by the microscope shows nothing noteworthy, unless much molecular matter in form of clear distinct particles or aggregated masses; but in this is no peculiarity.

The belly is mostly soft, doughy, and inelastic; sometimes distended and rather tight. Wind may be troublesome and very foetid. Appetite for food differs in different cases, being good, or ravenous, or bad. Heat of the body mostly natural; sometimes children are said to be hot at night, and especially so over the belly.

To diarrhoea alba add emaciation and cachexia, and we have a complete picture of the disease. At times the bowel complaint is overlooked: the wasting, weakness, paleness are what is noticed, and are thought to be due to another than the true cause. Ulceration of the intestines may be attended by all the symptoms of coeliac affection. In children, chronic ulceration of the intestines is often tubercular, sometimes syphilitic, seldom dysenteric. The diagnosis of ulceration turns upon a diarrhoea purulenta: the microscope discovers pus globules in the faeces. In rare cases the pus is so abundant that the stools consist of hardly anything else. But pus in the stools is not quite pathognomonic of ulceration; an abscess may open into the bowel: even apart from ulceration or abscess, a few pus globules may sometimes be found in the stools: still, for all practical purposes, the presence of pus in faeces may be deemed indicative of ulceration.

The course of the disease is always slow, whatever be its end; whether the patient live or die, he lingers ill for months or years. Death is a common end, and is mostly brought about by some intercurrent disorder; for instance, choleraic diarrhoea. Recovery is complete or incomplete. When recovery tends to be complete, a peculiar weakness of the legs is left long after all other tokens of disease have passed away, a weakness which shows itself in that the child is unable to jump. When recovery is incomplete, the illness drags on for years; the patient getting better on the whole, but being very subject to relapses of his complaint. While the disease is active, children cease to grow; even when it tends slowly to recovery, they are left frail and stunted.

To regulate the food is the main part of treatment. Cows' milk, which is recommended by Aurelian and some modern physicians in the case of the coeliac passion for hot climates, is not only not suited for children suffering from that disease, but is the least suited kind of food for them. Nothing more certain than that coeliac children cannot digest the hard curd of ruminants' milk. Asses' milk agrees with these patients very well, and they may take two, three or four pints of it daily. If asses' milk cannot be procured, we must make shift with cows' milk from which most or all of the curd has been removed; we must try whey, or cream mixed with water or scalded whey. The allowance of farinaceous food must be small; highly starchy food, rice, sago, corn-flour are unfit. Malted food is better, also rusks or bread cut thin and well toasted on both sides. No kind of fruit or vegetables may be given, except a tablespoonful or two of well-boiled mealy potatoes, mashed or rubbed through a sieve. Mutton and beef, raw or very underdone, pounded and rubbed through a wire sieve, should be given at the rate of from four to six tablespoonfuls daily. Even English beef, eaten raw, is now and then cause of tapeworm, much more so foreign beef. Broths and meat juices are allowed, also lightly boiled eggs and good fresh butter. A child, who was fed upon a quart of the best Dutch mussels daily, throve wonderfully, but relapsed when the season for mussels was over: next season he could not be prevailed upon to take them. This is an experiment which I have not yet been able to repeat. The disease being a failure of digestion, nothing seems more reasonable, at first sight, than to digest the patient's food artificially before it is given; but my experience has shown that peptonised milk and gruel are of little or no use in the treatment of the coeliac affection.

The diet recommended may seem to be scanty, but we must never forget that what the patient takes beyond his power of digestion does harm. The skin must be kept clean and warm; fresh air is necessary, muscular exercise not so. For drugs, carbonate of bismuth and aromatic chalk powder may be prescribed; also a small dose of compound decoction of aloes now and then. But if the patient can be cured at all, it must be by means of diet.

APPENDIX TWO

JOHN PAULLEY'S CASE REF. 59

"I was consulted in 1950 by a woman whose third child, a boy, 15 months old, had had coeliac disease for 7 months. Two weeks after he was born his brother, aged 2, was killed in tragic circumstances. The mother who was in full-time work, engaged a nurse shortly before the brother died, whereas the first 2 children she had managed herself with the help of a nursemaid. The nurse proved to be domineering, and was always making sly remarks about how well other people's children behaved or were dressed. She inferred that the accident was the mother's fault. Unlike the first 2 children who were breast fed, this last baby was put on a bottle early. The mother said this was due to the presence of the nurse, but one suspects it may have been due to lack of breast milk after the tragedy. The patient had overactive bowels and vomiting attacks from birth. When he was 8 months old the mother went on holiday without him, only to return to find him passing copious pale stools, which persisted till our consultation 7 months later. This consultation had a touch of melodrama. It had to be arranged in deep secrecy on the nurse's half day, in case she found out and disapproved, illustrating how far the unfortunate mother was dominated by this woman. Briefly I persuaded her to dismiss the nurse and to care for the child herself, taking him with her on her work as she had done with her first 2 children. I urged her to cuddle and play with the child, as she was by nature reserved. Within a fortnight a remission set in that still continues 6 years later. The boy is normal in size and weight, and only passes a pale stool when excited, as before a party. A gluten-free diet was never employed."

SECTION FOUR

INFLAMMATORY BOWEL DISEASE

CHAPTER THIRTY-FOUR

THE NINETEENTH CENTURY

In the spring of 1859, Miss Isabella Bankes, a lady in her early 40s, "who ordinarily enjoyed good health," began to complain of vomiting, diarrhoea, and a postprandial burning abdominal pain. After ten days, her husband, Dr. Thomas Smethurst, whom she had recently married even though he had a wife, summoned the local doctor who agreed that she had simple diarrhoea. Unfortunately she deteriorated, complained of a burning sensation in the epigastrium and soreness in the mouth and was unable to take any solid food. Her doctor began to suspect "that something of an irritant character was being administered", and his suspicion increased when a week later Isabella made a will leaving her small fortune (£1800) to her husband. After she had been ill for a month the doctor called in Dr. Bentley Todd (1809–60)[†] "the first physician of the day". Todd agreed with the diagnosis of irritant poisoning and had a stool examined by Dr. Alfred Swane Taylor (1806–80), Professor of Chemistry at Guy's Hospital and one of the fathers of forensic medicine. A small amount of arsenic was found. Two days later Isabella died and Dr. Smethurst was arrested and charged with her murder.[1]

The medical testimony at the trial was conflicting; ten doctors for the prosecution, including Todd, gave evidence to the effect that she was poisoned, and seven for the defence said that she had died from natural causes, probably dysentery of some kind. Professor Taylor admitted that the result of the test for arsenic had been a false positive. The judge was convinced that Dr. Smethurst was guilty and charged the jury to reach their opinion from the circumstantial evidence rather than the medical

---

[†]   Remembered today for his description of Todd's paralysis

evidence, which he regarded as unimportant. The jury took 40 minutes to reach a verdict of guilty.[2]

Reviewing the post mortem findings today, there seems little doubt that Miss Bankes had inflammatory bowel disease, probably Crohn's Disease, rather than irritant poisoning.[3] In the small intestine "nothing remarkable was observed until the lower end of the ileum was reached, when at about three feet from its termination in the caecum the mucous membrane commenced to exhibit an inflammatory response". In the large intestine "the mucous membrane was ulcerated from end to end". There were ulcers of all sizes, most commonly the size of a "sixpenny piece", and "mostly isolated though some had run together". In the rectum, descending, transverse colon, and ascending colon "this ulceration was tolerably uniform in amount". In the caecum "inflammation of the most acute and violent character was observed…"

The case was controversial and caused an outcry in the medical world at the time, notably from Dr. Samuel Wilks (1824–1911), assistant physician to Guy's Hospital. Wilks had worked in the department of morbid anatomy and had studied inflammation of the colon, so his opinion commanded respect. After the verdict against Dr. Smethurst, he wrote in the *Medical Times and Gazette* that "in all probability an irritant substance caused the ulceration, but the latter was not always distinguishable from the dysenteric form" (i.e. idiopathic colitis) "and consequently the prisoner should have had the benefit of the doubt on this point as on all others".[4] A memorial was sent to the Home Secretary from 30 medical men, headed by Sir Richard Quain (1816–98),[†] a prominent fellow of the Royal College of Physicians, and another by 29 barristers praying that the sentence (of death) be not executed. The Home Secretary, Sir George Cornewall Lewis, referred the medical details to Sir Benjamin Brodie (1783–1862) of St. George's Hospital. Sir Benjamin reported in favour of the defence: "though the facts are full of suspicion against Smethurst there is not absolute and complete evidence of guilt." As a result Dr. Smethurst was granted a free pardon. He was later convicted of bigamy and sentenced to hard labour for one year. During the second trial it emerged that Isabella Bankes was herself already married when she married Smethurst. Two years later in the probate court he succeeded in proving her will in his favour.

[†]   Best remembered for his editorship of the *Dictionary of Medicine*.

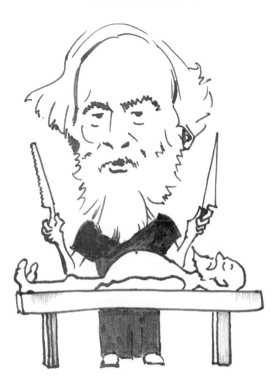

37 Wilks – Morbid anatomist.

Samuel Wilks' evidence had been crucial to the outcome of the case. He was one of the great Victorian physicians at Guy's Hospital; everything except politics and sport interested him though he used to say that the name Samuel was a handicap, because hardly anyone with that name was successful; indeed there were only three, namely, the prophet, Dr. Johnson and Mr. Weller Junior.[†/5] He followed in the footsteps of Bright, Addison and Hodgkin, and he built his reputation on his knowledge of pathology, being the first to undertake postmortem examinations on all who died in hospital. He wrote extensively on diseases of the nervous system and the pathology of syphilis and coined the name Hodgkin's disease, which had attracted little attention until he rediscovered it.

At the time of the Smethurst trial Wilks had just published his *Lectures on Pathological Anatomy delivered at Guy's Hospital during the Summer Sessions*

---

†   Curiously, he did not include Pepys whose diary was popular with the Victorian reading public.

1857–58, in which he differentiated ulcerative colitis from epidemic dysentery for the first time.[6] He wrote, "the term colitis is sometimes used to express this state, and the term dysentery as synonymous with it. Our language has been too indefinite and indeed incorrect in speaking of all infections of the lower intestine as dysenteric...dysentery being, in fact, only one variety of colitis." This was remarkably astute bearing in mind that the science of bacteriology was in its infancy.

He recognised two types of idiopathic colitis; the first was a simple inflammation of the colon with hyperaemia and increased mucous secretion like catarrh; "we occasionally find an inflammation in certain febrile and other disorders, as pyaemia, without any evident cause; patches of the colon being red, inflamed, and covered with tenacious mucus, or even adherent lymph." This was probably mucous colitis, an incidental finding at postmortem in patients with overwhelming infection or a spastic colon. He went on, "there are cases, however, of *simple idiopathic colitis,* though rare, and which may, indeed, be examples of acute dysentery, but such, in the absence of those peculiar features which are supposed to characterise that disease, can scarcely receive the name. For example, we have seen a case attended by discharge of mucus and blood where, after death, the whole internal surface of the colon presented a highly vascular, soft, red surface, covered with adherent mucus or adherent lymph, and here and there showing a few minute points of ulceration; the coats were also much swollen by exudation into the mucous and submucous tissues. The propriety of giving the name *acute dysentery* to such a case would depend much upon the opinion whether the disease can occur in London or not. Dysentery is a disease of tropical climates whereas simple ulceration of the lower intestine is a less severe and more chronic affection occurring in our own country."[†] He was describing ulcerative colitis as we know it today.

Apart from irritants or poison, Wilks could not explain how people contracted colitis and more than 25 years later, William Allchin (1846–1912), physician to the Westminster Hospital, had little to add when he described a further case of *Acute, extensive ulceration of the colon* in a young mother who died after an illness of less than three weeks.[7] She had colic and bloody diarrhoea with 17 to 22 stools per day and became

---

[†]   The second edition of the *Pathological Anatomy* (1875) was edited by Walter Moxon and is frequently cited as containing the first description of colitis.

emaciated and febrile with a tachycardia. There was moderate tenderness over the transverse and descending colon. She succumbed to exhaustion. At postmortem only the colon was abnormal and inflamed throughout its length. There were numerous large ulcers up to an inch in length all the way to the rectum. The mucosa was denuded in places. The bowel contained several ounces of dark, bloodstained, grumous feculent matter with masses of mucus. Allchin suggested that colitis was probably more common than people thought and often acute and fatal. Echoing Wilks, he wrote: "It is a pity that the term dysentery is not restricted to the true tropical malady." The cause was a complete mystery and another eminent physician, Hale-White, was equally at a loss.

In 1888 William Hale-White (1857–1949),[†] Assistant Physician to Guy's Hospital, reported eleven cases of *Simple ulcerative colitis* though they had little in common apart from ulceration of the colon.[8] Only one of the patients was actually under his care and most had died before he joined the staff, so he had to rely on postmortem data. Three of the patients, including his case, almost certainly died from acute total colitis, three had granular kidney or chronic Bright's disease and one had fungating endocarditis and cirrhosis. He emphasised that the ulceration was diffuse, not follicular (focal) in origin and was adamant that this disease was quite distinct from dysentery, "indeed the diagnosis was not even suggested during life".

Hale-White was senior physician at Guy's Hospital for nearly twenty years and was famous for his book, *Materia Medica, Pharmacy, Pharmacology and Therapeutics.* Known familiarly as *Hale-White,* it went through no fewer than 26 editions during his lifetime, tormenting generations of medical students. He can be credited for popularising the term ulcerative colitis and described it as such in the well-known *System of Medicine* edited by Sir Clifford Allbutt in 1896.

Confusion with dysentery continued despite, or indeed because of, the breathtaking advances in bacteriology during the last quarter of the nineteenth century. Year by year the cause of most of the great bacterial diseases was identified. Amoebic dysentery was discovered in 1875, typhoid in 1880 and bacillary dysentery in 1898 (by Shiga in Japan). Occasionally, an outbreak of dysentery occurred in Britain usually in an asylum. James Gemmel (1860–1920) reported an epidemic which he

---

[†] Son of the author known to literature as Mark Rutherford.

unfortunately called *idiopathic ulcerative colitis*, resulting in 118 deaths in the Lancaster County Asylum, and suggested that this condition, which had always been well known in asylums, was really dysentery.[9] In 1902 Simon Flexner (1863–1946) at the Rockefeller Institute in New York proved that epidemics of dysentery in institutions in America were caused by B. dysenteriae, a variant of the Shiga bacillus and later called Shigella Flexneri.[10] Two years later the distinguished bacteriologist John Eyre (1869–1944) at Guy's Hospital investigated an outbreak of dysentery in an asylum and found Shigella in six out of ten cases.[11]

Naturally ulcerative colitis was assumed to be infective in origin and hopes were high that the cause would soon be found. When efforts to isolate an organism were unsuccessful, various explanations were put forward. Sporadic disease was more difficult to investigate than an epidemic; cases commonly reached the chronic stage before examination was possible, and even in acute asylum cases the specific bacillus was frequently not isolated; yet the similarities with bacillary dysentery were so close that everyone believed that an elusive organism must be responsible.

Another problem was the precise meaning of the word colitis, which soon became a loose term for anyone with a chronic bowel disturbance. In particular there was a common disorder known as *muco-membranous colitis* that we would now call irritable bowel syndrome. This derived its name from the fact that patients passed the most impressive membranes during attacks. Mucus was excreted as membranous shreds, which sometimes formed tubular casts of the colon, and in extreme cases, the casts could be two or more feet in length and up to an inch in diameter.[12] Quite why these casts melted away during the twentieth century is difficult to say, but I suspect they were linked to the Victorians' penchant for purgatives. As the condition was not fatal, its nature was obscure because postmortem evidence was scanty.

CHAPTER THIRTY-FIVE

EARLY TWENTIETH CENTURY

Many patients with bowel symptoms were referred to St. Mark's Hospital for Diseases of the Rectum where a young surgeon, Percy Lockhart-Mummery (1875–1957), was rapidly making his name.

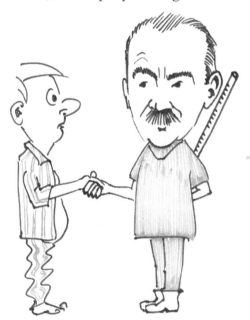

38 Lockhart-Mummery – OK, if you must.

Lockhart-Mummery was one of the pioneers of colectomy for cancer of the colon alongside Ernest Miles (1869–1947) at the Royal Cancer Hospital, and George Grey Turner (1871–1951) at Newcastle. Full of energy and enthusiasm, he would bound up the stairs for his operating session, so that few realised that he had had one of his legs amputated as a student (by Lord Lister). He wrote easily and well and contributed to 12 textbooks and at least 160 articles during his career.[1] He was also the first to use an electrically illuminated sigmoidoscope in this country, which had just been invented by Professor Hermann Strauss (1868–1944) of Berlin and was originally made of lead.[13] Lockhart-Mummery was clearly excited by the instrument because he wrote in 1904, "The human mind is so constituted that we always experience a certain pleasure when we have succeeded in obtaining access to some spot hitherto difficult or impossible to explore."[14] Inevitably he saw many patients with bloody diarrhoea and realised that a careful examination of the pelvic colon was essential in any patient with symptoms of colitis. "Serious errors in diagnosis," he wrote in 1905, "can thus often be avoided and definite information can be obtained on which a rational line of treatment may be based."[15] Absolutely, but for several years Lockhart-Mummery unintentionally added to the confusion about colitis, which he defined as chronic catarrh, congestion or ulceration of the mucosa (as seen by the naked eye of course, rectal biopsy came half a century later). He taught that colitis was simply a symptom or condition caused by a number of different diseases of the colon, and it is clear that he was muddling mucus colitis with ulcerative colitis as Wilks had done.

In his view, constipation was by far the commonest cause of colitis due to stagnation and trauma in the sigmoid colon. But cancer of the colon could also cause a colitis with which it was often confused, and conditions outside the bowel such as inflammation of the appendix or female genitals or uterine displacement were often responsible. Appendicitis was a particularly common association, perhaps by spread of inflammation, infection or the formation of adhesions and stagnation. He believed that these were all examples of secondary colitis. However, he did recognise a few patients with severe ulcerative colitis for which no cause could be found, which he called idiopathic or primary colitis.[16]

Most physicians were convinced that ulcerative colitis was a dysenteric infection and continued to search for the elusive organism. In 1909 Herbert Hawkins (1859–1940), an elegant and handsome physician to St. Thomas's Hospital and one of the leading teachers of his day, published a detailed analysis of 85 patients seen at the hospital during the previous 25 years.[17] He noted that a quarter of the patients had a

---

1   Before the second war, only Arthur Hurst surpassed this total with twelve books and 240 articles.

short illness lasting a few weeks and usually died. The illness was typical of dysentery except that it was acquired in England. The remaining three quarters of the patients, however, had a prolonged illness lasting months or even years and less than half of them died. Hawkins agonised over the cause and suggested that an unknown B. dysenteriae caused the first attack with subsequent infection by coliforms or pyogenic cocci perpetuating the disease.

He was rather pessimistic about treatment. Vaccines against Shigella were claimed by Shiga himself to reduce the mortality of bacillary dysentery, but the results in colitis were disappointing. The mainstays of treatment were bedrest, a bland diet and clearance of the colon to render it as aseptic as possible.

At first the colon was irrigated in the time-honoured fashion using enemata. Enemas have been used for thousands of years. For example, they were important in ancient Egypt where Iri, Keeper of the Royal Rectum, was presumably the pharaoh's enema expert.[18] A large variety of solutions were advocated for colitis including pints of warm water containing nitrate of silver, or a mixture of starch and laudanum, or the salts of various heavy metals, or creolin, or boracic acid. The list was long but often the patient was too weak or in too much pain to tolerate an enema. The alternative was to irrigate the colon from above. By the 1880s inguinal colotomy, as it was then called, was being used to relieve obstruction by cancer of the rectum.[19] Before long, attempts were made to use colotomy to clean the lower colon in patients with colitis. The results were bad because the extent of the colitis was pure guesswork and the colotomy was too low to be useful and frequently broke down. Then in 1902 an American surgeon, Robert Weir (1838–1927), introduced the technique of appendicostomy through which to irrigate the colitic bowel.[20] He had been President of the American Surgical Association in 1900 and in the same year received an honorary FRCS when the London college celebrated its centenary. His simple procedure was quickly adopted by British surgeons and remained in use for nearly 40 years. Daily irrigation via a small rubber tube in the appendix continued for three to six weeks and could be repeated for twelve months.[21]

Recognition of ulcerative colitis as an entity was slow because it was uncommon and, as we have seen, often confused with mucus colitis (irritable bowel syndrome). In any one year, only two or three cases were admitted to hospital so most physicians had almost no experience of the disease. Conscious of this, in 1909, a meeting was staged at the recently formed Royal Society of Medicine at which 288 cases were presented. These had been collected from the records of nine London Hospitals over a period of 25 years and included Hawkins' series at St. Thomas's, and Hale-White's patients at Guy's with the addition of twenty cases provided by Charles Cameron (1878–1958), author of *Mr. Guy's Hospital* (1954). Other eminent names involved were Frederick Price (1873–1957) at the Westminster Hospital, editor of *The Practice of Medicine* from 1922 to 1955; Bertrand Dawson (1864–1945), later Viscount Dawson of Penn, and Henry Tidy (1877–1960), later to be a founder member of the British Society of Gastroenterology, both at the London Hospital; Thomas Horder (1871–1955), later Lord Horder of Ashford, from St. Bartholemew's Hospital; Arthur Jex-Blake (1873–1957) at St. George's Hospital, a nephew of Sophia Jex-Blake who had been a key figure in the battle to open the profession to women; and Sidney Phillips (1851–1951) from St. Mary's Hospital, a successful treasurer of the Royal College of Physicians and a centenarian. It should be remembered that these physicians who all contributed cases were men of their time. Though astute clinicians, they were generalists living in the Edwardian era long before clinical science began to make its mark.

The meeting began with an address by William Allchin, now Sir William, who essentially agreed with Hawkins' experience at St. Thomas's Hospital.[22] During the discussion that followed, it was clear that this august body had little to add to what was already known. Most were satisfied with the term ulcerative colitis and agreed that the disease was not contagious but they could not explain it. Some thought it occurred as a result of tinned foods and the use of preservatives; some considered it to be a psychosomatic disease; and the majority believed it was infective in origin caused by an unknown organism related to the B. dysenteriae. They were all worried by the high mortality (50 per cent). The most important contribution came from Lockhart-Mummery who, again, extolled the importance of sigmoidoscopy, which no one else was using, and emphasised that a diagnosis of colitis based entirely upon symptoms was utterly fallacious.

In the absence of specific treatment, everyone agreed that rest and warmth were essential, and colonic lavage helpful. Hawkins thought that more of his patients might have been saved by an earlier recourse to colostomy and two experienced surgeons, George Makins (1853–1933) of St. Thomas's Hospital, and Walter Spencer (1858–1940) from the Westminster both favoured irrigation via a transverse colostomy. However, the St. Mark's surgeons, Lockhart-Mummery and Frederick Wallis (1859–1912), both strongly advocated appendicostomy rather than colostomy to ensure thorough cleansing of the whole colon.[23]

Lockhart-Mummery's exhortations to use the sigmoidoscope fell on deaf ears with the exception of Arthur Hurst (1879–1944) at Guy's Hospital who, ironically, was actually deaf. Hurst had been invited to take part in the discussion but had declined because, at that time, he said that he knew little about the disease. However, when he read the report of the meeting, he was instantly converted to the use of the sigmoidoscope, employing it whenever he suspected a patient might have disease of the colon. "Nobody," he said, "would think of treating a case of tonsillitis without looking at the tonsils; it is even less justifiable to treat a case of colitis without looking at the colon."[24] Nonetheless, sigmoidoscopy was considered a surgical procedure, and for decades it was the surgeon who generally dealt with the disease.

Hurst burst onto the scene with a typically robust description of muco-membranous colitis with which ulcerative colitis was so often confused. In 1910 he wrote, "Muco-membranous colitis occurs four or five times more frequently in women than in men...they are always neurotic, their abnormal mental condition dating from a period preceding the onset of the intestinal disorder. The disease is rare among hospital patients,[†] the few cases I have seen in hospital being among brain workers, whose occupation involved a mental strain which was too great for them. In many cases actual neurasthenia or hysteria is present, and all the patients tend to become depressed and hypochondriacal. They invariably take a great interest in their condition and make very minute examination of their excreta. The depressed condition of the nervous system in neurasthenia is generally associated with an abnormal irritability of the centres which influence visceral activity. This *faiblesse irritable*[§] is the condition which more than any other predisposes to muco-membranous colitis."[25]

Unlike Lockhart-Mummery, Hurst thought that the association with appendicitis had been exaggerated and he favoured counselling rather

---

†   As opposed to private patients
§   Feeble nervous disposition

than an exhaustive search for an underlying surgical cause. But he agreed that the constipation should be corrected.

CHAPTER THIRTY-SIX

BETWEEN THE TWO GREAT WARS
1918–39

Progress in the understanding of ulcerative colitis stagnated between the two world wars. Few physicians were interested in the disease because it was uncommon; only three to four cases were seen in a London teaching hospital in any one year. It continued to be confused with mucus colitis, and doctors, particularly physicians, were strangely reluctant to use the sigmoidoscope. A few enthusiasts kept the light burning, notably Hurst and Lockhart-Mummery. Nobody could improve on Hawkins' original theory that it was due to a chronic low-grade infection. In 1919, Hurst, in the belief that the disease was really an aberrant form of bacillary dysentery, tried the effect of intravenous injection of large doses of polyvalent antidysenteric serum. His first patient who was almost moribund responded miraculously, after which he was an enthusiastic believer in the treatment for many years.[26] But prolonged rest in bed for a year or more if necessary and a nutritious diet were the mainstays of his management. He also recommended that any focus of infection such as carious teeth should be removed to prevent a relapse (this was widely believed for many years).

Though a strong advocate of colonic lavage, Hurst gradually came to the conclusion that appendicostomy was of little or no value, and by 1920 he had abandoned the procedure. He thought effective lavage of the whole colon could be achieved with enemata alone. His favourite astringent was albargin, a preparation of silver nitrate, which Leonard Rogers (1868–1962), of tropical disease fame, had found most effective in dysentery.[27] Some of his patients were turned black with argyria as a result of prolonged treatment with this preparation. In contrast,

Lockhart-Mummery was enthusiastic about appendicostomy, and in 1923, in his book *Diseases of the Rectum and Colon,* he reported his success in 82 cases. Less than one out of five of those treated surgically (by appendicostomy) died compared with almost four out of five treated medically.[28] These results horrified Hurst who sprang to the defence of medical treatment, claiming that in his hands the mortality from ulcerative colitis was nearer ten per cent (a remarkably low figure at the time).[29]

However, even Hurst was only seeing three or four new cases of colitis each year whereas in America a few full-time hospital physicians were accumulating large numbers of patients. The best known was Arnold Bargen (1894–1976) at the Mayo Clinic who published his experience of no fewer than 693 cases (compared to Hurst's 40).[30] Bargen's huge experience enabled him to describe a number of the complications of colitis for the first time, including arthritis, cutaneous lesions and ocular disease. But his credibility was stretched when he isolated a diplococcus from the rectum of 80 per cent of his patients and claimed that he got good results using a vaccine prepared from it.[31] Other American physicians were unable to confirm his enthusiastic reports.

Unfamiliarity with the disease in Britain provoked a further discussion at the Royal Society of Medicine in 1926 led by Arthur Hurst. "No diagnosis," he said, "is made more frequently and with less justification."[32] Most cases of so-called colitis had symptoms that were purely functional, and much time and money was spent on vaccines, intestinal douches and visits to spas when nothing more than a little judicious psychotherapy was required. On the other hand, the same diagnosis was often made when a much more serious condition – cancer of the colon or rectum – was really present, and weeks or months were allowed to pass, by which time the chance of cure was lost.

In a similar vein, John Hern (1900–86), Medical Assistant at Guy's Hospital, published a review of 50 cases of ulcerative colitis in 1931.[33] Frustrated by widespread ignorance of the disease, his style was sardonic and he bore sole responsibility for his opinions, which, he said, may not have been orthodox; but I suspect that they had Hurst's approval. "Ulcerative colitis," he began, "has received official recognition in the terminology of the Royal College of Physicians but satisfaction felt by those who regard it as one of the most distinctive of all diseases is somewhat mitigated by the reflection that "intestinal sand" and "dilatation" are on the same footing, for they are found on the same list." He could accept a divergence of opinion on its cause and treatment, but he was upset by everyone's complete inability to diagnose it. Sigmoidoscopy was essential and he was among the first to emphasise the value of a barium enema in the diagnosis, which hitherto had only been used to exclude cancer.

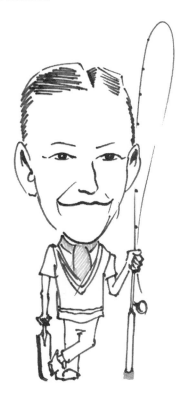

39 Hardy – Charm and gift for friendship.

One of the few physicians to heed this advice was Lionel Hardy (1887–1969) in Birmingham, a close friend and ardent admirer of Hurst whom he first met during service in the RAMC. He was a superb clinician but had a strong academic bias and trained many of the most notable medical and surgical gastroenterologists of the twentieth century. In 1933 he drew attention to the continuing high mortality of ulcerative colitis (33 per cent) particularly in acute cases during the first year of the disease.[34] While emphasising the need for prolonged and complete rest in bed for a minimum of six months, the treatment was so disheartening that he found it difficult to avoid the conclusion that those who recovered did so in spite of their treatment. The key thing was to help patients through their first attack.

Hurst agreed and showed that patients in his private hospital in Windsor Park[†] did much better than the patients in Guy's Hospital.[35] He believed that the mortality should not exceed five to ten per cent provided that the patient received adequate care for sufficient periods. As his private patients had identical treatment to the hospital cases, why was their prognosis so much better? A clue comes from the great centenarian physician Joseph Kirsner (1909–2012) in Chicago during his reflections on the treatment of ulcerative colitis at that time.[36] He was shocked by the death of a young woman with severe ulcerative colitis in 1936 and realised that he had not seen such a patient during his four years as a medical student and three years as an intern. Just as in Britain, most clinicians in America were still unaware of the disease.

Though specific treatment was unavailable, Kirsner ensured that his patients were well fed, nursed intelligently and caringly and supported by competent psychiatrists. In the 1930s the hypothesis that colitis was psychological in origin was popular. Kirsner recalls spending hours each day, including Saturday and Sunday, at the bedside of his patients offering support and encouragement. So perhaps Hurst's success was the result of the personal interest and support that he and his staff were able to give his private patients as much as it was to do with diet, rest, antiserum, tiny blood transfusions (250 millitres), or colonic lavage.

By this time ileostomy had become the favourite operation for ulcerative colitis in America. It was hoped that "resting the bowel" for a year or two would allow it to be restored to normal later. Healing was assumed to have occurred when water that had been flushed through the excluded colon from above was clean with no red corpuscles or pus cells in the deposit. Before a second operation was undertaken, the bowel was trained for several weeks by injecting some of the faeces discharged from the ileum through the distal ileostomy opening. The faeces were first diluted with water, and gradually made stronger, until finally the whole of the ileal contents were injected undiluted. If there was no untoward reaction it was safe to rejoin the divided ileum. But this was unusual. In fact most ileostomies were unsatisfactory with frequent complications

---

† New Lodge Clinic, which he opened in 1920 and closed down in 1939.

and patients hated them. One young woman in an American hospital told Hurst that she much preferred the ulcerative colitis to the ileostomy.[37] Many were poorly constructed causing recurrent obstruction, peristomal ulceration and infection and even necrosis of the abdominal wall. As colectomy was then very dangerous, these ill patients had to contend with a diseased colon as well as the miseries of their ileostomy.

CHAPTER THIRTY-SEVEN

CROHN'S DISEASE

a) Crohn's description

When Dr. Burrill B. Crohn (1884–1983) walked to the podium to read his paper on terminal ileitis to the Section on Gastro-Enterology and Proctology at the 83rd Annual Session of the American Medical Association in New Orleans on 13th May 1932, he had no idea that the disease would assume his name or that it would be as baffling today as it was then.

During the nineteenth century most circumscribed lesions of the intestine were assumed to be neoplastic, but in 1907 those two giants of early abdominal surgery from Leeds, Berkeley Moynihan[38] and Mayo-Robson,[39] presented several cases in which the original diagnosis of malignant disease of the colon was replaced by that of granuloma. Their concern, however, was simply to explain that these growths could be easily mistaken for cancer.

Crohn was head of the department of gastroenterology at Mount Sinai Hospital where there was already considerable interest in intestinal granulomas. A decade earlier two members of the staff, a physician, Eli Moschcowitz and a surgeon, A. O. Wilensky, had read a paper before the American Association of Pathologists and Bacteriologists in Washington in which they emphasised that there were many cases resembling ileocaecal tuberculosis that had negative bacteriology and were in reality simple non-specific granulomata.[40] They presented four cases and thought the lesion affected the colon, though the small intestine was involved in one case.

In 1925 Albert Ashton Berg (1872–1950), an experienced abdominal surgeon at Mt. Sinai Hospital, took on a young house surgeon, Leon Ginzburg (1899–1988), who soon became interested in granulomatous disease of the bowel. With his colleague, Gordon Oppenheimer (1900–74), a resident in pathology, Ginzburg identified a dozen patients with disease of the distal ileum "ending rather abruptly at the ileo-caecal valve", all of whom were operated on by Berg. At the same time Crohn was also studying the disease and sent two further patients with terminal ileitis to Berg for resection. Between them they had managed to isolate a subgroup of fourteen patients with terminal ileitis, a distinction made possible by the consistent anatomy, characteristic clinical course, typical complications and successful response to surgery. With Berg's help, Crohn obtained access to Ginzburg's work, which he expanded and planned to present as the single author at the New Orleans meeting. He was that year President of the American Gastroenterological Association. This upset Ginzburg and Oppenheimer and, after some shenanigans, it was agreed that they be added as co-authors in alphabetical order. Dr. Berg, of course, should have been the lead author, but it was not in his nature or custom to append his name to an article he had not written himself and anyway he was really more interested in antique furniture and rare folios.[41]

So it fell to Crohn to present their work. He began, "We propose to describe, in its pathologic and clinical details, a disease of the terminal ileum, affecting mainly young adults, characterized by a subacute or chronic necrotizing or cicatrizing inflammation. The ulceration of the mucosa is accompanied by a disproportionate connective tissue reaction of the remaining walls of the involved intestine, a process which frequently leads to stenosis of the lumen of the intestine, associated with the formation of multiple fistulas...the terminal ileum alone is involved...for in this disease the rectum and colon are never involved."

Later he stressed that the barium enema was always normal whereas the barium meal showed a definite delay in motility of the meal through the distal end of the small intestine.

He concluded, "Medical treatment is purely palliative and supportive... in general, the proper approach to a complete cure is by surgical resection."

By limiting his description to inflammation of the terminal ileum, Crohn had highlighted a specific entity that was readily identifiable and curable.

The paper was well received by a distinguished audience. Arnold Bargen from the Mayo Clinic had seen several cases and, "I am wondering whether the designation 'terminal' is adequately descriptive. To some it has conveyed the meaning of agonal. Perhaps the modifying adjective 'regional' or some other word suggesting its localized nature, instead of the end, would be more suitable." The paper was published later that year in the *Journal of the American Medical Association* under the title "Regional ileitis".[42]

Within a couple of years, several more reports appeared in America under such titles as "regional ileitis", "regional enteritis", and "chronic cicatrising enteritis: regional enteritis (Crohn)".[43] In some cases parts of the small intestine other than the terminal ileum were involved and lesions were found in the jejunum, duodenum and colon. This more widespread involvement of the intestine led Crohn and his colleagues to enlarge and amend their original concept, though, ironically, Crohn was one of the last to agree to the concept of "Crohn's colitis".[44] He continued to call the disease regional ileitis and was always modest about his role in the original description and would demur when "Crohn's disease" was mentioned, as it usually was by visitors from Britain. But "Crohn's disease" it had to be, if only to keep open all anatomical possibilities as it became clear that the disease was anything but limited to the ileum.

Eponyms are frequently controversial because others equally deserving have been omitted or because someone who first described the disease, instrument or procedure has been overlooked. Crohn's Disease is no exception. Ginzburg and Oppenheimer have reason to feel a bit miffed; years later Ginzburg sometimes introduced himself as "Al", explaining that Crohn et Al once wrote a paper together. But Crohn-Ginzburg-Oppenheimer's disease would have been cumbersome and probably abbreviated to CGO disease, which would have meant nothing. Alternatively there are those who think it should have been called Dalziel's disease, but surprisingly for a man so well versed in the literature, Crohn was apparently unaware of his work.

b) *Dalziel's Disease*

Kennedy Dalziel,(1861–1924), surgeon to the Western Infirmary, Glasgow, wrote an article entitled "Chronic Interstitial Enteritis" in the *British Medical Journal* in 1913.[45] He described how in 1901 he had seen a

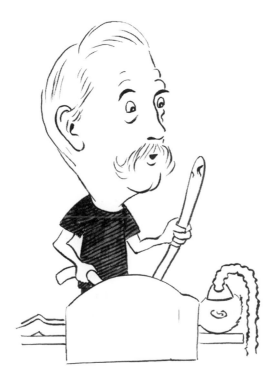

40 Dalziel – ileitis: – like an eel – in rigor mortis.

professional colleague with a history of two weeks' vomiting, colic and mild diarrhoea. At laparotomy he found "the whole of the intestines, large and small alike, contracted, rigidly fixed, so that when a loop was lifted from the abdomen it sprang back into its sulcus. That the wall of the whole intestine was chronically inflamed there was no doubt… nothing could be done and the patient died. We were not then familiar with the condition, and it was supposed to be tuberculous, though this was negatived by microscopic examination, the only information we obtained from the pathologist being that the condition was a chronic and inflammatory one." A few years later he saw a similar case, which was also inoperable. He then saw seven patients with localised disease of the jejunum, ileum or colon, all of whom underwent successful resection. The histology was typical of Crohn's Disease, ranging from acute to chronic inflammation and he thought the cases had much in common. "The affected bowel gives the consistence and smoothness of an eel in a state of rigor mortis," he wrote. Doubtless this was a common sight on the fishmonger's slab in those days. He concluded, "My friends the pathologists prefer to call it hyperplastic enteritis, and I regret that the aetiology of the condition remains in obscurity, but I trust that ere long further consideration will clear up this difficulty." He was knighted for his services to surgery in 1917.

c) *The string sign*

Personally I agree with John Kantor (1890–1947), the radiologist at Mount Sinai Hospital, who said, "Dr. Crohn deserves credit, as always for calling attention to this disease." It was only by focussing on the terminal ileum that he was able to avoid "the confusion that defies classification". Dalziel described the disease as we know it today, but it was Crohn and his colleagues whose careful clinico-pathological studies laid the basis for the modern understanding of the disease. Kantor, incidentally, described the classic "string-sign" of regional ileitis in 1934. The word was originally used to designate the spasm seen in irritable bowel, but it was so apt that he borrowed the name to describe the cotton string appearance seen in the terminal ileum in patients with Crohn's Disease.[46]

d) *Other early descriptions of Crohn's Disease in Britain*

Identifying isolated case reports of a disease before its formal recognition has long been an exercise enjoyed by medical historians, though usually of little more than academic interest. Ulcerative colitis is difficult because the symptoms and pathology are so non-specific. Bonnie Prince Charlie is said to have suffered from colitis on the grounds of his "bloody flux" but this is purely speculative. Crohn's Disease is more identifiable, though many cases were probably examples of intestinal tuberculosis. I have selected three reports worthy of note.

The first is a case reported in 1813 by two physicians, Charles Combe (1743–1817), obstetric physician and friend of William Hunter, and William Saunders (1743–1817) of Guy's Hospital, who had helped Sir George Baker (1722–1809) in his work on Devonshire colic.[†] They were both fellows of the Royal Society and Society of Antiquaries and were

---

† Lead poisoning

both 63 years of age when they reported before the Royal College of Physicians *A Singular Case of Stricture and Thickening of the Ileum.*[47]

Their patient, "of a very nervous and delicate habit, had been for many years troubled with complaints in the bowels, attended with costiveness and a quick pulse," Four months before he died he had an irregular intermittent fever, and his pain became so intense that "he refused taking any solid food, and subsisted entirely on jelly, broth, milk, etc. dreading the pain that succeeded even this kind of food". By the time he died, "he was more emaciated than any person we had ever witnessed". The body was opened by Dr. Combe who found "The lower part of the ileum, as far as the colon, was contracted for the space of three feet to the size of a turkey's quill. The colon had three constrictions. Wherever the intestines were constricted, the coats were very much thickened, and exhibited an appearance of inflammation."

The second case that may have been due to regional ileitis is mentioned by John Abercrombie of Edinburgh.[†] "A girl, aged 13, about a year before her death, began to be affected with pain of the abdomen and frequent vomiting. The bowels were at first natural, but soon became loose; and from this time she was almost constantly affected either with diarrhoea or vomiting…when I saw her about a week before she died, she was emaciated to the last degree…and complained of constant pain in the bowels, which was increased by pressure, but the abdomen was soft. On inspection (post mortem) the caput coli was dark coloured, hard and much thickened in its coats; internally, it was much eroded by ulceration; the disease extended, in the form of numerous small ulcers, about three inches along the ascending colon; and the valve of the colon was destroyed by the ulceration. The lower end of the ileum, to the extent of about eighteen inches, was distended, thickened in its coats, externally of a reddish colour and internally covered by numerous well-defined ulcers, varying in size from the diameter of a split pea to that of a sixpence. The lungs and all other viscera were healthy." Abercrombie carried out the post mortem himself and his excellent description of the gross pathology compensates for the lack of histology or bacteriology.[48]

Finally, Norman Moore (1847–1922) described a man of 47 with intestinal obstruction for a month. Moore was demonstrator in morbid

---

[†]   John Abercrombie see Section Two, p38 This quotation is taken from the 1830 (American) edition of his *Diseases of the Stomach* p284

anatomy at St. Bartholemew's Hospital at the time (1882) and must have seen some interesting surgical cases in his department. In this instance a colotomy was performed without relief and the patient died three days later. Post mortem examination revealed extensive ulceration above and below the ileocaecal valve, which was so contracted that it would just admit a large probe. No tubercle was discoverable. Microscopic sections showed that the thickening and contraction were due to long continued inflammatory changes. Unfortunately the colotomy had been fashioned two inches below the ileocaecal valve distal to the obstruction.[49] Moore had a distinguished career at St. Bartholemew's and at the Royal College of Physicians and is remembered today for his monumental *History of St. Bartholemew's Hospital.*

The concept of regional ileitis was slow to catch on in Britain after Crohn's description, partly because it was rare but mainly because it was a difficult diagnosis. Haematology and radiology were relatively unsophisticated before the Second World War and, as we have seen, even ulcerative colitis was frequently misdiagnosed or simply missed. Crohn's Disease was usually discovered at laparotomy for obstruction or suspected appendicitis as it can be today. Not surprisingly, the first reports after 1932 came from surgeons, and the disease was soon the subject of their discussion at meetings.

A report appeared in the *British Journal of Surgery* in 1933 in the short notes of rare or obscure cases section and was entitled "Granuloma of intestine. Stenosis of ileocaecal valve". It came from the unlikely pen of a surgeon practising in Folkstone called Hickman Walter Lancelot Molesworth (1892–1969), known to his friends as Moley, who described a woman of 30 with obstruction who had had an appendicectomy ten years earlier.[50] At laparotomy in July 1932 she had classical Crohn's Disease, though Molesworth would not have heard of Crohn whose paper did not appear until the following October. He was simply recording an unusual case and later probably dined out on his early description of a new disease, being a *bon viveur*, considerable athlete, first-class shot and fine fisherman. He was also an enthusiastic surgeon and once performed a successful partial cystectomy on one of his labradors.

Another provincial surgeon, Walter Jackman (1892–1964) in Bristol, described two cases of "localized hypertrophic enteritis as a cause of intestinal obstruction" in young women in 1934. They may have had Crohn's Disease though the pathologist found no evidence of a granulomatous infection, and Jackman was unaware of Crohn's description.[51]

Arthur Dickson Wright (1897–1976) was an outstanding surgeon at St. Mary's Hospital, Paddington, who "cut well, sewed well and whose patients got well". He was larger than life and is now best remembered for his wit and ability as an after-dinner speaker. Less well known is that he was probably the first person to mention the term Crohn's Disease in this country, choosing a meeting of the august Medical Society of London to present two cases in 1935. In his experience of seven cases most had presented as appendicitis and he recommended resection only if there were no complications; otherwise a short-circuit procedure was advisable. The prognosis was not entirely good as the disease tended to recur and some patients died. Several distinguished surgeons, including Zachary Cope (1881–1974), author, historian and poet, also from St. Mary's, had seen two or three cases and advised a short circuit.

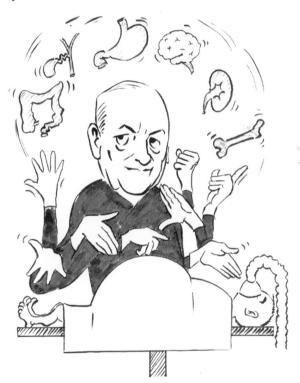

41 Dickson-Wright – Jack of all trades.

In addition, the physician-cum-pathologist, Frederick Parkes Weber (1863–1962), who collected everything from rare coins to rare diseases, had seen a case.[†] Someone in the audience suggested that occasionally a conservative approach was indicated, to which Dickson Wright replied, "All well-behaved surgeons feel that they must do something."[52]

The next year Harold Edwards (1899–1989), a surgeon at King's College Hospital and a future President of the British Society of Gastroenterology, presented a further case to the Medical Society. He thought his patient, an emaciated young woman aged 23, had tuberculous peritonitis, but undertook a laparotomy because of intense pain, and found a length of small intestine resembling a hosepipe. During discussion, Dickson Wright commented how extraordinary it was that such a clear cut, fairly common complaint had not been clearly described before Crohn's excellent paper. He also mentioned a patient aged 50 who was so emaciated that she weighed two stone twelve pounds (eighteen kilograms). At post mortem "the small intestine was greatly diminished in length due to fibrotic shrinkage", and again he stressed the high mortality of the condition.[53]

One of the fellows of the Medical Society who was especially interested in Dickson Wright's presentatation was Philip Manson-Bahr (1881–1966), physician to the Hospital for Tropical Diseases, London. Previously unaware of Crohn's Disease, he now realised that he had briefly witnessed a fatal case of the condition. The patient, a doctor aged 63, had been a medical missionary for 30 years until ill health kept him at home. In 1934 he was admitted to hospital with a fever and was thought to have amoebic hepatitis. He was difficult to manage and discharged himself, but two weeks later he was admitted to the Hospital for Tropical Diseases under Manson-Bahr's care, dehydrated and toxic with a thrombosis of the right calf. He was drowsy and occasionally violent, and as his uncooperative attitude was dominating the clinical picture he was transferred to the Maudsley Hospital for psychiatric management. There he was tube fed, but he remained very withdrawn and emaciated, vomited most days and was doubly incontinent. He deteriorated and died in February 1935. Post mortem examination showed thirteen inflammatory strictures in the small intestine. Manson-Bahr encouraged the two young psychiatrists who had been looking

---

[†]   Known for his descriptions of Rendu-Osler-Weber disease (familial telangiectasia) and Weber's disease (localised epidermolysis bullosa).

after the patient to write up the case. The report, by Robert Barbour (1904–89) and Aldwyn Stokes (1906–78), was published in 1936 and was the first full description of Crohn's Disease to appear in a widely read British journal (the *Lancet*) and included a comprehensive review of the literature. Their article was entitled "Chronic cicatrising enteritis, a phase of benign non-specific granuloma of the small intestine".[54] In it, Barbour and Stokes emphasised that the cicatrisation did not usually give rise to a gross form of obstruction and in the absence of a palpable mass the clinical picture was often indefinite and diagnosis difficult; a view with which we can all sympathise. If we add the complication of a severe mental illness, it is not surprising that the diagnosis can be overlooked.

e) Dr. Harmer and Dr. Bailey – a curious coincidence

At first surgical resection was invariably recommended but within a few years a more conservative policy was adopted when people realised that spontaneous resolution was possible, particularly in the acute stage of the disease. For example, William Gill (1908–76), surgical registrar at Guy's Hospital in 1937, recognised two cases of Crohn's Disease in patients suspected of appendicitis. He removed the normal appendix but left the inflamed ileum alone and both patients did well.[55] But this was a matter of great debate for many years, and an entertaining report supporting early resection came from two doctors with the disease, Michael Harmer (1912–98), a surgeon, and Joe Bailey (1915–97), a general practitioner.[56] Both underwent resection of the terminal ileum when they were medical students at St. Bartholemew's Hospital in 1936 and 1943, after which both enjoyed excellent health into ripe old age. At laparotomy, Harmer was thought to have ileocaecal tuberculosis but fortunately the surgeon, Harold Wilson (1880–1959) resected the offending bowel. Afterwards Wilson showed Harmer the pathology report saying, "Sonny, you had better read this, it's all Greek to me." It had been reported in detail by A. H. T. Robb-Smith who had read Crohn's paper and realised this was regional ileitis. His acumen spared the patient a year or more in a sanatorium, which undoubtedly would have been his fate if he had had tuberculosis. Joe Bailey presented with lassitude, abdominal pain and weight loss. A barium follow-through revealed the string sign. Later he obstructed and at laparotomy the assistant surgeon, who was none other than Michael Harmer, had no doubt that the diagnosis was

Crohn's Disease, which was resected. Bailey recalls how shortly before he obstructed he went for a forces medical, and in spite of his X-rays – string sign and all – he was passed A1 fit for service. Some months later, when he was completely recovered, the same army doctor pronounced him unfit for service anywhere.

f) First description of pathology of Crohn's Disease

An important British contribution just before the Second World War came from a pathologist, Geoffrey Hadfield (1889–1968), who was the first to define the precise histology of regional ileitis. Hadfield was well known for his teaching and successively held four chairs of pathology, at the Royal Free Hospital (1928), at Bristol (1933), at St. Bartholemew's Hospital (1934) and at the Royal College of Surgeons (1948). He showed that the lesion in Crohn's Disease began in the submucosa with lymphadenoid hyperplasia similar to tuberculosis but without caseation or acid fast bacilli. The lesion was often obscured by secondary infection and ulceration, but could usually be identified in the neighbouring lymph glands. He likened the process from a purely histological point of view to that seen in sarcoidosis.[57]

CHAPTER THIRTY-EIGHT

THERAPEUTIC BREAKTHROUGH OF IBD

During the Second World War, inflammatory bowel disease was low on the medical agenda. Many physicians and surgeons were on active service and research was naturally directed to the war effort. Colitis, it seemed, was still relatively rare, indeed Joseph Kirsner recalls that during three and a half years overseas' service he saw only two American soldiers with ulcerative colitis.[58]

Yet the war had a profound, if indirect, influence on the development of two new drugs that were to transform the treatment of inflammatory bowel disease. These were sulphasalazine and cortisone, synthesised in 1938 and 1948 respectively. Sulphasalazine was introduced during the war in Sweden, but few in Britain knew anything about it until long after the war was over. In contrast, rumours that Luftwaffe pilots, boosted with injections of adrenal cortex hormones, were able to fly at heights of over 40,000 feet, led to a major research programme in the United States to isolate cortisone, the new wonder drug. This was an era when several effective new compounds were being discovered by research chemists, such as antibiotics, antithyroid agents, oral hypoglycaemics and thiazide diuretics. Frequently, their discovery was serendipitous, and the diseases for which they were prescribed and their mode of action were far from understood at the time.

a) Sulphasalazine

The story of the discovery of sulphasalazine belongs to Dr. Nanna Svartz (1890–1986), Professor of Medicine at the Karolinska Hospital in Stockholm. Before the Second World War, she was convinced that rheumatoid arthritis was caused by an infection, probably with streptococci, and she knew, of course, that salicylates had a useful anti-inflammatory effect. She also believed that ulcerative colitis was caused by streptococci, so when Lionel Whitby (1895–1956) introduced sulphapyridine (M & B 693) into clinical use in 1938, she managed to obtain some samples of the drug from England, which she gave to patients with arthritis and colitis. Like others, she found that some of her colitics, but not arthritics, reacted favourably to sulfapyridine. However, in the belief that the inflammatory changes of the two diseases were similar and that the changes in ulcerative colitis began in the connective tissue of the submucosa, she was anxious to find a drug that would target this tissue. For some reason, she decided to combine salicylic acid with sulfapyridine, though quite why is obscure. There was certainly no evidence that either drug alone had a selective affinity for connective tissue, but presumably at the time she thought salicylic acid would carry the sulphapyridine to the site of the inflammation. The chemistry was difficult, but she was fortunate to obtain the help of Philip Willstedt, a chemist seconded from Berlin in 1938 by the pharmaceutical company, Pharmacia, to work with her at Stockholm University. Within weeks he produced a compound combining salicylic acid with sulfapyridine, which became known as salazopyrin. After experiments in mice, Svartz treated her first patient with ulcerative colitis in November 1940 with remarkable results. The patient, a young man aged seventeen, had had colitis for five years preventing him from attending school. On admission he had polyarthritis and hepatitis. He improved slightly with sulphapyridine but, after nine months in hospital, his colitis was still active. He was given sulphasalazine and responded rapidly. After discharge he was well and able to start work in a factory. Several other patients responded equally well, whereas the response in rheumatoid arthritis was much less impressive.[59]

Encouraged by these results, Svartz continued to study sulphasalazine, but her work remained unknown until after the war. By 1947 she had treated 124 colitics with remarkable success, particularly the milder cases.[60] She did not compare her patients with controls (this was before the time of double blind trials) but was in no doubt that the drug worked because most of the patients responded within a few days. Treatment had to be prolonged, a year or more, otherwise relapse was inevitable. Side effects were common but usually mild, and fewer than ten per cent of patients needed to stop the drug. She believed that the sulphapyridine component was the active agent and was able to exert its effect after its liberation from sulphasalazine in the submucosal connective tissue.

Once the war was over, Arnold Bargen at the Mayo Clinic introduced sulphasalazine to the United States, and by 1949 had given it to 300 patients with colitis.[61] He was enthusiastic: "Salicylazosulfapyridine is the most valuable drug that has been introduced for the treatment of ulcerative colitis in my lifetime." Others, including Lester Morrison in Los Angeles and Joseph Kirsner in Chicago, agreed and thought it had an antibiotic effect. However, in Britain, the drug only became available in 1955. A report in the *Brit. Med. J.* of the proceedings of the International Congress of Gastroenterology, held in London in July 1956, refers to sulphasalazine as an "apparently specific remedy", but the delegates must have been impressed by Svartz's series of 455 patients, most of whom were very well on maintenance therapy.[62] The slow adoption of sulphasalazine has several explanations. Colitis was still poorly understood by most doctors and the subject was accorded little importance in medical school; sulphasalazine was thought of as an antibiotic and several alternatives were available; the management of colitis was still largely in the hands of the surgeons who were more concerned about operative intervention; and, not least, the arrival of cortisone was dominating the picture.

b) Cortisone

Compound E was originally isolated from the adrenal gland in 1936 by Edward Kendall at the Mayo Clinic, but it was not until 1948 that a few grams of pure compound E, or cortisone, were obtained. Its effect on rheumatoid arthritis was miraculous and soon it was shown to be effective in a range of other, unexplained, inflammatory conditions. The first people to use it in ulcerative colitis were William Dearing and Philip Brown, physicians at the Mayo Clinic, in 1950, and the results were not encouraging.[63] Only one out of four young patients with moderate to severe chronic colitis given cortisone, 50 milograms twice daily for 35 days, became well, and none showed sigmoidoscopic improvement. Fortunately six patients in another study by Thomas Machella, assistant professor of medicine in Philadelphia, did better.[64] Meanwhile, Walter Palmer (1896–1993) and Joseph Kirsner in Chicago had begun a long series of studies of ACTH and various steroid preparations that showed how effective they could be.[65] Kirsner recalls that "the excitement and the anticipation of those early days among both patients and physicians can hardly be imagined. Despite attempts at controls, the generally high degree of expectation with this dramatically potent medication created an atmosphere of "success" and resulted in therapeutic responses obviously not exclusively attributable to the ACTH."[66] Indeed Arnold Bargen, with his huge experience of ulcerative colitis, went so far as to denounce cortisone in the treatment of colitis apart from a few specific indications. He was worried that cortisone was suppressing but not curing colitis and was worried by the side effects.[67]

The indications for its use had to be clarified but at the time nobody had a clear idea of the natural history and prognosis of colitis. It was this fact that first attracted the attention of Sidney Truelove (1913–2002), at the Nuffield Department of Clinical Medicine, Radcliffe

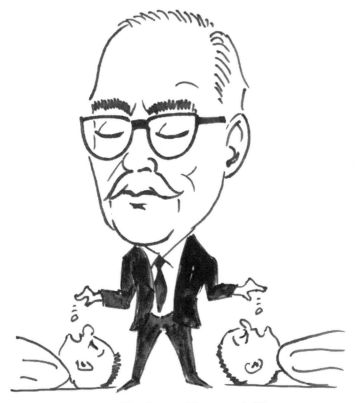

42 Truelove – Master triallist.

Infirmary, Oxford, whose name was to become indelibly associated with colitis.

After spending the war in the RAMC, Truelove joined Leslie Witts in Oxford as a general physician, but his interest soon turned to gastroenterology. He was well aware of the serious nature of ulcerative colitis and decided to review the fate of all the patients who had been admitted to hospital from 1938 to 1949.[68] What he found makes dismal reading; 20 per cent died during the first year of their disease with a further 10 per cent dying within five years. Half of those lucky enough to survive led very restricted lives. This was the state of affairs in 1950 shortly before cortisone was introduced, and it coincided with the stunning achievements of a statistician, Austin Bradford Hill (1897–1991), who had just proved that streptomycin combined with PAS (but not either drug alone) cured tuberculosis. Hill had achieved this using a new statistical method, the randomised controlled therapeutic trial, which was soon to become the sole arbiter of scientific truth. Truelove had already learnt the dark art of statistics during the war and realised that a randomised trial would be the only way to prove that cortisone was effective in ulcerative colitis.

The trial began in 1952. In order to obtain a significant result, Truelove and Witts were aware that they would need to recruit more patients than they had at their disposal. So they collaborated with several physicians from four other regions: North West London (Avery Jones), Birmingham (Lionel Hardy), Leeds (Geoffrey Watkinson) and Edinburgh (Wilfrid Card). Card (1908–85) was well chosen for his expertise as a statistician and mathematician, and ran the first gastrointestinal unit with "total collaboration between the disciplines (medicine and surgery) to the point of loss of personal sovereignty".[69]

The organisers were fortunate to have the help of Richard Doll (1912–2005), who had kept up his interest in gastroenterology with Avery Jones at the Central Middlesex Hospital, though he was now working with Bradford Hill on the link between lung cancer and smoking. Just over 200 patients entered the trial and they were randomised to receive cortisone or a placebo for six weeks. None of the physicians knew which treatment his patient had received. Most of the patients managed to complete the trial and those in the cortisone group fared much better than the others. Patients who were severely ill before treatment still did worse than patients with mild disease, but they nearly all showed some response to cortisone. Furthermore, the best response happened in the first attack of colitis, which was known to be the most dangerous. Consequently the mortality fell from 24 per cent in the control group to 7 per cent in the cortisone group.[70]

Before the trial, cortisone had been criticised because it was thought to be suppressing the symptoms of colitis while the underlying disease remained active, possibly with dire consequences. However, Truelove and Witts were able to show that the majority of patients in remission after cortisone had inactive disease. Admittedly a few did have active disease, but this applied equally to the control group, so the risk of suppressing the disease was probably unfounded.

The trial produced an unequivocal result despite the fact that only 200 patients were studied. This might seem a small number now, but was adequate because active treatment was being compared with placebo. Today attempts to prove that a new treatment is superior to an existing effective one require much larger trials backed by statistical analysis.

The trial highlighted the difficulty of assessing colitis and its response to treatment. In fact the Oxford definition of severe, acute colitis has never been bettered, despite its shortcomings (six or more bloody stools a day, fever, tachycardia, anaemia and raised sedimentation rate). Truelove used sigmoidoscopy as a key measure of activity, but 40 per cent of the patients did not have a second sigmoidoscopy after treatment. Physicians were still reluctant to use the instrument, as Truelove put it, either "for fear of provoking a recurrence", or (more likely) "because they failed to appreciate the desirability as part of the assessment of results". Truelove also realised that simply looking at the rectal mucosa with a sigmoidoscope was an inexact science prone to observer error and bias. Soon after the trial he showed that it was feasible and safe to obtain biopsies from the rectal mucosa. In one study, he found that more than half of his patients in apparent remission had abnormal sigmoidoscopies, and still more misleading, several with a normal-looking rectum had histological evidence of inflammation.[71] Biopsy would be essential in future.

The final lesson to come from the trial was that the benefit of cortisone was ill-sustained; relapses were common and surgery often necessary.

c) Surgery

Before the discovery of cortisone surgeons still dealt with most cases of colitis. The simple fact was that general practitioners referred their patients with rectal bleeding and diarrhoea to a surgeon because he was not only familiar with the diagnosis but offered hope of a cure. By the late 1940s it was clear that ileostomy alone did not work. Even when the colon had been "rested" for a year or more, closing the ileostomy was invariably followed by a flare-up of the colitis. Partial resection of the diseased bowel was tried for a while but recurrence of the colitis was inevitable. Gradually, despite the risks, surgeons began to remove the whole colon, initially as a two-stage procedure. An ileostomy was fashioned first and the colon excised a week or two later. The problem was not so much the colectomy, which, after all, surgeons had been doing for years, but the ileostomy.

Unlike colostomy, which was well tolerated, ileostomy was a disaster in itself for one reason: the contents of the small bowel are fluid, and it was impossible to contain these excretions. Leakage occurred constantly, soaking the dressings, so that the skin became ulcerated beneath what in effect became a faecal poultice. Peristomal ulceration, infection and even necrosis of the abdominal wall were not uncommon, and many patients developed relentless ulcerative enteritis and died. Surgery was frequently delayed until it was too late to save these emaciated patients. Then, in 1944, a young chemistry student with colitis living in Chicago, called Henry Koenig, changed everything.

Koenig needed a colectomy and ileostomy, and, encouraged by his surgeon Dr. Alfred Strauss (1881–1955), he managed to design a new receptacle to contain the ileal discharge. It consisted of a rubber pouch so thin as to be indiscernible even under tight-fitting clothes, and a glue to stick this to the skin. The bag could remain sealed to the skin for days with its contents being emptied at convenient moments during the day.[72] It worked brilliantly.[73]

News of Koenigs's invention soon spread. Lionel Hardy (1887–1969) visited Chicago in 1947 and brought a few samples back with him to Birmingham. He had many colitics under his care and was acutely aware of the failings of medical treatment. Ileostomy was still in vogue but miserable for the patients and in desperate need of refinement. Hardy had long felt that physician and surgeon working together were essential if patients with colitis were to be managed properly. He and his colleagues, Trevor Cooke (1911–87), and Clifford Hawkins (1915–91), his registrar at the time, were keen to experiment with the Koenig device and gave it to the newly appointed senior lecturer in surgery, Bryan Brooke (1915–98) to try out.[74] Here was an example of collaboration between physician and surgeon at its best. Cooke was a shy but determined man who was greatly respected by his surgical colleagues, Hawkins a man of excellent humour with plenty of drive and energy, and Brooke a talented and exuberant extrovert with natural ability. They enjoyed

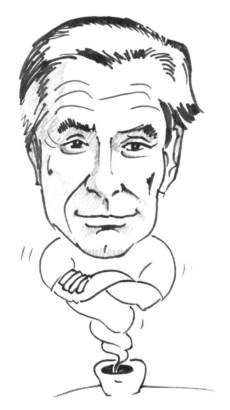

43 Brooke – Genie of spout ileostomy.

the support of their respective chiefs, Lionel Hardy, recently awarded a personal chair in gastroenterology, and Alan Stammers (1898–1982), professor of surgery, and they revelled in the exciting yet friendly ambience pervading the unit.

Brooke set about developing a stoma that would suit the adherent bag and the surgical technique to achieve a good fit. He realised that an ileostomy had to work perfectly if the surgical treatment of colitis was not to be discredited. A particular problem was stenosis at the stoma, and to get round this he devised an eversion ileostomy in which he evaginated the ileum and sutured the mucosa to the skin. This simple technique, described almost as an afterthought in an article in the *Lancet* in 1952, was highly successful and was later adopted worldwide.[75]

Meanwhile supplies of the ileostomy appliance were difficult to obtain due to currency restrictions. Undaunted, and despite a threat from the American manufacturer that they would be infringing his patent, Hardy and Brooke enrolled the help of the Dunlop company in Birmingham to manufacture the bag and the cement, which on analysis in the chemistry department of the university proved to be simple latex solution, laced with zinc oxide to give it a suitably medicinal appearance.

At first, Brooke fashioned a double-ended ileostomy leaving the colon *in situ*. This gave him the opportunity to hone his ileostomy technique and to gain experience of the new bag, but it also confirmed that resting the colon was ineffective. Thereafter he began to do a total colectomy, and almost overnight the outlook for these patients was transformed. Emaciated people regained weight, felt well and returned to normal life. Furthermore, the Koenig bag allowed surgeons to remove the colon as a matter of choice, before the patient was moribund, which meant the ileostomy and colectomy could be done as a one-stage procedure.

Bryan Brooke's ileostomy and the success of cortisone quickened interest in ulcerative colitis, as, for the first time, doctors had effective weapons with which to attack the disease. But treating a condition that was so capricious and inexplicable was never going to be easy, and few clinicians had much experience of it. By this time the National Health Service was well established with "specialists", as they were known, appointed to every district hospital. In fact, nearly all specialists, or consultants, were generalists, and gastroenterology was just one part of their job. Specialisation was still a long way off. The British Society of Gastroenterology was an exclusive organisation; in 1952 their council agreed that "it should be kept as small as possible and should consist only of people really interested and active in gastroenterology".[76] As a concession the number of ordinary members was increased that year to 65. So it was not surprising that Brooke's book *Ulcerative Colitis and its Surgical Treatment* had a profound impact on the profession when it appeared in 1954.[77] John Lennard-Jones recalls how, when he was a house physician, he was at the bedside of a patient with ulcerative colitis during a ward round, when his chief, Professor Max Rosenheim (1908–72), placed a copy of the book on the bed. It was opened at photographs showing the striking changes in a woman after surgical treatment. The team realised then how little they knew about the prognosis or management of colitis at that time.[78]

d) Medicine and surgery combined

The cortisone trial relied on the few centres already interested in colitis, such as Oxford, obviously, and Birmingham, but also Leeds where the young Geoffrey Watkinson(1921–96) was setting up a comprehensive gastroenterological service. As we have seen in an earlier chapter, Watkinson was heavily involved in researching the cause and treatment of peptic ulcer, but he also looked after a large number of patients with

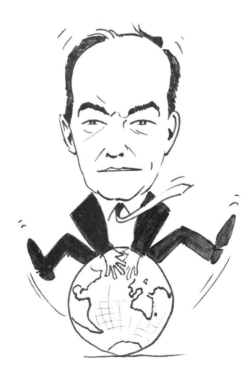

44 Watkinson – President of world organisation of gastroenterology.

colitis, which led Truelove and Witts to include Leeds in their trial. Just as this was completed, John Goligher (1912–98) moved to Leeds as the new professor of surgery in 1955. This was an inspired appointment as Goligher had been a consultant at St. Mary's Hospital, Paddington, and at St. Mark's Hospital for seven years and was an accomplished colorectal surgeon. His collaboration with Watkinson on a series of trials of surgery for peptic ulcer and ulcerative colitis continued for nearly fifteen years, long after Watkinson had moved from Leeds to York.

By 1960 Watkinson had almost 200 patients with colitis under his care, a remarkable personal series at the time. Most of these were mild to moderate cases, and he realised that preventing an attack of colitis was infinitely preferable to coping with a relapse; he was one of the first to use sulphasalazine as maintenance therapy in this country.[79]

At the same time, the favourable results from the topical use of hydrocortisone in skin and eye disease had prompted Truelove to apply steroids in the form of retention enemas to patients with distal colitis.[80] He and Watkinson both showed independently that hydrocortisone given as a rectal drip was more effective than saline given in the same way.[81] Later they joined forces to show that the best way of getting a speedy remission in severe attacks was to use a combination of local and systemic corticoid therapy.[82]

The problem facing surgeons was when to operate on a seriously ill patient in a relapse. Even a definition of "super-severe" colitis was well-nigh impossible, no criteria adequately defining the severity of the illness. Brooke wrote that a fulminating episode of colitis "beggared exact definition" but, in addition to all the criteria of Truelove and Witts, he suggested impending coma and serious alteration of blood chemistry.[83] Though cortisone was capable of inducing a remission, if it failed, surgery that had been postponed was now required in a critically ill patient.

For ten years Watkinson and Goligher tried not to operate until the patient had had a period of intensive medical treatment for at least ten days. With this plan they found that one third of the patients needed surgery (one-stage ileostomy and complete proctocolectomy) and twenty per cent died from sepsis or perforation. They blamed the high mortality on the delay in operating and began to operate much sooner if there was no response to medical treatment. As a result, more patients had a colectomy but only seven per cent died. Meanwhile, the results of conservative treatment also improved as time went by, particularly among the older patients. These trials were a model of their kind and succeeded because of the close cooperation between the medical and surgical departments.[84]

Goligher became President of the British Society of Gastroenterology shortly before his retirement in 1977, and Watkinson succeeded him as president a year later. By this time Watkinson had left York where circumstances beyond his control had led to tensions and the loss of the Leeds connection. Finding his position intolerable he moved in 1969 to Glasgow and became a key figure in the World Organisation of Gastroenterology.

Meanwhile Brooke founded the Ileostomy Association in 1956 and was elected its first president, but he was bitterly disappointed when he was not chosen to succeed Stammers in Birmingham who retired in 1962. The next year he was appointed the first professor of surgery at St. George's Hospital, but his senior colleagues found the presence of

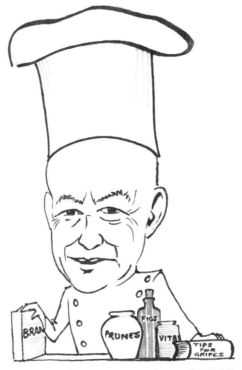

45 Avery Jones – Dietetic department – Central Middlesex Hospital.

an energetic and unconventional academic in their midst disquieting, and Brooke felt isolated and disillusioned. Fortunately his international reputation flourished and he was in steady demand at international meetings and as a visiting professor in America and Australia.

Unfortunately close cooperation between surgeon and physician was unusual in those days. Though matters were slowly improving, patients with colitis were still managed by general surgeons with minimal input from physicians.

Curiously the London consultants were no exception apart from Francis Avery Jones (1910–2000), physician to the Central Middlesex Hospital. His lifelong interest in nutrition had fuelled his concern for patients with ulcerative colitis who were dying of malnutrition and starvation, and he was the only physician in England to run a combined medical-surgical ward where he could take an active interest in the post-operative care of his patients. Taking after Hurst, he promoted the use of the sigmoidoscope keeping one concealed in his waistcoat and producing it with a flourish to startled physicians at every opportunity. For several

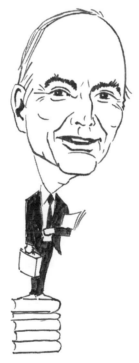

46 Lennard-Jones – Giant among gastroenterologists.

years he held an out-patient clinic at St. Mark's Hospital in an honorary capacity on Friday mornings. There he would see 40 to 50 patients with ulcerative colitis, so when Truelove and Witts began the cortisone trial, he was ideally placed to contribute cases and was closely involved in it.

When the results of that trial were discussed at the autumn meeting of the British Society of Gastroenterology in Oxford in 1955 (with Witts as president), the young John Lennard-Jones (born 1927) was a guest and was introduced to Avery Jones. Later he became his registrar at the Central Middlesex Hospital and began to see patients with ulcerative colitis and to assist Avery Jones with his weekly clinic at St. Mark's Hospital. At the time St. Mark's was run entirely by surgeons with no day-to-day medical gastroenterological care, so in his spare time Lennard-Jones voluntarily took over the care, at a junior level, of inpatients at the hospital, which he continued for seven years without a contract.

Inevitably he became involved in the management of fulminating colitis and decided to look at what had happened to 32 seriously ill patients treated between 1951 and 1959 at the two hospitals.[85] This was a critical decade because physicians were finding their way with cortisone, and surgeons were moving away from defunctioning ileostomy towards radical surgery. He was disconcerted to find that the overall mortality was 30 per cent. In essence he confirmed the problems highlighted by Goligher in Leeds and Brooke in Birmingham; large doses of cortisone could help but surgery should not be delayed. If it was, the risk of a fatal perforation was high. Furthermore, the patients who had a colectomy did better than those who had a diverting ileostomy. Close supervision by physician and surgeon was crucial, something that had not been available at the all-surgical St. Mark's Hospital until he arrived.

The exciting discoveries of cortisone and sulphasalazine and the feasibility of colectomy were paralleled by an apparent increase in the frequency of ulcerative colitis. It was certainly more common than people once thought and cases were appearing out of the woodwork for treatment especially at specialist centres. There was an air of optimism among clinicians but was this justified?

To answer this, Truelove extended his earlier study (p303) to look back at all the patients treated for colitis in Oxford from 1938–62. He was ably assisted by Felicity Edwards (born 1927) who had worked in Tom McKeown's (1912–88) social medicine department in Birmingham. They managed to trace every single case, 624 in all, a remarkable achievement in itself, driving around the Oxfordshire countryside in Truelove's Morris Minor calling on neighbours for any information on missing patients. Edwards and Truelove divided the study into two periods; 1938–52 (pre-cortisone), and 1952–62(post-cortisone) and used actuarial methods to analyse their data.[86] Several interesting facts emerged. Firstly, though the prognosis was much better in the cortisone era, ulcerative colitis was still a formidable disease with a high mortality (30 per cent) during attacks, especially if the colon was severely and extensively inflamed and the patient was over 60. Patients who survived could certainly expect further attacks; within twelve months, four out of every five patients had had a relapse, and the risk of death was much greater than normal for the rest of their lives. The second interesting feature was a decline in the number of severe attacks in the second period with a corresponding rise in mild cases, which in itself helped to improve the overall mortality. Lastly, and perhaps most striking, was the dramatic fall in deaths from moderate disease after 1952, which Truelove ascribed to improved supportive measures and cortisone in particular. In Oxford, a conservative approach was favoured at the time because early colectomy was considered to be too risky and delayed colectomy carried a 30 per cent mortality. As a result very few severely ill patients underwent emergency surgery during the period under review.

Thus the overall picture had improved since the arrival of steroids, but management of the seriously ill patient remained a challenge. Surgeons such as Goligher were pushing for earlier surgery, and Brooke in particular was concerned that persisting with steroids made the entire colon friable and prejudiced the results of surgery. This was a hard message for the naturally conservative physician.

The most fruitful approach appeared to be to prevent relapses from occurring at all, or at least minimise them, so rendering them more susceptible to steroids.

CHAPTER THIRTY-NINE

THE FIVE–AMINOSALICYLATES

Earlier I suggested that the introduction of sulphasalazine in Britain in 1955 was overshadowed by the dominance of cortisone. Despite the enthusiasm for sulphasalazine in America, doctors here had been impressed by the cortisone trial and were hoping that maintenance therapy with small doses of cortisone combined with rectal steroids would be effective. The chief protagonists were Truelove in Oxford and Watkinson in Leeds, but both found that small doses of cortisone given for months or even years were disappointing. Half of their patients relapsed and increasing the dose caused unacceptable side effects. Rectal steroids were more promising and most patients improved, but for obvious reasons their long-term use was unpopular and aesthetically unacceptable. Though Watkinson used sulphasalazine and found that half his patients remained in remission for periods up to six years,[87] he withdrew the drug after the patient had been in remission for six months. The concept of maintenance therapy for a disease that remitted for long periods was alien to most people (doctor and patient), especially if the drug in question had side effects or its mode of action was unknown.

a) Clinical trials at St. Mark's Hospital

In 1958 Avery Jones and Lennard-Jones began to experiment with sulphasalazine at St. Mark's Hospital, where there was a large clinic of patients with colitis at their disposal. They began by comparing sulphasalazine with cortisone in patients having a moderate attack of colitis and found that sulphasalazine, like cortisone, was certainly useful.[88] By this time the concept of the controlled trial was well established so they decided to conduct a formal trial of sulphasalazine alone, even though Witts had recently suggested that the use of a placebo was no longer justified as steroids were known to be effective in ulcerative colitis.[89] However, Lennard-Jones argued that steroids were dangerous and sulphasalazine would be used with more confidence if he could prove its value.

It was now that they were able to recruit the services of three honorary clinical assistants in medicine all working at St. Mark's Hospital. This curious state of affairs arose because, at that time, there were almost no research facilities in gastroenterology at the London teaching hospitals, whereas at St. Mark's Hospital, under the inspiration of Avery Jones, the opportunities for research were encouraged. All three young men were known to Avery; Hugh Baron (born 1931) had studied medicine at the Central Middlesex Hospital and was now completing his MD on gastric acid at the Middlesex Hospital with the support of George Hadley (1908–84). Alastair Connell (born 1931) and George Misiewicz (born 1930) were both research fellows at the Central Middlesex Hospital (not, it must be emphasised, at that time a teaching hospital) and visited St. Mark's Hospital to study colonic motility. All three were eager to be involved in the trial.

Svartz had already shown that the side effects of sulphasalazine were due to the sulphapyridine component, so they began by comparing the drug with a specially prepared compound, salicylazosulphadimidine which they thought might be less toxic.[90] The patients all had moderately active colitis, and it was soon clear that the sulphadimidine compound was ineffective, whereas, after four weeks, sulphasalazine was superior to placebo. Extraordinarily, this was the first randomised controlled trial of sulphasalaine, no less than twenty years after its introduction, and it was feasible because Lennard-Jones introduced a biometric approach to the assessment of ulcerative colitis. By grading the severity of the mucosal changes seen at sigmoidoscopy he was able to compare the response to treatment more objectively than before (quite novel in gastroenterology at the time).

Next, using this simple model of the so-called double-blind study (whereby neither doctor nor patient knew what was being prescribed), they proved that maintenance therapy for at least a year with sulphasalazine was highly effective, unlike maintenance with prednisone.[91] Furthermore the incidence of side effects from sulphasalazine was small (by comparison with steroids).

Subsequently, Truelove confirmed the benefit of maintenance treatment when he showed that his patients could be kept in remission for up to five years.[92] They not only felt well, but also had normal sigmoidoscopic appearances and rectal biopsies.

Francis Avery Jones was now the leading figure in British gastroenterology; and all three of the younger members of the St. Mark's group were destined to have eminent careers in gastroenterology and to become presidents of the British Society of Gastroenterology. Only Alastair Connell decamped, moving to the department of surgery in Belfast before emigrating to America to be Professor of Medicine in Cincinnati.

b) Unravelling the mode of action of sulphasalazine

Sulphasalazine became the drug of choice in ulcerative colitis, but no one knew how it worked and there was concern about its safety. Nanna Svartz always played down the side effects of the drug, but most clinicians in the United Kingdom found that ten to twenty per cent of their patients could not tolerate it. This had important implications for the Swedish manufacturers, Pharmacia, who were acutely aware of its huge potential (by 1975, 4,000 million tablets had been sold), so they once more asked their research department in Uppsala to study the metabolism of the compound that had baffled Svartz for so long. They were fortunate to have two biochemists, Hasse Schroder and Dag Campbell (of Scottish ancestry), whose brilliant studies managed to unravel its metabolism.

Using the technique of thin-layer chromatography to measure sulphasalazine and its metabolites, Schroder and Campbell studied ten healthy volunteers and showed that though the drug itself was absorbed to some extent, much more was absorbed as the metabolite, sulphapyridine.[93] Significantly, the appearance of the metabolite was delayed by two to three hours implying that it was absorbed further down the intestine. They deduced from this that most of the sulphasalazine reached the colon intact where it was split releasing its metabolites, sulphapyridine and 5-ASA. Schroder was aware that bacteria were able to cleave azo compounds and went on to show that this applied to the azo bond in sulphasalazine. For example he found that the colon of normal rats split the azo bond whereas the sterile colon of germ-free rats did not.

Quite independently, two Americans in Boston, delightfully named Peter Goldman and Mark Peppercorn, found exactly the same, but in addition they showed that most of the second major metabolite, 5-ASA, was not absorbed but was excreted in the faeces.[94] So it seemed that sulphasalazine was a means of delivering sulphapyridine and 5-ASA to the lumen of the colon where reduction of the drug by bacteria released the metabolites.

Schroder noticed that the level of sulphapyridine in his subjects was unpredictable so he approached David Price Evans, a quiet Welshman working in the department of medicine at Liverpool who was an authority on the genetics of drug metabolism. Evans had found that people varied in their ability to acetylate and excrete drugs such as isoniazid and sulfamethazine and could therefore be classed as slow or rapid acetylators. With Schroder he studied 27 healthy subjects and confirmed that this was also the case with sulphapyridine. Indeed they found that the adverse effects of sulphasalazine were not due to the drug itself but to the absorbed metabolite, sulphapyridine, particularly among slow acetylators who took longer to eliminate the drug.[95]

At much the same time, Pharmacia had asked Bill Sircus in Edinburgh to carry out further clinical studies of sulphasalazine in his patients. Sircus looked after a large number of people with inflammatory bowel disease and had just acquired a gastrointestinal research laboratory at the Western General Hospital sponsored by the Wolfson Foundation. This coincided with the appointment of Martin Eastwood (born 1935) who had an MSc in biochemistry and, incidentally, suffered lifelong subacute obstruction after an experiment during which he lost a nasogastric tube necessitating two laparotomies. He was joined by a bright young PhD student, Kiron Das, who later became Director of the Division of Gastroenterology at Mt. Sinai Hospital, New York. They worked well together, confirmed Schroder's work and found that among 88 patients with ulcerative colitis, the level of sulphapyridine in the blood was critical; below 20 ug/ml was ineffective and above 50 ug/ml was toxic. Patients varied according to whether they were fast or slow acetylators, and the group recommended that the dose of sulphasalazine should be reduced from the usual 4 grams per day to 2.5 grams per day in slow acetylators.[96] They published this suggestion in the *New England Journal of Medicine* in 1973 and thereafter received no more financial support from Pharmacia. In a further crucial study they looked at eight patients who had had a colectomy and, as expected, found that whereas the absorption of sulphasalazine was unaffected, very little sulphapyridine appeared in the blood, proving that colonic bacteria were necessary for the release of sulphapyridine from sulphasalazine.[97] For the first time they speculated on the possible role of 5-ASA in the colon but did not follow it up.

Similar experiments were carried out by Schroder and Price Evans in Liverpool who also suggested that the effect of sulphasalazine could be due to the intracolonic release of sulphapyridine or 5-ASA in high concentrations but again took things no further.[98]

The *coup de grace* came from Sidney Truelove who proved that 5-ASA was in fact the therapeutic moiety of sulphasalazine. He knew that he could not compare the effect of sulphasalazine with its metabolites in the colon if they were given by mouth because sulphapyridine and 5-ASA are completely absorbed from the small intestine. So he devised the simple but brilliant experiment to administer the three compounds topically in the form of retention enemas. With the help of Pharmacia he gave equivalent doses of each drug per rectum for two weeks to 62 patients with colitis and found that 5-ASA was far superior to sulphapyridine.[99]

Before long others had found that 5-ASA suppositories were useful in people with proctitis and also that high-dose 5-ASA enemas were effective in active distal colitis.[100] Unfortunately, 5-ASA is an unstable compound in solution turning an ominous brown colour and has to be made up freshly every three weeks. Furthermore enemas are not an ideal method of long-term maintenance therapy, though in the absence of an alternative, many patients with colitis were more than happy to put them up and to put up with them. Lastly, they are of limited value in patients whose colitis extends above the splenic flexure.

c) Olsalazine

In fact, no sooner had Truelove demonstrated that 5-ASA was the therapeutically active moiety of sulphasalazine than it occurred to him that it should be possible to synthesise an alternative compound that would deliver 5-ASA to the colon without the side effects of sulphapyridine. In due course, in collaboration with research chemists at Pharmacia, he came up with disodium azodisalicylate, consisting of two salicylate radicals linked by an azo bond, his so-called back-to-back

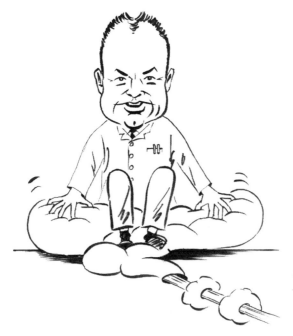

47 Travis – Suppressing colonic inflammation.

compound. This was a brilliant concept and he had high hopes that the drug would not only be safer but twice as effective as sulphasalazine.[101] The early trials, run by his senior registrar, Peter Willoughby (born 1948), were promising, and, after Truelove's retirement, the Oxford group now led by Derek Jewell spent several years championing the drug. A succession of research fellows including Warwick Selby,[102] G. D. Barr, Alan Ireland[103] and Simon Travis[104] showed that it was effective in ulcerative colitis and generally well tolerated but it had one drawback: nearly 30 per cent of patients developed diarrhoea forcing half of them to stop the drug.

d) Balsalazide

Meanwhile, in 1980, unaware of Truelove's work, Hugh Baron and John Lennard-Jones also conceived the idea of a prodrug similar to sulphasalazine but with an inert carrier molecule. Baron put their thoughts to Pharmacia who were not interested (naturally enough as they were busy developing olsalazine) so he turned to a research-based company, Biorex Laboratories, with whom he had worked on liquorice preparations for gastric ulcer. They were supportive and managed to synthesise a compound linking 5-ASA with 4-aminobenzoylalanine (4 ABA), which duly underwent extensive toxicology and pharmacokinetic studies.[105] All went well and eventually it was marketed as Balsalazide in 1990.[106] Subsequent large multicentre trials, notably one coordinated by Jonathan Green in Stoke-on-Trent, confirmed its efficacy and safety and possible superiority to alternative 5-ASA compounds.[107]

Astonishingly, neither of these drugs was widely prescribed in this country.

Olsalazine have one significant drawback in causing diarrhoea, but balsalazide did everything asked of it. So what was the problem? Simply that both drugs were forestalled by another drug, simple 5-ASA itself, or mesalazine, in a slow-release form that was highly effective.

e) Mesalazine

Slow-release mesalazine was the brainchild of John Rhodes (born 1935), a gastroenterologist in Cardiff. During the late 1970s he had been working on the delivery of peppermint to the colon to help people with irritable bowel syndrome. With his pharmacist, Brian Evans, who had a PhD in pharmacokinetics, Rhodes had been experimenting with various coatings for the compound (colpermin) when it occurred to him that they should see if they could do the same with 5-ASA. At this stage, 1981, his new senior registrar, Michael Dew, arrived to assist with the project, and things moved very quickly. They knew from the telemetry studies of Robert Bown that the pH of the intestinal juice rises steadily between the duodenum and the terminal ileum and found an acrylic resin, eudragit-S, that dissolves in an alkaline medium, making it an ideal coating for the delivery of compounds to the caecum. To test their hypothesis they coated some barium markers and sulphapyridine[†] with eudragit and followed their progress down the intestine of six volunteers radiographically.[108] After studying several thicknesses of eudragit they managed to produce a capsule that dissolved regularly in the distal ileum releasing sulphapyridine about twelve hours after ingestion. Next they gave the capsule, now containing 5-ASA instead of sulphapyridine to just

---

† They could not measure 5-ASA at the time.

6 patients with ulcerative colitis and were amazed and delighted by the result. All six patients stayed in remission. Further placebo-controlled trials followed with the support of the Boots Pure Drug Company[109] but Boots later withdrew believing that the market potential was too small. Rhodes then turned to Tillotts Laboratories who marketed colpermin, and they agreed to market the drug under the trade name Asacol.[110] The committee for the safety of medicines waved the drug through and by 1985 it was being widely prescribed.

Unlike olsalazine and balsalazide that were new compounds, mesalazine was already well known and did not have to endure the usual lengthy process of animal and human toxicology studies. By the time the prodrugs were launched, mesalazine, as Asacol, had been in use for three years and patients liked it. At one stage Asacol commanded 90 per cent of the salicylate market. Despite the theoretical advantages of balsalazide, which was a good product, innumerable clinical trials showed that there was little to choose between the salicylates in practice. A drug that is well established is difficult to dislodge, which has been the experience of another slow-release mesalazine preparation from Denmark, Pentasa. Here 5-ASA is coated with ethyl cellulose and released gradually throughout the small intestine and proximal colon. Many trials have shown that it is effective and aggressive marketing by Ferring has had a significant impact on sales.

CHAPTER FORTY

EPIDEMIOLOGY

a) Ulcerative colitis

The arrival of cortisone and the salicylates was not a moment too soon. More and more people seemed to be getting colitis and Crohn's Disease, though no one actually knew how common the diseases were.

Mortality figures for ulcerative colitis first became available in 1940 when the crude annual death rate in England and Wales was 1.5 per 100,000. This figure declined steeply to 0.9 in 1947 after which it levelled off for several years despite the introduction of steroids.[111] However, mortality rates cannot be used to calculate the frequency of a chronic disease such as ulcerative colitis because they reflect not simply the incidence of the disease but the efficacy of treatment.

Hospital records improved during the 1930s but the war interrupted their use for epidemiological research. Later, while interest in peptic ulcer became intense (the prevalence in middle-aged men was ten per cent in 1950), little notice was taken of ulcerative colitis until John Naish (1915–2009), a physician at Frenchay Hospital, estimated the frequency of colitis in the Bristol area.

Naish had seen a great deal of amoebic dysentery during war service with the Royal Navy. Afterwards, while registrar in Bristol, "where no one was interested in gastroenterology", he started a sigmoidoscopy clinic for the large number of servicemen returning home with chronic diarrhoea.[112] Very few had dysentery but he did see several cases of ulcerative colitis. He recalls how the mucosa, far from looking ulcerated as he expected, had the appearance of soggy pink blotting paper, "eczema of the colon", he called it. Gradually he accumulated

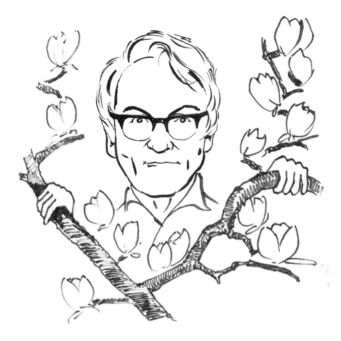

48 Naish – Algars Manor.

a large series of patients with colitis and Crohn's Disease and with the help of his registrar, Ted Houghton (1927–59), who lost his life in a climbing accident a few months later, Naish emphasised the familial nature of both conditions.[113] Colitis and Crohn's Disease occurred in the same family more often than if chance alone was responsible. To show this he needed to know the prevalence of colitis in the population as a whole. A search of the records revealed that 170 patients had been admitted for treatment of their colitis between 1953 and 1955. By assuming that at least a quarter of all colitics in the city were admitted once, he deduced that there might be 680 patients with ulcerative colitis living in Bristol (population 800,000), a prevalence of 85 per 100,000. Though highly speculative, this figure proved to be surprisingly accurate. An early member of the British Society of Gastroenterology, Naish was one of the group who were the first to describe lymphoma complicating coeliac disease. He also had a small farm and was interested in horticulture. On retirement he began to propagate magnolias and camelias; Algars Manor in Iron Acton is highly regarded in gardening circles and well worth a visit.

The first person to carry out a formal epidemiological study of ulcerative colitis was Donald Acheson (1926–2010) while in the Nuffield Department of Clinical Medicine, Oxford. Acheson had just returned from Washington DC, where, as Radcliffe Travelling Fellow, he had carried out the first surveys of ulcerative colitis in the United States using the comprehensive records of the veterans' administration.[114]

To gather data on every case of colitis in a community over a period of ten years (1950–60) was a daunting task and Acheson was well aware of the problems confronting him.

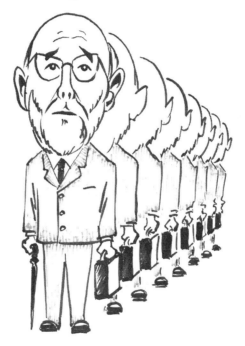

49 Acheson – CMO – and epidemiologist.

To start with, the diagnosis of ulcerative colitis was imprecise to say the least and he had to rely on the records and opinions of others. Furthermore his study would be retrospective and indirect as he put it. In other words he could only include people known to have colitis. This may sound obvious but meant that all those unaware of their disease or unprepared to seek advice were inevitably overlooked. Conversely some who were admitted to hospital several times would inflate the figures. Here Acheson was fortunate in that he was able to make use of the Oxford Record Linkage System, a remarkably complete diagnostic index of all patients admitted to hospital since 1938. This was obviously a huge help but he had to check the notes of every patient with symptoms remotely reminiscent of colitis including spastic colon. Only inpatients were recorded but fortunately Sidney Truelove had started a clinic for patients with ulcerative colitis in 1956, and before that most patients were admitted for sigmoidoscopy and therefore appeared on the index. Even so he wrote to all the physicians, surgeons and paediatricians as well as more than 200 general practitioners, and looked through the admission books of the private hospital, the local fever hospital and the geriatric hospital. During this work, Acheson was joined by a young research assistant, John Grimley-Evans (born 1936), and eventually they managed to trace over 600 cases, though half were rejected because the diagnosis was unsafe or the patient was not resident in the district.[115]

Their analysis of the results was a *tour de force* and set the standard for all future studies. Firstly the average incidence of ulcerative colitis in the population was 6 per 100,000, though during the decade of the study the incidence almost doubled. It was eight times more common than Crohn's Disease and the prevalence of both diseases together was 80 per 100,000, surprisingly close to the approximation of Houghton and Naish. Secondly colitis was slightly more common in women, rare in children and only twenty per cent had involvement of the whole colon. Thirdly while the disease was common in young adults, there was invariably a secondary peak later in life. They could not explain this but clearly felt it was an important clue to the aetiology. They also wondered if some of the later cases could have been examples of Crohn's colitis but found no evidence to support the suggestion.

Acheson left gastroenterology when he failed to get the post of first assistant with Avery Jones at the Central Middlesex Hospital. His research turned to the epidemiology of multiple sclerosis and later he was the first dean of the new medical school at Southampton. After that he was appointed Chief Medical Officer (CMO) for England and Wales. Grimley-Evans became a geriatrician in Oxford and was selected by Sir George Godber, then Chief Medical Officer, to head the first academic department of gerontology (or geratology as he preferred to call it) in Britain. Both men received knighthoods.

Thereafter further studies were carried out by clinicians able to take advantage of the local demography in circumscribed areas such as North East Scotland and the North Tees district.[116] Others came from larger centres, notably Cardiff, where a new breed of epidemiologically minded gastroenterologists was spawned. The Cardiff hospitals also had an excellent diagnostic index of inpatients dating back to 1926, and like Oxford but slightly later, a special colitis clinic established in 1965. This enabled John Rhodes, an unassuming but dedicated man with a prodigious output of publications and a reputation for guaranteeing that his registrar would obtain an MD, to conduct an impressive study of ulcerative colitis extending over two decades, 1968–77 and 1978–87. The first study was run by his senior registrar, Terry Morris (born 1947), and showed that the incidence of colitis was no longer increasing, though there were still two peaks in young and old people.[117] The second study confirmed the stable incidence of colitis and was an example of the collaboration Rhodes enjoyed with his colleagues and the help he gave young men in their careers.[118] Several people were involved including Robert Newcombe, a mathematician and statistician; Paul Smith (born 1936) from the nearby hospital in Penarth, an outrageous extrovert but astute clinician and later President of the British Society of Gastroenterology; Geraint Roberts (born 1941), a delightful radiologist, and John Mayberry (born 1952), a medical registrar rapidly making his name in gastrointestinal epidemiology.

Though the incidence of ulcerative colitis seemed stable, members of the Cardiff team were worried that they were underestimating the true incidence because many cases are silent. And indeed they were. When Mayberry moved to Nottingham as senior registrar he was able to take advantage of a screening programme for colorectal cancer in the community, using faecal occult blood testing, to look for asymptomatic inflammatory bowel disease. He found that hospital studies were underestimating the true prevalence of ulcerative colitis by about 30 per cent.[119]

(b) Crohn's Disease

As the frequency of ulcerative colitis stabilised, the incidence of Crohn's Disease took off. In the Oxford study, Acheson had found only 24 patients with regional enteritis in ten years, which he had felt were too few to merit further analysis. However, at the same time, a surgeon in Aberdeen, James Kyle (born 1925), was seeing several patients with Crohn's Disease who were to become the basis for a personal study lasting 30 years.

Kyle first became aware of Crohn's Disease when, as a medical student in Belfast in 1946, he was administering an anaesthetic for a case of suspected appendicitis. The surgeon delivered the ileum, which looked like a red sausage, realised it was Crohn's Disease and promptly replaced it, intact. This made a lasting impression on the young anaesthetist. After working in Charles Wells' department in Liverpool, he was appointed surgeon to Aberdeen Royal Infirmary, where his interest in the disease soon prompted his senior colleagues to give him their cases. "They were only too pleased to hand over these people with this terrible disease." Within five years of his appointment he had 65 patients with Crohn's Disease under his care.

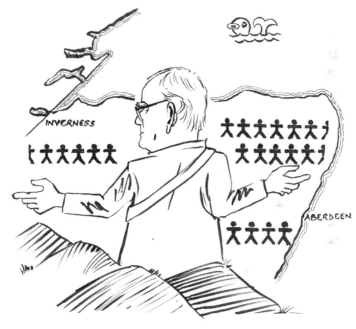

50 Kyle – surveying his fiefdom.

Kyle realised that the area around Aberdeen was ideally suited for an epidemiological study, being enclosed by the North Sea on one side and the Cairngorm Mountains on the other. He was fortunate too in having access to an excellent central records department with notes going back to 1938, and the same pathologist, Dr. S. W. B. Ewen, to review all the specimens. Over the years until his retirement in 1989, he recorded an inexorable rise in the incidence of Crohn's Disease from

1.3 to a staggering 11.6 per 100,000. Women always outnumbered men, and increasingly the disease affected the colon and rectum especially in older people. He also noticed an increase in familial cases and that people living in the city were more likely to get the disease than country folk. His comment in 1992 after a lifetime's study was perceptive: "In a disease that almost certainly has a multifactorial origin, a hereditary factor may play a background role in some families. When other factors, such as smoking, are superimposed on such a background, clinical disease may result; however, in most cases, the principle aetiological factor(s) remains unknown."[120]

The rise in Crohn's Disease was confirmed by the Hospital Inpatient Enquiry that records the number of discharges and deaths in England and Wales each year. After correction for the fact that an individual with Crohn's Disease might be admitted several times in any one year (which would inflate the figures), the disease more than trebled between 1960 and 1990. Noting the big increase in colonic disease, Michael Langman in Nottingham wondered if better diagnosis was partly responsible, especially since Crohn's Disease of the colon had been finally recognised as a distinct entity in 1960.[121]

Crohn's original achievement had been to highlight a specific disease, regional enteritis. Very soon, people were drawing attention to a combined form of ileitis and colitis, and Crohn himself later accepted that so-called right-sided or segmental colitis could occasionally be found in combination with ileitis. The first person, however, to suggest that segmental colitis, without involvement of the ileum, was a colonic form of Crohn's Disease was Charles Wells (1898–1989), Professor of Surgery at Liverpool, in a lecture to the Royal College of Surgeons in 1952.[122] But because Crohn himself would not sanction this extension of the entity called after him, Wells was content to describe it as a separate disease, and segmental colitis it remained. The waters were muddied further by Trevor Cooke and Bryan Brooke in Birmingham, who described yet another condition, non-specific enterocolitis, in which the ileum was inflamed, steatorrhoea was common and the proximal colon became secondarily involved.[123] With hindsight they may have been describing severe coeliac disease associated with ulcerative colitis.

The confusion was finally resolved by Hugh Lockhart-Mummery (1918–88) and Basil Morson (1918–2007) at St. Mark's Hospital. Lyn Lockhart-Mummery as he was known, the son of Percy Lockhart-

Mummery, was appointed resident surgeon at St. Mark's in 1951, a post that had been held by his father. At the time, the pathologist was Cuthbert Dukes (1890–1977), a legendary figure immortalised by his staging of colon cancer, the so-called Dukes classification.[124] Dukes was particularly interested in familial polyposis of the colon and had a register of 300 families with the condition. Many of these needed a colectomy and he had developed a special way of examining the operation specimens with the help of a remarkable technician, Dick Bussey (1907–91). Bussey had joined the staff as a laboratory assistant with no qualifications, but Dukes, recognising his potential, had encouraged him to obtain a degree and a PhD in his spare time, and eventually he became chief technician in the department. Quiet and methodical, Bussey pinned out the colectomy specimens with loving care on a long sheet of cork and immersed them in a bath of formalin where they were stored indefinitely.

When Basil Morson succeeded Dukes as senior pathologist in 1955, he and Lockhart-Mummery agreed that the classification of inflammatory bowel disease was a muddle (this had been brought home to Lockhart-Mummery during his MD on the subject) so they decided to do a

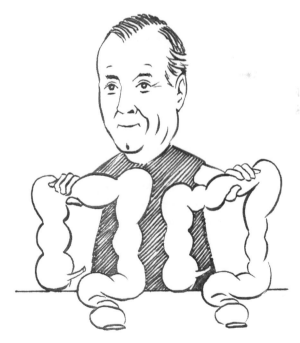

51 Lockhart-Mummery – UC or Crohn's disease?

detailed clinico-pathological study and were able to take advantage of Bussey's specimens and meticulous records. Their paper, published in the first volume of *Gut* in 1960, was a classic and established that Crohn's Disease (they preferred the eponym) could involve the colon exclusively.[125] They emphasised that they had never seen Crohn's Disease and ulcerative colitis in the same patient, in other words, anyone with regional ileitis and colitis had Crohn's Disease. They also drew attention to the frequency of anal lesions in Crohn's Disease that had not been previously recognised.

Their findings were confirmed by a pathologist, John Cornes (born 1926), a year later. Cornes had taken up pathology after being befriended by Cuthbert Dukes whom he met at a Quaker meeting in Trafalgar Square when he was a medical student. In due course he became senior registrar at the Gordon Hospital and often covered for Basil Morson at St. Mark's Hospital so he was well aware of his work. At the Gordon, he took the opportunity to re-examine hundreds of colectomy specimens provided by an enthusiastic surgeon, Stanley Aylett (1911–2003). Aylett was one of the few surgeons performing a total colectomy with ileo-rectal anastomosis on patients with ulcerative colitis. All these colons were preserved indefinitely in the laboratory in dustbins. With the help of his Danish technician, Mette Stecher, Cornes collected 45 examples of primary Crohn's Disease of the colon and rectum, which accounted for one in fifteen colectomies done for ulcerative colitis.[126] Later he was appointed senior lecturer in histopathology at Bristol but abandoned an academic career in order to spend more time with his family.

The recognition of Crohn's colitis certainly boosted the diagnosis of Crohn's Disease.

For example, John Rhodes in Cardiff followed the incidence of the disease from 1934 to 1990.[127] As expected there were very few cases in the 1930s (four) and only one new patient was diagnosed during the Second World War. After the war the frequency of all forms of the disease rose steadily until 1960 when the proportion of patients with colorectal disease increased rapidly, so much so that by 1990 it was commoner than the ileal form of the disease, especially in older people. Indeed during the course of 50 years the incidence of Crohn's Disease has risen more than fivefold.

CHAPTER FORTY-ONE

AETIOLOGY OF IBD

a) Genetic

The cause of colitis and Crohn's Disease remained elusive, which was very frustrating for the epidemiologists as they searched their data for a lead. One thing stood out; there seemed to be a genetic component. For years people had noticed that both diseases often occurred among members of the same family; in fact one of Burrill Crohn's original patients had a sister with ileitis, and in 1934 he suggested that the name familial ileitis might be used for the condition. Not infrequently a patient with ulcerative colitis had a relation with Crohn's Disease or vice versa. Of course these reports of two cases in a family merely showed that the clinician thought that the disease was too rare for this to happen by chance. This was why Naish tried to estimate the incidence in the population as a whole; if he knew this he could quantify the extra risk in families.

It was only when the true incidence of Crohn's Disease was known that its familial tendency could be proved. Taking advantage of the colitis clinic in Birmingham, John Fielding (1938–2002), senior registrar to Trevor Cooke, found that fifteen per cent of their patients had a relative with Crohn's Disease, far in excess of normal. This was the subject of his MD thesis in 1970 but was not published. In fact fifteen years later he did report a similar study in Dublin showing that siblings of patients with Crohn's Disease were 17 to 35 times more likely to get Crohn's Disease or, to a lesser extent, ulcerative colitis.[128]

Meanwhile it was the Cardiff group inspired by John Rhodes that first reported the high prevalence of inflammatory bowel disease in families.[129] John Mayberry simply asked all the patients with Crohn's Disease to complete a questionnaire about their family. Nine per cent had at least one relative (usually a sibling) with inflammatory bowel disease. Knowing the prevalence of colitis and Crohn's Disease in Cardiff, he calculated that the risk for a sibling developing one of these diseases was 30 times that for the population as a whole.

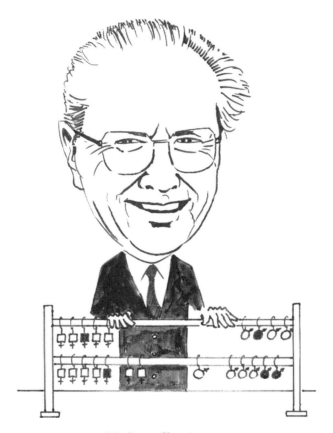

52 McConnell – Geneticist.

The doyen of gastrointestinal genetics in Britain during the second half of the twentieth century was Richard McConnell (1920–2003) in Liverpool. A friend and colleague of Sir Cyril Clarke (1907–2000), McConnell studied the genetics of peptic ulcer, coeliac disease, the gastrointestinal cancers and inflammatory bowel disease. No meeting about the hereditary basis of common gastrointestinal disorders could be considered complete without him. He lived through a time of remarkable progress in genetics and recalled that one of his more memorable discoveries was that one in five children in Liverpool were not related to the father.

McConnell confirmed and extended the Cardiff findings. Nearly one fifth of his patients with Crohn's Disease had a brother or sister with the disease, and almost as many patients with ulcerative colitis had a positive family history. Furthermore both diseases were often found in the same family.

McConnell realised that the disease should be fairly common among identical twins and indeed a few examples were reported, but, as he pointed out, isolated cases were not really of much value in deciding the extent to which heredity played a part. However, in 1982 he did pool the available case reports, which suggested that the inherited element in Crohn's Disease was stronger than that in ulcerative colitis.[130]

But it was not until 1988 that Gunnar Jarnerot in Sweden made use of the Swedish twin registry to prove that Crohn's Disease and, to a lesser extent, ulcerative colitis were much more likely to occur in identical (monozygotic) twins than non-identical (dizygotic) twins.[131] Unlike Sweden, England does not have a twin registry, but in 1995 Roy Pounder and Andrew Wakefield at the Royal Free Hospital took advantage of the growing membership of the National Association of Crohn's and Colitis (NACC) to look at the incidence in twins.[132] With the help of Richard Driscoll, Chairman of NACC, the Royal Free group found 150 twin pairs among the 16,000 members of the association. Nearly half were identical but, though several pairs had inflammatory bowel disease, the concordance rate was only seventeen per cent.

The familial frequency was too small to support a simple Mendelian pattern of inheritance due to a single gene, though there was one remarkable family in Southampton reported by Peter Morris in 1965 in which the mother and no fewer than five of her eight children had ulcerative colitis.[133] Morris (born 1934), an Australian graduate, thought an autosomal dominant gene was the most likely explanation. He was surgical registrar to Tom Rountree (1916–2007) in Southampton at the time and went on to distinguish himself in the field of transplant surgery in Oxford. Now Sir Peter, he later became President of the Royal College of Surgeons.

However, such families were exceedingly rare and Richard McConnell thought that a number of genetic loci must be involved in the inheritance of colitis. Unfortunately, locating these genes has been very difficult.

An early clue was provided by Donald Acheson while he was still a Radcliffe Fellow in America. During his study of huge numbers of United States army veterans he found that those with colitis and Crohn's Disease were more likely to have ankylosing spondylitis, a well known hereditary disease.[134] The discovery soon afterwards of the major histocompatibility complex on chromosome 6 caused great excitement, especially when Derrick Brewerton and his colleagues at the Westminster Hospital showed that there was a close association between ankylosing spondylitis and the HLA-B27 antigen.[135] Surely the HLA system would be concerned in inflammatory bowel disease too? After all, the genes in this complex are fundamental to the immune response and both Crohn's Disease and ulcerative colitis seemed to be caused by upsets of the immunological reaction to some insult.

Several groups with access to HLA typing began to look for an association with inflammatory bowel disease including McConnell's group in Liverpool, Peter Asquith and Pauline Mackintosh in Birmingham, Michael Langman in Nottingham and Rodney Harris, a medical geneticist in Manchester. HLA testing began in the early 1970s and, though some sort of association was found, the results were confusing and conflicting (unless the patient had ankylosing spondylitis in which case HLA-B27 was invariably found). Most series were too small to draw a definite conclusion, controls did not allow for ethnic differences, and the actual technique of HLA testing was not easy. Even so, a decade later, Michael Langman, Professor of Medicine in the department of therapeutics in Nottingham, carried out a meta-analysis of published results and was able to show that the risk of Crohn's Disease was increased in people with HLA-A2 allele, and decreased in people with HLA-A11.[136] This was encouraging particularly as, by this time, several more HLA antigens had been discovered and McConnell for example was finding a strong association between HLA-DR2 and ulcerative colitis.[137] But he was well aware of the shortcomings of his work. The HLA antigens that he was measuring were only associated with colitis because the corresponding alleles happened to be linked to the susceptible gene(s) (so-called linkage disequilibrium). Any number of these alleles could be involved, making it almost impossible to pin down the susceptible gene(s). This polygenic model of disease inheritance was thought to underlie a number of common disorders. McConnell refined this model to explain why patients with Crohn's Disease were more likely to have relatives with Crohn's Disease or ulcerative colitis than the other way round. He suggested that one genotype with perhaps ten to fifteen genes could confer susceptibility to all forms of inflammatory bowel disease; the "multiple loci-single-disease model". If a person had an incomplete genotype, ulcerative colitis was more likely; if the genotype was complete Crohn's Disease occurred. However, this assumed that Crohn's Disease and ulcerative colitis were a single disease entity, which was highly controversial. If, on the other hand, they were distinct diseases, or several diseases, as many people thought, far more genes might be involved, not just on chromosome 6 (HLA), but elsewhere; this theory, known as the "genetic heterogeneity model", was attractive and would explain the various subtypes of inflammatory disease.

In 1990 McConnell, now in his 70th year, wrote that further association studies of HLA system with inflammatory bowel disease would not be helpful.[138] Matters would have been bleak indeed were it not for the remarkable technical developments in molecular biology that now occurred, providing the tools for scientists to isolate and determine the structure of human genes. Even so the pathophysiology of inflammatory bowel disease was so complex that no one knew quite which chromosome(s) to target. The short arm of chromosome 6 was obviously one, but there were a number of other genes that were important in the regulation of the immune response. The most likely way to find them would be to show the same gene cropping up in a large number of families containing at least two close relatives with inflammatory bowel disease. Quite independently of each other, two groups in England did just this.

The first to get started were John Lennard-Jones and his colleagues in London. Lennard-Jones, now a highly respected figure at St. Mark's Hospital, was able to draw upon a large number of families with colitis or Crohn's Disease whose family trees had originally been studied twenty years earlier by his first research fellow, Michael Hinton (born 1934), but never published. The families were unusual in that all of them had at least three members with the disease.[139] From 1991 to 1994, 43 of these families were recruited by the senior registrar, John Lee, a Hong Kong Chinese graduate. The genetic studies were undertaken by Christopher Mathew, Professor of Medical and Molecular Genetics at Guy's Hospital. Initially they looked at genes at the HLA locus and drew a blank.[140] Undaunted they argued that their families with several affected individuals were unusual and might have a set of rarer, more highly penetrant genes than most patients with inflammatory bowel disease. By this time, a French team, led by Jean-Pierre Hugot, had also failed to find a link between the HLA region and Crohn's Disease. Convinced that there must be genes on another chromosome, the teams joined forces to increase the number of patients for study, and this time they concentrated on sibling pairs as being more representative of normal inheritance.[141] A genome wide search of 53 families struck gold when a locus susceptible to Crohn's Disease was found on chromosome 16, which they called IBD 1 (inflammatory bowel disease locus 1). Even though it accounted for only a small fraction of the known inheritance of Crohn's Disease, and the actual gene was yet to be found, this was indeed a breakthrough.

A year or so after Lennard-Jones began his family study, Derek Jewell began a similar study in Oxford. One would expect this knowing the reputation of the genetics department there, but for a number of reasons work on inflammatory bowel disease was slow to get underway. Jewell had been senior lecturer at the Royal Free Hospital where he had worked with George Janossy, an immunologist, on the immunological behaviour of intestinal lymphocytes. He returned to the Radcliffe Infirmary, Oxford in the mid-1970s and later succeeded Sidney Truelove on his retirement in 1978. Truelove was a hard act for anyone to follow and matters were not helped by the fact that the great man had fallen out with Sir George Pickering who was then the Nuffield Professor of Medicine. Unfortunately Jewell inherited this legacy and relations between the gastroenterology unit and the Nuffield department of medicine (led by the charismatic Sir David Weatherall) remained difficult. Jewell was interested in the immunology and pathogenesis of inflammatory bowel disease, not the genetics, and he was not encouraged when a small study he conducted with the department of surgery failed to find an association between HLA and colitis.[142] For his part, David Weatherall was rather dismissive of gastroenterology. However, the epidemiological evidence for a genetic predisposition became inescapable, and it was inevitable that the two sides would need to collaborate.

In 1987 John Bell, a Canadian, arrived back in the Nuffield department of medicine from California buzzing with his exciting work on HLA association with diabetes and rheumatoid arthritis. It so happened that Jewell's registrar, William Rosenberg (born 1958), was interested in molecular medicine, so Bell agreed to help him. Their first project was to clone and sequence the HLA DP locus in patients with coeliac disease, which showed that there was no association with these alleles (contrary to American reports, which were later retracted). Their next project was more productive and helped to unravel the genetic control of antigen receptors on the surface of T lymphocytes.

By this time, 1992, John Bell had succeeded David Weatherall as Nuffield professor of medicine and agreed with some reluctance to collaborate with Jewell and his new young research fellow, Jack Satsangi, in a large family study of HLA genes in inflammatory bowel disease. Satsangi (born 1965) was a bright and enthusiastic worker who was successively Jewell's SHO, registrar and lecturer. He grasped the nettle and really got things going. Meanwhile Rosenberg, who originally conceived the project, found himself caught between Bell and Jewell so he turned his attention to liver disease and the immunogenetics of haemochromatosis and hepatitis C, and later moved to the liver unit in Southampton.

Satsangi's first problem was to get hold of some families because, unlike St. Mark's Hospital with its long tradition of colorectal disease, Oxford had few families with inflammatory bowel disease. With the help of the National Association for Crohn's and Colitis (NACC), he was able to recruit 250 affected families from throughout the United Kingdom. A repository of clinical material was kept for genetic testing (DNA, plasma, and frozen lymphocytes), and clinical details were stored on a computer database. This became known as the Crohn's and Colitis Gene Bank. To this were added more than 400 out patients from the gastroenterology clinic who had no family history.

Like Lennard-Jones, Jewell realised that the term "inflammatory bowel disease" covered a multitude of sins. Clinically, it was a heterogeneous group of diseases that could behave in several ways, and it would be essential to take this into account when attempting to link them with a variety of underlying genes. Clearly different genes might be associated with different types of disease. During the course of their first genetic study, they examined this point and found that the majority of relatives did indeed have the same type of disease as each other. For example, two sisters might both have ileocaecal Crohn's Disease without, say, extraintestinal manifestations. This high "concordance rate" between family pairs suggested that close relatives had closely related susceptible genes.

The genetic studies were undertaken in the new Institute of Molecular Medicine (now the David Weatherall Institute) and at the Wellcome Trust Centre for human genetics in Oxford, directed by Mark Lathrop, a geneticist and friend of Bell from Canada who had been working in France. Initially they looked at the major histocompatibility complex and found that 28 out of 29 sibling pairs with ulcerative colitis shared the same class 2 alleles on chromosome 6, whereas those with Crohn's Disease did not.[143] However, when they compared unrelated colitics with controls, different HLA alleles were found. So here was strong evidence for genetic heterogeneity in inflammatory bowel disease; various HLA genes were important in the susceptibility to ulcerative colitis but not to Crohn's Disease. Like the London group, they predicted that in Crohn's Disease (and probably ulcerative colitis) important genes lay outside the HLA region. Unlike the London group they had used sibling pairs from the start thus avoiding the risk of finding rare and highly penetrant genes.

Using their growing bank of siblings with inflammatory bowel disease, the Oxford group undertook a genome-wide scan and confirmed the mutation gene on chromosome 16 that was linked to Crohn's Disease by Hugot and his colleagues.[144] This IBD 1 gene was similar to a gene found in non-obese diabetic mice and became known as NOD 2.[145] They also found evidence for the presence of susceptibility loci for both Crohn's Disease and ulcerative colitis on chromosomes 3, 7 and 12.[146] Other groups have subsequently reported further novel linkages. With such a heterogeneous disease associated with so much genetic heterogeneity, it has been suggested that as many as 700 sibling pairs may be required to allow fine mapping of susceptibility genes. The search continues and the size of the studies increases, now involving several countries in Western Europe who have formed an IBD international genetics consortium.

b) The environment

Besides drawing attention to the familial nature of inflammatory bowel disease, the epidemiologists had also shown that something else must be having an important influence on the disease. Genetic factors alone could not explain the big increase in the frequency of the disease over a mere 50 years, for example, and why should it be more common in cities than the countryside. Clearly something in the environment was at work, and this was supported by a study in Leicester by John Mayberry and Christopher Probert, who found that ulcerative colitis was much more common among immigrants from South Asia than it was among their countrymen at home.[147]

If the effort to find susceptible genes has been tedious, attempts to pinpoint external trigger factors has been equally frustrating. Unlike coeliac disease where gluten was known to be responsible, no one really knew where to look and people clutched at any straw that might lead somewhere.

(1) Atypical mycobacteria

The original view that ulcerative colitis was a form of bacillary dysentery was discarded in the early part of the twentieth century. Similarly with one exception everyone agreed with Crohn that his disease was not tuberculosis.

When Dalziel described his cases of chronic interstitial enteritis in 1913, he noted the similarity with Johne's disease, a chronic pseudotuberculous bacterial enteritis that had recently been described in cattle. He wrote, "The histological characters are so similar as to justify a proposition that the diseases may be the same." But he could not find atypical mycobacteria in his specimens. Recently his belief that Crohn's Disease may be caused by this mycobacterium has been championed by John Hermon-Taylor (born 1937), a surgeon at St. George's Hospital. He argues that the organism, mycobacterium avium paratuberculosis, is widespread and probably conveyed to humans in water supplies. It can lie dormant for years and cause disease in genetically susceptible people. It may be very difficult to culture unless amplified by the polymerase chain reaction and is resistant to conventional TB chemotherapy, but will respond to other antibiotics.[148]

However, Hermon-Taylor's view that this organism is the cause of Crohn's Disease remains controversial and unproved. So far Koch's postulates have not been met and, though the organism has been grown from individual cases of Crohn's Disease, it has also been cultured from people without the disease. Furthermore, though antibiotics may improve the disease, this may not be due to their effect on the specific organism but a more widespread antibacterial effect. In addition, one would expect that treating patients with anti-tumour necrosis factor would put them at risk of active and disseminated mycobacterial infection, but this serious complication has not been reported. Most people do not believe that mycobacterium paratuberculosis causes Crohn's Disease, but only a large study, with good controls, of the mycobacterial genome in many patients will settle the question once and for all.

(II) SMOKING

Almost every article on the aetiology of ulcerative colitis or Crohn's Disease over the last 50 years has begun by stating that the cause is unknown, which, of course, is true. Most of these articles have gone on to describe the latest association with some agent or event and seemingly no stone has been left unturned. If a medical student had been told that smoking was good for ulcerative colitis, or that possession of a hot water tap in childhood predisposed to Crohn's Disease, or that measles sometimes caused Crohn's Disease, he would probably think that he was having his leg pulled. Add to these an association with cornflakes for breakfast, the contraceptive pill, sugar intake or a history of appendicectomy, and we get some idea of the ingenuity of the profession in its attempts to find the cause. Many of these observations have been serendipitous and found by retrospective case control studies, which are always open to criticism, but there is no doubt that occasionally they come up with a winner. The association with smoking is a case in point.

In the mid-1970s, Anthony James (1921–2010), distinguished for his work on the physiology of gastric digestion (Chapter Seven, page 79) and now physician at Hillingdon Hospital in Middlesex, decided to investigate the breakfast habits of patients with Crohn's Disease on the assumption that food taken on an empty stomach is more likely to reach the areas usually affected by the disease. It was an ingenious idea and in a small study of 34 patients he actually found an association between Crohn's Disease and cornflakes eaters.[149] This surprising result triggered several papers on cereals and sugar intake and caught the attention of John Rhodes in Cardiff, who had known James when he was senior lecturer in medicine there. Rhodes asked his young research assistant, John Mayberry, to repeat the study on a larger scale using patients with ulcerative colitis as controls. He could

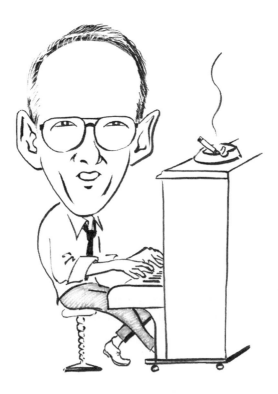

53 Rhodes – Smoking helps colitis.

not confirm James' findings but noticed that patients with ulcerative colitis tended to be non-smokers.[150]

Intrigued, Rhodes and his registrar, Anthony Harries, sent a questionnaire to all their patients with ulcerative colitis and Crohn's Disease asking about their smoking habits and found that it was indeed rare in people with ulcerative colitis. Only 8 per cent of the colitics were smokers compared with 44 per cent of controls.[151]

Reaction to their short report in the *British Medical Journal* in 1982 was immediate and widespread. Within days Harries had a phone call from a general practitioner in Newbury explaining that his wife could only control her colitis if she smoked. What should she do? Harries suggested the use of nicotine chewing gum, which did the trick.[152] Meanwhile several centres began to review their patients, notably Richard Logan and Michael Langman in Nottingham, now the Mecca of gastrointestinal epidemiology in Britain. They found that besides the tendency for patients with ulcerative colitis to be non-smokers,[153] their patients with Crohn's Disease were usually smokers.[154] This remarkable finding of "opposite associations" for smoking with inflammatory bowel disease now became the subject of intense scrutiny in the hope that it would explain an important pathogenic mechanism responsible for the two conditions.[155] Logan and Langman could not explain it, but made a highly prescient suggestion; they wondered if there might be a genetic predisposition to chronic inflammatory bowel disease and if so perhaps smoking determined which of the two diseases developed; this was in 1984.

Over the next few years cigarette smoke was found to affect most immune and inflammatory processes and to exacerbate experimental colitis in rats. During this time the polygenetic nature of inflammatory bowel disease was also being unravelled with the discovery of multiple linked loci for Crohn's Disease and ulcerative colitis. These genetic linkages could be shared between the two conditions and give rise to an intermediate form of colitis, or to examples of both diseases within a family. It occurred to Lennard-Jones and his group in London that smoking might be acting on a specific genetic background to influence whether the outcome was Crohn's Disease or ulcerative colitis. To test their hypothesis, the group, led by Andrew MacPherson at King's College Hospital, Stephen Bridger at St. Thomas's Hospital and John Lee at St. Mark's Hospital reviewed their large collection of sibling pairs.[156] As expected, two thirds of their pairs had Crohn's Disease or ulcerative colitis regardless of their smoking habits. However, in the remaining third, where one sib had Crohn's Disease and the other ulcerative colitis, smoking was confined to those with Crohn's Disease and non-smoking to those with ulcerative colitis. From this they concluded that though the genetic influence was all important, there were some cases where the risks between Crohn's Disease and ulcerative colitis were evenly balanced, and here smoking could displace the phenotype of chronic inflammatory bowel disease from ulcerative colitis to Crohn's Disease. So the apparent protection that smoking offered against ulcerative colitis was probably due to a shift of the condition towards Crohn's Disease.

(III) APPENDICECTOMY

Extraordinary as it may seem, appendicectomy in childhood is the only other factor that has been found to be important in inflammatory bowel disease.

In 1987 Michael Langman from Nottingham helped to organise the largest case control study looking for potential pathogens in the disease.[157] fourteen centres from nine countries were involved; the United States, Canada, Sweden, Denmark, Italy, the Netherlands, Britain and last but not least, Israel where the data was analysed. Two hundred patients with ulcerative colitis and 300 with Crohn's Disease, all under the age of 25, were interviewed personally. It was a considerable feat of organisation, taking two years to collect the data and at least as long to analyse it. A range of childhood factors was considered including allergies, family illness, stress, neonatal factors, food, vaccinations and childhood infections. Remarkably none of these were important but the investigators did note that significantly fewer appendicectomies were done in patients with colitis than controls. They had no ready explanation for this and indeed did not feel it was worth mentioning in their summary.

Elsewhere, however, people were intrigued and over the next fifteen years there have been at least eighteen independent studies showing that early appendicectomy protects people from ulcerative colitis or at least reduces the severity of the disease. No one has yet been able to explain why this should be but the popular theory is that the appendix contributes to the development and maintenance of the gut immune system. As David Sachar from Mount Sinai, New York said in an entertaining commentary in *Gut*, "Appendicectomy offers tantalising clues to the pathogenesis of inflammatory bowel disease. But Tantalus never did get to eat or drink the food and water surrounding him, and it seems we too are going to have to wait a little longer before satisfying our own hunger and thirst for understanding everything about inflammatory bowel disease."[158]

(IV) IMMUNE RESPONSE TO GUT FLORA IN INFANCY

One of the hypotheses tested by Langman and his colleagues in their study was the sheltered child hypothesis, also known as the hygiene hypothesis, which is quite different from the infectious hypothesis.

Instead of the child with inflammatory bowel disease becoming infected with a pathogen early on, a different sequence of events takes place; the child is overprotected, and only comes into contact with the common gut organisms later. This delayed exposure triggers an inappropriate immunological response, which then renders the bowel susceptible to disease. This has been used to explain paralytic poliomyelitis, which is

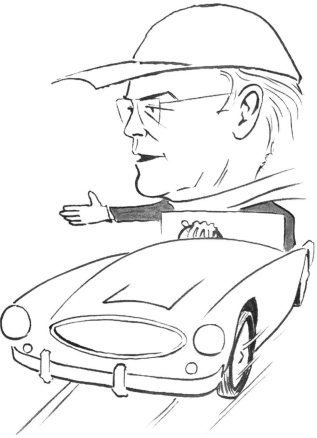

54 Hellier – Poop – poop!

inclined to attack well-to-do children who are exposed to the virus at a later stage.

They therefore looked at a whole series of factors such as age at entry to nursery, age at the start of bathing, number of playmates, pets, one-family house, shared or unshared bedroom, and so forth, but were unable to find any difference between patients and controls.

Nonetheless, the hypothesis was attractive since it would explain the inability to find a specific infective agent in the diseased gut as well as the much higher prevalence of inflammatory bowel disease in developed countries. So a year or two later, a small multicentre group of doctors decided to test the theory again. The group, which was the inspiration of Roger Grace, a surgeon in Wolverhampton, was formed in 1973 in order to record any information about new patients with inflammatory bowel disease that might be useful in a prospective study. The other three members were physicians, Tony Gent in Salisbury and Michael Hellier in Swindon (a future president of the BSG) who had both known Grace at St. Thomas's Hospital and Edwin Swarbrick in Wolverhampton. They accumulated 760 patients and, over the years, published several reports including, for example, a mortality study showing that the prognosis in Crohn's Disease was better than people thought, which had a favourable impact on the life insurance industry.

On this occasion, they were able to show that patients with Crohn's Disease were much more likely to have had a hot water tap and a separate bathroom in early childhood.[159] Good domestic hygiene, they thought, protected these patients from exposure to a full range of agents that programme the immune system of the gut during infancy. Later exposure to new agents triggered an inappropriate response, rendering the bowel susceptible to Crohn's Disease. Unfortunately this did not apply to patients with ulcerative colitis so a different mechanism must be at work in the two diseases.

CHAPTER FORTY-TWO

PATHOGENESIS OF IBD

a) Humoral immunity

When it became clear that an intestinal pathogen was not the cause of colitis or Crohn's Disease, people naturally cast around for another explanation. For years patients had reported that their colitis seemed worse if they consumed milk or its products, so in the early 1960s Sidney Truelove in Oxford decided to investigate this further. Though his results were inconclusive, his early work with antibodies was the beginning of an explosion of studies into the immunopathogenesis of inflammatory bowel disease.

Truelove collaborated with Keith Taylor (1924–2007), a lecturer working in Leslie Witts' department. Taylor had recently discovered that patients with pernicious anaemia had circulating antibodies to intrinsic factor and, like Truelove, was aware that several patients with ulcerative colitis were convinced that they were allergic to cow's milk.[160] So, with the help of Dr. Aschaffenburg, a scientist at the National Institute for Research in Dairying in Reading, who gave them purified milk proteins, they managed to demonstrate circulating antibodies to milk products, using a tanned red cell technique.[161]

Taylor saw himself as a gastroenterologist rather than an immunologist, though he went on to discover circulating antibodies to the cytoplasm of parietal cells in pernicious anaemia with Ian Roitt and Deborah Doniach, two distinguished immunologists.[162] He was approached by Avery Jones to join his new unit at the Central Middlesex Hospital and actually joined the Medical Research Council's external staff but never took up the appointment. Instead, he accepted an offer to set up a division of gastroenterology at Stanford University in the United States and left Oxford in 1963.

Meanwhile Truelove took on Ralph Wright (1930–90) who had come from South Africa for further postgraduate experience, and this was to be the beginning of his illustrious career in immunology. Together they ran a controlled trial allocating patients at random to a milk-free diet or a control group on a dummy diet for twelve months, and the milk-free patients did much better than the controls.[163] Furthermore several patients relapsed when they had milk again after the trial was over.

They extended the antibody tests but began to doubt their significance when they found no correlation between milk antibody titres and milk exclusion.[164] However, they did find an antibody to colonic epithelial cells obtained from patients by rectal biopsy, but it was infrequent and did not appear to be cytopathic so again they were not sure of its significance.[165]

Though Wright kept an interest in gut immunology, his future lay with the liver, and during a fellowship at Yale University in 1968 he showed that the newly identified hepatitis B virus was a cause of chronic liver disease.[166] Soon after his return to Oxford he was appointed to a chair at the new Southampton medical school.

Truelove's next research fellow was the young Derek Jewell (born 1941) whose name was to be synonymous with the immunopathogenesis of inflammatory bowel disease for the next 25 years. As circulating antibodies had no obvious pathogenetic action, Jewell now looked for another closely related immune mechanism of tissue injury, the deposition of antigen-antibody complexes. With the help of Ian MacLennan, an immunologist working in the field of rheumatology, he managed to demonstrate circulating immune complexes in patients with ulcerative colitis,[167] and he also took the opportunity to work with Keith Taylor in Stanford.

b) Cell-mediated immunity

While the Oxford workers were pursuing the humoral aspects of immunity, others were looking at cell-mediated immunity, particularly in Crohn's Disease. The histological similarities between Crohn's Disease and sarcoidosis had intrigued people for years, especially since Geoffrey

Hadfield's careful description in 1939.[†] He thought that a state of anergy existed in Crohn's Disease, particularly as the tuberculin test was often negative in these patients at a time when nearly everyone had a positive reaction.[168] However, John Fletcher and Michael Hinton at St. Mark's Hospital in a controlled trial in 1967 found no evidence to support his impression.[169]

The Kveim skin test was popular at this time in helping to make a diagnosis of sarcoidosis, and it occurred to Michael Willoughby (born 1935), a senior registrar in Birmingham, that patients with Crohn's Disease might also react positively to the Kveim antigen. Willoughby had reason to be interested in this because he himself had had sarcoidosis during his national service, and later one of his brothers developed Crohn's Disease and another sarcoidosis.[170] He discussed his idea with an indefatigable Yorkshireman, Donald Mitchell (born 1924), a chest physician working in John Squire's (1915–66) department of immunological chemistry. Unfortunately Squire died unexpectedly and Mitchell moved to the Medical Research Council's chest diseases unit at the Brompton Hospital. At the same time Willoughby fell out with Trevor Cooke and moved to Anthony Dawson's unit at St. Bartholemew's Hospital as a research associate. They got together and indeed found that 50 per cent of patients with Crohn's Disease had a positive reaction to Kveim antigen.[171]

They also made use of another in-vitro test of cell-mediated immune reactions in vogue at the time when they showed that Kveim antigen inhibited the migration of leucocytes taken from patients with Crohn's Disease.[172]

Yet another test of leucocyte function was the degree to which it responded or was "transformed" after stimulation by various plant mitogens. Several groups studied this in patients with colitis and Crohn's Disease with conflicting results. In fact all these tests were no more than an indicator that immune responses were associated with inflammatory bowel disease, but whether the response was cause or effect was impossible to say.

The subject was taken forward by Roy Shorter (1925–2008), an Englishman at the Mayo Clinic. Shorter qualified from the Westminster

---

[†] There was also a monograph *Morbus Crohn, Morbus Sarcoid* published by Israel Snapper, a Dutch Jew working in New York in 1935. Now scarce.

Hospital Medical School in 1948 and spent several years at St. Thomas's Hospital before emigrating to the United States in 1961 to take up a post as consultant in pathology in the Mayo Medical School, where he was appointed professor in 1974.

Shorter showed that lymphocytes from patients with inflammatory bowel disease exerted specific cytotoxicity against colon epithelial cells. He also showed that normal lymphocytes would do the same if they were exposed to an extract of E. coli first, suggesting that E. coli and colonic mucosa shared the same antigens.[173]

In 1972 he put forward a hypothesis for the aetiology and pathogenesis of non-specific inflammatory bowel disease.[174] First he drew attention to the fact that the gut had its own immune system that behaved differently from the systemic immune system. Patients destined to develop colitis were hypersensitive to bacteria normally present in the gut, and a cell-mediated immune reaction damaged the bowel wall. They became sensitised in infancy before the normal mucosal block was established when harmless bacteria could cross the mucosa, perhaps in association with cow's milk. He had some difficulty explaining why these lymphocytes did not damage the bowel immediately but suggested that they were immunosuppressed by anticolon antibodies also derived from the gut flora. This could be overcome later in life by exposure to a large dose of antigen from normal gut bacteria causing a chronic colitis. His hypothesis was highly speculative but drew attention to three important issues; firstly the idea that normal gut bacteria, not just pathogens, could trigger inflammatory bowel disease; secondly the concept of increased bowel permeability; and thirdly the cytotoxic role of lymphocytes on the colon, which was somehow controlled by other immune mechanisms. All three issues were to be the subject of considerable research over the next 30 years.

For many years people had been impressed by the colonic infiltration of neutrophil polymorphonucleocytes in inflammatory bowel disease. These cells are essential for the rapid removal of antigenic material from an inflammatory lesion before it progresses to a self-perpetuating state of chronic inflammation. One man who became particularly interested in neutrophils was Anthony Segal (born 1944), a young postgraduate from Cape Town. Segal originally intended to be a surgeon but after six months in the Accident and Emergency Department at Hammersmith Hospital he changed his allegiance to medicine. At first he had difficulty finding a registrar job but fortunately obtained a research post with Jonathan Levi at the Clinical Research Centre, Harrow in 1972. Shortly after his arrival an article in the *Lancet* on the nitroblue tetrazolium (NTB) test caught his attention.[175] This was a simple test of neutrophil function that was supposed to distinguish pyogenic infection from other inflammatory conditions, so it had clinical potential. In fact the test was unreliable but Segal modified it as a useful way to measure the phagocytic activity of neutrophils.[176] Now it so happened that dysfunction of the neutrophil causing a rare chronic granulomatous disease had recently been described with histological appearances that were almost identical to Crohn's Disease.[177] Could, Segal wondered, abnormal neutrophils be the cause of Crohn's Disease itself? Using his new test he examined the neutrophil phagocytic activity in 25 patients with Crohn's Disease and found that it was in fact normal.[178] However, he did find one significant abnormality, the migration of the neutrophils into areas of acute inflammation was poor. He showed this by creating "skin windows" on the forearms of his patients and measuring the migration of neutrophils into them.[179] The defective migration was probably due to an inadequate release of chemotactic mediators. A poor acute response delayed the clearance of micro-organisms as they crossed the mucosa. The build-up of these organisms promoted the arrival of macrophages and a chronic inflammatory process ensued. He went as far as to speculate that though treatment with immunosuppressive drugs such as steroids may temporarily relieve symptoms it may actually promote chronicity. Should we, he suggested, not heed the advice offered by George Bernard Shaw in *The Doctor's Dilemma* that, "There is at bottom only one genuinely scientific treatment for all diseases, and that is to stimulate the phagocytes."

The granulomas characteristic of Crohn's Disease had puzzled people for a long time. Granulomas arise when macrophages (monocytes) cannot degrade foreign material, either because it is indestructible (as in tuberculosis) or because the macrophage is incompetent in some way. The problem fascinated a young lecturer in medicine, Michael Ward (born 1945). Ward qualified in Birmingham and moved to the Western General hospital in Edinburgh to work with William Sircus and Martin Eastwood. He was a quiet and thoughtful man who spent many hours pondering the pathogenesis of Crohn's Disease and came to the conclusion that it arose from a genetically determined inability of the macrophage to degrade a variety of normal gut luminal constituents. He was assuming that there was an increase in mucosal permeability as Shorter had postulated. The frustrated macrophage released a variety of lysosomes causing tissue damage, which in turn stimulated further immune responses and ulceration. He reported his hypothesis in 1977 and much of it holds good today.[180] Sadly job prospects were poor at the time, so Ward emigrated to Australia where he is now Professor of

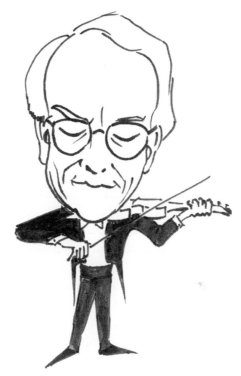

55 Jewell – Accomplished fiddler.

Medicine in Brisbane.

Segal and Ward had drawn attention to the role of phagocytes in Crohn's Disease and it was Derek Jewell who helped to establish the importance of the macrophage in inflammatory bowel disease. Jewell moved to the Royal Free Hospital in 1974 as senior lecturer in medicine in charge of luminal gastroenterology alongside Sheila Sherlock's liver unit. His arrival coincided with that of Humphrey Hodgson (born 1945) who had applied unsuccessfully for a lecturer's post on the liver unit. Hodgson must have impressed Sherlock because she magnanimously allocated him to her new senior lecturer (Jewell) with funds from a benefactor, Stanley Johnson. So Hodgson became the first of a series of Stanley Thomas Johnson Memorial fellows to work with Jewell, and in due course he succeeded Neil McIntyre (Sherlock's successor) as Professor of Medicine at the Royal Free in 1999.

A striking feature of the colonic mucosa in a patient with active inflammatory bowel disease is the considerable increase in plasma cells that secrete immunoglobulin. Hodgson and Jewell continued the work on circulating immune complexes and managed to provoke an acute form of proctitis in rabbits with immune complexes.[181] After two years, Hodgson was succeeded by Anthony Mee (born 1949) who managed to produce a chronic proctitis in rabbits that he had presensitised with colonic bacterial antigen.[182] But the case for immune complex mediation of inflammatory bowel disease was unconvincing, and Jewell and Mee turned their attention to the monocyte.

Circulating monocytes are the precursors of tissue macrophages, and were handy for study before biopsy material became readily available. Mee soon showed that monocytes from patients with inflammatory bowel disease had normal phagocytic activity, which did not support Ward's hypothesis.[183] He also found that activated monocytes secreted lysozymes, which presumably contributed to the inflammatory process.[184]

Mee moved on to the Central Middlesex Hospital as senior registrar with Misiewicz before taking up a clinical appointment in Reading. His place was taken by Jonathan Rhodes (born 1949) who had been Sherlock's registrar. Jewell and Rhodes re-examined the function of neutrophils and monocytes in vitro and found that both prednisolone and 5 aminosalicylic acid inhibited their motility by some means that was consistent with the anti-inflammatory action of these drugs.[185]

c) T lymphocytes

In 1980 Jewell left the Royal Free Hospital to succeed Sidney Truelove as consultant physician in the department of gastroenterology at the Radcliffe Infirmary, Oxford. He took with him a research fellow from Australia, Warwick Selby (born 1948), with whom he had been studying intestinal lymphocytes. By this time immunologists, especially George Janossy (born 1940) at the Royal Free Hospital, had found that

T lymphocytes could be subdivided into two main groups, so-called helper T cells that activated B lymphocytes or plasma cells to secrete immunoglobulin, and suppressor T cells that had an immunomodulatory role but could also be cytotoxic. Janossy and Selby had also noticed the helper T cells sought the company of HLA class 2 antigen-presenting cells in the lamina propria (sub-epithelium) of the gut whereas the suppressor T cells occupied sites in the epithelium itself (intraepithelial lymphocytes).[186] These functions were identified using the new technique of monoclonal antibody testing, which was about to revolutionise molecular biology. While still at the Royal Free Hospital, Selby, Janossy and Jewell showed that this distribution of T and B cells was the same throughout the stomach, small intestine and colon.[187]

They continued their studies in Oxford and using delicate techniques to isolate cells from colonic biopsies they confirmed that both types of lymphocyte were significantly increased in the mucosa of patients with inflammatory bowel disease.[188] This drew further attention to the gut's specialised immune system and emphasised the need in future to study what was happening in the mucosa rather than trying to draw conclusions from changes in peripheral blood. Perhaps, they speculated, the intraepithelial lymphocytes had an immunoregulatory role suppressing a systemic immune response to gut antigens, while the same antigens promoted a mucosal (lamina propria) immune response via the helper T cell.

When Humphrey Hodgson left the Royal Free Hospital in 1976, he was awarded a Radcliffe travelling fellowship and went to work on Isselbacher's unit at the Massachusset's General Hospital. Here he teamed up with Jack Wands who was carrying out some notable work on gut immunology, and they showed that the usual suppressor activity of intraepithelial lymphocytes was reduced in patients with active inflammatory bowel disease.[189] This fitted nicely with the concept of defective immunoregulation in colitis.

At the Royal Free Hospital, Leonard Poulter, an immunologist, and Janossy managed to develop monoclonal antibodies that could distinguish subpopulations not only of lymphocytes but also of macrophages.[190] Indeed the macrophage was clearly a key cell in the inflammatory process. Situated in the lamina propria, it was closely associated with lymphocytes, plasma cells and epithelial cells. So Roy Pounder (born 1944) who had succeeded Jewell at the Royal Free Hospital and his registrar, Miles Allison (born 1946), studied the cell intensively using these monoclonal antibodies,[191] while Jewell and Selby, now in Oxford, did the same.[192] Both groups found that patients with colitis had an increased number of macrophages and, remarkably, these were able to metamorphose and take on a variety of different tasks. Some continued their phagocytic activity while others became dendritic antigen-presenting cells, and in the case of Crohn's Disease many assumed an epithelioid appearance to form granulomas with lymphocytes.[193]

Isolating cells safely and reliably for study in vitro was a delicate process.

When Selby left Oxford to return to Australia, he was replaced by Peter Gibson (born 1952), another research fellow from Australia. Gibson helped Jewell to perfect a technique for the recovery of individual immune cells such as macrophages and lymphocytes from tissue biopsies, which helped to clarify their function in vitro.[194] Gibson used this technique to study a particular type of helper or effector lymphocyte known as a natural killer cell because of its ability to kill virus-infected cells without the need for activation by specific antigen first,[195] though in fact it was rarely found in colitis or Crohn's Disease.[196] He returned to Australia in 1984 to continue his research and is now Professor of Gastroenterology at Monash University in Victoria.

d) The role of cytokines

Gibson's place in Oxford was taken by Yash Mahida (born 1957), a Kenyan-born Liverpool graduate fresh from Misieiwicz's unit at the Central Middlesex Hospital. By now it was becoming clear that the mucosal immune response was controlled by a group of immunoregulatory molecules or cytokines that allowed the cellular components to communicate with each other. A new technique known as the polymerase chain reaction (the molecular biologists's answer to photocopying) had recently been discovered and was so sensitive that tiny peptides and even messenger RNA could be reproduced from minuscule biopsies and identified by monoclonal antibodies. Thus a few cells were sufficient to measure an individual cytokine protein or peptide and this was done using a highly sensitive and specific enzyme-linked immunosorbent assay (ELISA).

Mahida and Jewell were one of the first to study one of these molecules known as interleukin 1 (IL-1), a polypeptide produced by stimulated macrophages and thought to activate T cells. Using isolated mucosal mononuclear cells, they found that IL-1 was increased in patients with inflammatory bowel disease.[197] Mahida continued his research into the pathogenesis of inflammatory bowel disease, becoming especially interested in the protective role of epithelial cells in the colon and the part played by myelofibroblasts in tissue repair. In 1988 he moved to Nottingham where he is now Professor of Gastroenterology.

Over the next few years, a bewildering number of cytokines and chemokines (smaller peptides) were discovered using highly specific anti-cytokine monoclonal antibodies. Gradually a picture emerged of the remarkable way in which the gut immune system protects the body from gut organisms and other antigens if these manage to penetrate the mucosal barrier. This has been described as representing a state of "physiological inflammation".[198] The majority of our information has come from research in America, continental Europe and Japan, and the study of colitis has been helped by the discovery that a monkey, the cotton-top mandarin from South America, can acquire colitis spontaneously, the only animal with this doubtful privilege. As the complex interaction between epithelial cells, macrophages, lymphocytes and polymorphonucleocytes, variously stimulated and inhibited by a multitude of peptides, has become clearer (to those in the field at least), people have begun to find evidence of genetically determined dysregulation in the inflammatory response to gut antigens, which they believe will explain colitis and Crohn's Disease.

e) Lymphocytes again

Though our knowledge of cell signalling with various cytokines is far from complete, the helper or effector T lymphocytes have been subdivided into Th1 and Th2 subgroups according to the different cytokines that they produce. Th1 lymphocytes produce, among others, two cytokines known as tumour necrosis factor and interferon-y. Thomas MacDonald (see coeliac disease p230), then professor of the splendidly named Division of Infection, Inflammation and Repair at Southampton Medical School, who has spent years studying the behaviour of lymphocytes, believes like most that the tissue damage in Crohn's Disease arises from excessive Th1 responses or a failure to turn off such responses after infection in genetically susceptible people.[199] Ulcerative colitis on the other hand appears to involve Th2 responses with a different set of cytokines.

What stimulates the lymphocytes in the first place is still being unravelled. In the case of Crohn's Disease many think that the macrophage in genetically predisposed people is unable to respond normally to infection, which allows lymphocytes to accumulate and lose control. An alternative suggestion promoted by Tony Segal is that it is not the macrophage that is at fault but the neutrophil. Segal had never lost his enthusiasm for the neutrophil and had gone on to elucidate the defect in bactericidal activity of the neutrophil phagocyte in patients with chronic granulomatous disease.[200] For this work he had been elected a Fellow of the Royal Society, a rare honour for a

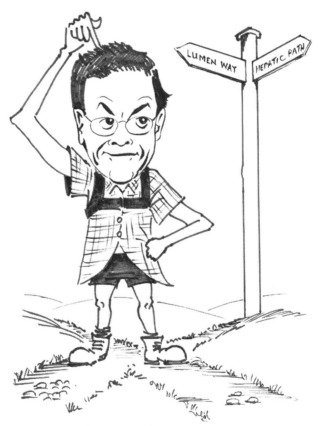

56 Hodgson – Which way, gut or liver?

gastroenterologist. Chronic granulomatous disease can cause colitis that is almost indistinguishable from Crohn's Disease so it was not surprising that Segal, now Charles Dent Professor of Medicine at University College in London, should discover that in Crohn's Disease there is a genetic failure to recruit neutrophils in response to infection because they fail to respond to interleukin-8, a cytokine produced by macrophages.[201] In his opinion this delay in the acute inflammatory response allows foreign material to accumulate within the mucosa and a chronic inflammatory response ensues.

The situation with ulcerative colitis is less clear and there is certainly no shortage of neutrophils as was demonstrated by Humphrey Hodgson. After his return from Massachusetts in 1980, Hodgson took a lecturer's post at the Hammersmith Hospital on Vinton Chadwick's (born 1952) gastroenterology unit. Here he was able to take advantage of the Medical Research Council's cell-labelling unit and the Nuclear Medicine Department to image the colon using indium-labelled neutrophils. He soon found that the technique was a simple way to quantify the activity of inflammatory bowel disease and calculated that in patients with ulcerative colitis over 60 per cent of the circulating granulocyte pool migrated to the inflamed gut.[202] As this was also a feature of bacillary dysentery, he speculated that bacterial chemotactic peptides (later shown to be cytokines) might be responsible. The problem was that like everyone else he could not identify an antigen. Frustrated after years studying inflammatory bowel disease, Hodgson defected to the liver and secured a senior lecturer's post back at the Royal Free Hospital in 1992, becoming Professor in 1999.

f) The mystery of the luminal antigen

However, the actual antigen or antigens responsible and how it/they manage to penetrate the mucosa continued to puzzle everyone. Most people agreed that something within the bowel lumen was necessary to trigger the inflammatory response. There were two lines of evidence for this assumption; firstly that diverting the faecal stream improved the inflammation in Crohn's Disease, and secondly that drastic changes to the diet were often beneficial.

Before colectomy became feasible, defunctioning ileostomy was widely employed by surgeons to "rest the bowel" of patients with ulcerative colitis, but the results were disappointing. However, when Sidney Truelove showed that corticosteroid enemas improved rectal inflammation, he encouraged his surgical colleagues in Oxford, Harold Ellis (born 1926 and Charles Webster (born 1927), to fashion a double-barrelled ileostomy on patients with an acute exacerbation of their disease. His intention was to defunction the colon and give the patients topical corticosteroids through the ileostomy. In fact those with ulcerative colitis did not respond, but a small group of patients with Crohn's Disease did.[203] The surgeons extended the study over several years and confirmed the benefit of faecal diversion in Crohn's Disease.[204] Presumably something in the faecal stream was important in the pathogenesis of Crohn's Disease, especially as most patients relapsed when the continuity of their bowel was restored. So together with Derek Jewell, now back in Oxford, three surgeons, Michael Kettlewell (born 1943), Emanoel Lee and their research fellow, Peter Harper (born 1952), tested this hypothesis by reintroducing faecal material into the defunctioned colon. More than half of the patients relapsed, but another group who were given a sterile ultrafiltrate of faecal material did not.[205] This suggested that bacteria or foreign proteins in the bowel lumen were somehow able to upset the mucosa.

This theory was supported by reports that patients with Crohn's Disease responded well to a liquid elemental diet, which contains all essential nutrients but supplies nitrogen in the form of amino acids instead of protein. The first person to carry out a controlled trial of an elemental diet in Crohn's Disease was Jonathan Levi (1933–99), a gastroenterologist at Northwick Park Hospital. He teamed up with his erstwhile research fellow, Tony Segal, who was then senior lecturer in the department of haematology at University College Hospital, though still primarily a gastroenterologist. The research was led by Colm O'Morain (born 1946) who was Levi's senior registrar and later to be Professor of Gastroenterology at Trinity College, Dublin. They found that an elemental diet was just as effective as high doses of prednisolone in acute Crohn's Disease.[206] The patients responded too quickly for it to be merely a nutritional effect, and Levi suggested that they improved because the protein-free diet did not provoke the mucosal immune response characteristic of the disease.

Their findings were confirmed by Humphrey Hodgson and Vinton Chadwick at the Hammersmith Hospital,[207] and by Anne Ferguson and Richard Logan in Edinburgh.[208] However, workers at the Mayo Clinic reported good results with a feed containing egg albumin[209] and subsequently Jonathan Rhodes, by now reader in medicine at the university department of medicine in Liverpool, also found a good response to protein feeds.[210] This somewhat undermined Levi's "low allergenic load" theory, but left people wondering why liquid feeds worked. No one knew, but a combination of low residue, good nourishment and alterations in antigenic load seemed likely. Rhodes studied one stoical patient for four years with various feeds and food challenges without reaching a firm conclusion. Nonetheless liquid feeds have slowly gained support in Britain, especially among paediatricians whose patients have special reason to avoid steroids. For example Ian Sanderson, a research fellow at St. Bartholemew's Hospital, used a liquid diet to treat children with active Crohn's Disease.[211] Sanderson was funded by CICRA (Crohn's in Childhood Research Appeal), a charity inspired by John Walker-Smith (1936), Professor of Paediatric Gastroenterology at St. Bartholemew's Hospital whom he later succeeded. The diet certainly worked but was so unpalatable that most children preferred to receive it through an intragastric tube. Fortunately it was only needed for two to three months by which time the disease was in remission.

Unfortunately none of these measures helped patients with ulcerative colitis, but it was now generally assumed that in both types of inflammatory bowel disease the antigen came from normal microflora in the colon. After all there are up to ten times more bacteria there than there are cells in the body and over 400 bacterial species, half of which have yet to be cultured.[212]

CHAPTER FORTY-THREE

MEASLES

The concept of a specific infection was still attractive and became the Holy Grail of a group at the Royal Free Hospital led by Roy Pounder and Andrew Wakefield. As we have seen Pounder succeeded Jewell in 1980. He was well known for his studies of H2-receptor antagonists in the treatment of peptic ulcer and could be guaranteed to entertain any audience with his witty presentations. He had been secretary of the British Society of Gastroenterology and was founding co-editor of Alimentary Pharmacology and Therapeutics (from 1987). In due course he became Professor of Medicine at the Royal Free and University College Medical School and Clinical Vice-President, Royal College of Physicians.

While working on the role of monocytes and macrophages in colitis Pounder had been impressed by the extensive distribution of Crohn's Disease and wondered if an underlying vasculitis could be responsible. In 1986 he took on a research fellow, Andrew Wakefield (born 1951), a man of considerable energy and enthusiasm, formerly a surgeon but now pursuing a career in gastroenterology who was later promoted to reader by the Royal Free School of Medicine and director of the inflammatory bowel disease study group at the hospital.

With the help of their colleagues in pathology they devised an elegant technique to outline the blood supply of the terminal ileum and colon taken from patients with Crohn's Disease, perfusing the vessels with heparin/saline and casting them in resin.[213] Detailed examination of the specimens showed that the patients did indeed have a focal vasculitis causing patchy infarction of the gut. This explained the segmental nature of the disease and occurred before the mucosa became ulcerated, suggesting that it was a primary process.

Occasionally granulomas were seen in the blood vessels indicating an interaction between immune cells such as monocytes and macrophages and vascular endothelial cells, which can cause intravascular coagulation. Pounder happened to know that his wife, Christine Lee, who was director of the Haemophilia Centre at the hospital, could not recall seeing a case of inflammatory bowel disease in any of her patients. The group looked into this intriguing observation and found that inherited disorders of coagulation such as haemophilia protected people from inflammatory bowel disease.[214] Conversely most people with inflammatory bowel disease had an excess of various thrombotic agents, notably factor VII.[215] So it seemed that an immune response in the mesenteric vessels of people with a hypercoagulable state was especially likely to cause colitis.

But what, they wondered, lay at the heart of the granuloma? What triggered the whole process in the first place? This of course was what everyone wanted to know and Pounder and Wakefield thought it might be the measles virus. This was a reasonable suggestion for several reasons. Firstly measles is an enteropathic virus; it causes Koplik's spots in the mouth and occasionally bloody diarrhoea during acute infection. Secondly Wakefield had done some research with Anders Ekbom, a noted epidemiologist in Sweden, showing that children born after an epidemic of measles were more likely to acquire Crohn's Disease later.[216] The rapid rise in Crohn's Disease since the Second World War could, they suggested, be due to the fact that these children now survived infancy whereas before they died. Some had an incomplete response to the virus and failed to clear it, becoming carriers. If so they should be able to find it.

The group examined their specimens again and found particles compatible with measles virus within the vascular endothelium.[217] They used the best techniques available including electron microscopy and immunohistochemical techniques, but unfortunately were unable to demonstrate the virus genome using the polymerase chain reaction (PCR). Nonetheless they felt they were onto something despite a large postal questionnaire that they sent to members of the National Association of Crohn's and Colitis, which did not confirm Wakefield's earlier survey in Sweden.[218]

The incidence of Crohn's Disease continued to rise even though measles was disappearing, so the team next wondered if measles vaccination might be a risk factor too. To find out Nick Thompson, the registrar on the firm, recalled that he was still a participent in a Medical

Research Council trial of the effectiveness of live measles vaccine given to children in 1964. Each year the recipients were asked by post if they had subsequently contracted measles and dropped out of the trial if they had. It was a relatively simple matter to add a further question the following year: "Had they had, or been told by a doctor that they had, Crohn's Disease or ulcerative colitis?" Unfortunately the control group who had not been vaccinated could not be used because they had either caught measles or been vaccinated later. Instead they used a surrogate control group drawn from the National Child Development Study of children born in March 1958, who of course had not been vaccinated and they found that the vaccinated group were more likely to have Crohn's Disease or ulcerative colitis.[219] Though excited by their findings they were careful to point out that the study only showed an association between measles vaccination and inflammatory bowel disease; the one was not causing the other.

The study was rightly criticised by several epidemiologists who pointed out that the control group was not really comparable.[220] Later a careful case-control study from Dorset led by Jonathon Snook (born 1956) in Poole found no evidence to support the vaccination hypothesis.[221] Virologists also criticised the theory because there was no proof that measles virus had yet been isolated in the gut. Accordingly the Chief Medical Officer, Kenneth Calman, who had been alerted to the anticipated outcome of the study by Wakefield, concluded that there was no need to change the immunisation policy.[222] He will have felt vindicated in this assumption when Philip Minor, a virologist working at the National Institute for Biological Standards in Potters Bar, was unable to find measles virus genome in any form of colitis using a highly sensitive PCR system.[223]

Undaunted Wakefield and Pounder continued their research with the help of an enthusiastic statistician, Scott Montgomery, and showed that inflammatory bowel disease throughout Europe was much commoner where there was a low infant mortality.[224] Whatever the reasons for this, it was in keeping with their original hypothesis that survival in infancy was a key factor in the aetiology of inflammatory bowel disease.

At the same time Wakefield began to receive telephone calls from a number of highly articulate parents convinced that their children had developed bowel symptoms and autism after immunisation with the recently introduced measles, mumps and rubella vaccine. He was not a paediatrician so he sought the help of John Walker-Smith, Simon Murch and Michael Thompson, three paediatric gastroenterologists who had moved to the Royal Free Hospital after their unit at St. Bartholemew's Hospital was closed in 1995. Colonoscopy revealed that most of these children had a non-specific colitis and what they called ileo-lymphoid-nodular hyperplasia. The early results were published in the *Lancet* in 1998 and the possibility of a link with MMR was mooted, though wisely the authors added, "We do not prove an association between MMR vaccine and the syndrome described."[225] The paediatricians felt quite strongly about this as they were naturally committed to the vaccination programme and knew that proof of measles had not yet been found in the gut.

The article might not have attracted much publicity but at a subsequent press conference Wakefield surprised his colleagues by suggesting that children should be offered the three vaccines individually, with an interval of a year between each dose. This was "news" and provoked a media frenzy leading to a fall in uptake of vaccination. Public health doctors, virologists and paediatricians were dismayed and Wakefield, a charismatic character who has been described as a man of utter sincerity and honesty, was hounded out of the Royal Free Hospital and moved to America. Whatever the shortcomings of his research, the press conference and his remarks were unfortunate if not foolish. In fact a virologist in Dublin, John O'Leary, has subsequently found evidence of measles genome in the tissue of these children with autism, though this does not in itself prove anything.[226] Others are endeavouring to reproduce the Dublin results. The whole MMR controversy has been well described in two books, one by Richard Horton,[227] editor of the *Lancet* and the other by Michael Fitzpatrick,[228] a general practitioner and father to a son whose autism began to manifest itself a few months after receiving the MMR vaccine. Both authors are supporters of the vaccine. Recently a damning report by a journalist, Brian Deer, has appeared in the *Brit. Med. J.* suggesting that Wakefield's original article was fraudulent.[229]

Most people are highly sceptical that measles has a role in Crohn's Disease but Roy Pounder still believes that there is something in it. In his view the virus is just one part of a combination lock; after perinatal exposure to measles, a genetically prone child with, say, the NOD 2 deletion, which facilitates penetration of the bowel wall, together with an inborn hypercoagulable state, later decides to smoke and hey presto! Crohn's Disease ensues. He likens the role of measles to helicobacter pylori and peptic ulcers; just as ulcers were well controlled with acid suppression but not cured until antibiotics were used to kill the organism, so inflammatory bowel disease can be helped with anti-inflammatory and immunomodulatory agents but if measles was the antigen an antiviral would be the elusive cure.

CHAPTER FORTY-FOUR

COLONIC MUCUS

To reach the mucosa, bacteria have to avoid the clutches of an immunoglobulin, IgA, which is secreted exclusively in the intestine by plasma cells. They also have to penetrate the epithelium, which is protected by a thick layer of mucus. As mucus has been the subject of intensive study, a digression on the subject is warranted.

Most clinicians if asked what they could tell you about mucus would probably reply with a diffident smile that you cannot do without it. Few know much about its structure, though it is fascinating stuff.

One of the first people to study the secretion of mucus was Howard Florey (1898–1968), one of the greatest doctors of the twentieth century, Nobel Laureate, President of the Royal Society and immortalised for his work on penicillin during the Second World War. In his Croonian lecture to the Royal Society in 1954 he spoke of mucus as a slimy secretion essential for the protection of many parts of the body, and he described its secretion from the goblet cells in the gut.[230]

Florey was Professor of Pathology in Oxford, and for many years only a handful of biochemists dotted around the country showed any interest in mucus. They studied animal and human material, especially saliva, and secretions from the bronchi, gut and genital tract; they were a dedicated band of individuals but their work was largely ignored by the profession.

A good example was Jacob Schrager (1914–81), a Ukrainian Jew. He fled his homeland in 1934 and settled in Britain, "the land of liberty", after reading a Hebrew translation of Thomas Carlyle's biography of Oliver Cromwell. After qualifying in Belfast he trained in biochemistry and was appointed county pathologist to Wigan. There, backed by generous grants from the Medical Research Council, he poured his knowledge of carbohydrate chemistry into the study of mucus and showed that its viscoelastic property arose from the arrangement of its sugars.[231]

The study of mucus was a gel of a problem. Glycoproteins are extremely difficult to purify or analyse by conventional techniques (they clog chromatographic columns for a start), and a laboratory was doing well if it obtained results from as few as six patients a year. It took ages to build up a database which was the problem facing John Clamp (born 1927) working in the Department of Medicine in Bristol with Professor Alan Read (1926–93), a personal friend who gave him great support. Clamp had a degree in biochemistry as well as medicine and was advised to study glycoproteins for a PhD. This led him into the field of mucus which became his lifetime interest, and in due course he was awarded a personal chair in experimental medicine within the department. A shy man, he wrestled with the structure of mucus glycoproteins for years and managed to show that the carbohydrate side chains are attenuated in patients with inflammatory bowel disease, thus weakening the protective effect of mucus.[232] He studied material scraped from resected colons and tissue from colonic biopsies. Fortunately one of his MD students, Robin Teague (1944), who obtained these biopsies, was among the first to use a colonoscope in Britain.[233]

An alternative approach to the study of mucus was histochemical, a method championed by Isabel Filipe (born 1934), a graduate of the Faculty of Medicine in Lisbon. She had worked with Tony Pearce at the Hammersmith Hospital and later joined Ian Dawson (1921–95),† Professor of Experimental Pathology at the Westminster Hospital, who was interested in diagnostic enzyme histochemistry. They were among the first to observe that mucus secretion was severely depleted in patients with ulcerative colitis whereas it was normal in Crohn's Disease.[234] In 1973 Dawson moved to the new Nottingham medical school and Filipe next collaborated with Brian Gazzard (born 1941) on the gastroenterology unit. They showed that mucus from patients with ulcerative colitis was not only depleted but also structurally unsound, rendering it susceptible to bacterial attack, a finding that agreed with Clamp's biochemical analysis.[235] Filipe was appointed senior lecturer to the department of pathology, Guy's Hospital, where she later made use

---

†   His book on gastrointestinal pathology with Basil Morson, popularly known as Morson and Dawson, was a classic text.

of the fact that lectins bind to glycoproteins. Using specific lectins, she managed to identify individual mucins histochemically, considerably simplifying the laborious biochemical methods of the time.[236] In the early '90s she was offered a professorship at Lisbon University but did not take the post. Quiet and unassuming, some felt her work was unappreciated and she retired in 1995 when the changes at Guy's Hospital left her with no means to continue her research.

One of the few gastroenterologists excited by mucus at the time was

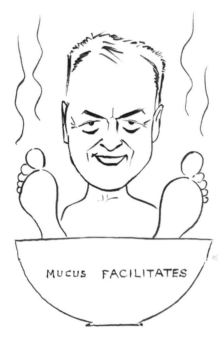

57 Rhodes – Easing our way.

Avery Jones, and in 1976 he chaired an international conference on the subject. Not surprisingly most of the delegates were biochemists and the meeting made no impact on clinicians. However, it did stimulate the board of the *British Medical Bulletin* to devote an issue to mucus two years later. At the time, Jonathan Rhodes (born 1950) was a registrar at the Royal Free Hospital where the indomitable Professor Sheila Sherlock ran a journal club. Every so often, each member of the staff was expected to expound on a topic of their choice provided that it had nothing to do with their own research. To avoid awkward questions it was generally wise to choose a subject with which no one was familiar. Rhodes happened to come across the *British Medical Bulletin's* review and was able to impress everyone, including himself, by what he found out about mucus. Fascinated he began to study it, particularly in relation to inflammatory bowel disease, first in Birmingham when he was senior registrar to Robert Allan and Elwyn Elias, and subsequently in Liverpool as senior lecturer, reader and Professor of Gastroenterology. Apart from his own research on the structural changes to mucus in colitis, Rhodes has been instrumental in bringing mucus to the attention of clinicians and convincing them that it is physiologically important.

Two young biochemists who attended the original mucus conference in 1976 will have caught Rhodes' attention. Adrian Allen (born 1942) and Tony Corfield (born 1947) both worked with Paul Kent, a noted carbohydrate chemist in Oxford who stimulated their interest in mucins. In due course Allen became Professor of Physiology in Newcastle and studied gastric mucus. He developed a simple but accurate way to measure its thickness in the stomach, and subsequently used his method in the colon to show conclusively that the mucus layer is thin in ulcerative colitis but normal or even thickened in Crohn's Disease.[237]

Corfield joined John Clamp in 1981 and has been in Bristol ever since. He now heads the Mucin Research Group in the Dorothy Hodgkin laboratory in the Division of Medicine there. Advances in molecular biology, and particularly the use of lectins and anticarbohydrate antibodies, have recently transformed the ability to detect specific mucins and to relate them to individual genes. These genes have been identified and appropriately labelled as MUC 1, MUC 2, etc. Corfield and his group have found that mutations of the MUC genes affect the carbohydrate structure of mucus, predisposing people to severe ulcerative colitis.[238] This could explain the disparity between Europeans and Asians with ulcerative colitis; John Mayberry and Christopher Probert found that though colitis was common among the Asian community living in Leicester, it was usually quite mild.[239] Later, when Probert moved to Bristol, he teamed up with Corfield to show that Asian colitics have normal mucus, which presumably protects them from the more severe forms of the disease.[240]

Meanwhile Rhodes and his team in Liverpool had shown that the carbohydrate structure of glycoproteins can also be altered if a group of enzymes known as glycosyl transferases are defective. This, they realised, may predispose patients not just to colitis but to cancer of the colon. According to Rhodes, these attenuated glycoproteins are more likely to bind to lectins found in the bowel lumen; these in turn cause the colonic mucosa to proliferate and increase the risk of cancer.[241] It is this association with cancer that has stimulated so much interest in mucus today.

The concept that weak and thin mucus predisposes patients to ulcerative colitis was attractive and would also explain why the distal colon, which is exposed to a heavier bacterial load, is more inflamed than the proximal colon.

To sum up (very simplistically), ulcerative colitis could be the result of a normal inflammatory response to recurrent and persistent invasion by the normal flora of the colon. Crohn's Disease, on the other hand, might arise from a genetically determined abnormal inflammatory response to occasional attack by the flora in the gut.

CHAPTER FORTY-FIVE

CARCINOMA COMPLICATING ULCERATIVE COLITIS

The Americans were the first to recognise that cancer could complicate ulcerative colitis. Crohn (1884–1983) in New York described an ulcerating invasive adenocarcinoma in the rectum of a patient with long-standing colitis as far back as 1925.[242] Shortly afterwards the evergreen Arnold Bargen (1894–1976) reported fifteen cases from his huge series of 700 patients at the Mayo Clinic.[243] Both men deserve credit for spotting what was, and still is, a rare complication of a relatively uncommon disease. Hurst could only recall three cases in his experience, which he thought were coincidental.[244] However, after the Second World War, Bargen suggested that patients with colitis were 30 times more likely to get bowel cancer,[245] though Kirsner in Boston calculated the risk to be 8-fold.[246]

In Britain, two great characters, William Bashall Gabriel (1893–1975) and Cuthbert Esquire Dukes (1890–1977), were the first to draw attention to the subject. Apart from the possession of memorable middle names, they were close colleagues at St. Mark's Hospital for more than 30 years. Gabriel, a surgeon, joined the staff in 1920 and established the cancer follow-up department in 1922, the first of its kind in the United Kingdom. The wealth of information obtained from these records has been the foundation of most of the publications emanating from St. Mark's ever since.[†] Dukes meanwhile became the first pathologist at St. Mark's in 1922 and began his classical study on the pathology of cancer of the colon and rectum that was to bring him international fame.

[†] His book *Principles and Practice of Rectal Surgery* was affectionately known as "St. Mark's Gospel according to the Archangel Gabriel".

370

In 1950, Gabriel presented two cases of carcinoma complicating ulcerative colitis to the Royal Society of Medicine,[247] and two years later Dukes included these in a report on the pathology of thirteen cases.[248] He was impressed by two features of these carcinomas; firstly they looked unusual and could be easily missed by the unaided eye "because in this altered soil growth proceeds in an unfamiliar way"; secondly they seemed highly malignant and carried a poor prognosis. He was firmly of the opinion that the cancer did not arise from pseudopolyps (as Bargen had suggested) and that it frequently developed without any sign of a polyp.

Another pathologist, Ian Dawson (1925–95), later disagreed with Dukes. In a retrospective survey of nineteen cases from the Gordon Hospital for Diseases of the Rectum in 1959, he decided that these carcinomas probably did arise from polyps and pseudopolyps.[249]

By this time there had been several reports of carcinoma complicating ulcerative colitis; these were reviewed by Geoffrey Slaney (born 1922), then senior lecturer in surgery in Birmingham (and later to be President of the Royal College of Surgeons) and Bryan Brooke.[250] They also looked back at their own patients and found that nearly seven per cent had developed cancer with the figure rising to seventeen per cent in those who had had colitis for ten years or more. Worryingly the colitis was often quiescent and conventional follow-up including radiological checks was ineffective because by the time a lesion was detected it was usually too late for a cure. The surgeon and the patient were faced with a most difficult decision – should prophylactic colectomy be undertaken and if so when?

Their views were echoed by Felicity Edwards and Sidney Truelove who drew on their great series of Oxford patients which, it will be recalled, amounted to 624 colitics seen between 1938 and 1962. Twenty-two of these patients had developed cancer, they were younger than average and most had died. They stressed that the risk was greatest in people with total colitis, especially when it had been present for twenty years and felt there was a place for elective colectomy.[251]

Another clinician to examine the problem was Ian MacDougall (1918–96) who was research assistant at the Gordon Hospital for Diseases of the Rectum. MacDougall knew that patients with total colitis seemed more likely to develop cancer so he did a careful retrospective survey of all the patients with colitis at the hospital from 1947 to 1963 and compared their rate of bowel cancer with the incidence in the South

East of England.[252] Three facts stood out; firstly the risk of cancer was much higher (30-fold) in patients with total colitis; secondly patients with distal colitis were not at risk; and finally patients with a rectal stump after colectomy for total colitis were still at risk of cancer in the stump. He, too, came to the "almost irresistible conclusion" that patients with total colitis for more than ten years should have a prophylactic colectomy. MacDougall kept his connection with the Gordon Hospital, which he found invaluable long after he was appointed physician to the East Hertfordshire group.

Shortly after, two other surveys showed much the same. In Leeds, the complications of ulcerative colitis seen in the colitis clinic run by Watkinson and Goligher were analysed in 1966 by a young research assistant on the surgical unit, Tim de Dombal (1937–95). Eight patients with total colitis developed a carcinoma over a period of eight years and five died.[253] The death rate was eleven times that expected. As their patients got cancer despite the most careful supervision, and the risk of cancer after ten years was so high (estimated as 40 per cent after 25 years), the Leeds group felt that the "drastic step of excisional surgery" was fully justified. De Dombal later became Director of the Clinical Information Science Unit at Leeds University, and was awarded a personal chair in this specialty. He was one of the first to encourage computerised data collection and retrieval to improve the accuracy of diagnosis. For over twenty years he was Chairman of the World Congress of Gastroenterology Research

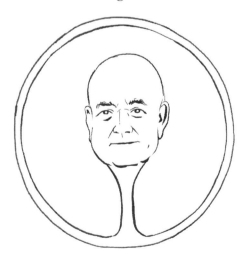

58 Dukes – Pioneering pathologist.

Committee and directed multinational surveys worldwide. He died prematurely awaiting a triple bypass operation.

The other survey came from St. Mark's Hospital, which, as we have seen, was famous for its records department. For example it was the excellence of their research records, long before computers came on the scene, that helped Cuthbert Dukes and his technician Dick Bussey to unravel the family curse of familial polyposis of the colon. In 1966, Michael Hinton (born 1934), MRC research fellow with Lennard-Jones and incidentally the first medical registrar at the hospital, also took advantage of the records to unearth 32 patients with colitis and carcinoma treated over the previous eighteen years.[254] What worried him and Lennard-Jones was that, with recent progress in medical treatment, a growing number of high-risk patients with extensive colitis were quite fit and anxious to avoid surgery. Well over half these people would not develop cancer for three decades. Was there any way that an individual patient could be identified before he got cancer?

It was now that Basil Morson (1918–2007) published his seminal paper on rectal dysplasia (pre-cancer) with his Chinese research assistant, Lillian Chang.[255] Morson knew of course that the detection of pre-cancerous lesions was an effective method of cancer control, citing carcinoma of the cervix as a good example. He was also aware that Dukes had already identified dysplasia as a risk factor in colitis, sometimes associated with small polypoid lesions. He now found that dysplasia was just as likely in flat mucosa without obvious polyps. This was a critical discovery for two reasons; firstly, the mucosa appeared normal to the naked eye so random biopsies were necessary to spot any changes, and secondly, dysplasia in the rectum indicated dysplasia elsewhere in the colon and sometimes an actual carcinoma. In all, Morson and Chang examined more than 200 colons during their study and found that ten per cent of patients with total colitis had rectal dysplasia. Moreover, patients without pre-cancer in the rectal biopsy showed no evidence of pre-cancer or cancer in the subsequent colectomy specimen.

So here, it seemed, was a test that could identify individual colitics at particular risk of a carcinoma. This was just what Lennard-Jones was looking for and he at once (1966) began a long-term prospective follow-up programme of patients with extensive colitis.[256] He wanted to know if it was safe and reasonable to manage them conservatively as long as they remained well without evidence of severe dysplasia in the rectal mucosa. He reported his results at intervals and felt sufficiently encouraged to keep going for 22 years. By the end of the study 401 patients had entered the programme and only 25 had refused to attend. As expected he found that the risk of developing cancer increased as the years went by.

Ultimately twenty patients were found with severe dysplasia and all of them agreed to have a colectomy. Of these, twelve had dysplasia or pre-cancer in the colectomy specimen, and would probably have got cancer later, and six actually had a carcinoma. This was disturbing but all of them were caught early and did well. Another 76 patients had milder dysplasia and eight of these developed cancer that was unexpected. Five patients who left the programme developed carcinomas and three of them died.[257]

By comparison with various surgical series of unselected patients, Lennard-Jones' figures were good. Several cancers were avoided and most of the others were cured. Moreover two thirds of the patients still had their colons. But the effort was considerable and the St. Mark's group were dedicated. Lennard-Jones himself inspired his colleagues with his wisdom, compassion and capacity for hard work, and throughout the study he was supported by three key people. The first, naturally, was Basil Morson; the second was Jean Ritchie (1923–2005) who kept superb clinical records. Ritchie trained as a radiotherapist and came to St. Mark's with a research fellowship to study the health of people with ileostomies. She settled in, abandoned radiotherapy and never left. Promoted to senior research fellow and later director of the research records department, she began a card index system for the colitis clinic, and though she never actually saw a patient she knew their histories inside out.

The third member of the team was Christopher Williams (born 1938), who came to St. Mark's as a registrar in 1969 intending to write an MD on the immunology of colitis. It so happened that Alan Parks (1920–82), later Sir Alan, consultant surgeon and future President of the Royal College of Surgeons, had recently returned from Tokyo with a colonoscope. The surgical registrars were too busy to grapple with it, so Parks gave it to Williams who used it for the first time in December 1970. He soon realised that he had a challenge on his hands but a combination of skill and determination saw him become the foremost colonoscopist in the country. Serendipity played its part; he recalls how, late one evening, after a two-hour struggle, he wearily withdrew the instrument only to see it unravel itself and slide into the caecum. A new technique was born. After two years he and his equally raw Japanese colleague, Tesu Muto, later to be a leading surgeon in Tokyo, had managed their first 100 examinations together. What they found altered the management of 30 per cent of the patients and colonoscopy was here to stay. In 1974 the decision was taken to include regular colonoscopy in the surveillance programme. Williams devoted his life to colonoscopy; he was a generous and inspiring teacher and an enthusiastic raconteur with an endless supply of alimentary anecdotes.

St. Mark's colitis clinic was a rarity when Lennard-Jones began his surveillance study. In most hospitals, patients were more likely to come under the care of surgeons and few were followed up once they were in remission. Gastroenterology was still practised by general physicians and it was not until flexible endoscopes appeared that the specialty came into its own. Even then colonoscopy was slow to catch on; it was technically demanding and most who tried it were enthusiasts randomly drawn from surgeons, physicians and radiologists. Formal training came years later, so the procedure was frequently incomplete and painful, tarnishing its reputation. Many gastroenterologists during the 1970s continued to rely on sigmoidoscopy and barium enema to assess colitis.

But there were other concerns. In 1972, two pathologists, David Evans (born 1937) and David Pollock (born 1932) from the Hammersmith and London Hospitals respectively, described four patients with ulcerative colitis and carcinoma who did not have rectal dysplasia.[258] Subsequently Morson and his research fellow, Bob Riddell (born 1945), found the same and realised that the changes could be patchy and easily missed.[259] To get round this they recommended multiple rectal biopsies, but I suspect few clinicians actually did this. Riddell subsequently emigrated to McMaster University, Canada, where he spent years agonising over the significance of dysplasia. In 1983, he brought together an international group of pathologists who recommended a standardised description of it that was accepted worldwide.[260]

CHAPTER FORTY-FIVE

CANCER SCREENING

Meanwhile, at the General Infirmary in Leeds, John Goligher (1912–88) was having second thoughts about automatic colectomy in patients with long-standing colitis, quite apart from the fact that he found rectal dysplasia to be an unreliable marker.[261] His medical colleague, Geoffrey Watkinson, had left the colitis clinic in 1968, and for some years it had been supervised by Goligher and his surgical team without the help of a physician. When Tony Axon (born 1941) was appointed as consultant gastroenterologist in 1975, he was invited to sit in on the clinic for two years until Goligher's retirement after which he took it over. Axon had learnt his gastroenterology at St. Thomas's Hospital with Brian Creamer (1924–2005) and was an accomplished colonoscopist. Soon after his arrival in Leeds, he showed that several patients with no evidence of dysplasia in the rectum did have dysplasia in the colon and two had unsuspected carcinomas.[262] He was not particularly excited by his findings, but he was asked to speak against cancer surveillance at a debate in Baltimore arranged by Riddell. To his chagrin his seconder, Roger Haggitt,† a well known pathologist in Boston, far from speaking against the motion, spoke in favour of surveillance and they lost the debate. Consequently Axon felt he should continue his surveillance programme, which he did for a further twelve years. He followed 160 patients with annual colonoscopies but only picked up one patient with an early carcinoma.[263] He did in fact come across seven other patients with cancer and colitis but they were discovered independently, not because of the programme. Furthermore 25 per cent of the patients defaulted. Axon argued that

---

†   Tragically, Haggitt was murdered a few years later by a disgruntled research fellow who felt he had not supported him sufficiently.

whereas all patients with colitis should be followed up indefinitely, the case for colonoscopic surveillance was not convincing, and the costs could be channelled into a more effective cancer prevention scheme. He abandoned his programme in 1990.

Others with similar results disagreed; it was all a matter of opinion. Anthony Hoare (born 1941), a gastroenterologist in a district hospital (Wycombe General), undertook a similar surveillance programme of 313 patients for ten years.[264] The data was analysed by his registrar, Hywel Jones (born 1951) when computers were in their infancy. They found two asymptomatic patients with early carcinomas and none of the patients who stayed in the programme died. Unfortunately a quarter of the patients defaulted and five of these developed carcinomas, three of whom did die. Nonetheless Hoare thought the considerable effort and cost were worthwhile and recommended surveillance.

Some form of surveillance for colorectal cancer in colitis became part of routine clinical care during the 1980s, though clinicians were still divided on its effectiveness. What was the real risk of cancer in these patients and what happened to them? Was screening really worthwhile? One person who tried to answer these questions was Bob Allan (born 1941) in Birmingham.

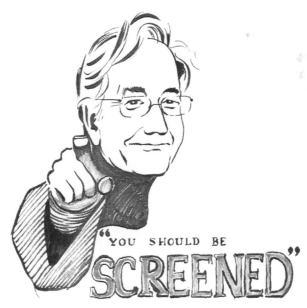

59 Allan – Yes to cancer screening.

Allan was a Birmingham man through and through; he qualified there and while house physician to Clifford Hawkins he was inspired by Lionel Hardy (1887–1969), a friend of Arthur Hurst and founder member of the BSG, who was a patient on the ward with peripheral vascular disease for several months. In due course he became senior registrar to Trevor Cooke (1912–87) and later succeeded him at the General Hospital in 1977. Allan was interested in the natural history of inflammatory bowel disease and capitalised on the huge series of patients with ulcerative colitis accumulated by Cooke from 1940 to 1976. He was fortunate to be able to collaborate with the Cancer Epidemiology Research Unit, particularly Patricia Prior, a meticulous statistician. He also took on a research registrar, Sylvia Gyde (born 1938), from general practice, who was to spend eight years on his unit before leaving to become Director of Public Health in North Birmingham.

They began by looking back at Cooke's patients, a retrospective cohort of almost 700 patients, and, using actuarial analysis, they calculated that the relative risk of cancer in these people was eight per cent after 25 years, much lower than earlier estimates.[265] As this group of patients with cancer and colitis was also thought to have a worse prognosis than those with cancer alone, they next looked at a group of patients without colitis and found that their five-year survival was in fact the same.[266] This agreed with a study at St. Mark's Hospital where Jean Ritchie and Lennard-Jones had also found that both groups had a similar prognosis.[267]

The cancer risk seemed very variable and Allan and Gyde realised that this was due to selection bias inherent in any series drawn from specialised hospitals. If they were to advise patients on the relative merits of surgery and conservative treatment, they felt they had to know the real cancer risk in patients with colitis in a given district. To get enough patients for a large retrospective study, they joined forces with two other centres, Stockholm County and Oxford. This made sense because the Scandinavians were noted for their good epidemiology and in Oxford they could draw on Truelove's cases. Gyde visited the Radcliffe Infirmary once a week to sift through the records. Eventually they managed to review what had happened to more than 800 patients after a minimum of eighteen years.[268] Altogether 29 patients had developed cancer, and the relative risk was seven per cent at twenty years, still significantly higher than in people without colitis. These people needed screening.

They also noticed that almost all the cancers occurred in middle age, no matter how long a patient had had colitis. In other words, the pattern was similar to cancer in the general population but the risk was at a higher level. Perhaps their susceptibility to cancer was genetically determined and nothing to do with the inflammatory process itself? Perhaps, too, it would be more rational to base screening on the age of the patient rather than the duration of his disease, though this would not actually alter the workload.

Cancer surveillance continued at Birmingham despite a blistering broadside two years later from, of all people, Sylvia Gyde. By now she was working in the field of public health and had become concerned about the cost effectiveness of screening. In a leading article in *Gut* (when, incidentally, Bob Allan was editor) she drew attention to the difference between surveillance (good clinical follow-up) of which she approved and screening (regular colonoscopy), the benefits of which were unproven.[269] She was worried by the poor sensitivity and specificity of dysplasia as a marker in screening and called for a randomised controlled trial or failing that a better marker for screening purposes. "One thing is certain," she concluded, "we should not go on as we are." At the same time Michael Langman, an influential gastroenterological epidemiologist in Birmingham, wrote a progress report on cancer screening in *Gut*.[270] In his view this was needed but the current methods were unsatisfactory. Proof of benefit was lacking and better tests were needed.

Anti-screeners were also quick to point out that taking four biopsy specimens from each ten-centimetre segment of colon was not merely time-consuming but a blind procedure with a very poor yield.

These articles will have been widely read by gastroenterologists only too happy to abandon screening if it was a waste of time and effort. Not surprisingly, Lennard-Jones sprang to its defence.[271] "To undertake a controlled trial," he wrote in a letter to *Gut*, "would be daunting, if not impossible, and probably unethical at this stage. Furthermore there were now several clinical studies, including an excellent one from Stockholm County, in which there had been no deaths and the removal of 3 localised tumours (all Dukes A)." He admitted that low-grade dysplasia was not as benign as he had first thought. It was an evolving situation in which clinician and pathologist were learning from one another. Most people now agreed that significant dysplasia was usually associated with a visible lesion; and the tropical-sounding acronym, DALM (dysplasia-associated lesion or mass), first coined by Riddell in 1981, came into vogue.

So why did people continue with screening? Simply because to do nothing gave the unlucky patient no chance. But what people did varied widely. In 2000, John Mayberry and his research fellow, Jayne Eaden (born 1969), carried out a national audit of the surveillance practices of gastroenterologists in Britain and found that though most clinicians were doing something, screening was haphazard.[272] Concerned by this, they next did a meta-analysis of 116 studies of cancer in colitis and confirmed the known risks of cancer, indicating the need to screen this high-risk group.[273] Accordingly, in 1992, Eaden and Mayberry, on behalf of the British Society of Gastroenterology, published guidelines that formerly recognised the importance of screening. These laid down (but not in tablets of stone) what they considered to be best practice at the time, which of course included regular colonoscopy and multiple blind biopsies after eight to ten years of disease.[274]

The guidelines illustrated the controversy surrounding the subject because the St. Mark's team, the leading protagonists of screening, complained that the evidence was insufficient to justify regular colonoscopy on every patient with extensive colitis.[275] This was asking too much of many district general hospitals, and patients should be given the choice after appropriate counselling. They were also concerned about the benefits during routine colonoscopy of taking multiple random biopsies because they themselves had recently failed to find dysplasia in 3,000 surveillance biopsies. The whole issue of screening was as contentious as ever.

In fact, even as the guidelines were being published, the St. Mark's group were revising their approach to screening. The hospital had moved from its old site in City Road to Harrow in Middlesex where there was a fine, state-of-the-art endoscopy unit with research and teaching facilities funded by the Wolfson Foundation. Christopher Williams had been joined by another endoscopy physician, Brian Saunders (born 1964), and Alastair Forbes (born 1958) had succeeded Lennard-Jones on his retirement from clinical work in 1992. Colonoscopy by well trained practitioners was now a quick procedure, taking on average twenty minutes, a far cry from the early '70s.

In 2001, Forbes and Saunders took on a research fellow, Matthew Rutter (born 1970), who looked back at the long surveillance programme undertaken by Lennard-Jones and found that it had probably saved the lives of three quarters of the patients with cancers.[276] It had been well worthwhile though the effort and expense had been considerable. Rutter also noted that as time went by, the ability to see dysplastic lesions had steadily improved, especially after the introduction of high-resolution videoendoscopy. But several "flat" lesions were still being missed.

The group then hit on the idea of spraying the whole colon with a dye, indigo carmine, in order to highlight the lesions that were otherwise invisible.[277] Pancolonic chromendoscopy, as they called it, was a great advance making it easy to identify lesions for biopsy. Clearly this was much more efficient than taking random biopsies. But there was more. Rutter and his colleagues were able to refine the screening procedure further with the discovery that colitics with "healed", pristine colons were no longer at risk of dysplasia and could be removed from the programme. So a smaller number of patients required screening, and those that did would have targeted biopsies and be much more likely to benefit. The case for screening seemed inescapable.

CHAPTER FORTY-SEVEN

CARCINOMA COMPLICATING CROHN'S DISEASE

The first case of a cancer of the colon complicating "regional ileitis" was described in 1948 by Warren and Sommers, two pathologists in New York.[278] Several more reports soon followed, particularly from America, but it was many years before people accepted that cancer was indeed a complication of Crohn's Disease. Why? First, Crohn's Disease was relatively rare and the number of cases was so small that meaningful analysis was almost impossible. Second, before 1960 people with Crohn's colitis were thought to have ulcerative colitis, so they would have been reported as such. Third, some population-based studies of Crohn's Disease overlooked the tremendously increased cancer risks shown in their own data by failing to analyse small subsets of their population that were actually at risk.

In Britain, the first reports came from well-known centres with large series of patients, as one would expect. In 1968, John Goligher in Leeds reported two cases[279] followed by Truelove in Oxford with another three cases,[280] there were four examples at St. Mark's Hospital[281] and Trevor Cooke in Birmingham found six patients with adenocarcinoma among 295 cases seen over a period of more than 30 years though only one of these was in the colon.[282] No one felt confident that these cancers were anything more than coincidental, though David Pollock (born 1931), pathologist at the London Hospital, thought the risk was significant after he had reported two more cases with his surgical colleague, Alan Parks, and reviewed the literature.[283]

The first statistical estimate of colorectal cancer complicating Crohn's Disease came from Roy Shorter's group at the Mayo Clinic in 1973.[284]

They found eight cancers of the colon and rectum among nearly 450 young patients with Crohn's Disease, which was twenty times that expected for the population of Minnesota. Even so their report had little impact on clinicians at the time because the numbers were small and the disease still rare. It was not until Crohn's Disease became common that people finally recognised the cancer risk.

The Birmingham group, led by Bob Allan (born 1941), deserve much of the credit and, as with their work on the cancer risk in ulcerative colitis, they were fortunate to have the services of Patricia Prior, a statistician from the cancer epidemiology research unit at the university.[285] It is easy to see why it had been difficult to quantify the cancer risk earlier. Allan had more than 500 patients at his disposal, but in order to eliminate selection bias inherent in any specialist hospital series, only 300 who were local residents were eligible. He came up with just eight cancers (six colon, two rectum), all in a smaller group of 125 patients who had had extensive colitis for many years.[286] This was similar to ulcerative colitis except that two thirds of the Crohn's group had had a colectomy for troublesome symptoms long before they were at risk. Even so Allan and Prior calculated that the risk was eighteen-fold despite the small numbers. They then compared this risk with their earlier studies on ulcerative colitis and found that it was the same in both diseases. So the argument for screening patients with ulcerative colitis was now the same for Crohn's colitis.[287]

A final comment; in general carcinomas of the small and large bowel tend to arise in areas affected by active Crohn's Disease, so one might have expected cancer of the lower rectum or anus to be common in these patients. However, surprisingly few cases have been reported. Lennard-Jones found only twelve patients at St. Mark's Hospital over a period of 53 years, all of whom had severe anorectal disease.[288] Considering that a high proportion of patients attending St. Mark's Hospital actually have anorectal disease, one can assume that a gastroenterologist working in a district general hospital will see one, or maybe two, cases in the whole of his career.

CHAPTER FORTY-EIGHT

TREATMENT OTHER THAN STEROIDS AND 5–AMINOSALICYLATES

(a) Diet

Though the introduction of steroids transformed the outlook for people with acute colitis, not everybody responded and many patients still needed colectomy. Unfortunately these people were usually so ill and undernourished that major surgery was hazardous; even at a specialist hospital such as St. Mark's Hospital, Lennard-Jones found the mortality after colectomy was 25 per cent.[289]

During the 1960s and '70s the concept of "bowel rest" was popular. Doctors hoped that the inflamed intestine would heal more quickly if relieved of mechanical trauma, intestinal secretions and the antigenic challenge of food. So patients survived, and sometimes did not survive, on infusions of saline and five per cent dextrose that provided salt and water but precious little else. The arrival of solutions containing amino acids, sugars and lipids was an exciting advance, and, in Philadelphia, Samuel Dudrick suggested that these solutions were safe and possibly beneficial to patients with inflammatory bowel disease.[290] Michael Clark (born 1932) who worked in Philadelphia for a time in the mid-60s recalls that Dudrick had three indications for using parenteral nutrition, "patients who cannot eat, will not eat or cannot eat enough".

In Britain intravenous feeding was slow to catch on; doctors were suspicious, if not sceptical of its value and it was tricky to manage (intensive care units were still a thing of the future). But there were enthusiasts, particularly on the new renal units, who were dealing with wasted, hypercatabolic patients in renal failure, often following major surgery. Gradually, in the early 1970s, the message spread and parenteral nutrition began to be used in patients with severe inflammatory bowel disease. Here surely was the ideal way to rest the bowel and feed the patient at the same time. Two groups of patients were thought to benefit; those with extensive Crohn's Disease who were cachectic, and those with severe colitis needing surgery. Unfortunately the benefits in Crohn's Disease appeared to be short-lived and stopping parenteral nutrition inevitably led to a relapse. There were problems too with infection and venous access. In Oxford Truelove reviewed his results and could only conclude that "parenteral nutrition appeared to add little to the acute management of colitis".[291]

A controlled clinical trial to prove its value was needed but this was difficult for two reasons; acute colitis needing inpatient treatment was uncommon so sufficient numbers would be hard to come by, and assessing the response to treatment objectively was surprisingly difficult. Nevertheless two centres did manage it.

(b) Bowel rest (laid to rest)

In Leeds, the professor of surgery, John Goligher, retired in 1977 and Tony Axon, recently appointed as a much needed gastroenterologist there, took over his famous colitis clinic. Goligher's senior lecturer in surgery, Graham Hill, was particularly interested in the nutrition of the surgical patients and now joined forces with Axon and two registrars, Richard Dickinson and Michael Ashton, to look at the need for bowel rest. Dickinson (born 1946) had become interested in colitis while working on the infectious diseases unit in Edinburgh. He once said that fever doctors thought that anyone with diarrhoea had dysentery of some sort whereas gastroenterologists assumed that they had inflammatory bowel disease. He was interested in the role of pathogenic E. coli and joined Tony Axon to study this. Michael Ashton (born 1948) was research assistant in the university department of medicine when Axon arrived in Leeds. His interest was in the pancreas but he acted as the independent assessor of the patients' progress during the trial. This combined surgical and medical team compared two groups of patients with acute colitis and concluded that there was no advantage in adding parenteral nutrition to the standard medical regimen.[292] Dickinson, after a spell in

Cambridge, settled in Hinchingbrooke Hospital, Huntingdon. Ashton took an appointment in Sunderland, later moving to the Chesterfield and North Derbyshire Hospital.

The other study was led by Lennard-Jones at St. Mark's Hospital who, appreciating the difficulty of obtaining sufficient patients with severe colitis collaborated with Robert Colin's group at the Hôpital Charles-Nicolle, in Rouen. Lennard-Jones' interest in nutrition was stimulated by his old chief, Francis Avery Jones, who was possibly the only gastroenterologist of his generation to recognise the importance of a good diet in health and disease. His research fellows at St. Mark's Hospital were Jeremy Powell-Tuck and Paul McIntyre. Powell-Tuck (born 1948) had done much to improve the technical aspects of intravenous feeding. He had introduced the technique of central venous catheterisation for long-term parenteral nutrition and had developed a

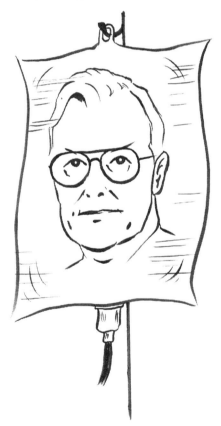

60 Allison – Doyen of clinical nutrition.

single disposable bag to replace the assortment of bottles then in use. He showed that for parenteral nutrition to work a team approach was necessary, including pharmacist, dietician and nurse all dedicated to the subject.[293] It was not cheap but in due course a few patients with intestinal failure managed to live at home on their feeds. In fact the first patient came from the Isle of Wight and was under the care of an enthusiastic nephrologist, Professor Harry Lee (born 1935), who was one of the pioneers of parenteral nutrition. The two teams from England and France found that patients given intravenous feeding and bowel rest did no better than those who ate normally.[294] Their trial dealt a mortal blow to the bowel rest theory, though it did show that cachectic patients who were unable to eat were helped by parenteral nutrition. Indeed the patients with Crohn's colitis all responded so well that they did not require colectomy. Not long afterwards another large study from Jeejeebhoy and Tremaine's group in Toronto confirmed that bowel rest was unnecessary in Crohn's Disease.[295]

(c) Enteral feeding

By now enteral feeding was gathering pace, much to the relief of many who flinched at the rigours and risks of intravenous feeding. Treating patients with a liquid diet began in the late 1960s but was slow to catch on partly because "bowel rest" was in vogue, partly because intravenous feeding was more glamorous and mostly because the feeds were so unpalatable.

Water soluble, chemically designed diets were first devised for the American space programme in the early 1960s for sanitary reasons but the astronauts hated them. However, the diets were the forerunners of elemental diets that are used today. Initially the idea was to improve nutrition during periods of active disease and in Britain one of the first to publish a study showing this was Ivan Johnston (1929–2004), Professor of Surgery in Newcastle who had a lifelong interest in nutrition. Some of his patients with Crohn's Disease managed to swallow an elemental diet for almost a year and all regained their usual weight.[296] This said almost as much for his powers of persuasion as it did for the benefit of the diet.

Many patients with severe inflammatory bowel disease were anorexic and literally could not stomach the diets. One person who made a study of this was Simon Allison (born 1938), a diabetologist in Nottingham.

Aghast at the quality of meals served in hospital when he was a research fellow, he himself had sometimes cooked meals for the patients. Some years after his appointment in Nottingham, he was asked in 1978 to see a young woman with Crohn's Disease with a view to providing terminal care. She had had a colectomy and ileostomy twenty years before and had relapsed in 1972 with fistulae, pelvic abscesses and electrolyte depletion, and was a chronic invalid.[297] Allison arranged an intensive course of sip feeding (twenty millilitres every fifteen mins) over three weeks which in itself was a remarkable achievement. As her weight increased her appetite recovered and it became unnecessary to force her to feed. Soon she was back to her normal weight and remained well for several years. This stimulated his concept of primary and secondary anorexia. Disease causes a primary loss of appetite with a consequent fall in weight. Beyond a certain point, a secondary anorexia supervenes similar to that seen in anorexia nervosa.

Tube feeding was the obvious way to treat the secondary anorexia, but until the mid-1970s this meant passing a large bore tube (such as Ryle's) into the stomach. This was uncomfortable for the patient, inflamed the oesophagus and encouraged reflux. The situation was transformed by a gastroenterologist in Ealing, Hugh McMichael (born 1937), son of Sir John McMichael, the legendary professor of medicine at the Hammersmith Hospital. He was studying the physiology of carbohydrate absorption and found the Ryle's tube unsatisfactory, so in 1975 he obtained a reel of portex tubing, stiffened it with a Seldinger wire and the soft, fine bore naso-gastric tube was born.[298] The McMichaels had a way with fine tubes; Hugh's father was the first to pass a catheter into the heart in 1944.

Allison[299] and Powell-Tuck[300] soon adopted this tube and found that it was best to feed patients overnight with a concentrated feed using a pump to deliver it slowly to avoid diarrhoea. The patients were free to eat during the daytime and felt better physically and happier in themselves.

Meanwhile David Silk (born 1944) who was rapidly making his reputation as a nutritionist at the Central Middlesex Hospital, refined the soft bore tube and used it to study many permutations of chemically defined diets over the next few years.[301] Ultimately he showed that most patients requiring enteral nutrition did well on a polymeric (whole protein) feed and not so well on an elemental (amino acid) feed. Perhaps a few patients with Crohn's Disease of the small bowel needed something in between these diets and did better with nitrogen derived from short chain peptides rather than whole protein.[302]

Apart from its nutritional value, the elemental diet proved to be a valuable research tool. I have already described how Colm O'Morain, Tony Segal and Jonathan Levi at the Clinical Research Centre, Harrow, used elemental diets to induce a remission in Crohn's Disease, showing that it was as effective as prednisolone and that the effect was not simply due to better nutrition.[303] They monitored the response to treatment by a simple activity index devised by Richard Harvey (born 1940), a gastroenterologist in Bristol, and his research registrar, Jane Bradshaw (born 1952) who was later appointed gastroenterologist to Brighton.[304] This was easy to use and reflected mucosal inflammation, but it was non-specific and could be misleading. So research workers needing conclusive evidence of improved absorption turned to Ian Menzies (born 1929), chemical pathologist at St. Thomas's Hospital, who was able to measure intestinal permeability.

Menzies first became interested in intestinal permeability at Great Ormond Street Hospital working on the absorption of disaccharides. He moved to St. Thomas's Hospital in 1965 where with the support of Brian Creamer he gradually perfected tests to measure absorption using various sugars as markers. Years ahead of his time, he found himself in great demand by those studying small bowel diseases, including the paediatric gastroenterologists Ian Sanderson and John Walker-Smith at the Institute of Child Health. Earlier I mentioned how they had achieved an excellent clinical response in children using liquid diets; now Menzies was able to use his sugar markers to show that intestinal permeability improved as the children recovered.[305]

Menzies also worked closely with Levi's group at Northwick Park Hospital which was affiliated to the Medical Research Council's Clinical Research Centre employing about 1200 scientists. One of these was Ingvar Bjarnason (born 1951), who arrived from Iceland in 1981 to study absorption with Tim Peters (born 1941). He was looking for a new substance to measure permeability and quite by chance stumbled across Norman Veall who was head of the radioisotopes division. Veall suggested Cr-labelled edetic acid and within months a new test appeared complementing Menzies' use of sugar markers.[306/307]

In 1985 Levi appointed a new young registrar, Kathy Teahon (born

1957), fresh from Galway, who was impressed by the ability of the elemental diet to help patients with Crohn's Disease. She worked closely with Bjarnason, Peters and Levi and showed that permeability correlated well with disease activity and, incidentally, was normal in patients' relatives showing that permeability was not a primary or genetic defect in Crohn's Disease.[308]

The British climate and sense of humour clearly suited the droll Bjarnason; he originally came here for three years but stayed and is now Professor of Gastroenterology at King's College Hospital. Known as Mr. Permeability in the 1980s, he became Mr. Calprotectin in the 1990s.

Workers in Oslo had found that the protein, calprotectin, was the main cytosolic protein of neutrophils and that it was resistant to degradation by intestinal bacteria. Saverymuttu, Hodgson and Chadwick at the Hammersmith Hospital had used their technique of neutrophil scanning to show that inflammation in the colon subsided as patients responded to dietary treatment, but their test was impracticable for routine use. As calprotectin was easy to measure in faeces and as Hodgson had shown that there was a ten–fold excess of neutrophils in active Crohn's Disease, its potential as a test to discriminate between normal and inflamed bowel was promising. Bjarnason teamed up with his erstwhile colleague Kathy Teahon, now a consultant gastroenterologist in Nottingham, and friends in Reykjavik and Oslo to show that measurement of stool calprotectin was indeed a simple, sensitive and specific indicator of bowel inflammation and could be useful as a screening test in differentiating Crohn's Disease from irritable bowel syndrome.[309]

Whereas liquid diets, elemental or not, were useless in patients with ulcerative colitis, there was now good evidence that they induced remissions in Crohn's Disease. Yet few centres adopted the diet approach for the simple reason that it required enthusiasm and determination by doctor and patient to persevere with it.[310] Few hospitals had the dedicated nutrition teams that were so necessary and doctors found it much simpler to prescribe steroids. Even paediatricians who were particularly keen to avoid steroids had difficulty in persuading their young patients to try a diet that was so unpalatable.

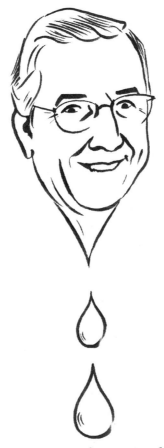

61 Hunter – Elimination diets.

d) Exclusion diets

If ultimately they were to use these diets clinicians needed to know if they could postpone or prevent further attacks of Crohn's Disease, and in due course reports of their long-term benefit appeared. Three centres in Britain were committed to the treatment and their results raised the thorny issue of food intolerance.

The person best known for his work on food intolerance was John Hunter, a gastroenterologist in Cambridge. Hunter (born 1940) trained as a hepatologist at King's College Hospital but on his appointment to Addenbrooke's Hospital he discovered that most of the patients in his clinic had irritable bowel syndrome (apart from a few alcoholic dons).

Undaunted he treated them with fibre, which was in vogue at the time, but this made them worse. Cambridge patients are particularly critical of their treatment apparently. So his dietician, Elizabeth Workman, suggested they try a low-fibre diet instead with some striking successes. At this stage Hunter was joined by a new senior house officer, Virginia Alun Jones, who embraced the subject wholeheartedly, stayed on as a research fellow, wrote her MD and was co-author with Hunter of an excellent book, *Food and the Gut*, published in 1985.[311]

Encouraged by the success of the low-fibre diet they wondered if intolerance to certain foods might be important and in a carefully conducted experiment found that it was.[312] They were the first to admit that the detection of specific intolerance was tedious and required six to eight weeks of single-minded concentration on a diet that was very restricted. They were fortunate to have the support of the Dunn Clinical Nutrition Centre in Cambridge. They also pointed out that none of their patients had a food allergy in the immunological sense after innumerable tests by Robin Coombs (1921–2006), a distinguished immunologist, were negative.

In the late 1970s they happened to treat an eighteen-year-old girl with presumed irritable bowel syndrome, who in fact had granulomatous proctitis and she got better. Intrigued they went on to treat 77 patients with Crohn's diseae over the next five years inducing remission with parenteral nutrition or an elemental diet, E028. The diet was supplied by a company anxious for them to try their product – "it tastes much better than vivonex, Doctor". Once in remission most of the patients persevered with the exclusion regimen and did well for several months or even years.[313]

Aware that this treatment, which they presented at the Twelfth International Congress of Gastroenterology in 1984, would excite controversy and public interest fanned by the media and women's magazines, and anxious not to be the butt of every gastroenterologist besieged by patients wishing to try the diet, Alun Jones and Hunter ran a small controlled trial, which showed that seven out of ten patients on the exclusion diet were still in remission after six months compared with none of the ten on an ordinary diet.[314] Yet again they emphasised that the dietary approach required full co-operation between patient, doctor and dietician and that many people were unsuitable for this type of treatment.

Hunter wondered how certain foods, commonly cereals, dairy products, caffeine, yeast and citrus fruits upset patients with Crohn's Disease and irritable bowel syndrome and came to the conclusion that ordinary bacteria in the colon were responsible. Dietary manipulation altered the substrate available for fermentation by bacteria, which in turn changed the composition of the colonic flora. This maintained the benefit of the elemental diet that had induced the remission in the first place. Altering the bacterial load in the colon removed, or reduced, the stimulus for an inflammatory response by the mucosa.[315]

To give credence to his work, Hunter next organised a multi-centre controlled trial with his colleagues in hospitals around East Anglia.[316] This was a daunting prospect and he knew that many patients would drop out, but it would at least reflect the experience of other gastroenterologists less dedicated to the dietary approach. Indeed, out of a possible 224 patients, 88 were not enrolled for one reason or another: 136 patients entered the trial, but 43 refused to continue the diet and a further 15 did not respond. Thus only 76 patients, one third of the original group, were available for randomisation. Admittedly those who took an exclusion diet fared better than the others, though by the end of two years there was little to choose between them, relapses occurring in about two thirds of the patients in both groups. Hunter concluded ruefully that diet did not provide the final answer to Crohn's Disease but it did point the way to further research. If he could discover the mechanism underlying food intolerance it might help us to understand the pathogenesis of Crohn's Disease.

Meanwhile Tony Levi in Northwick Park Hospital, Harrow, had continued to use elemental diets. By 1988 he had treated more than 100 patients over a period of ten years and Kathy Teahon looked back at the results.[317] Most of the patients had responded to the diet and nearly half of these were still in remission after three years, at least as good as conventional treatment. Teahon emphasised the safety of the treatment, but reading between the lines, the dedication required by all concerned to achieve these excellent results was enormous.

Lastly, in Sheffield, Derek Holdsworth decided to try the dietary approach to Crohn's Disease. Holdsworth (born 1933) qualified in Leeds and was attracted to gastroenterology while working as registrar to Michael Atkinson (born 1925) and Geoffrey Watkinson (1921–96) when they were senior lecturers in Leeds. Moving to the Royal Free

Hospital he wrote his MD on monosaccharide absorption under the tutelage of Anthony Dawson and continued his research as senior lecturer at St. Bartholemew's Hospital. In 1969 he was appointed consultant physician to the Royal Hallamshire Hospital in Sheffield, where despite a heavy clinical load he maintained an active clinical research programme throughout his career. Unassuming and modest, he built up a large colitis clinic and was the first to describe hyposplenism in ulcerative colitis.[318]

His interest in absorption led him into the nutrition field but it was a young lady with steroid-resistant Crohn's Disease who stimulated his dietary approach to the disease. She requested a second opinion from Hunter in Cambridge and did extraordinarily well on an exclusion diet. Impressed, Holdsworth decided to re-examine the case for liquid feeds and ran a series of controlled trials. With his research fellow, Mustafa Giaffer (born 1951) from Libya, he showed that whole protein (polymeric) feeds were not quite as effective as amino acid (elemental) feeds in treating acute Crohn's Disease.[319] But they were cheaper and more palatable so he took matters further and with his new research fellow, John Mansfield (born 1961), found that a protein hydrolysate (oligopeptide) diet was equally as good as the amino acid diet but cheaper and more palatable.[320] In this carefully designed study he demonstrated the response by scanning the colon after labelling it with technetium labelled leucocytes. Finally, with his senior registrar, Paul Cann (born 1953), he followed this up with a longer trial in which he showed that an exclusion diet was helpful in a few patients, though the majority relapsed within a few months, especially those with Crohn's Disease of the colon.[321] Cann, Giaffer and Mansfield were appointed as gastroenterologists to Middlesbrough, Hull and Newcastle respectively.

The practicalities and the unpredictability of these diets have inhibited most clinicians from using them. But they are more than mere jungle juice and everyone agrees that they can be beneficial. Hunter believes that they alter the bacterial flora of the colon thus reducing the inflammatory process of Crohn's Disease in some way, and his research continues.

e) Azathioprine

The use of azathioprine in colitis and Crohn's Disease spluttered into life in the 1960s and on reflection it is remarkable that it survived. Even today how the drug works is not understood. The compound was prepared as an anti-neoplastic derivative of 6-mercaptopurine in 1960 and a year later was thought to have immunosuppressive properties. No one knew if colitis was caused by a disturbance of immunity but an Australian, Dr. R. H. Bean, used azathioprine as an immunosuppressant in 1962 and three years later concluded that it might occasionally be useful in acute severe colitis, though he was careful to point out its dangers.[322] Soon after, Kirsner in Chicago reported its potential in ten patients.[323]

In 1964 Francis Avery Jones had under his care a girl of nineteen with severe colitis unresponsive to steroids. She refused surgery so with some trepidation he gave her azathioprine. Within a month she developed severe marrow depression and died from a fulminating chest infection.[324] This was an inauspicious start and in 1968 Geoffrey Watkinson in York reviewed the literature and concluded that "the results in 25 patients (worldwide) to date have been far from impressive".[325] It is possible that British interest could have stopped there but for two unlikely and very different people.

The first was Richard Arden Jones (1910–95), a general physician in a small district hospital in Newmarket. Towards the end of his career, for reasons I do not know, he treated twelve patients with all grades of colitis for several months claiming excellent results in all of them.[326] He used high doses of azothioprine (not less than five mg/kg) because he thought that some leucopoenia was necessary to obtain a good response. Fortunately he got away with it.

The second was the mercurial Bryan Brooke (1915–98), Professor of Surgery at St. George's Hospital. One morning in 1968, on a ward round, Brooke was discussing the nature of Crohn's Disease with his senior registrar, Des Hoffman from South Africa, and the house surgeon, Edwin Swarbrick (born 1945). Brooke thought that the granulomatous reaction, so similar to that seen in tuberculosis, could be a manifestation of hypersensitivity, akin in some ways to tissue rejection. He was also aware that azathioprine helped to prevent rejection of transplanted organs. He had several cases of severe fistulating Crohn's Disease on the ward and had run out of therapeutic options, so Hoffman suggested that they might try azathioprine. Brooke jumped at the idea and Michael Clarke (born 1932), who often attended his round, recalls Brooke's response when asked why he was using the drug. "Imuran?" he would reply. "Why, it's immuno logical!" All the original six patients given the drug responded dramatically and 5 returned to work.[327] Encouraged Brooke went on to treat a further 32 patients who were less ill with satisfactory results.[328]

But not everyone was happy. Trevor Cooke (1911–87) in Birmingham, with huge experience of treating Crohn's Disease, wrote in a letter to the *Lancet* that "Professor Brooke was to be congratulated for his courage – or admonished for his rashness – in using azathioprine so freely".[329] Cooke felt that most of the patients would have done just as well with conventional treatment. Not enough was known about the cause and immunological aspects of Crohn's Disease to justify the routine use of the drug and he was worried that it might increase the risk of cancer. He personally had only used azathioprine when the risks of the disease far outweighed those of the drug.

Nonetheless clinicians were beginning to use the drug cautiously and clearly a controlled trial was needed; not an easy matter in such a variable and unpredictable disease. However, Michael Clarke, now senior lecturer at St. Bartholemews's Hospital and fresh from St. George's Hospital, persuaded Tony Dawson (1928–97), head of the gastroenterology unit at the hospital, that they should do one. Dawson agreed and gave the project to his MRC research fellow, Michael Willoughby (born 1935) and the new registrar, Parveen Kumar (born 1942). They collected 22 patients with moderate to severe Crohn's Disease and showed unequivocally that patients who had needed steroids could be kept in remission on azathioprine alone.[330] Willoughby was so impressed that throughout his career as gastroenterologist at the Lister Hospital in Stevenage he argued that any patient ill enough to need steroids should automatically receive azathioprine. In his view prednisolone was a much more dangerous drug.

Yet most clinicians continued to use the drug sparingly, concerned by the occasional case of unpredictable neutropoenia and the possible risk of cancer. Though useful in maintaining remission, no one knew for how long it should be given. In 1978 Tony Dawson joined forces with Lennard-Jones at St. Mark's Hospital in another trial, which showed that patients who stopped it nearly all relapsed within a year.[331] Yet as recently as 1995 a survey showed that almost half the gastroenterologists in Britain were using azathioprine for less than two years.[332] Consultants with more experience of the drug treated patients with milder disease and used larger doses for longer periods. Fortunately, everyone will have been reassured by a survey from St. Mark's Hospital showing that there was no risk of malignancy as late as nine years after treatment with azathioprine.[333]

Returning to ulcerative colitis, after Arden Jones' paper to the Royal Society of Medicine, Sidney Truelove in Oxford realised better than anyone that it was imperative to test azathioprine under the strict conditions of a controlled trial. Accordingly, with the help his young research assistant, Derek Jewell, he studied 80 patients and after a year of treatment the results were disappointing or at least equivocal.[334] They did at least show that the drug was of no help in acute attacks, which was useful. On the other hand they had the distinct impression that azathioprine could reduce the relapse rate but their results just failed to achieve statistical significance. They concluded that there might be a place for azathioprine in patients unresponsive to sulphasalazine who were unsuitable for proctocolectomy.

This rather dampened enthusiasm for a while until John Lennard-Jones ran another small trial eight years later, which showed that azathioprine was significantly superior to placebo in controlling colitis.[335] But, like Truelove, he felt that its use should be restricted to patients with troublesome disease.

Matters rested there with clinicians using azathioprine when there was no alternative, until Christopher Hawkey, Professor of Gastroenterology in Nottingham, reviewed the situation. Together with Richard Logan, a gut-orientated senior lecturer in clinical epidemiology and his research fellow, Barney Hawthorne (born 1960), he showed that many of the patients with chronically active disease could achieve complete remission with azathioprine and stop steroids.[336] Encouraged by this, Hawthorne set up a multicentre trial to establish, once and for all, the case for azathioprine in treating ulcerative colitis. He enlisted help from four other centres noted for their interest in colitis.[337] These were Lennard-Jones at St. Mark's Hospital, Tony Axon in Leeds, Ed Swarbrick in Wolverhampton (who, it will be recalled, first used azathioprine when he was Bryan Brooke's house surgeon twenty years earlier) and Brian Scott in Lincoln. Sixty-seven patients who had been taking azathiopine for at least six months were randomised to stay on it or to switch to a placebo. A year later twice as many patients on the placebo had relapsed. The case was made; azathioprine should be used more often in patients with poorly controlled colitis and for a minimum of two years.

Finally, in 2002, an older Derek Jewell, now Professor of Gastroenterology at the Radcliffe Infirmary presented a fascinating review of his experience with azathioprine over 30 years.[338] During this time more than a third of his patients with inflammatory bowel disease had been treated with azathioprine with remission in nearly 90 per cent of those with ulcerative colitis and 64 per cent of those with Crohn's Disease (especially colonic disease), which were remarkable figures.

Within the last few years several new designer drugs have been introduced but among "immunosuppressants", azathioprine has won its place.

CHAPTER FORTY-NINE

MODERN SURGERY

Despite the best efforts of surgeons in specialist units, emergency colectomy on patients with severe acute colitis was still a dangerous undertaking in the 1960s and '70s. General surgeons in district hospitals dealt with one or two patients each year so their experience was limited, intensive care facilities were unusual and nutritional support was in its infancy. Admittedly steroids were having a favourable impact but frequently patients were treated by physicians for too long before being referred for surgery. At least there was no argument about the appropriate operation, ileostomy and proctocolectomy, usually as a one-stage procedure.

The same applied when it came to patients with chronic colitis who needed elective colectomy because medical treatment had failed or to pre-empt cancer. But needless to say most people, especially the young, dreaded the prospect of a permanent ileostomy despite the advances in stoma care.

With this in mind Stanley Aylett, a surgeon at the Gordon Hospital, began to undertake colectomy without an ileostomy, simply joining the ileum to the rectum. Aylett (1911–2003) was a remarkable man with supreme confidence in his surgical ability, partly learnt while operating in the field throughout the Second World War, for which he received the *Croix d'honneur* and a military MBE. After demobilisation he was appointed to the Westminster and Gordon Hospitals where in 1952 he did his first colectomy and ileo-rectal anastomosis. Within six years he had performed 100 of these operations with only one failure and 90 of his patients were back at work.[339] He believed that the inflamed rectum settled spontaneously after colectomy or could be treated easily by medical means if not. Not surprisingly, as his reputation grew, patients flocked to his clinic, which had the aura of a family gathering and was supervised by his outpatient sister, Kay Page (later to be his second wife).

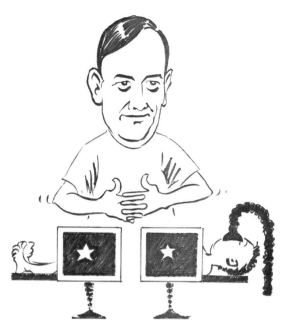

62 Aylett – Magical continuity.

Many surgeons attempted his operation but few could emulate him. Most found that their patients were bedevilled by recurrent or continued proctitis. It was even suggested that Aylett's great charm seduced his patients into belittling their problems.

One of the few who did succeed was Oswald Lloyd Davies (1905–87), surgeon to the Middlesex and St. Mark's Hospitals and notable for his sphincter-preserving procedure during anterior resection of the rectum. He did several colectomies with ileo-rectal anastomoses with what seemed good results. His senior registrar, Peter Jones (born 1920) was so impressed that when he was appointed reader, and later professor, in paediatric surgery and consultant surgeon in Aberdeen he undertook the procedure himself for many years with excellent results, particularly in children and young people.[340] Why did he succeed where others failed? Like Aylett he was a gifted surgeon but he was also careful to select suitable patients with severe colitis and a relatively normal rectum, including many young people with Crohn's Disease. Not surprisingly he found it much easier to convince children of the need for surgery once they knew that they would not have a bag (his youngest patient was eight years old). He recognised that the disease could recur and that removal of the rectum may be needed later, but by then a youngster would have completed his education, married and had children and so be more amenable to an ileostomy.[341]

Another of Lloyd-Davies' senior registrars, Peter Hawley (born 1932), also adopted the technique successfully and after his appointment to St. Mark's Hospital as many as one third of the patients needing colectomy were having an ileorectal anastomosis. Careful follow-up was crucial, particularly as cancer could arise in the rectal stump, but like Peter Jones, he felt that the operation was ideal for young people even if the rectum had to be excised some years later.[342]

As I have indicated others were less impressed and had bad results with the technique. The Birmingham school, influenced by Bryan Brooke, were in favour of a permanent ileostomy and men such as Geoffrey Slaney (born 1922) and Gilroy Bevan (born 1922), who were senior registrars with Brooke, avoided the Aylett operation. The chief protagonists, Brooke and Aylett, enthralled audiences with heated exchanges on the subject. The same applied at Leeds where John Goligher persevered with colectomy and ileostomy. Many were daunted by the risk of a bowel leak after joining diseased rectum to the ileum.

The other concern was the continuing risk of cancer in the rectum and anyone lost to follow-up was particularly vulnerable.[343] Yet as the medical management of colitis improved, urgent surgery in ill patients became less frequent and the demand for elective surgery simply to prevent cancer developing in patients with inactive or mild disease increased. Most of these patients were quite well and naturally reluctant to have an ileostomy. Surgeons needed an alternative and it came with the development of an ileo-anal pouch devised by Alan Parks (1920–82).

Parks was a Rockefeller student at the Johns Hopkins Hospital, Baltimore during the Second World War and completed his undergraduate training at Guy's Hospital in 1947. His interest in the lower bowel began early and his research was prolific. Papers on haemorrhoidectomy, fistula-in-ano, pelvic-floor physiology, pharmacokinetics of the intestinal musculature and techniques of colo-anal anastomosis followed each other in steady succession. He joined the staff of St. Mark's Hospital in 1959, the only consultant surgeon to be appointed without having been a resident there. He gathered around him experts, including neurophysiologists and pharmacologists, and perfected the technique of ileo-anal anastomosis with a reservoir (Park's pouch), the direct result of his painstaking work on submucosal dissection and his knowledge of pelvic physiology. Later he became President of the Royal College of Surgeons but died while in office.

The Park's pouch was quickly adopted by surgeons throughout the kingdom and America. The first restorative proctocolectomy, as it became known, was done by Parks and his senior registrar, John Nicholls (born 1944) in 1976[344] and within fifteen years well over 450 patients had had the operation. By 1990 over half the elective procedures undertaken at St. Mark's Hospital were restorative proctocolectomies.[345] It was not a substitute for colectomy and ileostomy in patients with acute disease but many of these were suitable for a restorative operation later, either an ileoanal pouch or an ileorectal anastomosis. Though the complication rate of the pouch procedure was high, it was little worse than that of routine total colectomy, and the patients, who were all young (average age 30 years), thought it was well worthwhile.

Coloproctology became a specialty in its own right and many thought there was little more that surgeons could achieve even though their operations were a major undertaking and carried a significant morbidity. Few could have guessed that within a few years colectomy would be transformed not by colorectal surgeons but by people skilled in the art of laparoscopy.

Laparoscopy had been used for simple diagnostic purposes by gynaecologists since the 1970s, though their instruments were relatively primitive and the procedure excited little interest from abdominal surgeons. One exception was Alfred Cushieri (born 1938), later Sir Alfred. Cushieri, who qualified in Malta, became interested in the potential of laparoscopy in the early 1970s when he was senior lecturer and reader in surgery at the University of Liverpool. At the time it was believed that good surgery could only be done through large incisions so he had to learn the basic skills of laparoscopy from the gynaecologists. One was Patrick Steptoe (1913–88), a remarkable NHS gynaecologist in Oldham with no academic pretensions, who subsequently worked with Dr. Edwards, an embryologist in Cambridge on in vitro fertilisation culminating in the birth of the first test-tube baby Louise Brown. Steptoe advised Cushieri to visit another gynaecologist, Professor Kurt Semm (1927–2003) in Kiel, Germany, who was a pioneer in operative laparoscopy. Recently Cushieri told me that the time he spent with Semm was seminal to his career. On his return he was appointed

Professor of Surgery in Dundee, giving him a position of authority with which to pursue his research. But his ideas were ahead of his time and he had to proceed cautiously. Semm had been in trouble with his peers in Germany; for example, during a lecture on laparoscopic enucleation of an ovarian cyst someone in the audience had unplugged the projector stating that this type of surgery was unethical. On another occasion his colleagues persuaded him to undergo the indignity of a brain scan on the assumption that only a person with brain damage would contemplate surgery through a laparoscope. Fortunately Cuschieri managed to build up a strong department of academic surgery with financial support from the Wellcome Foundation and the Medical Research Council. Even so he had to turn to the German company, Karl Storz, to develop the instruments he needed as there was no alternative in Britain. He was essentially an upper gastrointestinal surgeon and at the time there was great interest in dissolving gall stones chemically, led by Ian Bouchier, Professor of Medicine in Dundee at the time. So he naturally turned his attention to the gall bladder and reported the first series of experimental laparoscopic cholecystectomies in pigs to the first world congress in Berlin in 1980.[346] It was another five years before a German surgeon, Erich Muhe, did the first laparoscopic cholecystectomy in man, though his achievement went unrecognised and he too was vilified locally for his efforts.[347] But in 1987 the French surgeon Philippe Mouret did a cholecystectomy while performing a laparoscopy on one of his gynaecology patients. This might also have been forgotten had not the patient come to the attention of another surgeon, Francois DuBois, who was particularly interested in minimally invasive surgery. DuBois sought out Mouret and continued to develop and perfect his technique. In May 1988 he performed his first laparoscopic cholecystectomy, presented the work to his colleagues and awoke interest in Europe.[348] Other surgeons including Cuschieri in Scotland and Douglas Olsen in America followed suit,[349] and with the rapid development of new technology especially video endoscopy, the procedure quickly caught the imagination of enthusiasts. By 1990 for example there were no fewer than 45 surgeons in the west of Scotland practising laparoscopic cholecystectomy.[350]

Initially most physicians and surgeons were reluctant to support laparoscopic surgery because they thought it was dangerous. Many gynaecologists could recall frightening cases of perforation or haemorrhage during examination of the pelvis. Goodness knows what might happen if the practice became widespread among surgeons. Such was the situation prevailing at the Central Middlesex Hospital when a young Irish-rained Armenian, Ara Darzi (born 1960), later Lord Darzi, arrived from Dublin as the new senior surgical registrar on the famous gastrointestinal unit of Avery Jones, George Misiewicz and company. The great men were highly concerned when Darzi suggested he might do a laparoscopic cholecystectomy on one of their patients, but Darzi had been to Philippe Mouret's unit in Lyons and with his colleagues in Dublin already had 100 cases under his belt.[351] Fortunately they agreed and all went well. A year later Darzi was appointed as the first consultant in endoscopic surgery in Britain. Two years later, in 1993, he moved to the academic surgical unit at St. Mary's Hospital, Paddington, and became tutor in minimally invasive surgery to the Royal College of Surgeons. Like Cuschieri in Dundee, his department began to tackle most areas within the abdomen, perfecting fundoplication, cardiomyotomy, splenectomy, and all forms of colectomy.[352] The last of these, colectomy, upset the established colorectal surgeons at St. Mark's Hospital who refused to accept it as a viable alternative to their open procedures.

So it was that in Britain as elsewhere general abdominal surgeons rather than colorectal surgeons were the first to become proficient in laparoscopic techniques, and they were not necessarily from teaching hospitals. One was Roger Motson (born 1946), a surgeon in Colchester General Hospital who visited France in 1988 to practise the procedure on pigs. At that time he did not believe that it would be possible to perform a colectomy laparoscopically but in 1994 he began to perform laparoscopic ileo-caecal resections on patients with Crohn's Disease and after eleven years has more than 125 procedures to his credit.[353] He has extensive experience of laparoscopic colectomy, especially for cancer of the colon, and has been impressed by the advantages of this approach. Patients no longer need five days' preparation of their bowel by lavage or a cocktail of antibiotics; the operation is done under an epidural anaesthetic; the patient is mobilised within hours and encouraged to eat almost immediately and is normally fit to leave hospital within two to three days. Motson has done much to promote laparoscopic colectomy and in 2002 he was awarded a personal chair at the University of Anglia in recognition of his efforts.

Another to adopt the laparoscopic approach was Robin Kennedy (born

1953), working in a small district hospital in Yeovil. Kennedy too was first and foremost an upper gastrointestinal surgeon with particular interest in pancreatic disease. However, before his arrival in Yeovil in 1992 he had been the recipient of two travelling research fellowships in France where he had become proficient in laparoscopic cholecystectomy. In 1993 he began to tackle the colon and by 2005 had performed 350 colectomies of all types including 100 for benign conditions such as diverticular disease and inflammatory bowel disease. He has confirmed Motson's work showing the advantages of laparoscopy and has built a team who run an enhanced recovery programme ensuring early discharge from hospital.[354] For this he was chosen hospital doctor of the year in 2004.

Initially, therefore, it was the surgeon with experience of laparoscopic work who undertook colectomy and the thoroughbred colorectal surgeon missed out. By the time laparoscopic colectomy was accepted as the procedure of choice many more senior coloproctologists found it difficult to adapt. Only recently have younger colorectal surgeons taken on the technique, happily performing restorative proctocolectomies and ileo-anal anastomoses nationwide that would amaze and doubtless earn the approval of Alan Parks and Stanley Aylett.

The cause of inflammatory bowel disease remains elusive despite extensive research, but we have come a long way in the last 200 years. On 11th April 1817 Lord Byron wrote to Thomas Moore from Venice:

> "My late physician, Dr. Polidori, is here on his way to England, with the present Lord Guilford and the widow of the late Earl. Dr. Polidori has, just now, no more patients, because his patients are no more. He had lately three, who are now all dead – one embalmed. Lord Guilford died of an inflammation of the bowels: so they took them out, and sent them (on account of their discrepancies) separately from the carcass, to England. Conceive a man going one way, and his intestines another, and his immortal soul a third! Was there ever such a distribution? One certainly has a soul, but how it came to allow itself to be enclosed in a body is more than I can imagine. I only know if once mine gets out, I'll have a bit of a tussle before I let it get in again to that or any other."[355]

Unfortunately the discrepancies were never made public.

REFERENCES

SECTION FOUR

1   Parry L. A. 1928 Dr. Smethurst's lucky escape. In *Some Famous Medical Trials*, reprinted 2000 by Beard Books, Washington DC 193–207

2   Willoughby Lyle H. 1935 The case of Dr. Smethurst in *King's and Some King's Men* . Oxford Union Press London 64–66

3   Fielding J. F. 1985 "Inflammatory" bowel disease. *Brit. Med. J.* i 47–48

4   Wilks S. 1859 Morbid appearance in the intestines of Miss Bankes. *Med. Times & Gazette* 19, 2, 264–265

5   Hale-White W. 1935 *Great Doctors of the Nineteenth Century*. E Arnold & Co. London p236

6   Wilks S. 1859 *Lectures on Pathological Anatomy delivered at Guy's Hospital during the summer sessions* 1857–58 London, Pater Noster Row: Longmans, Brown. Green, Longmans, Roberts

7   Allchin W. H. 1885 Case of acute extensive ulceration of the colon. *Trans. Path. Soc. London.* 36: 199–202

8   Hale-White W. 1888 On simple ulcerative colitis and other rare intestinal ulcers. *Guy's Hosp. Reports.* 14: 131–162.

9   Gemmell J. F. 1898 *Idiopathic Colitis (Dysentery)*. London, Balliere, Tindall, and Cox ppviii- 140

10 Vedder E. B., Duval C. W. 1902 The etiology of acute dysentery in the United States. *J. Exp. Med.* 6: 181–205

11 Eyre J. W. H. 1904 Asylum dysentery in relation to B. dysenteriae. *Brit. Med. J.* i 1002–04

12 Hurst A. F. 1910 A clinical lecture on muco-membranous colitis. *Clinical Journal* 36: 263–267

13 Strauss, H. 1903 Zur Methodik der Rectoskopie. *Berlin Klin. Wschr.* 48, 1100–04

14 Lockhart-Mummery J. P. 1904 The diagnosis of tumours in the upper rectum and sigmoid flexure by means of the electric sigmoidoscope. *Lancet* i 1781–83

15 Lockhart-Mummery J. P. 1905 Remarks on the value of the sigmoidoscope in the diagnosis between primary and secondary colitis. *Brit. Med. J.* ii 1630–31

16 Lockhart-Mummery, J. P. 1907 The causes of colitis with special reference to its surgical treatment. *Lancet*, i, 1638–43

17 Hawkins H. P. 1909 An address on the natural history of ulcerative colitis and its bearing on treatment. *Brit. Med. J.* i 765–770

18 Porter R. 1999 in *The Greatest Benefit to Mankind*. Fontana Press. London 3: p49

19   Allingham W. 1888 Inguinal colotomy. In *Diseases of the Rectum* by W. Allingham. London 5th edition 313–328

20   Weir R. 1902 A new use for the useless appendix in the surgical treatment of obstinate colitis. *Med. Rec.* 62: 201–202

21   Wallis, F. C. 1909 The surgery of colitis. *Brit. Med. J.* i, 10–13

22   Allchin W. H. 1909 Ulcerative colitis. Symposium and discussion of 314 cases reported by the London Hospitals. *Proceedings of the Royal Society of Medicine* II med. sec. 59

23   Ulcerative colitis 1909 Symposium and discussion. *Proceedings of the Royal Society of Medicine.* Vol 2, Part 2, Medical Section, 59–151

24   Hurst A. F. 1926 Diagnosis and treatment of colitis. *Lancet* ii 1151–54

25   Hurst A. F. 1910 op. cit. ref. 12

26   Hurst A. F. 1926 Diagnosis and treatment of colitis. *Lancet* ii p1153

27   Hurst A. F. 1921 Ulcerative colitis. *Guy's Hosp. Reports* 71 26–41

28   Lockhart-Mummery J. P. 1923 *Diseases of the Rectum and Colon.* Balliere, Tindall & Cox. London p429

29   Hurst A. F. 1925 Is medical or surgical treatment indicated for ulcerative colitis? *Guy's Hosp. Reports* 75: 48–50

30   Bargen J. A., Weber 1929 *Collected Papers Mayo Clinic* xxi 209

31   Bargen J. A., Logan A. H. 1925 The etiology of chronic ulcerative colitis: experimental studies with suggestions for a more rational form of treatment. *Arch. Int. Med.* 36: 818–829

32   Hurst A. F. 1926 A discussion on the diagnosis and treatment of colitis. *Lancet* ii 1151–54

33   Hern J. R. B. 1931 Ulcerative colitis. *Guy's Hosp. Reports* 81: 322–373

34   Hardy T. L., Bulmer E. 1933 Ulcerative colitis. A survey of ninety-five cases. *Brit. Med. J.* ii 812–815

35   Hurst A. F. 1935 Prognosis of ulcerative colitis. *Lancet* ii 1194–96

36   Kirsner J. B. 1985 Inflammatory bowel disease at the University of Chicago – the first 50 years: some personal reflections. *Amer. J. Gastroenterol.* 80: 219–228

37   Hurst A. F. 1935 Ulcerative colitis. *Guy's Hosp. Reports* 85: 317–355

38   Moynihan B. G. 1907 Mimicry of malignant disease in the large bowel. *Edin. Med. J.* 21: 228–236

39   Mayo Robson A. W. 1908 An address on some abdominal tumours simulating malignant disease and their treatment. *Brit. Med. J.* i 425–428

40   Moschcowitz E., Wilensky A. O. 1923 Non-specific granulomata of the intestine. *Amer. J. Med. Sci.* 66: 48–66

41   Ginzberg L. 1986 Regional enteritis: historical perspective. *Gastrenterology* 90: 1310–11

42   Crohn B. B., Ginzberg L., Oppenheimer G. D. 1932 Regional ileitis: a pathologic and clinical entity. *J. Amer. Med. Assoc.* 99: 1323–29

43   Harris F. I., Bell G. H., Brunn H. 1933 Chronic cicatrizing enteritis. Regional ileitis (Crohn). A new surgical entity. *Surg. Gynae. Obstet.* 57:637–645

44   Crohn B. B. 1934 Broadening conception of regional ileitis. *Amer. J. Dig. Dis. & Nutr* i 97

45   Dalziel T. K. 1913 Chronic interstitial enteritis. *Brit. Med. J.* ii 1068–70

46   Kantor J. L. 1934 Regional (terminal) ileitis: its roentgen diagnosis. *J. Amer. Med. Assoc.* 103: 2016–2021

47   Combe C., Saunders W. 1813 A singular case of stricture and thickening of the Ileum, read at the College July 4th 1806. *Med. Trans. Coll. Phys. London.* 4: 16–21

48   Abercrombie J. 1830 *Pathological and Practical Researches on Diseases of the Stomach, the Intestinal Canal, the Liver, and Other Viscera of the Abdomen.* Part III, Sect II 284–285

49   Moore N. 1882 Stricture of intestine at the ileo-caecal valve. *Trans. Pathol. Soc.* 34: 112–3

50   Molesworth H. W. L. 1933 Granuloma of intestine. Stenosis of ileo-caecal valve. *Brit. J. Surg.* 21: 370–372

51   Jackman W. A. 1934 Localised hypertrophic enteritis as a cause of intestinal obstruction with a report of two cases. *Brit. J. Surg.* 21: 112–3

52   Wright A. D. 1935 Two cases of coeliac disease. *Trans. Med. Soc. Lond.* 58: 94 -96

53   Edwards H. 1936 Specimen of coeliac disease. *Trans. Med. Soc. Lond.* 59: 87–88

54   Barbour R. F., Stokes A. B. 1936 Chronic Cicatrising Enteritis. A phase of benign non-specific granuloma of the small intestine. *Lancet* i 299–303

55   Gill W. G. 1939 Regional ileitis (Crohn's disease) 5. Two cases of acute regional ileitis reated conservatively. *Guy's Hosp. Reports* 89: 77–79

56   Harmer M., Bailey A. G. S. 1986 Crohn's disease: two fortunate young men. *Lancet* ii 94–96

57   Hadfield G. 1939 The primary histological lesion of regional ileitis. *Lancet* ii 773–775

58   Kirsner J. B. 1985 op. cit. ref. 36 p221

59   Svartz N. 1942 Salazopyrin, a new sulphanilamide preparation B. Therapeutic results in ulcerative colitis. *Acta. Med. Scand.* 110: fasc 6 580–598

60   Svartz N. 1948 The treatment of 124 cases of ulcerative colitis with salazopyrine and attempts at desensitisation in cases of hypersentiveness to sulfa. *Act. Med. Scand. Suppl.* 206 465

61   Bargen J. A. 1949 Treatment of ulcerative colitis with salicylazosulfapyridine (salazopyrine) *Med. Clin. North America* 33: 935

62   Svartz N. 1956 The treatment of ulcerative colitis. *Gastroenterologia*, Basel. 86: 683–688

63   Dearing W. H., Brown P. W. 1950 Experience with cortisone and ACTH in chronic ulcerative colitis. *Proc. Staff Meet. Mayo Clin.* 25: 486–488

64   Machella T. E., Hollan O. R. 1951 The effect of cortisone on the clinical course of chronic regional enteritis and chronic idiopathic ulcerative colitis. Amer. J. Med. Sci. 221: 501–507

65   Kirsner J. B., Palmer W. L. 1951 Effect of corticotrophin (ACTH) in chronic ulcerative colitis. *J. Amer. Med. Assoc.* 147: 541–549

66   Kirsner J. B. 1985 op. cit. ref. 36 p222

67   Bargen J. A. 1956 Report on his experience of ulcerative colitis to the Internat. Congress of Gastroenterology. *Lancet* ii 185.

68   Rice-Oxley J. M., Truelove S. C. 1950 Ulcerative colitis: course and prognosis. *Lancet* i 663–666

69   Sircus W. 1984 Medical-surgical collaboration and practice of gastroenterology. *Postgrad. Med. J.* 60: 725–732

70   Truelove S. C., Witts L. J. 1955 Cortisone in ulcerative colitis. Final report on a therapeutic trial. *Brit. Med. J.* ii 1041–48

71   Truelove S. C., Richards W. C. D. 1956 Biopsy studies in ulcerative colitis. *Brit. Med. J.* i 1315–18

72   Strauss A. A., Strauss S. F. 1944 Surgical treatment of ulcerative colitis. *Surg. Clin. N. Amer.* 24: 211–224

73   Dennis C. 1945 Ileostomy and colectomy in chronic ulcerative colitis. *Surgery* 18: 435–452

74   Hardy T. L., Brooke B. N., Hawkins C. F. 1949 Ileostomy and ucerative colitis. *Lancet* ii 5–9

75   Brooke B. N. 1952 The management of an ileostomy including its complications. *Lancet* ii 102–4

76   Sladen G. E. 1987 in *History of the British Society of Gastroenterology 1937–87* ed J. H. Baron BMA p16

77   Brooke B. N. 1954 *Ulcerative Colitis and its Surgical Treatment.* Livingstone Edin. & Lond.

78   Lennard-Jones J. E. 1997 Inflamed passions; an interview with T. T. MacDonald. *Gut* 40 (Suppl. 2) S17

79   Watkinson G. 1961 Medical management of ulcerative colitis. *Brit. Med. J.* i 147–151

80   Truelove S. C. 1958 Treatment of ulcerative colitis with local hydrocortisone hemisuccinate sodium. A report of a controlled therapeutic trial. *Brit. Med. J.* ii 1072–77

81   Watkinson G. 1958 Treatment of ulcerative colitis with topical hydrocortisone hemisuccinate sodium. A controlled trial employing restricted sequential analysis. *Brit. Med. J.* ii 1077– !082

82   Truelove S. C., Watkinson G., Draper G. 1962 Comparison of corticosteroid and sulphasalazine therapy in ulcerative colitis. *Brit. Med. J.* ii 1708–11

83   Brooke B. N. 1956 Outcome of surgery for ulcerative colitis. *Lancet* ii 532–536

84   Goligher J. C., Hoffmann D. C., deDombal F. T., 1970 Surgical treatment of severe attacks of ulcerative colitis, with special reference to the advantages of early operation. *Brit. Med. J.* ii 703–706

85   Lennard-Jones J. E., Vivian A. B. 1960 Fulminating ulcerative colitis: recent experience in management. *Brit. Med. J.* ii 96–102

86   Edwards F. C., Truelove S. C. 1963 The course and prognosis of ulcerative colitis. *Gut* 4: 299–315

87   Watkinson G 1961 op. cit. ref. 79 p150

88   Lennard-Jones J. E., Longmore A. J., Newall A. C., Wilson C. W. E., Jones F. A. 1960 An assessment of prednisone, salazopyrin and topical hydrocortisone hemisuccinate used as an out-patient treatment for ulcerative colitis. *Gut* 1: 217–222

89   Witts L. J. 1960 in *Controlled Clinical Trials* (edited by Bradford Hill) Oxford p.10

90   Baron J. H., Connell A. M., Lennard-Jones J. E., Jones F. A. 1962 Sulphasalazine and salicyl-azo-sulphadimidine in ulcerative colitis. *Lancet* i 1094–96

91   Misiewicz J. J., Lennard-Jones J. E., Connell A. M., Baron J. H., Jones F. A. 1965 Controlled trial of of sulphasalazine in maintenance therapy for ulcerative colitis. *Lancet* i 185–9

92   Dissanayake A. S., Truelove S. C. 1973 A controlled therapeutic trial of long-term maintenance treatment of ulcerative coitis with sulphasalazine (salazopyrin). *Gut* 14: 923–926

93   Schroder H., Campbell D. E. S. 1972 Absorption, metabolism and excretion of salicyl-azo-sulfapyridine in man. *Clin. Pharmacol. Therap.* 13: 539–551

94   Peppercorn M. A., Goldman P. 1973 Distribution studies of salicyl-azo-sulfapyridine and its metabolites. *Gastroenterology* 64: 240–245

95   Schroder H., Price-Evans D. A. 1972 Acetylator phenotype and adverse effects of sulphasalazine in healthy subjects. *Gut* 13: 278–284

96   Das K. M., Eastwood M. A., McManus J. P. A., Sircus W. 1973 Adverse reactions during salicyl-azo-sulfapyridine therapy and the relation with drug metabolism and acetylator phenotype. *New England Journal of Medicine.* 289: 491–495

97   Das K. M., Eastwood M. A., McManus J. P. A., Sircus W. 1974 The role of the colon in the metabolism of salicyl-azo-sulphapyridine. *Scand. J. Gastroenterol.* 9: 137–141

98   Leukonia R. M., Schroder H., Price-Evans D. A. 1973 Pharmacokinetics and azo-link cleavage of salazopyrin in man. *Gut* 14: A426

99   Azad Khan A. K., Piris J., Truelove S. C. 1977 An experiment to determine the active therapeutic moiety of sulphasalazine. *Lancet* ii 892–895

100   Campieri M. et al. 1981 Treatment of ulcerative colitis with high dose 5–aminosalicylic acid enemas. *Lancet* ii 270–271

101   Willoughby C. P., Aronson J. K., Agback H., Bodin N. O., Truelove S. C. 1982 Distribution and metabolism in healthy volunteers of disodium azodisalicylate, a potential therapeutic agent for ulcerative colitis. *Gut* 23: 1081–87

102   Selby W. S., Barr G. D., Ireland A., Mason C. H., Jewell D. P. 1985 Olsalazine in active ulcerative colitis. *Brit. Med. J.* 291 1373–75

103   Ireland A., Mason C. H., Jewell D. P. 1988 Controlled trial comparing olsalazine and sulphasalazine for the maintenance treatment of ulcerative colitis. *Gut* 29: 835–837

104   Travis S. P. L., Tysk C., deSilva H. J., Sandberg-Gertzen H., Jewell D. P., Jarnerot G. 1992 Optimum dose of olsalazine for maintaining remission in ulcerative colitis. *Gut* 35 1282–86

105   Chan R. A., Pope D. J., Gilbert A. P., Sacra P. J., Baron J. H., Lennard-Jones J. E. 1983 Studies of two novel sulfasalazine analogs, Ipsalazide and Balsalazide. *Dig. Dis. Sci.* ns28 609–615

106   McIntyre P. B., Rodrigues L. A., Lennard-Jones J. E., Barrison I. G., Walker J. G., Baron J. H., Thornton P. C. 1988 Balsalazide in the maintenance treatment of patients in ulcerative colitis, a double-blind comparison study with sulphasalazine. *Alimentary Pharmacology and Therapeutics* 2: 237–243

107   Green J. R. B., Lobo A. J., Holdsworth C. D., Leicester R. J., Gibson J. A., Kerr G. D., Hodgson J. H. F., Parkins K. J., Taylor M. D. and the Abacus Investigator Group. 1997 Balsalazide is more effective and better tolerated than mesalazine in the treatment of acute ulcerative colitis. *Gastroenterology* 114: 1–10

108   Dew M. J., Hughes P. J., Lee M. G., Evans B. K., Rhodes J. 1982 An oral preparation to release drugs in the human colon. *Br. J. Clin. Phar.* 14: 405–408

109   Dew M. J., Hughes P. J., Harries A. D., Williams G., Evans B. K., Rhodes J. 1982 Maintenance of remission in ulcerative colitis with oral preparation of 5–aminosalicylic acid. *Brit. Med. J.* ii 1012

110   Dew M. J., Harries A. D., Evans B. K., Rhodes J. 1983 Treatment of ulcerative colitis with oral 5–aminosalicylic acid in patients unable to take sulphasalazine. *Lancet* ii 801–803

111   Crude annual mortality rate from ulcerative colitis (I. S. C. 572.2) for England and Wales, 1940–62 Quoted by J. G. Evans and E. D. Acheson *Gut* 1965 6: p322

112   Naish J. M. 2003 Personal communication

113   Houghton E. A. W., Naish J. M. 1958 Familial ulcerative colitis and ileitis. *Gastroenterologia* (Basel) 89: 65–74

114   Acheson E. D. 1960 The distribution of ulcerative colitis and regional enteritis in United States veterans with particular reference to the Jewish religion. *Gut* I: 291–293

115   Evans J. G., Acheson E. D. 1965 An epidemiological study of ulcerative colitis and regional ileitis in the Oxford area. *Gut* 6: 311–324

116   Devlin H. B., Datta D., Dellipiani A. W. 1980 The incidence and prevalence of inflammatory bowel disease in North Tees District. *World J. Surg.* 4: 183–193

117   Morris T., Rhodes J. 1984 Incidence of ulcerative colitis in the Cardiff region. 1968–77 *Gut* 26: 846–848

118   Srivastava E. D., Mayberry J. F., Morris T. J., Smith P. M., Williams G. T., Roberts G. M., Newcombe R. G., Rhodes J. 1992 Incidence of ulcerative colitis in Cardiff over 20 years: 1968–87. *Gut* 33: 256–258

119   Mayberry J. F., Ballantyne K. C., Hardcastle J. D., Mangham C., Pye G. 1989 Epidemiolocal study of asymptomatic inflammatory bowel disease: the identification of cases during a screening programme for colorectal cancer. *Gut* 30 481–483

120   Kyle J. 1992 Crohn's disease in the Northeastern and Northern Isles of Scotland: an epidemiological review. *Gastroenterology* 103: 392–399

121   Miller D. S., Keighley A. C., Langman M. J. S. 1974 Changing patterns in epidemiology of Crohn's disease. *Lancet* ii 691–693

122   Wells C. 1952 Ulcerative colitis and Crohn's disease. *Ann. Roy. Coll. Surg. (Eng.)* 11: 105–120

123   Cooke W. T., Brooke B. N. 1955 Non-specific enterocolitis. *Quart. J. Med.* ns24: 1–22

124   Dukes C. 1932 The classification of cancer of the rectum. *J. Path. Bact.* 35: 323–332

125   Lockhart-Mummery H. E., Morson B. C. 1960 Crohn's disease (regional enteritis) of the large intestine and its distinction from ulcerative colitis. *Gut* I: 87–105

126   Cornes J. S., Stecher M. 1961 Primary Crohn's disease of the colon and rectum. *Gut* 2: 189–201

127   Thomas G. A. O., Millar-Jones D., Rhodes J., Roberts G. M., Williams G. T., Mayberry J. F. 1995 Incidence of Crohn's disease in Cardiff over 60 years: 1986–90 an update. *Eur. J. Gastroenterol. & Hepatol.* 7: 401–405

128   Fielding J. F. 1986 The relative risk of inflammatory bowel disease among parents and siblings of Crohn's disease patients. *J. Clin. Gastroenterology* 8: 655–657

129   Mayberry J. F., Rhodes J., Newcombe R. G. 1980 Familial prevalence of inflammatory bowel disease in relatives of patients with Crohn's disease. *Brit. Med. J.* i: 84.

130   McConnell R. B. 1983 Ulcerative colitis – genetic features. *Scand. J. Gastroenterol. Suppl.* 88: 18:14–16

131   Tysk C., Lindberg E., Jarnerot G., Floderus-Myrhed B. 1988 Ulcerative colitis and Crohn's disease in an unselected population of monozygotic and dizygotic twins. A study of heritability and the influence of smoking. *Gut* 29: 990–996

132   Thompson N., Driscoll R., Pounder R. E., Wakefield A. J. 1996 Genetics versus environment in inflammatory bowel disease: results of a British twin study. *Brit. Med. J.* 312: 95–96

133   Morris P. J. 1965 Familial ulcerative colitis. *Gut* 6: 176–8

134   Acheson E. D. 1960 An association between ulcerative colitis, regional enteritis and ankylosing spondylitis. *Quart. J. Med.* 29: 489–499

135   Brewerton D. A., Hart F. D., Nicholls A., Caffrey M., James R. C. O., Sturrock R. D. 1973 Ankylosing spondylitis and HL-A27. *Lancet* i 904–907

136   Biemond I., Burnham W. R., d'Amaro J., Lanbman M. J. S. 1986 HLA-A and-B antigens in inflammatory bowel disease. *Gut* 27: 934–941

137   McConnell R. B. 1983 op. cit. ref. 129

138   McConnell R. B. 1990 Genetics of inflammatory bowel disease. In *Inflammatory Bowel Disease* ed. Allan R. N., Keighley M. R. B., Alexander Williams J., Hawkins C. F. Edinburgh, Churchill Livingstone p11–13

139   Lee J. C. W., Lennard-Jones J. E. 1996 Inflammatory bowel disease in 67 families each with three or more affected first-degree relatives. *Gastroenterology* 111: 587–596

140   Naomi I., Lee J. et al. 1996 Analysis of the contribution of HLA genes to genetic predisposition in inflammatory bowel disease. *Amer. J. Hum. Genet.* 59: 226–233

141   Hugot J-P., Laurent-Puig P. et al. 1996 Mapping of a susceptibility locus for Crohn's disease on chromosome 16. *Nature* 379: 821–823

142   Cottone M., Bunce M., Taylor C. J., Ting A., Jewell D. P. 1985 Ulcerative colitis and HLA phenotype. *Gut* 26: 952–954

143   Satsangi J., Welsh K. I., Bunce M., Julien C., Farrant J. M., Bell J. I., Jewell D. P. 1996 Contribution of genes of the major histocompatibility complex to susceptibility and disease phenotype in inflammatory bowel disease. *Lancet* i 1212–17

144   Parkes M., Satsangi J., Lathrop G. M., Bell J. I., Jewell D. P. 1996 Susceptibility loci in inflammatory bowel disease. *Lancet* ii 1588 (L)

145   Hugot J-P., Chamaillard M. et al. 2000 Association of NOD 2 leucine-rich repeat variants in susceptibility to Crohn's disease. *Nature* 411: 599–603

146   Satsangi J., Parkes M., Louis E. et al. 1996 Two stage genome-wide search in inflammatory bowel disease provides evidence for susceptibility loci on chromosomes 3,7 and 12. *Nat. Genet.* 14: 199–202

147   Probert C. S. J., Jayanthi V., Pinder D., Wicks A. C., Mayberry J. F. 1992 Epidemiological study of ulcerative proctocolitis in Indian migrants and the indigenous population of Leicestershire. *Gut* 33: 687–693

148   Hermon-Taylor J., Barnes N., Clarke C., Finlayson C. 1998 Mycobacterium paratuberculosis cervical lymphadenitis, followed five years later by terminal ileitis similar to Crohn's disease. *Brit. Med. J.* i 449–452

149   James A. H. 1977 Breakfast and celiac disease. *Brit. Med. J.* i 943–945

150   Mayberry J. F., Rhodes J., Newcombe R. G. 1978 Breakfast and dietary aspects of Crohn's disease. *Brit. Med. J.* ii 1401

151   Harries A. D., Baird A., Rhodes J. 1982 Non-smoking: a feature of ulcerative colitis. *Brit. Med. J.* i 706

152   Roberts C. J., Digger R. 1982 Non-smoking: a feature of ulcerative colitis. *Brit. Med. J.* ii 440

153   Logan R. F. A., Edmond M., Somerville K. W., Langman M. J. S. 1984 Smoking and ulcerative colitis. *Brit. Med. J.* i 751–753

154   Somerville K. W., Logan R. F. A., Edmond M., Langman M. J. S. 1984 Smoking and Crohn's disease. *Brit. Med. J.* ii 954–956

155 Thomas G. A. O., Rhodes J., Green J. T. 1998 Inflammatory bowel disease and smoking – a review. *Amer. J. Gastroenterol.* 93: 144–9

156 Bridger S., Lee J. C. W., Bjarnason I., Lennard-Jones J. E., MacPherson A. J. 2002 In siblings with similar genetic susceptibility for inflammatory bowel disease, smokers tend to develop Crohn's disease and non-smokers develop ulcerative colitis. *Gut* 51: 21–25

157 Gilat T., Hacohen D., Lilos P., Langman M. J. S. 1987 Childhood factors in ulcerative colitis and Crohn's disease. An international cooperative study. *Scand. J. Gastroenterol.* 22: 1009–24

158 Sachar D. B. 2002 Appendix redux. *Gut* 51: 764–765

159 Gent A. E., Hellier M. D., Grace R. H., Swarbrick E. T., Coggon D. 1994 Inflammatory bowel disease and domestic hygiene in infancy. *Lancet* i 766–767

160 Truelove S. C. 1961 Ulcerative colitis provoked by milk. *Brit. Med. J.* i 154–160

161 Taylor K. B., Truelove S. C. 1961 Circulating antibodies to milk protein in ulcerative colitis. *Brit. Med. J.* ii 924–929

162 Taylor K. B., Roitt I. M., Doniach D., Couchman K. G., Shapland C. 1962 Autoimmune phenomena in pernicious anaemia: gastric antibodies. *Brit. Med. J.* ii 1347–52

163 Wright R., Truelove S. C. 1965 A controlled therapeutic trial of various diets in ulcerative colitis. *Brit. Med. J.* ii 138–141

164 Wright R., Truelove S. C. 1965 Circulating antibodies to dietary proteins in ulcerative colitis. *Brit. Med. J.* ii 142–4

165 Wright R., Truelove S. C. 1966 Autoimmune reactions in ulcerative colitis. *Gut* 7: 32–40

166 Wright R., McCollum R. W., Klatskin G. 1969 Australia antigen in acute and chronic liver disease. *Lancet* ii 117–121

167 Jewell D. P., MacLennan I. C. M. 1973 Immune complexes in inflammatory bowel disease. *Clin. Exp. Immunol.* 14: 219–226

168 Blackburn G., Hadfield G., Hunt A. H. 1939 Regional ileitis. *St. Barts. Hosp. Rep.* 72: 181–224

169 Fletcher J., Hinton J. M. 1967 Tuberculin sensitivity in Crohn's disease. A controlled study. *Lancet* ii 753–754

170 Willoughby J. M. T., Mitchell D. N., Wilson J. D. 1971 Sarcoidosis and Crohn's disease in siblings. *Amer. Rev. Resp. Dis.* 104: 249–254

171 Mitchell D. N., Cannon P., Dyer N. H., Hinson K. F. W., Willoughby J. M. T. 1969 The kveim test in Crohn's disease. *Lancet* ii 571–573

172 Willoughby J. M. T., Mitchell D. N. 1971 In-vitro inhibition of leucocyte migration in Crohn's disease by a sarcoid spleen suspension. *Brit. Med. J.* ii 155–7

173 Shorter R. G., Cardoza M., ReMine S. G., Spencer R. S., Huizenga K. A. 1970 Modification of in-vitro cytotoxicity of lymphocytes from patients with chronic ulcerative colitis or granulomatous colitis for allogenic colonic epithelial cells. *Gastroenterology* 58: 692–698

174 Shorter R. G., Huizenga K. A., Spencer J. 1972 A working hypothesis for the aetiology and pathogenesis of non-specific inflammatory bowel disease. *Dig. Dis.* 17: 1024–32

175 Wollman M. R., David D. S., Brennan B. L., Lewy J. E., Stenzel K. H., Rubin A. L., Miller D. R. 1972 The nitroblue tetrazolium test. *Lancet* ii 289–291

176   Segal A. W., Peters T. J. 1975 The nylon column dye test: a possible screening test of phagocytic function. *Clin. Sci. Mol. Med.* 49:591–596

177   Ament M. E., Ochs H. D. 1973 Gastrointestinal manifestations of chronic granulomatous disease. *New England Journal of Medicine.* 288: 382–387

178   Segal A. W., Loewi G. 1976 Neutrophil dysfunction in Crohn's disease. *Lancet* ii 219–221

179   Senn H. 1972 *Fektalswehr bei Homoblastosen.* p.36 Berlin

180   Ward M. 1977 The pathogenesis of Crohn's disease. *Lancet* ii 903–905

181   Hodgson H. J. F., Potter B. J., Skinner J., Jewell D. P. 1978 Immune-complex mediated colitis in rabbits: an experimental model. *Gut* 19: 225–232

182   Mee A. S., McLaughlin J. E., Hodgson H. J. F., Jewell D. P. 1979 Chronic immune colitis in rabbits. *Gut* 20: 1–5

183   Mee A. S., Szawatakowski M., Jewell D. P. 1980 Monocytes in inflammatory bowel disease: phagocytosis and intracellular killing. *J. Clin. Pathol.* 33: 921–925

184   Mee A. S., Jewell D. P. 1980 Monocytes in inflammatory bowel disease: monocyte and serum lysosomal enzyme activity. *Clin. Sci.* 58: 295–300

185   Rhodes J. M., Bartholemew T. C., Jewell D. P. 1981 Inhibition of leucocyte motility by drugs used in ulcerative colitis. *Gut* 22: 642–647

186   Janossy G.,Tidman N., Selby W. S., Thomas J. A., Grainger, Kung, Goldstein G. 1980 Human T-lymphocytes of inducer and suppressor type occupy different microenvironments. *Nature* 288: 81– 84

187   Selby W. S., Janossy G., Jewell D. P. 1981 Immunohistological characterisation of intraepithelial lymphocytes of the human gastrointestinal tract. *Gut* 22: 169–176

188   Selby W. S., Janossy G., Bofill, Jewell D. P. 1984 Intestinal lymphocyte subpopulations in inflammatory bowel disease: an analysis by immunohistological and cell isolation techniques. *Gut* 25: 32–40

189   Hodgson H. J. F., Wand J. R., Isselbacher. 1978 Decreased suppressor cell activity in inflammatory bowel disease. *Clin. Exp. Immunol.* 32: 451–458

190   Poulter L. W., Campbell D. A., Munro C., Janossy G. 1986 Discrimination of human macrophages and dendritic cells in chronic inflammatory bowel disease. *Scand. J. Immunol.* 21: 401–407

191   Allison M. C., Cornwall S., Poulter L. W., Dhillon A. P., Pounder A. P. 1988 Macrophage heterogeneity in normal colonic mucosa and inflammatory bowel disease. *Gut* 29: 1531–38

192   Selby W. S., Poulter L. W., Hobbs S., Jewell D. P. 1983 Heterogeneity of HLA-DR positive histiocytes in human intestinal lamina propria: a combined histochemical and immunohistological analysis. *J. Clin. Pathol.* ol. 36: 379–384

193   Mahida Y. R., Patel S., Gionchetti P., Vaux D., Jewell D. P. 1989 Macrophage subpopulations in lamina propria of normal and inflamed colon and terminal ileum. *Gut* 30: 826–834

194   Gibson P. R., Hermanowicz A., Verhaar H. J. J., Ferguson D. P. J., Lopez Bernal A., Jewell D. P. 1985 Isolation of intestinal mononuclear cells: factors released which affect lymphocyte viability and function. *Gut* 26: 60–68

195   Gibson P. R., Dow E. L., Selby W. S., Strickland R. S., Jewell D. P. 1984 Natural killer cells and spontaneous cell-mediated cytotoxicity in the human intestine. *Clin. Exp. Immunol.* 56: 438–444

196   Gibson P. R., Jewell D. P. 1986 Local immune mechanisms in inflammatory bowel disease and colorectal carcinoma. Natural killer cells and their activity. *Gastroenterology* 90: 12–19

197   Mahida Y. R., Wu K., Jewell D. P. 1989 Enhanced production of interleukin 1–B by mononuclear cells isolated from the mucosa with active ulcerative colitis and Crohn's disease. *Gut* 30: 835–838

198   Shanahan F. 2000 Mechanisms of immunologic sensation of intestinal contents. *Amer. J. Physiol.* 278: G191–G196

199   MacDonald T. T., Monteleone G. 2001 Interleukin-12 and Th1 immune responses in Peyers patches. *Trends Immunol.* 22: 244–247

200   Segal A. W. 2005 How neutrophils kill microbes. *Ann. Rev. Immunol.* 23: 197–223

201   Segal A. W., Loewi G 1976 op. cit. ref. 177

202   Saverymuttu S. H., Camilleri M., Rees H., Lavender J. P., Hodgson H. J. F., Chadwick V. S. 1986 Indium-111 granulocyte scanning in the assessment of disease extent and disease activity in inflammatory bowel disease. *Gastroenterology* 90: 1121–28

203   Truelove S. C., Ellis H., Webster C. U. 1965 Place of a double barrelled ileostomy in ulcerative colitis and Crohn's disease of the colon: a preliminary report. *Brit. Med. J.* i 150–3

204   Harper P. H., Truelove S. C. Lee E. C. G., Kettlewell M. G. W., Jewell D. P. 1983 Split ileostomy and ileocolostomy for Crohn's disease of the colon and ulcerative colitis: a 20 year survey. *Gut* 24: 106–113

205   Harper P. H., Lee E. C. G., Kettlewell M. G. W., Bennett M. K., Jewell D. P. 1985 Role of the faecal stream in in the maintenance of Crohn's colitis. *Gut* 26: 279–284

206   O'Morain C., Segal A. W., Levi A. J. 1984 Elemental diet as primary treatment of acute Crohn's disease: a controlled clinical trial. *Brit. Med. J.* i 1859–62

207   Saverymuttu. S. H., Hodgson H. J. F., Chadwick V. S. 1985 Controlled trial comparing prednisolone with an elemental diet plus non-absorbable antibiotics in active Crohn's disease. *Gut* 26: 994–998

208   Logan R. F. A., Gillon J., Ferrington C., Ferguson A. 1981 Reduction of gastrointestinal protein loss by elemental diet in Crohn's disease of the small bowel. *Gut* 22: 383–387

209   Greenberg G. R., Fleming C. R., Jejeebhoy K. N., Rosenberg I. H., Sales D.,Tremaine W. J. 1988 Controlled trial of bowel rest and nutritional support in the management of Crohn's disease. *Gut* 29: 1309–15

210   Raouf A. H., Hildrey V., Daniel J., Walker R. J., Krasner N., Elias E., Rhodes J. M. 1991 Enteral feeding as the sole treatment for Crohn's disease: controlled trial of whole protein v amino acid based feed and a case study of dietary challenge. *Gut* 32: 702–707

211   Sanderson I. R., Udeen S., Davies P. J. W., Savage M. O., Walker-Smith J. A. 1987 Remission induced by an elemental diet in small bowel Crohn's disease. *Arch. Dis. Child* 61: 123–7

212   Shanahan F. 2002 Crohn's disease. *Lancet* i p65

213   Wakefield A. J., Sawyer A. M., Dhillon A. P., Pittilo R. M., Rowles P. M., Lewis A. A. M., Pounder R. E. 1989 Pathogenesis of Crohn's disease: multifocal gastrointestinal infarction. *Lancet* ii 1057–62

214 Thompson N. P., Wakefield A. J., Pounder R. E. 1995 Inherited disorders of coagulation appear to protect against inflammatory bowel disease. *Gastroenterology* 108: 1011–15

215 Hudson M., Chitolie A., Hutton R. A., Smith M. S. H., Pounder R. E., Wakefield A. J. Thrombotic vascular risk factors in inflammatory bowel disease. *Gut* 38: 733–737

216 Ekbom A., Wakefield A. J., Zack M., Adami H. O. 1994 Perinatal measles infection and subsequent Crohn's disease. *Lancet* ii 508–510

217 Wakefield A. J., Pittilo R. M., Sim R., Cosby S. L., Stephenson J. R., Dhillon A. P., Pounder R. E. 1993 Evidence of persistent measles virus infection in Crohn's disease. *J. Med. Virol.* 39: 345–353

218 Thompson N. P., Pounder R. E., Wakefield A. J. 1995 Perinatal and childhood risk factors for inflammatory bowel disease: a case control study. *Eur. J. Gastroenterol. & Hepatol.* 7: 385–390

219 Thompson N. P., Montgomery S. M., Pounder R. E., Wakefield A. J. 1995 Is measles vaccination a risk factor for inflammatory bowel disease? *Lancet* i 1071–74

220 Farrington P., Miller E. 1995 Measles vaccination as a risk factor for inflammatory bowel disease. *Lancet* i 1362

221 Feeney M. A., Clegg A. J., Winwood P. J., Snook J. A. 1997 A case-control study of measles vaccination and inflammatory bowel disease. *Lancet* ii 764 -766

222 Calman K. C. 1995 Measles vaccination as a risk factor for inflammatory bowel disease. *Lancet* i 1362

223 Afzal M. A., Minor P. D., Begley M.L., Armitage E., Ghosh S., Ferguson A. 1998 Absence of measles-virus genome in inflammatory bowel disease. *Lancet* i 646–647

224 Montgomery S. M., Pounder R. E., Wakefield A. J. 1997 Infant mortality and the incidence of inflammatory bowel disease. *Lancet* i 472–473

225 Wakefield A. J., Murch S. H., Anthony A., Linnell J., Casson D. M., Malik M., Berelowitz M., Dhillon A. P., Thompson M. A., Harvey P., Valentine A., Davies S. E., Walker-Smith J. A. 1998 Ileal-lymphoid-nodular hyperplasia, non-specific colitis, and pervasive developmental disorder in children. *Lancet* i 637– 641

226 Uhlmann V., Martin C. M., Sheil S. O., Pilkington L., Silva I., Killalea A., Murch S. B., Walker-Smith J. A., Thomson M., O'Leary J. J. 2002 Potential viral pathogenic mechanism for new variant inflammatory bowel disease. *J. Mol. Pathol.* 55: 84–90

227 Horton R. 2004 *MMR: Science and Fiction. Exploring the Vaccine Crisis.* Granta Books ISBN 1 86207 764 9

228 Fitzpatrick M. 2004 *MMR and Autism: What Parents Need to Know.* Routledge ISBN 0 415 32179 4

229 Deer, B. 2011 How the case against the MMR vaccine was fixed. *Brit. Med. J.* 342 77–82 and 136–142

230 Florey H. M. 1955 Mucin and the protection of the body. *Proc. Roy. Soc. Lond.* 143: 144–8

231 Schrager J., Oates M. D. G. 1978 Relation of human intestinal mucus to disease states. *British Medical Bulletin* 34: 79–82

232 Clamp J. R., Fraser G.,Read A. E. 1981 Study of the carbohydrate content of mucus glycoproteins from normal and diseased colons. *Clin. Sci.* 61: 229–234

233 Teague R. H., Fraser D., Clamp J. R. 1973 Changes in monosaccharide content of mucus glycoproteins in ulcerative colitis. *Brit. Med. J.* i 645–646

234 Filipe M. I., Dawson. 1970 The diagnostic value of mucosubstances in rectal biopsies from patients with ulcerative colitis and Crohn's disease. *Gut* 11: 229–234

235 Ehsanullah M., Filipe M. I., Gazzard B 1982 Mucin secretion in inflammatory bowel disease: correlation with disease activity and dysplasia. *Gut* 23: 485–489

236 Filipe M. I., Ramanchandra S. 1995 The histochemistry of intestinal mucins: changes in disease. In *Gastrintestinal and Oesophageal Pathology*. ed. Whitehead R. 2nd edition, Edinburgh: Churchill Livingstone, 73–95

237 Pullan R. D., Thomas G. A. O., Rhodes M., Newcombe R. G., Williams G. T., Allen A., Rhodes J. 1994 Thickness of adherent mucus gel on colonic mucosa in humans and its relevance to colitis. *Gut* 35: 353–359

238 Corfield A. P., Myersclough N., Longman R., Sylvester P., Arul S., Pignatelli M. 2,000 Mucins and mucosal protection in the gastrointestinal tract: new prospects for mucins in the pathology of gastrointestinal disease. *Gut* 47: 589–594

239 Probert C. S. J., Jayanthi V., Pinder D., Wicks A. C., Mayberry J. F. 1992 Epidemiological study of ulcerative proctocolitis in Indian migrants and the indigenous population of Leicestershire. *Gut* 33: 687–693

240 Probert C. S. J., Warren B. F., Perry T., Mackay E. H., Mayberry J. F., Corfield A. P. 1995 South Asian and European colitics show characteristic differences in colonic mucus glycoprotein type and turnover. *Gut* 36: 696–702

241 Rhodes J. M. 1996 Unifying hypothesis for inflammatory bowel disease and associated colon cancer: sticking the pieces together with sugar. *Lancet* i 40–44

242 Crohn B. B., Rosenberg H. 1925 The sigmoidoscopic picture of chronic ulcerative colitis (non-specific). *Amer. J. Med.* 170: p226

243 Bargen J. A. 1928 Chronic ulcerative colitis associated with malignant disease. *Arch. Surg. Chicago.* 17: 561–576

244 Hurst A. F. 1935 Ulcerative colitis. *Guy's Hosp. Reports* 85: 317–355

245 Sauer W. G., Bargen J. A. 1949 Chronic ulcerative colitis and carcinoma. *J. Amer. Med. Assoc.* 141: 982–985

246 Goldgraber M. B., Humphreys E. M., Kirsner J. B., Palmer W. L. 1958 Carcinoma and ulcerative colitis: a clinical-pathologic study II Statistical analysis. *Gastroenterology* 34: 840–846

247 Gabriel W. B. 1950 Chronic ulcerative colitis with pseudopolyposis terminating in diffuse colloid carcinoma of the colon. *Proceedings of the Royal Society of Medicine* 43: 680–682

248 Counsell P. B., Dukes C. E. 1952 The association of chronic ulcerative colitis and carcinoma of the rectum and colon. *Brit. J. Surg.* 39:485–495

249 Dawson I. M. P., Pryse-Davies J. 1959 The development of carcinoma of the large intestine in ulcerative colitis. *Brit. J. Surg.* 47: 113–128

250 Slaney G., Brooke B. N. 1959 Cancer in ulcerative colitis. *Lancet* ii 694–698

251 Edwards F. C., Truelove S. C. 1964 The course and prognosis of ulcerative colitis. Part IV Carcinoma of the colon. *Gut* 15: 15–22

252 MacDougall I. P. M. 1964 The cancer risk in ulcerative colitis. *Lancet* ii 655–658

253 deDombal F. T., Watts J. McK., Watkinson G., Goligher J. C. 1966 Local complications of ulcerative colitis: stricture, pseudopolyposis and carcinoma of colon and rectum. *Brit. Med. J.* i 1442–47

254   Hinton J. M. 1966 Risk of malignant change in ulcerative colitis. *Gut* 7: 427–432

255   Morson B. C., Pang L. S. C. 1967 Rectal biopsy as an aid to cancer control in ulcerative colitis. *Gut* 8: 423–434

256   Lennard-Jones J. E., Misiewicz J. J.,Parrish J. A., Ritchie J. K., Swarbrick E. T. 1966 Prospective study of outpatients with extensive colitis. *Lancet* i 1065–67

257   Lennard-Jones J. E., Melville D. M., Morson B. C., Ritchie J. K., Williams C. B. Precancer and cancer in extensive ulcerative colitis: findings among 401 patients over 22 years. *Gut* 31: 800–806

258   Evans D. J., Pollock D. J. 1972 In-situ and invasive carcinoma of the colon in patients with ulcerative colitis. *Gut* 13: 566–570

259   Riddell R. H., Morson B. C. 1979 Value of sigmoidoscopy and biopsy in detection of carcinoma and premalignant change in ulcerative colitis. *Gut* 20: 575–580

260   Riddell R. H., Goldman H., Ransohoff D. F., et al. 1983 Dysplasia in inflammatory bowel disease: standardised classification with provisional clinical applications. *Hum. Pathol.* 14: 931–968

261   Cook M. G., Goligher J. C. 1975 Carcinoma and epithelial dysplasia complicating ulcerative colitis. *Gastroenterology* 68: 1127–36

262   Dickinson R. J., Dixon M. F., Axon A. T. R. 1980 Colonoscopy and the detection of dysplasia in patients with longstanding ulcerative colitis. *Lancet* ii 620–622

263   Lynch D. A. F., Lobo A. J., Sobala G. M., Dixon M. F., Axon A. T. R. 1993 Failure of colonoscopic surveillance in ulcerative colitis. *Gut* 34: 1075–80

264   Jones H. W., Grogono J., Hoare A. M. 1988 Surveillance in ulcerative colitis: burdens and benefit. *Gut* 29: 325–331

265   Prior P., Gyde S. N., Macartney J. C., Thompson H., Waterhouse J. A. H., Allan R. N. 1982 Cancer morbidity in ulcerative colitis. *Gut* 23: 490–497

266   Gyde S. N., Prior P., Thompson H., Waterhouse J. A. H., Allan R. N. 1984 Survival of patients with colorectal cancer complicating ulcerative colitis. *Gut* 25: 228–231

267   Ritchie J. K., Hawley P. R., Lennard-Jones J. E. 1981 Prognosis of cancer in ulcerative colitis. *Gut* 22: 752–755

268   Gyde S. N., Prior P., Allan R. N., Stevens A., Jewell D. P., Truelove S. C., Lofberg R., Brostrom O., Hellers G. 1988 Colorectal cancer in ulcerative colitis: a cohort study of primary referrals from three centres. *Gut* 29: 206–217

269   Gyde S. N. 1990 Screening for colorectal cancer in ulcerative colitis: dubious benefits and high costs. *Gut* 31: 1089–92

270   Weil J., Langman M. J. S. 1991 Screening for gastrointestinal cancer: an epidemiological review. *Gut* 32: 220–224

271   Lennard-Jones J. E. 1991 Screening for colorectal cancer in ulcerative colitis. *Gut* 32: 722–723

272   Eaden J. A., Ward B., Mayberry J. F. 2000 How British gastroenterologists screen for colonic cancer in ulcerative colitis: an analysis of performance. *Gastrointest. Endosc.* 52: 153–8

273   Eaden J. A., Abrams K. R., Mayberry J. F. 2001 The risk of colorectal cancer in ulcerative colitis: a meta analysis. *Gut* 48: 526–535

274   Eaden J. A., Mayberry J. F. 2002 Guidelines for screening and surveillance of asymptomatic colorectal cancer in patients with inflammatory bowel disease. *Gut* 51 Suppl. V v10–v12

275 Forbes A., Gabe S., Lennard-Jones J. E., Wilkinson K. 2003 Screening and surveillance for asymptomatic colorectal cancer in inflammatory bowel diseae. *Gut* 52: 769

276 Rutter M. D., Wilkinson K. H., Rumbles S., Forbes A., Saunders B. P. 2003 How effective is cancer surveillance in ulcerative colitis? *Gut* 52 Suppl. 1 A66

277 Rutter M. D., Saunders B. P., Schofield G., Forbes A., Price A. B., Talbot I. C. 2004 Pancolonic indigo carmine dye spraying for the detection of dysplasia in ulcerative colitis. *Gut* 53: 256–260

278 Warren S., Sommers S. C. 1948 Cicatrizing enteritis (regional enteritis) as a pathological entity. *Amer. J. Pathol.* 24: 475–501

279 Sheil F. O'M., Clark C. G., Goligher J. C. 1968 Adenocarcinoma associated with Crohn's disease. *Brit. J. Surg.* 55: 53–58

280 Perrett A. D., Truelove S. C., Massarella G. R. 1968 Crohn's disease and cancer of the colon. *Brit. Med. J.* i 464–468

281 Hywel Jones J. 1969 Colonic cancer and Crohn's disease. *Gut* 10: 651–654

282 Fielding J. F., Prior P., Waterhouse J. A. H., Cooke W. T. 1972 Malignancy in Crohn's disease. *Scand. J. Gastroenterol.* 7: 3–7

283 Darke S. G., Parks A. G., Grogono J. L., Pollock D. J. 1973 Adenocarcinoma and Crohn's disease: a report of 2 cases and analysis of the literature. *Brit. J. Surg.* 60: 169–175

284 Weedon D. D., Shorter R. G., Ilstrup D. M., Huizenga K. A., Taylor W. F. 1973 Crohn's disease and cancer. *New England Journal of Medicine* 289: 1099–1103

285 Gyde S. N., Prior P., Macartney J. C., Thompson H., Waterhouse J. A. H., Allan R. N. 1980 Malignancy in Crohn's disease. *Gut* 21: 1024–29

286 Gillen C. D., Andrews H. A., Prior P., Allan R. N. 1994 Crohn's disease and colorectal cancer. *Gut* 35: 651–655

287 Gillen C. D., Walmsley R. S., Prior P., Andrews H. A., Allan R. N. 1994 A comparison of the colorectal cancer risk in extensive colitis. *Gut* 35: 1590–92

288 Connell W. R., Sheffield J. P., Kamm M. A., Ritchie J. K., Hawley P. R., Lennard-Jones J. E. 1994 Lower gastrointestinal malignancy in Crohn's disease. *Gut* 35: 347–352

289 Lennard-Jones J. E., Vivian A. B. op. cit. ref. 85

290 Dudrick S. J., Wilmore D. W., Vars H. M., Rhoads J. E. 1968 Long term total parenteral nutrition with growth, development and positive nitrogen balance. *Surgery* 64: 134–142

291 Truelove S. C., Willoughby C. P., Lee E. C. G., Kettlewell M. G. W. 1978 Further experience in the treatment of severe attacks of ulcerative colitis. *Lancet* ii 1086–88

292 Dickinson R. J., Ashton M. G., Axon A. T. R., Smith R. C., Yeung C. K., Hill G. L. 1980 Controlled trial of intravenous hyperalimentation and total bowel rest as an adjunct to the routine therapy of acute colitis. *Gastroenterology* 79: 1199–1204

293 Powell-Tuck J., Nielson T., Farwell J. A., Lennard-Jones J. E. 1978 Team approach to long term intravenous feeding in patients with gastrointestinal disorders. *Lancet* ii 825–828

294 McIntyre P. B., Powell-Tuck J., Wood S. R., Lennard-Jones J. E., Lerebours E., Hecketsweiler P., Galmiche J-P., Colin P. 1986 Controlled trial of bowel rest in the treatment of severe acute colitis. *Gut* 27: 481–485

295 Greenberg et al. 1988 op. cit. ref. 209

296 Goode A., Hawkins T., Feggetter J. G. W., Johnston I. D. A. 1976 Use of an elemental diet for long-term nutritional support in Crohn's disease. *Lancet* i 122–4

297 Allison S. P. 1986 Some psychological and physiological aspects of enteral nutrition. *Gut* 27 Suppl. 1 18–24

298 McMichael H. B. 1979 Physiology of carbohydrate, electrolyte and water absorption. *Research & Clin. Forums.* I 25–28

299 Allison S. P., Walford S., Todovoric V., Elliott E. T. 1979 Practical aspects of nutrition support. *Research & Clin. Forums.* 1 49–57

300 McIntyre P. B., Wood S. R., Powell-Tuck J., Lennard-Jones J. E. 1983 Nocturnal nasogastric tube feeding at home. *Gut* 24: A 488

301 Jones B. J. M. 1986 Enteral feeding: techniques of administration. *Gut* 27: Suppl. 1: 47–50

302 Rees R. G. P., Hare W. R., Grimble G. K., Frost P. G., Silk D. B. A. 1992 Do patients with moderately impaired gastrointestinal function requiring enteral nutrition need a pre-digested nitrogen source? A prospective crossover controlled clinical trial. *Gut* 33: 877–881

303 Op. cit. ref. 205

304 Harvey R. F., Bradshaw J. M. 1980 A simple index of Crohn's disease activity. *Lancet* i 514–515

305 Sanderson I. R., Boulton P., Menzies I. S., Walker-Smith J. A. 1987 Improvement of abnormal lactulose/rhamnose permeability in active Crohn's disease of the small bowel by an elemental diet. *Gut* 28: 1073–76

306 Bjarnason I., Peters T. J., Veall N. 1983 A persistent defect of intestinal permeability in coeliac disease demonstrated by a 51Cr-labelled EDTA absorption test. *Lancet* i 323–5

307 Bjarnason I., O'Morain C., Levi A. J., Peters T. J. 1983 Absorption of 51 chromium–labelled ethylene diamine tetra acetate in inflammatory bowel disease. *Gastroenterology* 85: 318–322

308 Teahon K., Smethurst P., Levi A. J., Menzies I. S., Bjarnason I. 1992 Intestinal permeability in patients with Crohn's disease and their first degree relatives. *Gut* 33: 320–323

309 Tibble J., Teahon K., Thjodleifsson B., Roseth A., Sigthorsson G., Bridger S., Foster R., Sherwood R., Fagerhol M., Bjarnason B. 2000 A simple method for assessing intestinal inflammation in Crohn's disease. *Gut* 47: 506–513

310 Payne-James J. J., Silk D. B. A. 1990 Use of elemental diets in the treatment of Crohn's disease by gastroenterologists. *Gut* 31: 1424

311 *Food and the Gut.* 1985 edited by Hunter J. O. & Alun Jones V. Addenbrooke's Hosp. Cambridge. Eastbourne: Balliere Tindall.

312 Alun Jones V., McLaughlan P., Shorthouse M., Workman E., Hunter J. O. 1982 Food intolerance: a major factor in the pathogenesis of irritable bowel syndrome. *Lancet* ii 1115–17

313 Alun Jones V., Dickinson R. J., Workman E., Freeman A. H., Hunter J. O. 1984 Controlled trial of diet in the management of Crohn's disease. Abstract of 12th Internat. Cong. *Gastroenterology.* 943

314 Alun Jones V., Dickinson R. J., Workman E., Wilson A. J., Freeman A. H., Hunter J. O. 1985 Crohn's disease: maintenance of remission by diet. *Lancet* ii 177–180

315 Hunter J. O. 1991 Food allergy – or enterometabolic disorder? *Lancet* ii 495–496

316 Riordan A,M., Hunter J. O., Cowan R. E., Crampton J. R., Davidson J. R., Dickinson R. J., Dronfield M. W., Fellows I. W., Hishon S., Kerrigan G. N. W., Kennedy H. J., McGouran R. C. M., Neale G., Saunders J. H. B. 1993 Treatment of active Crohn's disease by exclusion diet. East Anglian Multicentre Controlled Trial. *Lancet* ii 1131–34

317 Teahon K., Bjarnason I., Pearson M., Levi A. J. 1990 Ten years' experience with an elemental diet in the management of Crohn's disease. *Gut* 31: 1133–37

318 Ryan F. P., Smart R. C., Holdsworth C. D., Preston F. E. 1978 Hyposplenism in inflammatory bowel disease. *Gut* 19: 50–55

319 Giaffer M. H., North G., Holdsworth C. D. 1990 Controlled trial of polymeric versus elemental diet in treatment of active Crohn's disease. *Lancet* i 816–818

320 Mansfield J. C., Giaffer M. H., Holdsworth C. D. 1995 Controlled trial of oligopetide versus amino acid diet in treatment of active Crohn's disease. *Gut* 36: 60–66

321 Giaffer M. H., Cann P., Holdsworth C. D. 1991 Long-term effects of elemental and exclusion diets for Crohn's disease. *Alimentary Pharmacology and Therapeutics.* 5: 115–125

322 Bean R. H. D. 1966 Treatment of ulcerative colitis with antimetabolites. *Brit. Med. J.* i 1081–84

323 Bowen G. E., Irons G. U., Rhodes J., Kirsner J. B. 1965 Precautionary early experiences with immunosuppressive medication (Azathioprine) in ulcerative colitis. *Gastroenterology* 48: 807–808

324 Jones F. A., Lennard-Jones J. E., Hinton J. M., Reeves W. G. 1986 Dangers of immunosuppressive drugs in ulcerative colitis. *Brit. Med. J.* i 1418

325 Watkinson G., de Dombal F. T. 1968 The management of ulcerative colitis. *Scot. Med. J.* 13: 133–143

326 Arden Jones R. 1969 Immunosuppressive therapy in ulcerative colitis. *Proceedings of the Royal Society of Medicine. Sect. of Proctology.* 499–501

327 Brooke B. N., Hoffmann D. C., Swarbrick E. T. 1969 Azathioprine for Crohn's disease. *Lancet* ii 612–614

328 Brooke B. N., Javett S. L., Davison O. W. 1970 Further experience with azathioprine for Crohn's disease. *Lancet* ii 1050–53

329 Cooke W. T. 1970 Azathioprine in Crohn's disease. *Lancet* ii 1195–96

330 Willoughby J. M.T., Kumar P. J., Beckett J., Dawson A. M. 1971 Controlled trial of azathioprine in Crohn's disease. *Lancet* ii 944–947

331 O'Donoghue D. P., Dawson A. M., Powell-Tuck J., Bown R. L., Lennard-Jones J. E. 1978 Double-blind withdrawal trial of azathioprine as maintenance treatment for Crohn's disease. *Lancet* ii 955–957

332 Stack W. A., Williams D., Stevenson M. et. al. 1999 Immunosuppressive therapy for ulcerative colitis: results of a nation-wide survey among consultant physician members of the British Society of Gastroenterology. *Alimentary Pharmacology and Therapeutics.* 5: 569–575

333 Connell A. M., Kamm M. A., Dickson M., Balkwill A. M., Ritchie J. K., Lennard-Jones J. E. 1994 Long-term neoplasia risk after azathioprine treatment in inflammatory bowel disease. *Lancet* 343: 1249–52

334 Jewell D. P., Truelove S. C. 1974 Azathioprine in ulcerative colitis: final report on controlled therapeutic trial. *Brit. Med. J.* ii 627–630

335 Kirk A. P., Lennard-Jones J. E. 1982 Controlled trial of azathioprine in chronic ulcerative colitis. *Brit. Med. J.* i 1291–92

336 Hawthorne A. B., Logan R. F. A., Hawkey C. J. 1989 Azathioprine in resistant ulcerative colitis. *Gastroenterology* 96: A201

337 Hawthorne A. B., Logan R. F. A., Hawkey C. J., Foster P. N., Axon A. T. R., Swarbrick E. T., Scott B. B., Lennard-Jones J. E. 1992 Randomised controlled trial of azathioprine withdrawal in ulcerative colitis. *Brit. Med. J.* ii 20–22

338 Fraser A. G., Orchard T. R., Jewell D. P. 2002 The efficacy of azathioprine for the treatment of inflammatory bowel disease: a 30 year review. *Gut* 50: 485–489

339 Aylett S. 1959 The surgery of diffuse ulcerative colitis including a review of 100 cases of colitis treated by total colectomy and ileo-rectal anastomosis. *Postgrad. Med. J.* 35: 67– 74

340 Jones P. F., Munro A., Ewan S. W. B. 1977 Colectomy and ileo-rectal anastomosis: report on a personal series, with a critical review. *Brit. J. Surg.* 64: 615–623

341 Jones P. F., Keenan R. A. 1986 The place of colectomy with ileo-rectal anastomosis in inflammatory bowel disease. *Ann. Chir. et Gynae.* 75: 75–81

342 Jones P. F., Bevan G., Hawley P. R. 1978 Ileostomy or ileorectal anastomosis for ulcerative colitis? *Brit. Med. J.* i 1459–63

343 Baker W. N. W., Glass R. E., Ritchie J. K., Aylett S. O. 1978 Cancer of the rectum following colectomy and ileorectal anastomosis for ulcerative colitis. *Brit. J. Surg.* 65: 862– 868

344 Parks A. G., Nicholls R. J. 1978 Proctocolectomy without ileostomy for ulcerative colitis. *Brit. Med. J.* ii 85–88

345 Melville D. M., Ritchie J. K., Nicholls R. J., Hawley P. R. 1994 Surgery for ulcerative colitis in the era of the pouch: the St. Mark's Hospital experience *Gut* 35: 1076–1080

346 Cuschieri A. 1980 Laparoscopy in general surgery and gastroenterology. *Brit. J. Hosp. Med.* 24: 252–258

347 Litynski G. 1996 Erich Muhe – a surgeon ahead of his time. The first laparoscopic cholecystectomies. In: *Highlights in the History of Laparoscopy*. Frankfurt: Bernert.

348 Litynski G. 1996 Mouret, Dubois, and Perissat. The French connection. In: *Highlights in the History of Laparoscopy*. Frankfurt: Bernert.

349 Litynski G. 1996 The American spirit awakens. In: *Highlights in the History of Laparoscopy*. Frankfurt: Bernert

350 Fullerton G. M., Bell G., and the west of Scotland laparoscopic cholecystectomy audit group. 1994 Prospective audit of the introduction of laparoscopic cholecystectomy in the west of Scotland. *Gut* 35: 1121–26

351 Grace P., Quereshi A., Darzi A., et al. 1991 Laparoscopic cholecystectomy: 100 consecutive cases. *Irish Med. J.* 84: 12–14

352 Darzi A., Lewis C., Menzies Gow N. et al. 1993 Laparoscopic assisted surgery of the colon: operative technique. *Endosc. Surg. Allied Technol.* 1: 13–15

353 Motson R. W., Kadirkamanathan S. S., Gallegos N. 2002 Minimally invasive surgery for ileo-colic Crohn's disease. *Colorectal Dis.* 4 (2): 127–131

354 King P. M., Blazeby J. M., Ewings P., Franks P. J., Longman R. J., Kendrick A. H., Kipling R. M., Evans L. B., Soulsby M. J., Kennedy R. H. 2005 Open versus laparoscopic surgery for colorectal cancer: a randomised study embedded within an enhanced recovery programme. Submitted to *Brit. J. Surg.*

355 "Days like these 11 April 1817" compiled by Ian Irvine for the *Independent* 17 April 2005

SECTION FIVE

FUNCTIONAL BOWEL DISEASE

"When I use a word," Humpty Dumpty said in rather a scornful tone, "it means just what I choose it to mean, neither more nor less."[1] So what I wonder would he have meant by functional disease? Probably nothing more or less than a disease caused by disordered function. Fair enough, but we would add that the disturbed function is unexplained. We have not yet found the cause for it.

Indigestion and bothersome bowels have preoccupied healthy people for centuries. It is natural to blame some dietary indiscretion for an upset tummy, a fact well known to medical men who have used it to their advantage for years, long before they understood the process of digestion.

Hippocrates (420–350 BC) likened the stomach to an oven in which food was mixed and heated (concoction). Abnormal concoction caused indigestion and an imbalance of the four humours (blood, phlegm, bile and black bile) leading to general ill-health. He also knew that the function of the liver was to secrete choler or yellow bile and believed that an excess of bile made people feel choleric or bilious. The stomach and liver were essential to good health.

Later Greek authorities, notably Erasistratus (circa 330–255 BC), took a more mechanical view of digestion and thought the stomach ground and crushed ingested food (trituration). Indeed if the stomach continued grinding after the food had been finely milled, a person felt hungry. For centuries these two theories of digestion, concoction and trituration, went unchallenged and served as a useful basis for dietary advice.

CHAPTER FIFTY

DYSPEPSIA IN THE SEVENTEENTH CENTURY

People with functional diseases are concerned, if not consumed, by their symptoms but are unlikely to die. They must have been ideal patients to treat before the modern era of sophisticated diagnosis and investigation. A typical seventeenth-century herbal, for example, contains any number of remedies for every conceivable problem. Most of these were ineffective so that recipes for, say, fever, jaundice, wasting, or obstructed urine were useless. But potions for anorexia, wind, nausea, colic and constipation, symptoms that today we would regard as typical of dyspepsia or an irritable bowel, had at least a sporting chance of success.

The term dyspepsia was first used in England by Robert Lovell (1630–90), an almost forgotten naturalist and physician in Coventry. In 1661 when he was a still a student at Oxford, Lovell wrote a two-volume tome on the natural history of animals and minerals in which he says, "imbecility of the stomach is a vice of the concocting faculty, by reason of which, it concocteth not at all, slowly, or depravedly; it's called apepsy, bradypepsy or dyspepsy".[2] In keeping with Hippocratic theory dyspepsia in this sense was the cause of many chronic diseases, not merely a collection of vague abdominal symptoms.

Lovell's great contemporary, Thomas Sydenham (1624–89), also believed in the doctrine of the humours and would have agreed. He himself suffered from gout and believed it was caused by "indigestion or an impaired concoction of matters, both in the parts (organs) and the juices of the body."[3] Like Lovell he was not thinking of indigestion or dyspepsia (a term he did not use) in the modern sense but rather as a cause of putrid humours that pervaded the body.

Sydenham was the most influential physician of his day and his clinical description of gout is a classic but he also had a shrewd understanding of functional disease. Born in Dorset, the son of a country gentleman and staunch Puritan, he fought on the side of Parliament during the English Civil War (1642–51) when he was involved in several bloody skirmishes and was lucky to survive.

After the war he began to practise medicine but had little time for the sterile traditions of medical scholarship. Instead he kept careful notes on his patients, collected case reports and built them into disease histories. As a result he realised that psychological illness was far more common than people thought. Many of his patients had anxiety states or depression collectively known as hysteria in his day. Hysteria had hitherto been explained as "uterine suffocation" caused by corrupt menstruation. Sydenham discarded this view when he found that males were also susceptible to psychological symptoms. He suggested, instead, that there was an imbalance of the "animal spirits" (nervous energy) perhaps arising from a sudden burst of anger or fear. These spirits upset mind-body relationships and allowed the accumulation of putrid humours, especially bile, in the most vulnerable organs, particularly those concerned in the purification of the blood such as the liver and spleen. A variety of psychological symptoms ensued, which might include abdominal pain, vomiting and diarrhoea, typical of functional bowel disease. Sydenham called the disorder hysteria if women were afflicted and hypochondriasis when it occurred in men. It is worth noting that he thought of hypochondriasis as a physical condition meaning pain in the lower abdomen, even if it was stress-related. He also emphasised that "the greatest caution must be used in the diagnosis of hysteria, lest the symptoms be confounded with those of some other disease like it" and he singled out "bilious colic".[4]

Sydenham's ability to spot psychological illness allowed him to reassure his patients, gain their confidence and keep his therapy simple. He was perhaps over fond of laudanum for pain relief (Sydenham's Laudanum was in use for a century or two after his death) but fresh air, exercise and a moderate diet were essential. He recommended bleeding and purging to purify the blood, followed by remedies to fortify it such as iron. But nothing did so much "to comfort and strengthen the Blood and Spirits as riding on horseback every day for a long while; since by this kind of exercise the lower belly is most strongly moved, in which the vessels for excretion (to drain the impurities of the blood) are situated".[5]

Horse-riding had other benefits. There is an amusing story of a deception practised by Sydenham in order to get a wealthy patient to undertake a long journey in the saddle. After attending him for several months without alleviating his symptoms, Sydenham frankly told him that he was unable to render any further service. But he added that a

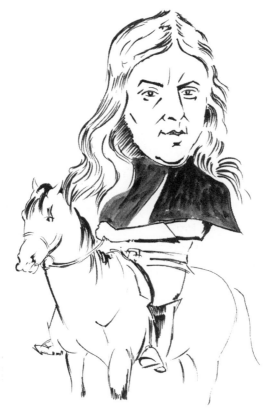

63 Sydenham – Riding is good for you.

certain Dr. Robertson of Inverness had performed several remarkable cures in this particular malady. Armed with Sydenham's letter of introduction, the patient set out for Inverness where he lost no time in seeking Dr. Robertson. To his dismay he learned that there was no physician of that name in the city. Returning to London the gentleman vented his indignation on Sydenham for having sent him on such a long and fruitless journey. "Well," inquired Sydenham, "are you any better in health?"

"Yes, I am now quite well, but no thanks to you."

"No," added Sydenham, "but you may thank Dr. Robertson for curing you. I wished to send you on a journey with some objective interest in view. I knew it would be of service to you; in going you had Dr. Robertson and his wonderful cures in contemplation, and in returning, you were equally engaged in scolding me."[6] We are not told the nature of the patient's complaint, but presumably he had a functional disorder.

CHAPTER FIFTY-ONE

DYSPEPSIA IN THE EIGHTEENTH CENTURY

a) Biliousness

During the eighteenth century another concept crept into use alongside dyspepsia, namely biliousness. Bile was one of the four fluids that played a key role in humoral theory and was well known to the ancients. Usually an excess of bile was the problem as hinted by Sydenham in the case of hysteria.

In 1711 its role was given a considerable boost by John Woodward (1665–1728), Professor of Physick at Gresham College, Cambridge. Woodward was a self-confident, successful and industrious man, and he was convinced that digestive balance was the key to good health. Influenced by his own troubled digestive system, he maintained that a whole variety of disorders were caused by an excess of "biliose salts" in the stomach. As Goulstonian lecturer at the Royal College of Physicians he spoke *on the Bile and its uses*, giving his talks an air of scientific authority by experiment (from personal experience of attempts to treat his own indigestion) and dissection.[7/8]

Unfortunately Woodward was an irascible man and felt compelled to publish again in 1718 in response to a commentary on the treatment of smallpox written by a well known London physician, Dr. John Freind (1675–1728).[9] Freind believed that the evils of the disease should be evacuated by purging whereas Woodward felt they should be vomited. Woodward used his response to reiterate his view that "The great Wisdom and Happiness of Man consists in a due Care of the Stomach and Digestion".[10] Again he emphasised that everything depended upon keeping the right balance of biliose salts in the stomach. Too much, as in the case of smallpox, and there was but one relief – the bilious matter had to be ejected.

Woodward even hinted that Freind was killing his patients and his arrogance led to a long and acrimonious dispute that did neither side much credit. Satire in Georgian England was rife at the time and the contentious Woodward was an obvious target. The following year his theories were ridiculed by one of the leading wits of the time, Dr. John Arbuthnot (1667–1735), with *The Life and Adventures of Don Bilioso de L'Estomac*. Written in the manner of Cervantes, fun is made out of Woodward's biliose salts, though the humour is rather marred by coarseness.[11] The only beneficiary was biliousness itself, a new term that was to catch the imagination of the public and rank alongside dyspepsia to this day.

b) The English malady

Sydenham's influence continued well into the eighteenth century long after his death. Chronic non-specific functional disorders began to attract attention and became highly fashionable thanks to the efforts of an anglicised Scot, George Cheyne (1671–1743).

Cheyne studied in Edinburgh under Archibald Pitcairn (1652–1713), from whom he got his iatro-mechanistic theories that were then competing with the philosophy of the humours. Moving to England he settled in Bath where he wrote several books for the general public on health matters. His most influential book, *The English Malady* (1733) dealt with what we would now call psychiatric disorders.[12]

Cheyne discarded the humoral theory and saw the body as an infinite number of tubes conveying blood, air, chyle and other juices to the liver, muscles and various organs. The vessels required the widest possible bore and had to remain unclogged. Unfortunately these tubes readily became blocked by swellings, inflammation and other obstructions and the chief culprits were improper diet, rich food and too much alcohol. In addition the state of the nerves was vital. Cheyne was no anatomist and likened the nerves to a well tuned musical string, which, when plucked, would vibrate and so convey the right signal between the brain, the intestines and the limbs. The nerves' job was to convey sensation and motion throughout the body. If they lost their tone, the body failed

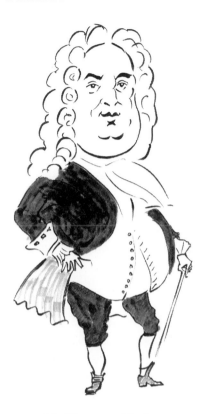

64 Cheyne – 32 stone.

to function properly causing pain and mental distress. Clogged tubes, viscid fluids and lax nerves caused a languid, sluggish body and feelings of lethargy and gloom. He felt able to explain practically all the chronic diseases with his remarkable theory including Sydenham's hysteria and hypochondriasis.

Though Cheyne had not a shred of evidence for his ideas, he was highly successful for two reasons. Firstly he linked his English malady to the trappings of success and high society; it was the archetypal malady of the elite. Not surprisingly his views quickly became socially acceptable and the intelligentsia, who were particularly susceptible, delighted in comparing each other's flatus or vapours (irritable bowel symptoms). This led some to criticise Cheyne for encouraging a morbid interest in non-existent diseases and the term hypochondria began to assume its modern meaning. The second reason for his success was that his treatment was straightforward and similar to Sydenham's. People should abandon high living and revert to a simple bland diet and thin fluids to unclog their tubes. All forms of evacuation were called for to rid the body of surplus bile, slime, faeces etc. Emetics and phlebotomy would both help and, of course, a variety of purgatives. Finally something to restore tone and elastic force to the nerves was needed and among his favourites were bitters, chalybeats and bark (quinine). He also believed in the bracing effects of Bath waters.

Cheyne's regimen illustrates how, despite the changing theories of disease during the seventeenth, eighteenth and much of the nineteenth century, treatment hardly altered. There were almost no therapeutic advances during this period anyway. Physicians and quacks alike were supremely adept at justifying their management within the context of current medical theory, be it humoral, iatro-chemical, iatro-mechanical or simply "the soul's attempt to counter threats to its well-being posed by morbific matter".

In Cheyne's time views on digestion were certainly confused. Some believed that there was an acid ferment in the stomach but that chemical activity alone was insufficient and that there must be an invisible spiritual agency at work.[13] Others rejected the need for a spiritual influence and held that digestion was simply a process of fermentation aided by saliva and pancreatic juices.[14] Still others regarded digestion as the result of a mechanical trituration (grinding) of the food within the stomach.[15]

c) Physiology of digestion

During the eighteenth century several serious minded investigators tried hard to unravel the process of digestion, which was still centred exclusively on the stomach. The methods they used to obtain and examine gastric juice were ingenious to say the least and worth recalling.

The first to suggest that the gastric juice might be acid was a Swiss, Jean Viridet (1655–1736), who studied a specially fattened pig. He poured a litmus-like solution, "solutio heliotropii", down its throat, killed it and found the blue colour preserved in the oesophagus but an intense red solution in the stomach. Viridet admitted that there were occasions when the oesophagus might contain acids due to regurgitation of the stomach contents. "We experience it by an acid in the mouth. The condition is not a natural one," he added.[16] His remarkable conclusions were followed by some equally impressive investigations by a Frenchman, Rene Reaumur (1683–1757).

Reaumur was a bachelor with a large private income and devoted his life to experiments and investigation in subjects ranging from natural history to meteorology. He became known as the Pliny of the eighteenth century. He had a pet kite which, according to the habit of this species, would vomit after a time anything it could not stomach. Reaumur constructed some glass and metal tubes, open at both ends, put food inside them and gave them to the kite to swallow. When they were returned, the food inside was softened, bitter to the taste and acid.[17] Unfortunately his attempt to show gastric digestion in vitro failed because he did not do the experiment at body temperature. Reaumur's work on birds was extended by other eighteenth-century investigators, particularly Lazaro Spallanzani.

Spallanzani (1729–99) is usually referred to as Abbe Spallanzani, for he became an ordained priest, though his interests remained more terrestrial than celestial. He studied an astonishing variety of animals and devised methods of attaching pieces of meat or other foods to strings. He also used himself and was able to procure gastric juice by self-induced vomiting while in the fasting state. From in vitro experiments at body temperature he was able to demonstrate the solvent quality of gastric juice, his most important observation. Oddly he reported that the juice was neither acid nor alkaline, but neutral. He also showed that trituration of the food aided digestion and that this was effected by the gastric muscles.[18/19]

d) Nervous indigestion

Despite Cheyne's vague understanding of the nervous system, he gave his book a subsidiary title, *A Treatise of Nervous Diseases of All Kinds*, thereby introducing the concept of functional disorders as nervous in origin, though he still placed the pathology firmly in the body not the mind.

The importance of the nervous system was brought to light by the brilliant work of the Swiss polymath, Albrecht von Haller (1708–77) in Göttingen,[20] who showed that irritability or contractility was an inherent property of muscle fibres whereas sensitivity was the exclusive attribute of nerve fibres. His work was seized upon by William Cullen (1710–90), who had recently been appointed Professor of Chemistry and Medicine at the University of Edinburgh. Cullen was the most influential teacher in the English-speaking world. He interpreted life itself as a function of nervous power, and, by extension, construed all disease as ultimately "nervous". In this he agreed with his colleague Robert Whytt (1714–66), Professor of Medicine at Edinburgh[21] who had said some years before that, "In a certain view, almost the whole of the diseases of the human body might be called nervous."[22.]

Cullen's influence on perceptions of dyspepsia was crucial. In 1769 he published his elaborate classification of diseases[23] that was inspired by taxonomies being developed at the time by various botanists (notably Linnaeus). In fact many of his diseases weren't diseases at all but merely a list of symptoms. Cullen divided diseases into four classes, of which the most interesting were the nervous diseases or neuroses, a word he invented meaning "affections of sense or motion which are without pyrexia". The neuroses were in turn subdivided into four orders, one of which, called the adynamiae, consisted of hypochondriasis, dyspepsia, syncope and chlorosis. The meaning of dyspepsia had now changed and included "anorexia, nausea, vomiting, inflation, belching, rumination, cardialgia, gastrodynia, more or fewer of those symptoms at least concuring, for the most with a constipation of the belly, and without any other diseases either of the stomach itself, or of any other parts".[24] The old terms apepsy and bradypepsy had dropped out of use and dyspepsia was being subsumed into a new framework of physiology based on nervous function.

Cullen justified including dyspepsia among the neuroses at some length on the basis that the stomach's motility became highly disorganised in nervous conditions. While admitting that the symptoms of dyspepsia could be secondary to another cause, such as ulcer or tumour, he also thought they constituted a disease entity in its own right. This could often be recognised in conjunction with other conditions through the process of sympathy. The stomach was second only to the brain in its connection with the nervous system, and with no organ was the power of sympathy so apparent.

e) Abdominal sympathy

From ancient times, it had been assumed that disturbances in one part of the body could have consequences elsewhere in the body, a phenomenon referred to as sympathy of the parts. The great anatomist and surgeon, John Hunter(1728–93), in particular drew attention to the concept of abdominal sympathy. Though he published little on the subject, his students were left in no doubt about his views. For instance, James Parkinson (1755–1824) in his notes taken in shorthand of Hunter's lectures in 1785, recorded him as saying that "in disease we find the brain seems to be intimately connected with the stomach, and vice versa; and that it has a kind of intelligence of what passes on in the rest of the body... . The stomach is affected by the injuries of several parts which have no connection with it in the nourishment of the body."[25] This notion was to have considerable influence on early nineteenth-century views of indigestion.

John Hunter's views on digestion were important. In 1772, well before Spallanzani began his experiments, he wrote on the digestion of the stomach after death. In effect he was explaining post mortem changes in the stomach for the first time. He wrote "...observing that the half-digested parts of the stomach were similar to the half-digested food, it immediately struck me that it was the process of digestion going on after death; and that the stomach, being dead, was no longer capable of resisting the powers of that menstruum which itself had formed for the digestion of its contents." He concluded that "these appearances throw considerable light on the principles of digestion; they shew that it is not mechanical power, nor contractions of the stomach, nor heat, but something in the coats of the stomach, which is thrown into its cavity, and there animalises the food, or assimilates it to the nature of blood." In a footnote he added, "I constantly found that there was an acid, but not a strong one, in the juices contained in that viscus in a natural state."[26]

Hunter's paper on digestion was republished in 1784 as an appendix to a translation of Spallanzani's work by Thomas Beddoes (1760–1808). Beddoes also included a second appendix recording *Experiments concerning digestion translated from the inaugural dissertation of Dr. Stevens.* This is a translation from the Latin of a thesis *De Alimentorum Concoctione* submitted by Stevens in 1777 when he was a medical student in Edinburgh aged 22. He was the first to apply Reaumur's experiments to human beings and certainly the first to perform an in vitro digestion successfully, though he was probably unaware of Reaumur's work. His first experiments "were made at Edinburgh upon a Hussar, a man of weak understanding, who gained a miserable livelihood, by swallowing stones for the amusement of the common people, at the imminent hazard of his life. He began this practice at the age of seven, and has now followed it twenty years. His stomach is so much distended, that he can swallow several stones at a time; and these may not only be plainly felt, but heard, whenever the hypogastric region is struck." Stevens simply replaced the stones with perforated silver hollow spheres containing different foods, which the obliging soldier swallowed and subsequently rejected. He concluded that the gastric juice was acid and wrote: "These experiments throw great light on digestion. They shew, that it is not the effect of heat, trituration, putrefaction, or fermentation alone, but of a powerful solvent, secreted by the coats of the stomach, which converts the aliment into a fluid, resembling the blood." This process was known as assimilation. His final comment reveals how far ideas on digestion had come since Cheyne's time, yet how little was known about the liver: "The food, when dissolved, is expelled from the stomach, and being mixed with the bile and pancreatic juice in the duodenum, is changed into a mild blood and inodorous liquid, which is denominated chyle. The chyle is absorbed by numberless vessels, and is carried by the thoracic duct into the subclavian vein, in order to repair the constant waste of the body."[27]

Denis Gibbs has pointed out that Hunter elevated the stomach to a very high level in the hierarchy of importance of the different organs in the body.[28] This was because he perceived the unique nature of animal life to arise through a process of what he termed assimilation, animalisation and vivification of inanimate matter. He regarded the stomach as the vitalising link in the chain of development of animal life. It is not surprising that his followers treated the problems of the stomach so seriously as it was almost 100 years before the metabolic role of the liver was recognised. Throughout the first half of the nineteenth century people believed that the only job of the liver was to produce bile from blood.

f) Bile

Curiously, though the ancients knew about bile, they were unaware of gall stones. They were first described in the German literature in the sixteenth century but Sydenham appears to have known little about them, though he did refer to bilious colic on occasion. The first English account was by a Chelmsford practitioner, Thomas Coe (1704–61) and it makes refreshing reading. After reviewing the literature and indulging in a diatribe against quackery, he describes the formation of gall stones and how they cause colic and obstructive jaundice if they escape from the gall bladder. He thought biliary colic was as common as renal colic and should not be confused with nervous spasms. He wrote, "This notice of a jaundice from nervous spasms has been, perhaps, too much grounded on Sydenham's account of an hysteric or hypochondriac colic; which he describes in a manner very much resembling a fit of the stone in the biliary ducts. But as he seems to have known nothing at all of these concretions, since he never mentions them once in his writings, it seems highly probable that he confounded the two diseases, and that, whenever he met with a patient under a fit of the stone in the biliary ducts, he imputed it merely to a nervous cause." [29]

Coe's enlightened views on the biliary tract did not include fanciful ideas about the functions of the liver whose job was, he thought, simply to produce bile. In contrast, twenty years later, an Aberdonian, William Grant (died 1786), with a successful London practice, published a depressingly moral and highly speculative treatise on what he called the atrabilious temperament (atrabilis, the mythical fourth humour, black bile). This he contended was the underlying cause of many chronic distempers such as gout, paralysis and cases of apoplexy. It arose from the liver in people who "live much on the diseased flesh of pampered animals, fatted in stalls, without air or exercise, till they become foul, soft, and leucophlegmatic", whereas "the labouring and common people, such as the tough hungry Scots, are almost exempted" because of their lenten fare. Luxurious eating gradually overwhelmed the liver and, harking back to a mixture of humoral and mechanical theory, Grant held that "the texture of solids was destroyed, secretions and excretions interrupted, obstructions formed and new humours and salts produced." So biliousness affected the whole constitution and, however, far fetched (and perhaps prejudiced) his views on the pathology of decadence may have been, they certainly promoted awareness of this ill-defined concept.[30]

In contrast to Grant's theory of excessive bile, others saw biliousness as a deficiency of bile. One such was a surgeon, John Andree (1749–1833), whose father, a Huguenot physician by the same name, had founded the London Hospital. The younger Andree was not as successful as his father, which I suspect did nothing for his own indigestion. He made the most of his infirmity by writing about it in a book that sold well. In the preface he begins, "Bilious diseases are among the most common of the chronic distempers of the inhabitants of England, and therefore merit the peculiar attention of medical practitioners. During twelve years, I had too much reason to lament the imperfect state of this part of medical knowledge, having been nearly so long subject to a bilious disorder, undescribed by any authors, and opprobrious to my own, and learned friends' kind medical aid." He goes on to give his credentials, "Failing in the requisite knowledge of these kind of diseases, in the common course of medical learning, my next recourse was to anatomical investigation; by embracing every opportunity of examining the parts affected, by dissection of many who had been afflicted by such disorders. Having flattered myself that some of the opinions contained in the following pages will tend to the relief of mankind in such diseases, I felt it a duty incumbent on me to submit them to the public inspection in this, far from perfect state, satisfying myself with 'mens sibi, conscia recti'."[31]

The book is highly speculative and the turgid rhetoric contributes nothing of note. It is tempting to deride Andree's ingratiating style and obscure ideas but he is typical of his time. On the strength of anatomy alone, he tried to divide biliousness into three types; redundancy of bile causing diarrhoea, diminished secretion of bile causing anorexia, and misplaced bile causing jaundice; an impossible task without the benefit of clinical chemistry and current concepts of metabolism.

An overview of dyspepsia during the eighteenth century was satirically portrayed by a physician practising in Bath, James Makittrick Adair (1728–1802). Adair's medical writings enjoyed a good reputation on the continent, and his MD thesis on the subject of yellow fever was authoritative. In 1790, he published a collection of essays dealing with such subjects as *The dangerous effects of Hot and Crowded Rooms; The Cloathing of Invalids; Lady and Gentleman Doctors; and Quacks and Quackery*. The last is a particularly corrosive contribution to medical literature in which the quarrelsome Adair displays his gift for vindictiveness. He refers to several respectable doctors by name who are in his opinion "mountebanks", "water-castors", and "vendors of nostrums". One suspects that the law of libel in the eighteenth century was something of a dead letter. It is his essay on *Fashionable diseases* that concerns us and some of what he has to say has a familiar ring.[32]

"Fashion has long influenced the great and opulent in the choice of their physicians...but it is not so obvious how it has influenced them also in the choice of their diseases. This I shall endeavour to explain.

"Patients are generally prompted by curiosity to enquire of their medical guide, what is their disease? But an explicit answer is not always either convenient or practicable; because the doctor is sometimes ignorant of it himself; or candidly confessing his ignorance, which would not be always consistent with good policy; he gratifies his patients by a general term, which may, or may not, be expressive of the disease."

At the beginning of the century, says Adair, "spleen, vapours, or hyp[†] was the fashionable disease" but things have changed:

"Upwards of thirty years ago, a treatise on nervous diseases was published by my quondam learned and ingenious preceptor Dr.Whytt, professor of physic at Edinburgh. Before the publication of this book, people of fashion had not the least idea that they had nerves; but a fashionable apothecary of my acquaintance, having cast his eye over the book, and having been often puzzled by the enquiries of his patients concerning the nature and causes of their complaints, derived from thence a hint, by which he readily cut the Gordian knot – 'Madam, you are nervous!' The solution was satisfactory, the term became fashionable, and spleen, vapours, and hyp were forgotten."

But this was just a passing fad:

"Some years after this, Dr. Coe wrote a treatise on biliary concretions, which turned the tide of fashion: nerves and nervous diseases were kicked out of doors, and bilious became

---

† Hypochondriasis

the fashionable term. How long it will stand its ground cannot be determined.

"From a well grounded opinion that Bath waters are very beneficial in colics produced by gall-atones, and other cases of defective bile, a very considerable proportion of the patients who resort to that place (Bath), go with a strong prepossession that their complaints are bilious; insomuch that instead of my patients giving me a detail of their symptoms, by which I might judge of the nature of the disease, the answer generally was, 'Doctor, I am bilious.'"

g) Dyspepsia

In fact nervous diseases were anything but a passing fad. Both Cheyne's and Cullen's theories were taken up and enlarged upon as the eighteenth century drew to a close and were given credence by the discovery in the 1780s of the eighth pair of nerves (later reclassified as the tenth

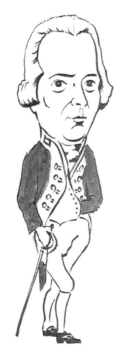

65 Trotter – Admiral of the fleet.

cranial nerves or vagi). Rather than the straightforward excess theory epitomised by Woodward and Grant, biliousness began to be seen as a disease of civilisation, reminiscent of the kind of nervous malady discussed by Cheyne.

The concept was elegantly promoted by another Scotsman, Thomas Trotter (1761–1832), poet, playwright, physician to the fleet and medical reformer. In his book *A View of the Nervous Temperament* published in1807, Trotter begins, "The last century has been remarkable for the increase of a class of diseases, but little known in former times, and what had slightly engaged the study of physicians prior to that period. They have been designated in common language, by the terms Nervous; Spasmodic; Bilious; Indigestion; Stomach complaints; Low spirits; Vapours, etc."[33]

Trotter believed that nervous disorders were not just confined to the upper classes but extended to the newly sensitised middle classes; indeed they now accounted for two thirds of the diseases of mankind, in this country at least, thanks to Britain's vast wealth. "Nervous feelings, nervous affections or weak nerves, though scarcely to be resolved into technical language, or reduced to a generic definition, are in the present day, terms much employed by medical people, as well as patients, because the expression is known to comprehend what cannot be so well explained." A host of depressive symptoms "accompanied more or less with dyspeptic symptoms, are the leading characteristics of nervous disorders; to be referred in general, to debility, increased sensibility, or torpor of the alimentary canal".

Stressing the importance of the great sympathetic nerve (as well as the vagus) in its connections with the gut, Trotter reminds us that the stomach, intestines and liver, and all the viscera subservient to digestion have an innate sympathy with the nervous system. "The effect of violent passions on the chylopoietic viscera, is to destroy the appetite, disturb digestion, invert the peristaltic motion of the stomach and bowels and render the alvine discharges variable and irregular." Here we see the forerunner of the irritable bowel. "The biliary secretion is also inconstant, and perhaps altered in quality; the hepatic, cystic and common ducts may be affected into spasms, inverted and obstructed, thus jaundice, and vomiting of bile are no infrequent attendants of violent emotions." In his view the commonest cause of a violent passion was prolonged grief, which is fair enough, but other causes included certain novels and melodramas perhaps in sympathy for his fellow playwrights.

Despite his comments on biliary secretion he is sceptical about the use of the word bilious. "The term belongs to common language; as such I have adopted it in my title; but it is not correct in a medical nomenclature. Some members of the profession, to improve our vernacular idiom, have thought proper to give these ailments the name of liver complaints as that organ is said to be their seat; but this term is equally undefined in a scientific view, as that of stomach complaints, so long applied to diseases of the digestive powers. The phrase Bilious derives its origin from that tinge of the skin so often observed in dyspeptic persons, who also occasionally pass bile both upwards and downwards. Now Bile appearing in these forms, being a natural secretion made by the liver, is to be considered as the effect, rather than the direct cause of indisposition. In the present day, a dyspeptic person no sooner complains of pain in the right hypochondrium, than the liver is said to be diseased; and a bilious suffusion of the surface is considered an infallible symptom of the same viscus being affected; and the mercurial process is immediately commenced. It is disgusting to hear this phraseology so common in the mouths of medical people."

On the other hand Trotter was fully conversant with gall stones and the dangers of biliary colic which "in common language, some people call a bilious or nervous attack".

Trotter, like Hunter, believed in the supreme importance of the stomach and his influence was considerable. "The stomach is an organ endowed by nature with the most complex properties of any in the body; and forming a centre of sympathy between our corporeal and mental parts, of more exquisite qualification than even the brain itself... . In those disorders whose seat is the nervous system, it particularly suffers." Other writers of the time expressed the same sentiments.[34]

CHAPTER FIFTY-TWO

DYSPEPSIA IN THE NINETEENTH CENTURY

a) Dyspepsia and universal sympathy

John Hunter's views on universal sympathy were championed by one of his students, John Abernethy (1764–1831), surgeon to St. Bartholemew's Hospital. Abernethy founded the medical college at the hospital and was the first surgeon to be interested in physiology as well as anatomy. He had an enquiring mind, was well up in the chemistry of his period and conducted his own postmortem examinations, a practice that was just becoming acceptable in Britain.[35] He was an inspiring lecturer and wrote extensively, so his influence was considerable. He believed that just as external injuries acting on the nervous system could upset the digestive system (through sympathy) so the reverse could be true. Disorders of the stomach and bowels frequently underwrote all manner of conditions through sympathy including weakness and irritability of the nervous and muscular system, inflammation of the liver, shortness of breath, feeble pulse, delayed healing of skin ulcers and abscesses, etc., etc. Furthermore the digestive disturbance was easy to overlook as the symptoms were often minimal or suppressed. As each could influence the other, a vicious circle arose between cause and effect.

His diagnosis of indigestion, particularly among patients who thought their digestion was normal, was based on his view of the normal processing of food by the gut. There were three stages. Digestion took place in the stomach where food was converted to chyme. Chylification occurred in the small intestines and this was followed by a third process in the large intestines where the residue underwent a sudden change into faeces.

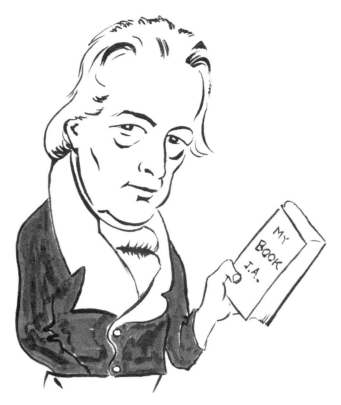

66 Abernethy – Dr – 'My book'.

The key to disorder of the stomach, apart from the usual rumblings and flatulence, was the state of the tongue. A dry, furred tongue reflected a poorly secreting stomach. Impaired chylification could be assumed by subtle changes in the colour of the stool, in extreme cases becoming almost white as the supply of bile dried up.

Constipation allowed chemical decomposition of the stool to occur within the colon with the release of ammonia that was in turn capable of irritating it.

Finally he stressed that "the duration of the affection, without fatal consequences, shows that it is a disorder of functions, and not a disease of structure. Dissections confirm the opinion".

Abernethy linked indigestion to gastric and bilious disorders "as it appeared to him on the most attentive examination". His treatment was logical; reduce the quantity and frequency of meals and keep the food simple, use mercury in moderation to augment the biliary secretion and give gentle laxatives to clear the colon without overstimulating it.

He published his extreme and eccentric views in a famous book, *Surgical Observations, Part 2*, in 1806,[36] and it reappeared as a single volume in 1809.[37] He liked to quote from his book at every opportunity and, at the end of a consultation, instead of issuing a prescription, he would give his patients details of his book on a slip of paper, advising them to read page 72 (section on treatment). Unsurprisingly, the book went into at least eleven editions, and Abernethy was caricatured in the popular press as *Dr. My Book*.[38]

Abernethy promoted his ideas on gastric sympathy with zeal bordering on the obsessional. One of his pupils, Thomas Pettigrew (1791–1865), who became the first surgeon to be appointed at the new Charing Cross Hospital, refers to this in an anecdote he included in a biography of Abernethy:

> "I was once consulted by a lady for a common affection of one of the bursae mucosae of the knee-joint, which had been occasioned by a blow received on the edge of a step. She went to Mr. Abernethy, and was about to show the affected part, when he rudely exclaimed, 'I don't want to see your knee, Ma'm. Allow me!' And he pressed his fist with force upon her stomach. She called out, and he declared her digestive organs to be at fault. The treatment she received occasioned her to have an attack of hysterics, in the alarm at which, I was called in. She was afterwards under my care, and recovered completely without taking a single dose of medicine. The case was strictly local. This is indeed a sad perversion of judgement...but it was his hobby."[39]

Hobby or not, he was not the only person with unusual views. Wilson Philip (1792–1851), a London physician interested in the physiology of the gut and a prolific writer, believed that indigestion was a common cause of pulmonary phthisis.[40] Not many shared this opinion, which was soon discredited.

b) Dyspepsia and sensibility

In the early nineteenth century, the stomach assumed even greater significance as the seat of physical and mental disorders with the concept of sensibility. This term, meaning an increased susceptibility to physical or mental stimuli, had recently caught the imagination of the literati. Several late eighteenth-century novels had been written around the subject though it was mocked by Jane Austen in *Sense and Sensibility*. Nevertheless, it was applied to the stomach by Trotter and later taken up by James Johnson (1777–1845), an erstwhile naval surgeon, who believed that the stomach and bowels could acquire a morbid sensibility allowing the simplest of foods to upset people. By the time Johnson elaborated his views he was a successful London physician, editor of the prestigious *Medico-Chirurgical Review* and physician extraordinary to William IV.

According to Johnson the stomach could be rendered morbidly sensible by physical and moral stimuli, which included everything from the weather, pollution, and luxurious food to stress and anxiety of all kinds. With regard to stress,

> "there is but one path along which this cause can travel from the organ of thought to the organs of digestion; but the number of airy sprites, and the velocity with which they glide along the silvery pneumo-gastric conductors, baffle all calculation! ... A single look, and a very few words from the tyrant monarch, gave the ambitious Wolsey a fit of indigestion, which terminated the Cardinal's life!"†

A morbidly sensible stomach responds to food with a typical attack of indigestion that in turn upsets other organs sympathetically, especially the nervous system and liver. These then repay with interest the injuries they have sustained from the stomach. "The gastric fluid, so much under the influence of the nerves, becomes impaired; the hepatic secretion vitiated, and the indigestion becomes more intense."[41]

This may seem convoluted, but Johnson went further. He believed that a morbid sensibility of the nerves of the stomach and bowels could trigger symptoms in other organs through sympathy even in

---

† He had dysentery and may have compounded this with an overdose of purgatives.

the absence of gastric symptoms. This applied especially in the case of mental afflictions. Someone, say, who had lost his business experienced languor, sadness and fear, but these were mediated through the stomach not the nervous system. Pursuing this argument he concluded that hypochondriasis was usually the result of a morbidly sensitive but often silent stomach.

Johnson's theory led to simple treatment. Both indigestion and hypochondriasis should respond to diet. Only a bland diet would allow the morbid sensibility of the nerves of the stomach and bowels to recover, otherwise all the normal stimuli and stresses of life would perpetuate the condition, be it dyspepsia, biliousness, irritation of the bowels or indeed hypochondriasis.

Not surprisingly he thought it was very common. "It knocks at the door of every gradation of society, from the cabinet minister, planning the rise and fall of empires, to the squalid inhabitant of St. Giles or Saffron Hill, whose exterior exhales the effluvia of filth, and interior those of inebriating potations. No moral attributes, no extent of power, no amounts of wealth, are proofs against this wide-spreading evil. The philosopher, the divine, the general, the judge, the merchant, the miser, and the spendthrift, are all, and in no unequal degree, a prey to the Proteian Enemy."

c) Dyspepsia and William Beaumont

The two concepts of sympathy and sensibility dominated thought on dyspepsia for much of the nineteenth century. Even the remarkable studies on gastric juice by William Beaumont (1785–1853), the American army surgeon, failed to change attitudes for some years. As every medical student knows, in 1822 a French Canadian trapper, Alexis St. Martin (1804–87), was accidentally shot in the stomach but miraculously survived and was left with a gastric fistula. Beaumont treated his wound and looked after him in his own home for two years by which time "he was able to walk and help himself a little".[42] In return St. Martin agreed to let Beaumont study his stomach between 1825 and 1833, though there were several interruptions because the cantankerous fellow often absconded.

Beaumont not only described the mucous membrane and the movements of the stomach but also confirmed recent work by the great English chemist, Prout (1785–1850), proving that hydrochloric acid was the important acid of the gastric juice. He also noted the effect of various foodstuffs upon gastric flow, and the influence of mental disturbances on the secretion of gastric juice. However, he left one misconception: that gastric secretion did not occur unless food was present in the stomach.

Though Beaumont was primarily concerned with the physiology of digestion he took the opportunity to draw some conclusions about dyspepsia. He constantly referred to the injurious effects on the stomach of tea and coffee when taken in excess, and the pernicious influence of alcoholic drinks on digestion. Furthermore, "The system requires much less than is generally supplied to it. The stomach disposes of a definite quantity. If more be taken than the actual wants of the body require, the residue remains in the stomach and becomes a source of irritation and produces a consequent aberration of function, or passes into the lower bowel in an undigested state, and extends to them its deleterious influence. Dyspepsia is oftener the effect of over-eating and over-drinking than of any other cause." This was music to the ears of the Victorian physician whose wealthy patients often ate colossal meals.

Beaumont published his findings in Plattsburgh, upstate New York, in 1833.[43] In Britain during the same decade there was a growing movement to promote popular education in many subjects, including health, hygiene, anatomy and contemporary notions of physiology. Digestion and diet were favourite subjects for consideration in both public lectures and books, and it was by these means that Beaumont's work first became known to the British public. In 1836 the sanitary reformer, Thomas Southwood Smith (1788–1861), a founder member of the Society for the Diffusion of Useful Knowledge and an eloquent writer, expounded his views on physiology in his book, *The Philosophy of Health*, in which he included mention of Beaumont's experiments.[44]

Beaumont's work also came to the attention of a well-known physiologist and popular writer, Dr. Andrew Combe (1797–1847) of Edinburgh. This was largely because Combe's brother, William, lived in New York State and was an intimate friend of a Dr. McCall in Utica, New York, who knew Beaumont. Andrew Combe had a gift for popular exposition and a mission to inform and educate. In a book on the physiology of digestion, also published in 1836, he included a detailed account of Beaumont's work with an accompanying woodcut of the famous fistula.[45] Later, in 1838, Combe also edited the Edinburgh edition of Beaumont's book with numerous notes and comments of his own.[46]

Beaumont's work was exciting, and, naturally, subsequent authors interpreted what he had seen in the fistula to explain their own views on dyspepsia, though these did not always agree with the facts. Thanks to the importance accorded to the stomach there was no shortage of books on indigestion, which was said to be "the prevailing malady of civilised life".[47] A typical example was that written by George Chaplin Child *On Indigestion and Certain Bilious Disorders Often Conjoined With It*. Child (1800–75?) was Physician to the Westminster General Dispensary and his views reflect prevailing thought on indigestion. He believed that indigestion could be brought on in four ways. Firstly it could follow a debauch causing acute inflammation of the stomach. Beaumont had observed this on several occasions, though occasionally the stomach looked inflamed when St. Martin felt perfectly well. This was difficult to explain but ideas about inflammation and gastritis were still rudimentary and based on what the eye could see. Microscopical histology was still in its infancy. Child's second cause was indigestion from habitual overindulgence, which fitted nicely with Beaumont's view. His third cause harked back to Johnson's sensibility in which the stomach was predisposed to indigestion from some weakening disease such as anaemia, depression or liver disorder. This also included hysteria to which women were particularly prone. The fourth type arose from faulty action in the liver. Child tried hard to distinguish various forms of biliousness but his ideas were confused and speculative. People were in his view bilious if they had sick or bilious headaches, nausea, or vomit containing bile. However, he did admit that it was often hard to say whether the liver or the stomach be most at fault. "Hence it happens that each case is apt to be viewed according to the peculiar bias of the practitioner – with some, it is 'all stomach'; with others, it is 'all liver'."[48]

Reading Child's book I was struck by the huge attention he pays to the history and symptoms of indigestion. There are no fewer than 38 pages given to the description of abdominal pain and 17 comparing gastric and bilious headache. This reflects the lack of investigations at his disposal that we take for granted today. He had no thermometer, no haematology, no blood chemistry and of course no X-rays. Inflammation was beginning to receive intense study under the microscope but Virchow was yet to expound his cellular theory of life and disease.

d) Three eminent Victorian physicians and dyspepsia

Sir Thomas Watson

If Cullen was the most celebrated teacher of the eighteenth century, Sir Thomas Watson was among the best of the nineteenth century. Watson (1792–1882) had a distinguished career as physician to King's

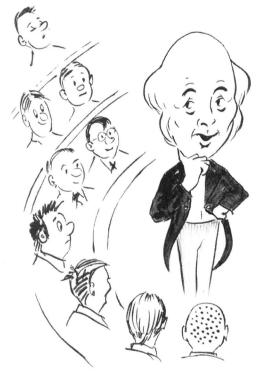

67 Watson – Lecturer supreme.

College, London, President of the Royal College of Physicians and physician to Queen Victoria, being created a baronet in 1866. His popular lectures were published in two volumes that ran through five large editions. The chapter on dyspepsia is lucidly written and summarises what students were taught at the time. He begins by stating that, "We are more often consulted about the disorders that belong to eating and drinking, than perhaps about any others; and I know of no medical topic concerning which there is afloat, both within and beyond the profession, so much ignorant dogmatism and quackery." Unlike Chaplin

Child he had little time for biliousness. "It is pretty evident that the state of the biliary functions can have no direct influence in the production of mere dyspepsia... . The effort of vomiting, however induced, will, if often repeated, be attended with the expulsion of yellow bile. The fallacy I now point out has been one cause of the notion that is prevalent among patients, and the public – and not unfrequently perhaps among practitioners – that dyspepsia very commonly depends upon a disordered state of the biliary organs."

On the other hand he had sympathy for the hypochondriac. "One of the worst occasional concomitants of dyspepsia is that peculiar state of the mind to which I just now alluded under the term hypochondriasis... . Now when the attention of the hypochondriac is thus morbidly fixed upon the states and sensations of his digestive organs (as it is very apt to be) the patient becomes a plague to his physicians as well as to himself." He goes on: "Our task is hardest of all when the patient's anxiety relates to his own complaints; when he is morbidly engrossed by his bodily feelings, and despondent about his recovery. The management of the mind of a hypochondriac is peculiarly nice and difficult. It will not do to treat him as if his ailments were imaginary. He disbelieves you, contemns your judgement, and deserts you: to be fleeced perhaps by some villainous quack. You must hear what he has to say; shew an interest in his case; and prescribe for him: assuring him that you understand his malady, that it is curable, and that he will be cured provided he follows your directions."[49]

GEORGE BUDD

The effect of nervous influences on digestion was taken up by George Budd, one of the first two physicians to be appointed at King's College Hospital. Budd (1808–82) had already made his name with his book on diseases of the liver published in 1845; now, ten years later, he published his lectures on disorders of the stomach. He reiterated the views on sympathy of his predecessors and devoted a chapter to *Deficient secretion of gastric juice – slow and imperfect digestion*. There were several causes including excessive fatigue and great mental excitement that were well known. He also refers to Beaumont's work, "in the case of St. Martin, Dr. Beaumont had ocular proof that the depressing passions of fear and anger lessen the secretion of the gastric juice. Feebleness of digestive power, arising from this cause, is often seen in men of excitable temperament who suffer anxiety, or who overstrain their minds in the pursuit of wealth or other objects of ambition."

Furthermore the secretion of gastric juice may be only relatively deficient as in the case of the middle and upper classes. "The stomach can digest food enough to nourish the body, but not enough to satisfy the pampered appetite." He agreed with Beaumont that the quantity of juice required for digestion was proportional to the quantity of food. The juice became saturated and could dissolve no more. So overeating can overtax even a normal stomach. "Indigestion brought on in this way is the natural penalty for the violation of a natural law, or, as a humorous writer has termed it, 'the remorse of a guilty stomach'."[50]

He goes on to suggest that the result of insufficient gastric juice is to slow digestion. Food may remain undigested for several hours causing uneasiness in the pit of the stomach followed by cramp as it enters the pyloric orifice. Here he recalled the cramp felt by St. Martin when Beaumont inserted a thermometer into his pylorus. Lastly undigested food lying around in the stomach was liable to unnatural fermentation with distension and the evolution of foul belchings.

Budd also believed that gastritis was an important cause of dyspepsia but emphasised the difficulty of proving this. Firstly pure gastric juice from an inflamed stomach that might have shed some light on the underlying inflammation was difficult to obtain as it was normally contaminated with mucus or food. Secondly gastritis was rarely fatal so evidence from post mortem examination was not available. He had to admit that knowledge of the inflammatory diseases of the mucous membrane of the stomach was extremely limited.

Once again he drew on the observations of Beaumont who had had the rare opportunity of seeing much of what took place in the stomach. Acute gastritis, by which he meant aphthous patches, red spots and occasional bleeding together with very little proper secretion and ropey mucus, often occurred after the ingestion of ardent spirits or indigestible food. Recovery was quick but, if the patient had no symptoms, a good appetite and continued to eat and drink as usual, repair was interrupted and chronic gastritis supervened. This was somewhat speculative and diagnosed on clinical grounds by constant epigastric tenderness, pain in the stomach, occasional vomiting after meals and a white, furred tongue.

WILLIAM BRINTON

Dyspepsia due to gastritis was also promoted by William Brinton (1823–67), physician to St. Thomas's Hospital and an authority on gastric diseases (see peptic ulcer). By the time his *Lectures on the Diseases of the Stomach* appeared in 1859, Virchow had published his cell theory and the microscope had revealed the layout of the glands within the gastric mucosa.[51] Brinton made use of post mortem material to describe the microscopic appearances of acute gastritis in cases of poisoning and delirium tremens. Building on Beaumont's evidence of naked eye inflammation seen in life, he suggested that subacute or chronic gastritis was probably common and frequently a cause of some varieties of dyspepsia. But he was careful to emphasise that dyspepsia could be purely functional with no apparent underlying pathology and conversely that gastritis could be symptomless.

Brinton reflected on the meaning of dyspepsia. "Dyspepsia – equivalent to difficulty of digestion – is evidently a wide word. One step towards its conversion into a definition we may perhaps take, by pointing out what it evidently implies: namely, not only that a certain amount of digestion is (though with difficulty) effected, but that this difficulty is not due to any serious structural lesion." He then goes on to ask, "How far is dyspepsia a gastric disease? In other words, considering that the function of the stomach is but a part (however large or essential) of the total digestive process, how far are disturbances of this process in general to be referred to the stomach? ... Doubtless there are many derangements of other parts of the alimentary canal equally entitled to the name of indigestion... . Constipation, where really specific to the malady, and not (as it often is) a mere secondary result of the habits of the patient, belongs rather to intestinal than to gastric dyspepsia; a fact in which it resembles the opposite (and less frequent) variety attended by diarrhoea."[52] Here we are witnessing the first description of functional bowel disease as an entity.

He has something pertinent to say about diagnosis. "Since dyspepsia represents, not so much a single and substantive disease, as a variety of ailments; and is characterised, not so much by the presence of certain symptoms, as by the absence of structural lesions; the diagnosis of the malady in general, and of any case in particular, are opposed by analogous difficulties. As the progress of scientific Medicine has gradually revealed the morbid anatomy of the digestive canal, and thus detected structural diseases with increasing accuracy, the vague (but useful) term 'dyspepsia' has acquired a continually more restricted meaning." He predicted that "the aggregate of maladies called dyspepsia must undergo successive subtractions...into special maladies, and to the removal of this term from our nosology". So most people who had recurrent abdominal symptoms would one day be found to have structural abnormalities, and the word dyspepsia would be left to describe the minority in whom "special maladies" could not be demonstrated. In fact, as Denis Gibbs has pointed out, it is the terminology rather than the clinical manifestations that have changed.[53] Many people with dyspepsia in the nineteenth century would now be categorised as suffering from irritable bowel syndrome. Brinton would be surprised to learn that, despite ever increasing refinements in diagnostic methods, functional bowel disease is still the commonest cause of recurrent abdominal symptoms.

Brinton's advice on treatment was both wise and circumspect. Diet and regimen were the mainstays of management. "In the vast majority of cases, drugs do not cure dyspepsia. They mitigate its symptoms, they diminish its effects; but they hardly touch (if we may draw such a distinction) its nature or its essence." He was at pains to remind his students that dyspepsia was often mild and remitting by nature and that it typically affected the rich and gullible. It was therefore tailor made for quacks and their phoney cures. Indeed physicians often believed their remedies were effective when they were not. "A person suffering from dyspepsia takes a certain remedy. He recovers. Therefore he is cured by it. So runs the popular conclusion. But the conscientious physician can accept no such flattering or delusive estimate of his remedy." Was the recovery spontaneous? Was it due to the concomitant diet and regimen? He even hints that a form of drug trial would be valuable by suggesting that the efficacy of a given drug could be confirmed by the results of interrupting, omitting, and repeating its administration.

e) Three eminent Victorian dyspeptics

CHARLES DARWIN

Brinton believed that undue intellectual exertion and mental anxiety were common causes of dyspepsia. One of his most famous patients was Charles Darwin (1809–82) who suffered bitterly from indigestion for thirty years. Darwin consulted most of the leading physicians and surgeons of his day but none of them ever found anything organically wrong. Initially he consulted Sir James Clark (1788–1870), physician to the young Queen Victoria, who urged him "to knock off all work and go and live in the country".[54] Darwin was an anxious man and was agitated by pressures of work with his journal. Shortly after, he saw Sir Henry Holland (1788–1873), the society physician and a personal friend, who told him his illness was not quite dyspepsia and nearer suppressed gout. Holland prescribed colchicum and endorsed his move to the country. Darwin's flatulence and occasional vomiting continued and aware that some patients had been helped by hydropathy, he read a book written by a Dr. Gully on the subject.[55] Gully's water regime was based on the idea that chronic disorders were caused by a faulty supply of blood to the viscera and that applying cold water to the skin would improve the circulation. Gully recognised that Darwin's dyspepsia was a mixture of physical debility, despondency and gloom, and was happy to hold his stomach responsible. This was exactly the kind of malady that his hydropathic establishment claimed to cure.

Darwin had some faith in Gully and for a time he felt slightly better, but his stomach ailments were never cured. In 1863 he was visited at his home in Kent by Brinton whom he described as "one of the most cheery and skilful physicians of the day".[56] At the time he was troubled by palpitations and pain around his heart, but Brinton could find little physically wrong declaring that neither his brain nor heart was primarily affected by his chronic illness.

Darwin's chronic ill health has fascinated many experts over the years and most think that his dyspepsia was psychosomatic. In 1943, Douglas Hubble suggested that he had Da Costa's syndrome,[57] now known as hyperventilation syndrome, a view that was supported by Sir George Pickering in 1974.[58] In the same year a former president of the Royal College of Surgeons, Sir Hedley Atkins, also examined the records with special attention to the gastric symptoms.[59] He concluded, "We are not only thrown back on a diagnosis of neurosis, but we can muster an unequalled array of evidence in a positive way in favour of it." This was also the opinion recently of the psychiatrist John Bowlby (1907–90). Bowlby was the originator of what is now known as "attachment theory". Separation from the mother in early childhood often had dire results and could be mitigated by forming ties of attachment with fellow human beings, with serious consequences if these were severed. He studied attachment in other species, and his interest in biological theory and in the effects of bereavement led to his interest in Darwin.[60] In his biography of Darwin he assigns the scientist's chronic ill health and recurrent anxiety and depression to the early death of his mother. Victorian physicians such as Brinton would have called this nervous indigestion and seen Darwin as worn out by mental strain and particularly prone to nervous irritation that deranged the gut.

THOMAS HUXLEY

Several eminent Victorians suffered from dyspepsia. In his book, *Biographical Clinics*, George Gould (1858–1933), an American ophthalmologist and medical editor, discussed many well-known figures who were chronically ill for much of their lives with dyspeptic complaints.[61] One was Thomas Huxley (1825–95), a good friend of Darwin, who thought he was poisoned when he was fourteen years old while assisting at a postmortem examination. Though he soon recovered, he believed that the poison had permanently injured him for he said "...from that time my constant friend, hypochondriacal dyspepsia, commenced his half-century of co-tenancy of my fleshy tabernacle". Huxley's letters show how debilitating dyspepsia could be. He explained that it wasn't his brain but his stomach that was to blame. Phrases like "...being worried to death with dyspepsia and the hypochondriacal bedevilments that follow its train" are found in his letters to his friends. Rest, travel, special diets, and care with alcohol and tobacco provided only temporary relief. For much of his life Huxley was treated by his schoolmate and contemporary, Sir Andrew Clark (1826–93), who was a friend and doctor to many of the scientists and thinkers of the time, including Darwin in his later years. Clark spent his early career in pathology, but later became a successful clinician and President of the College of Physicians. He was a man of serious turn of mind and for relaxation turned to theology and speculative philosophy. He was popular because he avoided purgings, leechings and blood lettings and emphasised the importance of dieting and travel to cure dyspeptic ailments. His instructions specified what Huxley was to "...eat, drink, and avoid, how much he was to sleep and rest, how little to talk and walk, etc.".". He also recommended what Huxley called "Clark's pills", which contained strychnine, or a mixture of quinine and strychnine. Huxley had faith in Clark, though the two men were quite different in character. Huxley's humour never left him even in his darkest moments. Referring to an intended visit to Penzance, he wrote: "I am possessed by seven devils – not only blue, but of the deepest indigo – and I shall try to transplant them into a herd of Cornish swine." And a few days later he wrote: "I am convinced that the prophet Jeremiah (whose works I have been studying) must have been a flatulent dyspeptic – there is so much agreement between his views and mine."[62]

THOMAS CARLYLE

No one scrutinised his dyspepsia so incessantly or lugubriously as did Thomas Carlyle (1795–1880). His problems began when he was a student in Edinburgh with dyspepsia "like a rat gnawing at the pit of his stomach". The next three years were the "most miserable of his life" though he continued to suffer for another forty years. As he grew "sicker and sicker" he began to consult doctors and described an eminent Edinburgh physician as "a long hairy-eared jackass who ordered him to give up his dear nicotine and take to mercury".[63] Whether prescribed by doctors or self-inflicted, there can be little doubt that a great part of Carlyle's digestive difficulties came from dosing himself with castor oil for his constipation. He often described himself as bilious and linked this with nervousness, sleeplessness and general gloom. He was always worse after writing or correcting proofs, and felt better after some fresh air and exercise. Like Darwin, Carlyle went to Malvern for its water cure, and became the guest of Dr. Gully. Unlike Darwin, he concluded that hydropathy was worse than useless. He avoided doctors for years but in old age he submitted to occasional visits.

Writing in the British Medical Journal after his death, Sir Richard Quain (1816–98) said, "The late Mr. Carlyle was a patient of mine. As all the world knows he was a man of great judgement and great power of observation. With regard to himself, the only remedy I could ever get him to take was grey powder.[†] He lived to 82 or 83. Grey powder was his favourite remedy when he had that wretched dyspepsia to which

†   Mercury with chalk.

he was a subject, and which was fully accounted for by the fact that he was particularly fond of very nasty gingerbread. Many times I have seen him sitting in the chimney corner smoking a clay pipe and eating this gingerbread. He overcame the difficulties incident to this habit by his grey powder, which did him much good."[64]

Late Victorian view of dyspepsia

In fact Carlyle found that continued and prolonged exercise helped him more than anything. A large part of his life was spent in riding horseback (he spoke of one of his horses having carried him 20,000 miles). Horse riding, so popular with Sydenham in the seventeenth century, was thought to be superior to other forms of exercise. Lord Palmerston (1784–1865) once remarked that "the outside of a horse is the best thing for the inside of a man"; and as late as 1885 Sir Thomas Lauder Brunton was justifying this view in his Lettsomian lectures to the Medical Society of London.

Brunton (1844–1916) was lecturer on material medica at St. Bartholemew's Hospital and is best remembered for showing that amyl nitrate relieves the pain of angina pectoris. He published a large number of papers on pharmacological and physiological subjects and thought that biliousness and indigestion were distinct but closely related conditions.

A bilious patient suffered from dull, heavy, and languid feelings, a disinclination to exertion, mental or bodily, an irritable or peevish temper, failing appetite, muddy complexion, dingy conjunctiva and headache.

By this time it was known that the liver was not a mere secreter of bile but the site of essential metabolic processes such as the synthesis of peptides and formation of glycogen. The importance of the portal venous system in conveying products of absorption to the liver was also appreciated as was the entero-hepatic circulation. The liver not only secreted bile but also re-excreted bile absorbed from the duodenum.

Brunton linked indigestion and biliousness by assuming that the products of imperfect digestion could upset the liver causing obstruction in the hepatic capillaries. The resulting congestion of the liver caused venous congestion of the stomach and intestines; this further interfered with digestion, which in turn reacted upon the liver once more. He

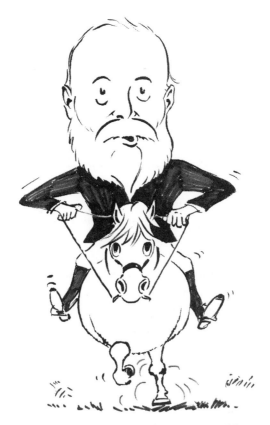

68 Brunton – Squeezing his congested liver.

also thought that biliousness could arise if the bile itself became too thick or viscid by the action of certain products of digestion upon its secretion.

Simple fasting was the best cure but drugs were often needed. Fasting allowed time for matters to right themselves and was perfect for those overindulging at Christmas time. Unfortunately many Victorian gentlemen indulged themselves on a regular basis and were disinclined to stop. For them a blue pill and black draught were the answer. The blue pill was mercury, which not only reduced the secretion of bile by the liver but also acted as an effective duodenal purgative, eliminating secreted bile before it could be reabsorbed into the circulation. Black draughts were various salt-based laxatives, which added to the cathartic effect of mercury.

If the bile was thought to be thick and viscid, anything that assisted its flow through the ducts into the intestine was beneficial, especially a brisk horse-ride in the morning, which he believed was better than any amount of mercury or laxatives. In his Lettsomian lectures he suggested that riding a horse compressed the liver between the diaphragm and the abdominal muscles, squeezing the bile out of it.[65]

In a similar vein, Brunton wrote at length on indigestion as a cause of nervous depression. He believed that peptones and other products of digestion were not always properly eliminated by the liver and circulated to the brain causing irritability, melancholy, forgetfulness and headache. For some reason that he found difficult to explain this was most likely among brain workers in office jobs. A good holiday made them better because the body was somehow more efficient at eliminating waste, perhaps through sustained exercise. But this was not a long-term or practical solution. Once again they needed to curb their diet, especially of meat, take more exercise, and clear out the liver and gut with mercurials and purgatives. Inadvertently, Brunton was helping to popularise the already widespread belief in habitual purgation and even colonic lavage. Anyone with a headache or general malaise could justify the use of a laxative.

Brunton relied heavily on Beaumont for his views on dyspepsia, which were still quite theoretical. Meanwhile in Germany physicians were studying the stomach with the help of gastric tubes. Adolf Kussmaul (1822–1902) was one of the first to treat pyloric obstruction by lavage through a tube.[66] He inspired many others to intubate the stomach for research purposes, notably Wilhelm Leube (1842–1912), who introduced the test meal to measure gastric acid,[67] and Carl Ewald (1845–1915), who studied gastric motility.[68] Their work formed the basis for a new classification of nervous dyspepsia by Franz Riegel (1843–1904) and this was promoted in Britain and America by William Osler in his book *Principles and Practice of Medicine*. In the chapter on diseases of the digestive system, neuroses of the stomach merited seven pages, with another eleven on gastritis and only nine on peptic ulcer. (Duodenal ulcer was still thought to be rare in 1901 when this edition of the book was published.)[69]

Osler divided nervous dyspepsia into three types; motor, secretory and sensory. The motor neuroses included ten sub-varieties such as eructations, rumination, spasms and so on. The secretory neuroses described a stomach producing too much or too little acid, and the

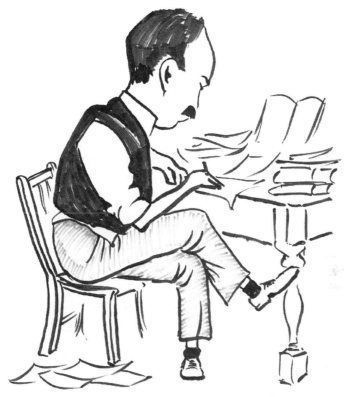

69 Osler – Thoughts on dyspepsia.

sensory neuroses referred to sensations of pressure, burning or pain. They usually overlapped, though the sensory disturbances were predominant. Precise diagnosis necessitated intubation, which was hardly practical in every case. The diagnosis was made by failing to detect abnormal pathology.

In the same chapter Osler discussed the causes and symptoms of chronic gastritis. The diagnosis relied on a combination of postmortem material and analysis of gastric contents obtained by intubation, both of which were unreliable. He recognised three types: simple gastritis, mucus gastritis and atrophic gastritis. The symptoms were similar to those of nervous dyspepsia, except that the patient did not have a nervous constitution. Unfortunately many patients with gastritis were neurasthenic and likewise many patients with nervous dyspepsia did not appear to be anxious. It was all very confusing even for a man of Osler's experience and must have been baffling for the student. To this should be added the constant worry that the patient might have an underlying peptic ulcer, cancer or gall stones. Radiology was not yet available.

Fortunately treatment, assuming the patient had simple dyspepsia, was relatively straightforward and much the same as it had been for centuries. Patients with nervous dyspepsia required counselling, rest, a change of air and sometimes antacids. However, if the patient had a supersecretory stomach, gastric lavage with alkaline solutions or nitrate of silver was recommended. If pain was very severe, opium or even chloroform could be used.

The commonest causes of chronic gastritis were bolting down food or overeating or both. Often all that was required was to count to a certain number before swallowing each mouthful. People habitually ate too much and, said Osler, it was probably true that a greater number of maladies arose from overeating than from excessive drinking. Otherwise treatment was similar to that of nervous dyspepsia.

CHAPTER FIFTY-THREE

MUCOMEMBRANOUS COLITIS IN THE NINETEENTH CENTURY

Unlike dyspepsia, functional bowel disease did not attract much attention until the late nineteenth century. The colon never enjoyed the status of the stomach, which for years had been considered equal in importance to the brain. This is not to say that people did not take a keen interest in their bowels, but the colon itself was seen as a tube that merely stored and evacuated the waste products of digestion. It was "simply a sewer canal".[70] The usual fear was that any delay in evacuation would risk illness from auto-intoxication. This was nothing new. One of the oldest treatises on medicine in existence, an Egyptian papyrus dating from the fourteenth century BC gives directions for the preparation of enemata. Enemata were in common use among the ancient Egyptians; Herodotus (443 BC) wrote that "they clear themselves on three consecutive days in each month by emetics and enemata, for they think that all disease comes to man from his food".[71] As indeed did many of their successors, and purging the gut by one means or another has continued ever since.

William Cullen had been one of the first to make a list of disorders of the colon and to recognise that these could be functional. In his classification of neuroses written in 1769, he referred to an order called spasmi which he divided into several genera including colica and diarrhoea. Colic was caused by spasm of the natural functions, giving rise to twisting pains round the navel and spasms of the abdominal muscles. Diarrhoea could be idiopathic with the passage of frequent stools and need not be infective. An example was diarrhoea crapulosa following a debauch.[72]

Cullen had little time for postmortem evidence to support his clinical observations, unlike John Abercrombie (1780–1844), a remarkable physician in Edinburgh who carried out his own autopsies.[†] In his book *Pathological and Practical Researches on Disease of the Stomach, the Intestinal Canal, the Liver and other Viscera of the Abdomen*, Abercrombie emphasised the importance of examining patients with abdominal pain. He belonged to a new breed of physician who sought the diagnosis by history and examination, and correlated the findings with an autopsy in the event of death. For example he observed that patients with simple colic did not object to abdominal palpation whereas those with inflammation, such as peritonitis or enteritis, were exquisitely tender.[73]

Abercrombie also noted a chronic affection of the bowel causing protracted bad health, with obscure and undefined symptoms "such as a superficial observer is apt to consider as hypochondriacal. A painful feeling of distension is often complained of, though no actual distension can be perceived." He was describing a condition that was to assume prominence throughout the nineteenth century and early part of the twentieth century. "The motions are sometimes natural, but frequently they are mixed with mucus in a very concrete or tenacious state, assuming various forms, as irregular crusts of aphthae, or masses of a rounded or tubular form, which are apt to be mistaken for worms. The affection is often extremely tedious and untractable; and it is difficult to say what treatment is most beneficial."[74] He did not try to explain it or give it a name.

About the same time John Howship (1781–1841), assistant surgeon to St. George's Infirmary, London, wrote a small and very readable book on the subject of spasmodic stricture of the colon.[75] He recognised that the complaint was due to "a deficient freedom of relaxation in some part of the intestinal canal", and both as a diagnostic test and a therapeutic measure advocated gradual distension of the bowel with a large warm gruel enema. Howship was a highly regarded surgeon who had the misfortune to die of a haemorrhage from an abscess of his leg caused by chronic disease of the tibia.

Abercrombie and Howship were almost certainly describing the same condition which was common in constipated young women said to be neurotic. It became known as mucous colic or muco-membranous colitis.

---

† See chapter on peptic ulcer, page 64

The name originated because the colon was thought to be inflamed causing the production of coagulable lymph, which formed a fibrinous membrane. The membrane was evacuated in shreds, which sometimes formed tubular casts of the colon. In extreme cases these could be two or more feet in length. Impressive as these membranes were, Sir Thomas Watson lecturing in the 1840s doubted that they were really composed of fibrin.[76] Like Abercrombie he thought they were more likely to be formed by viscid mucus, and this was subsequently proved to be the case by Andrew Clark (1826–93) early in his career when he was curator of the museum at the London Hospital. In collaboration with a young Jonathan Hutchinson (1828–1913), best remembered for his description of the deformity and notching of the teeth in inherited syphilis, he presented a case to the Pathological Society of London in 1857. The patient, a lady aged 49, complained of pain in the left iliac fossa with alternating constipation and diarrhoea and the regular passage of "brown, thick skins, four or five inches long". Treatment had been ineffective. Examination of the membrane under the microscope and by chemical analysis showed it was simple mucus with no evidence of fibrin.[77]

Clark described his findings with the help of Samuel Wilks (1824–1911), assistant physician to Guy's Hospital, who had long recognised the importance of morbid anatomy in diagnosis. Indeed in the same year Wilks had described idiopathic ulcerative colitis as a distinct entity for the first time.[78] The condition described by Hutchison and Clark was a secondary colitis commonly seen in melancholics. However, Wilks clearly thought that there was an inflammatory component to mucomembranous colitis as he called the disease pellicular (thin skin) or diphtheritic colitis, likening the membrane to that found in diphtheria.[79]

It is worth noting that this was the period, the mid-nineteenth century, when medicine began to enter the modern era. Students were taught to examine their patients thoroughly; the microscope was transforming pathology; Virchow was proclaiming his cellular theory of life and disease; clinical thermometry was being introduced, and soon the germ theory of infectious diseases would be established through studies such as those by Koch and Pasteur, which indisputably linked a specific organism with a specific disease.

The discovery of micro-organisms naturally led doctors to hope that colitis in its various forms would be caused by a specific infection, but unfortunately repeated attempts to find a pathogen failed. So the terms colitis, ulcerative colitis, mucous colitis, membranous colitis, muco-membranous colitis and mucous colic were used interchangeably and confusion reigned.

As is often the case when the cause of a disease remains elusive many thought muco-membranous colitis was a neurotic disorder. But this did not explain every case and other theories were put forward. One suggestion, popular in America, was that it was secondary to disease of the vermiform appendix. The appendix was beginning to attract the attention of surgeons now that it was possible, thanks to Lister, to enter the abdomen without killing the patient. In 1886 a physician Reginald Fitz (1843–1913) in Boston, realised that abscesses in the right iliac fossa were due to appendicitis and not to inflammation around the caecum (typhlitis) as people thought. His advice to remove the inflamed appendix was rapidly taken up in the United States.[80] At the same time people began to wonder if inflammation of the appendix could be linked with colitis. Within a decade a surgeon in Philadelphia, John Deaver (1855–1931), hinted that appendicitis could cause "inadequate digestion in the large bowel, colitis etc.".[81] Two years later, in 1898, another paper from Philadelphia entitled *The Importance of Chronic Irritability of the Colon, with Mucous Stools as a Symptom of Appendicitis* attracted wide attention.[82]

However, the idea of appendicitis as a cause of muco-membranous colitis never caught on in Britain; admittedly many patients with colitis had their appendix removed but this was because surgeons were terrified that they might miss an inflamed appendix. This was understandable in the era before saline transfusions and antibiotics, when late diagnosis of appendicitis was usually fatal.

Another potential cause of muco-membranous colitis that caught the imagination of the profession and lasted several years was a condition known as visceroptosis. By the late nineteenth century most doctors accepted that many of the abdominal organs could be compressed and displaced by poor posture, slack abdominal muscles, tight wasted corsets or simple neurasthenia. Moveable kidney was particularly common but the stomach, transverse colon, liver and spleen were all at risk of dropping or drooping within the abdomen. At first the diagnosis was entirely clinical, by palpation of the abdomen, and most believed that the condition was symptomless and harmless. But some thought it caused abdominal pain and neurasthenia and it became known as Glenard's disease after a Frenchman, Frantz Glenard (1848–1920), who wrote extensively on the subject.[83] He had a good imagination and initially suggested that the transverse colon could bow under the weight of faeces causing kinks of the nearby flexures. The falling colon brought the stomach down with it. Later he proposed that disturbed liver function altered bowel function and somehow displaced the colon. Finally he proposed that enteroptosis could cause muco-membranous colitis. This set the cat among the pigeons with surgeons able and anxious to find a surgical cure for colitis. They were further encouraged at operation when they discovered to their surprise that the organs were often much lower in the living subject than they were in the preserved cadaver of the dissecting room. Soon they were hitching up drooping colons wholesale.

The discovery of X-rays in 1895 gave further support to the diagnosis of visceroptosis and its link to mucous colitis. Using radio opaque bismuth salts Walter Cannon (1871–1945), the great Boston physiologist, showed in cats that antiperistalsis occurred in the proximal colon.[84] Before long people were linking mechanical interference of peristalsis with enteroptosis and colitis. Later when bismuth was replaced by barium, the concept of visceroptosis was strengthened as radiologists began to see dropped stomachs and transverse colons routinely in apparently healthy people. Most continued to believe it was harmless and Osler cautioned physicians not to lay too much stress on the disorder. "It is well never to tell the patient that a kidney is movable: the symptoms may date from a knowledge of the existence of the condition."[85]

But some, including, as we shall see, the influential Arbuthnot Lane (1856–1943), believed that angulation caused by adhesions (common in enteroptosis) led to chronic intestinal stasis and mucous colitis.[86]

Even Arthur Hurst writing in 1910 initially thought that visceroptosis, including movable kidney, co-existed with muco-membranous colitis, though he came up with another explanation. "The association is not a result of kinking at the flexures of the colon, but is due mainly to the fact that the weakness of the abdominal muscles, which permits the viscera to drop, is a common cause of dyschezia (inability to defaecate completely). This view receives support from the benefit derived in cases of muco-membranous colitis associated with visceroptosis from temporary rest in the horizontal position."[87] He later rejected this idea as the concept of visceroptosis became discredited.

CHAPTER FIFTY-FOUR

EARLY TWENTIETH CENTURY

a) Dyspepsia

By the end of the nineteenth century, the stomach had lost its place as the hub around which the body functioned. People now realised that digestion and absorption took place primarily in the small intestine, and surgeons had shown that it was possible to live without a stomach. Doctors and patients were also less inclined to link depression and melancholy with disorder of the liver. Hypochondriasis did not originate under the ribs and hysteria had nothing to do with the womb. The dilemma posed by George Sand in her memoirs was no longer relevant: "Whether it is the bile which has made me melancholy, or the melancholy which has made me bilious; this would resolve a great metaphysical and physiological problem, which I will not take up."[88] Neuroses, neurasthenia, hysteria, hypochondriasis and melancholy were disturbances of the mind, not the stomach or liver. Unfortunately the general perception of mental disease still left much to be desired, there was little sympathy for hysterics and hypochondriacs, and the very word neurotic was used derisively.

Functional disease was giving way to organic disorders. An editorial in the *Lancet* in 1902 put the case cogently explaining how for many years a connection between chronic dyspepsia and definite organic disease had hardly been suspected. Such cases were unlikely to be detained in hospital for any length of time and rarely came to a postmortem. But now that some definite structural change could be found, it could confidently be stated that in the vast majority of cases of severe chronic dyspepsia the disease was not merely functional but had an organic basis. It was remarkable, concluded the *Lancet*, how often a simple healed gastric ulcer was found to be the cause.[89] This could well have been written by no less a man than the surgeon, Berkeley Moynihan of Leeds (1865–1936), who was operating on two patients a week. Indeed within a few years he would be promoting duodenal ulcer over gastric ulcer as the likeliest cause of dyspepsia.

Surgeons operating on the stomach were helped by the recent discovery of X-rays and the use of the bismuth meal to outline the stomach. At first only gross pathological changes could be detected such as obstructions and giant ulcers. However, this did not deter a man with as much confidence and self-belief as Moynihan, who felt able to make a confident diagnosis of duodenal ulceration from the history alone.[90]

Aware of this new disease, pathologists began to find evidence of ulcers. Previously, small scars indicative of a healed gastric ulcer were overlooked or thought to be insignificant and the duodenum was not even examined. From the turn of the century the rise of peptic ulcer was dramatic so that by 1950 ten per cent of working men were said to be affected.

Unfortunately, despite enthusiastic investigation with X-rays and various forms of test meal for excess acid, unexplained dyspepsia was at least as common as peptic ulceration. This was bad news for patients without an ulcer who were either dismissed as neurotic or neurasthenic, or told that they had reflex dyspepsia caused by a mild form of appendicitis or cholecystitis. Once again the appendix was singled out, this time by the British not the Americans. Chronic appendicitis was first put forward as a cause of dyspepsia in 1896 by Rutherford Morison (1853–1939), a well-known surgeon in Newcastle. But it was not until 1910, when Moynihan introduced the term "appendix dyspepsia", that people took notice.[91] Not everyone agreed with him; Anthony Bowlby (1855–1929), a surgeon at St. Bartholemew's Hospital who was later to be knighted for distinguished service during the Great War, complained of the vagueness of the clinical picture that had been drawn. He predicted that "one result of the results of Mr. Moynihan's paper will be that many 'dyspeptic' people will undergo operations for the removal of the appendix, and the great majority of them will be none the better". Others supported Moynihan; Sir Clifford Allbutt (1836–1925), a leading physician of the day and editor of the famous *System of Medicine,* wrote: "May we not ask ourselves if there is not something in it – perhaps a great deal – immature, fragmentary if you please, yet with a core of important truth?" There wasn't, but with two such powerful backers and Arthur Hurst's support,[92] innumerable dyspeptic people had their appendix removed unnecessarily for supposed appendix dyspepsia over a period of at least thirty years. Hurst was impressed by what he called Bastedo's sign, described by a New York physician, Walter Bastedo (1873–1952) in 1911.[93] Insufflation of the colon with air caused severe pain in patients with sensitive colons and this was taken as indicative of chronic appendicitis at the time.[94]

If the appendix was exonerated the gall-bladder frequently took the blame instead. Chronic cholecystitis was suggested by persistent tenderness in the right hypochondrium, especially on deep inspiration. Even if a cholecystogram, which became available in the 1920s, showed the gall bladder was normal, it was removed on clinical suspicion.[95]

Perhaps it is not surprising that physicians, surgeons and research workers found peptic ulcer disease much more interesting than functional dyspepsia. Though common and often exceedingly troublesome to the victim, non-ulcer dyspepsia was trivial in its physical effects, there was no obvious pathology, the mechanism was ill understood and the treatment unsatisfactory.

b) Mucous colitis

By contrast, interest in the colon accelerated, though there was still much confusion and misinformation about the wretched organ. In 1906 Herbert Hawkins (1859–1940), an urbane and highly regarded physician at St. Thomas's Hospital, wrote an admirably descriptive paper based on the study of 35 cases of enterospasm, drawing particular attention to the frequent confusion of the disease with appendicitis.[96] He emphasised spasm of the colon could be the cause of very severe abdominal pain and, echoing Bowlby's warning about needless surgery, added, "They (visceral neuroses) are at this moment particularly worthy of study, owing to the advance of abdominal surgery, not because they are amenable to surgical treatment, but rather because they need protection." Three years later Hawkins published another paper, this time on the subject of ulcerative colitis, which he clearly distinguished from so-called mucous colitis or spasm. This coincided with a celebrated meeting held at the Royal Society of Medicine at which the surgeon,

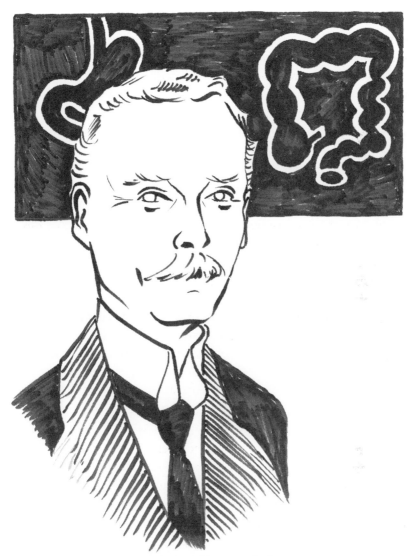

70 Hawkins – Suave and elegant.

Percy Lochhart-Mummery (1875–1957), extolled the virtues of the electrically illuminated sigmoidocope for the first time.

Arthur Hurst (1879–1944) was invited to take part in the discussion at the meeting but declined because he felt he knew little about ulcerative colitis at the time. This was a pity as Hurst was one of the few physicians to appreciate the importance of the sigmoidoscope. For years most physicians were only too happy to delegate the colon to the surgeons;

bowel disease was a messy subject and physicians saw themselves as elegant men in tailored suits wielding a stethoscope and fountain pen rather than a tail-end torch.

Hurst, an enthusiastic and likeable man, was carrying out some fundamental research at Guy's Hospital into the movement of food along the alimentary tract using the new discovery of X-rays.[97] In 1907 he traced the passage of the "bismuth meal" through the stomach and small intestine to the colon and established a timetable that was accepted as the normal standard for decades. At one stage he was joined by a young surgeon from Melbourne, Alan Newton (1887–1949), later Sir Alan, President of the Royal Australian College of Surgeons, who had come to work in London. Newton spent part of his time at Guy's Hospital where he studied the movements of the colon and the ileo-caecal sphincter.[98]

Hurst went on to study constipation. There were two causes; the first was spastic constipation due to poor relaxation of segments of the colon, and the second was what he called dyschezia from an inability to defaecate completely. This could vary from a mild inconvenience to complete inability to defaecate. He recalled how he once saw a lady, who for six years had had to dig the faeces from her rectum every day with her fingers. There were several reasons for inefficient defaecation;

1 habitual disregard of the call to defaecation,
2 inefficiency of the voluntary muscles that normally take part in defaecation,
3 the assumption of an unsuitable posture during the act,
4 weakness of the defaecation reflex, and
5 hysteria.[99]

Hurst was also among the first to study the sensibility of the gut. By introducing very hot or cold water into the stomach or colon through a tube he showed that the whole of the alimentary tract from the upper end of the oesophagus to the junction of the rectum with the anal canal was completely insensitive when simply touched. The stomach and colon were also insensitive to thermal stimuli but the oesophagus and anal canal appreciated heat and cold. This may have seemed self-evident to people, but until he carried out his experiments there was no scientific evidence for the view commonly held on the subject. He made good use of his observations on a man who for 30 years had complained of a burning sensation inside his abdomen which had become intolerable. Hot food aggravated it, so he drank iced water at all hours of the day and in desperation frequently gave himself ice-cold enemas. After blindfolding him, Hurst poured very hot and cold water through a tube into his stomach and up his colon and the man experienced no sensation of any kind. "His sensibility was in fact normal, and the feeling of heat and the relief from cold drinks and enemas were the result of auto-suggestion."[100]

Formerly people thought that acid produced a burning sensation in the stomach but Hurst showed that hydrochloric acid caused no sensation in it of any kind. However, he was misled in concluding that the oesophagus even when inflamed was insensitive to acid, something that he found difficult to explain in view of the everyday experience of heartburn among his patients.[101]

Using balloons Hurst and his colleagues also studied the sensation of fullness and pain in the alimentary canal. If a balloon was inflated slowly in the oesophagus it caused a feeling of fullness but if inflated rapidly it caused pain. The same applied in the colon if a balloon was inserted through a colostomy opening. Hurst also managed to induce a sense of fullness and pain in the stomach by inflating it with air through a tube connected to a manometer.[102] From this he concluded that visceral pain was caused by tension exerted on the muscular coat of the alimentary canal.

Thanks to his research and radiological studies, Hurst was able to speculate on the pathogenesis of muco-membranous colitis. Like Hawkins he thought that mucous colic and mucous colitis were varieties of the same condition. The key problem was an abnormal nervous system causing spastic constipation. Retention of faeces in an individual, predisposed by an abnormally irritable nervous system as found in hypochondriasis, led reflexly to local over-activity of the motor and secretory fibres of the colon, causing painful spasms, pockets of wind and over-secretion of mucus and mucous casts. He compared the condition to asthma with bronchospasm, excess mucus and Curschmann's spirals.[103] The seat of the spasm and the production of excessive mucus lay in the distal colon.

Treatment of the condition as Osler pointed out was very unsatisfactory. Measures directed to the nervous condition were the most important.[104] Hurst agreed and said that the patient should be encouraged to think as little as possible about his illness, and be forbidden to make minute daily examinations of his excreta. A healthy lifestyle was important thereby avoiding undue fatigue. The constipation required treatment by a generous mixed diet containing porridge, wholemeal bread and plenty of fruit and green vegetables. Enemata were often necessary but as time went by Hurst became increasingly outspoken against purgatives and douches, which in themselves irritated the colon.

The frequent failure of medical treatment encouraged the surgeons to do their bit. The first operation was a colotomy in the right inguinal fossa to relieve constipation. This was said to have been successful in several cases of great obstinacy, though it is hard to imagine how any chronic illness could justify the misery of a colotomy. Subsequently appendicectomy came into vogue despite misgivings by Hawkins and Hurst[105] followed by various procedures to hitch up dropped colons (and surgeons' bank balances).

One of the most remarkable facts about muco-membranous colitis was that during the First World War the membranes disappeared, not to be seen again. Mucus casts became a thing of the past despite the fact that colon spasm, with which they were associated, remained as common as ever.

Hurst had taken advantage of a new technique, X-rays in his case, to study the gut. Research on patients was quite unusual at the time and his findings were highly relevant to functional bowel disease. Unfortunately the First World War put a stop to any work that was not considered important to the war effort and patients with gastric and colonic neuroses were low on the medical agenda if they were on it at all.

After the war, clinical research was supported by the Medical Research Committee (later Council) and by new academic professorial units springing up in London teaching hospitals. Sadly, though the science of physiology dominated research at the time, this did not encompass functional bowel disease. Spastic colons did not interest professors of medicine, and even if they had, the influence of their units was small. Unlike America, where the professor was also chief of service in his hospital, English professors had little influence outside their own unit. London hospitals were largely staffed by part-time consultants in general medicine who devoted the rest of their time to private practice.

Though some of the surgical academic units studied the gut as a whole, most were consumed with the measurement of gastric acid and its link with peptic ulcer. With the inexorable rise of gastric and duodenal ulcer and the inadequacy of medical treatment, surgeons believed that the cure lay in their hands. Understandably patients with "non-ulcer dyspepsia" did not interest them. Similarly patients with colicky abdominal pain, constipation or diarrhoea initially found their way to a surgeon in case they had cancer of the colon. Once cancer had been excluded they were usually sent back to the general practitioner with a reassuring pat on the back to cope as best they could. Spastic colons did not excite professors of surgery either.

The most useful information about the colon came from the radiologists before the dangers of excessive radiation were fully appreciated. Foremost among these was Alfred Barclay (1876–1949) in Manchester who followed up Hurst's early work with cinematographic studies of the bowel.[106] He described how the so-called haustral contractions of the colon mix and churn the contents but do not propel them forwards, and he also noted that these contractions ceased immediately before a mass movement of the bowel moved the contents on. In other words the colon was often more active in patients with constipation as was later rediscovered when manometry became available.

Between the two world wars and for some years afterwards colitis remained poorly understood by most doctors. Ulcerative colitis was still considered to be a rare disease and often confused with mucous colitis and spastic colon. Medical students received little if any teaching about colitis despite the efforts of Arthur Hurst and a few of his colleagues to get the message across.

This is not to say that the colon was ignored by everybody, far from it; there were some who could hardly leave the wretched organ alone. In 1921 Arthur Hurst gave an address *on the sins and sorrows of the colon* to the Harrogate Medical Society.[107] He began by stating that the sins of the colon were its diseases. But he wondered whether it was not more sinned against than sinning, for what with attacks from above with purges, attacks from below with douches, and frontal attacks by the surgeon, its sorrows were numerous and real.

c) Intestinal autointoxication

A brief diversion on the concept of intestinal intoxication helps to explain why the colon was under attack at the time. Throughout the nineteenth century, sluggish bowels were seen as the foremost medical problem of civilisation in Europe and America. A popular health manual warned in the 1850s, "daily evacuation of the bowels is of the utmost importance to the maintenance of health".[108] Ironically this view was encouraged by the new germ theory of disease in the last quarter of the nineteenth century. Pasteur had shown that germs caused putrefaction of animal and vegetable material outside the body. Lister followed this up by using carbolic acid to suppress wound infection because he had seen it used in the city of Carlisle to prevent putrefaction in its sewage dump. Surely, the argument went, within the body was not the colon a veritable sewage pit teeming with bacteria, a cesspit that in people with constipation, was not being emptied? Self-poisoning from one's own

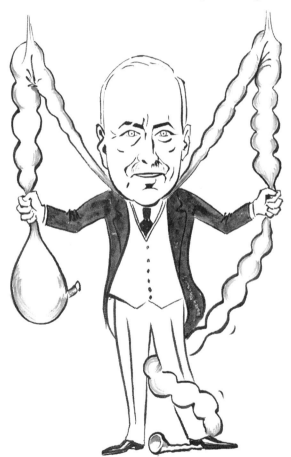

71 Lane – 'Colon, semi-colon, full stop'.

intestinal wastes, or intestinal autointoxication as it was called, was put forward as the cause of all manner of diseases.

The makers of laxatives, irrigation equipment, electrical stimulants and other devices made the most of people's fears. Hundreds of brands of bowel cleansers were marketed with lurid advertisements emphasising the dangers of constipation. But the most worrying cure for autointoxication was colectomy, which was strongly advocated by a renowned surgeon at Guy's Hospital, Sir William Arbuthnot Lane (1856–1943). Fortunately colectomy in the first decade of the twentieth century was so hazardous that most surgeons were deterred from following his example. But Lane was a consummate surgeon with a reputation as the only man in London who could open the abdomen safely. He believed that once the colon was overloaded it became kinked by the crystallisation of the abnormal forces acting on it (Lane's kink), exacerbating the original constipation. This led to the process of what he called chronic intestinal stasis. He denounced the assumption that a daily bowel action was sufficient to stay healthy. Such an assumption, he said, resulted in "constipation for twenty-four hours".[109] Stasis could, in Lane's view, cause problems ranging from general debility to rheumatoid arthritis, tuberculosis, or cancer. He removed literally hundreds of entire colons from patients with constipation. Not surprisingly his theory was widely opposed and in 1913 the operative treatment of chronic intestinal stasis was formally rejected by his colleagues at a meeting held at the Royal Society of Medicine.[110] Nonetheless the practice continued in some places until after the Second World War.[111]

d) Spastic colon

Some including a physician in Birmingham, Theodore Stacey Wilson (1861–1949), still believed that simple spasm of the colon caused a host of physical and mental disturbances. Wilson was an exponent of thorough physical examination and had a bee in his bonnet about the colon. Whatever the patient's complaint he would examine the abdomen with infinite care and as often as not find that the colon was palpable and tender.[112] This was not in his view caused by faeces or gas but by thickening of the bowel wall due to rigidity of its muscle. Though useful in drawing people's attention to mucous colitis he went too far. In a remarkable book, *Tonic Hardening of the Colon*,[113] he described his eccentric view that severe and prolonged spasm of the colon caused not just severe abdominal pain but, by a reflex nervous reaction, anything from angina to neurasthenia, depression and suicide. The true cause of these problems could be easily overlooked unless one took the trouble to palpate the abdomen where the hardened colon could be felt. This was reminiscent of the nineteenth-century beliefs of Abernethy, Philip and Johnson, and his devotion to outmoded theories did not endear Wilson to his colleagues.

Writing at about the same time, John Ryle (1889–1950) at Guy's Hospital published in 1928 a review of what he called spastic colon based on 50 cases of his own.[114] He noted Stacey Wilson's contribution but felt that he attributed too long a list of physical and mental disturbances to the direct agency of tonic hardening. Ryle was an outstanding clinician and his paper was later included with 33 other essays and lectures under the title of *The Natural History of Disease*.[115] This medical classic was reprinted by the Keynes Press in 1988 and contains a wealth of clinical description as relevant today as it was when first published in 1936.

Ryle and Hurst thought as one on gastro-intestinal diseases, though it was left to the extrovert Hurst to deplore the misconceptions about colitis. In a clinical lecture delivered at Guy's Hospital in 1930, he spoke about mythical maladies, among which he included mucous colitis.[116] Visceroptosis was still in vogue so Hurst began by dismissing gastroptosis, pelvic caecum and dropped colon as "diseases" we owed to the radiologist. "Just as some people have long noses and others have short noses, some have long stomachs and others have short stomachs, which are nothing more than normal variations from the average." They did not cause constipation and had nothing to do with mucous colitis. He next emphasised that mucus was secreted by the colon to protect it from mechanical and chemical irritants. Its appearance around a hard stool or a soft stool after an aperient was normal. Yet doctors still gave the presence of mucus as the reason for diagnosing mucous colitis. Colitis meant inflammation of the colon with loose bloody stools. As mucus was always present in true colitis there was no point in speaking of mucous colitis, quite apart from the fact that the term was almost invariably used for a condition in which the patient was suffering from inefficient defaecation. Naturally he added that the sigmoidoscope was essential in making the diagnosis, though he knew that his words were falling on deaf ears where physicians were concerned.

To hammer the point home Hurst referred to a recent case. A woman of 45 became exhausted as a result of severe puerperal sepsis. Mucous colitis was diagnosed without a single stool being seen and without a sigmoidoscopy; she had twelve intestinal douches in London, followed by a course at Plombières (a spa in eastern France). She then developed abdominal pain as well as fatigue and was told she would have to remain in bed for six months. He found nothing at all the matter, discontinued the douches, her bowels worked normally, and with encouragement she soon recovered.

Warming to his theme Hurst again warned against douching. Mucous colitis was best treated with wholesome neglect. He was supported in his views by an influential Paris physician, Albert Matthieu, who said that he had seen more cases of colitis come from Plombieres than ever went there. Europeans got the message and by 1930 patients were drinking and bathing in spa water instead of having it injected into their colons. Unfortunately, as lavage became less popular in France it became more fashionable in England. For example, a colon laundry, as an American author called it, was established in London for what was referred to as the new indoor sport of washing out the intestines.[117]

Hurst died in 1944, by which time he had founded the Gastro-Enterological Club, later the British Society of Gastroenterology. This was a small select club and at first there were only forty members including one surgeon. The Second World War started two years after its foundation and for many years it was left to the Americans to promote research into functional bowel disease. In Britain general practitioners referred patients with disorders of the colon to the surgeons who were well aware of the psychogenic component. The disordered mind and disordered colon of the neurotic played upon each other. It was as simple as that. For example in his presidential address to the Royal Society of Medicine in 1951, Sir Heneage Ogilvie (1887–1971) suggested that proctologists might translate the old adage "Mens sana in corpore sano" into "normal defaecation brings a contented mind" and normal defaecation in turn comes from equanimity and common sense. "Sanum e sana mente nascitur corpus."[118]

CHAPTER FIFTY-FIVE

DYSPEPSIA IN THE MID-TWENTIETH CENTURY

a) Gastritis

The onset of the Second World War focussed attention on dyspepsia because soldiers with a peptic ulcer were automatically invalided out of the service. In March 1941 at the height of the London blitz, Colonel Letheby Tidy (1877–1960) led a discussion at the Royal Society of Medicine on the subject of dyspepsia in the forces. Henry Tidy, later Sir Henry, physician to St. Thomas's Hospital and consultant to the army, was a man of commanding and aristocratic bearing with an encyclopaedic knowledge of medicine. He was a founder member in 1937 of the Gastro-Enterological Club and served as its chairman in 1943.

At the RSM meeting, he began by making the point that though dyspepsia in the army was very common, it was no more common than in civilian life. Half the hospital patients had an ulcer and these could be discharged unless their skills made them indispensable to the war effort. The rest had gastritis and/or functional dyspepsia, which he grouped together. Though these men were assumed to be psychoneurotic they were not malingerers but rapidly became exaggerators if they were over-investigated and treated. In peacetime such patients usually managed to stay at work with occasional days off but this did not suit army routine. The symptoms in patients with functional dyspepsia were more obstinate and more continuous than in peptic ulcer and when a dyspeptic soldier returned to his unit it was difficult for the medical officer to keep him fit for duty; indeed many had to be discharged.

There was a third group, transient dyspepsia, that was more frequent than the other two groups together. Tidy gave an example:

"A healthy man when he joins the army is placed in a new environment and often develops dyspepsia after a month or so when he reports sick. An experienced medical officer recognises the condition, reassures the man and explains it to him and gives him a bottle of medicine. This last is essential as otherwise he would be branded as a malingerer which he is not and knows that he is not. He may report sick twice in the following fortnight, once in the next and then no more is heard of him. He has become acclimatized. But a medical officer not so experienced, or lacking self-confidence, may send the man to hospital for a specialist opinion. This is the first mistake. The specialist should return him at once to his unit, but he may make the further mistake of admitting him to hospital for investigation which proves negative. The symptoms respond readily to hospital treatment and the man is sent back 'cured' to the Training Centre. But though the symptoms have been removed the man has not been acclimatized and the cycle starts over again and he is admitted to hospital for a second time. It is almost true to say that a recruit who has been twice admitted to hospital within a short time for the same complaint will not subsequently get rid of the symptoms. His chance of making a useful soldier has been taken away and, further, he can claim that in the Army he developed chronic dyspepsia from which he had never suffered previously."[119]

During the discussion of Tidy's paper, it emerged that many doctors did not know what to do about soldiers with X-ray negative dyspepsia. These men tended to drift in and out of reception stations and hospitals without any definite decisions about diagnosis, treatment and disposal being made. Dr. Charles Newman (1900–89), a future president of the British Society of Gastroenterology, had carried out a survey of dyspepsia among men evacuated from the British Expeditionary Force in 1940.[120] He felt the non-ulcer group often drew the short straw. Many doctors regarded gastric patients as an unsatisfactory class, with no physical signs, uncongenial personalities, likely to need long and dull treatment and a tendency to relapse. Special units should be established to deal with and make definite decisions about these doubtful cases.

The participants also discussed the significance of gastritis in soldiers without an ulcer. By this time a few enthusiasts were able to examine the stomach with a semi-flexible gastroscope, though the technique was tricky and the view limited to the lesser curve of the stomach and the upper part of the posterior wall. The procedure was distinctly uncomfortable for the patient so it was not undertaken lightly. The usual indication was severe unexplained dyspepsia in looking for a gastric ulcer or cancer missed by the radiologist. Gastritis was a naked-eye diagnosis as biopsy was not yet possible. Reginald Payne (1896–1967), a surgeon at the British Postgraduate Medical school at Hammersmith Hospital, had gastroscoped the doubtful cases collected by Dr. Newman and found that a few had patchy gastritis, but the numbers were small and he was unsure of its significance. On the other hand Stanley Hartfall (1899–1982) and Arthur Hurst from Guy's Hospital both felt that gastritis was an important diagnosis. With his customary optimism, Hurst stated that gastritis could be cured by a short period in hospital on strict diet with hydrogen peroxide lavage first thing in the morning. Such cases could return to duty and were unlikely to relapse. On the other hand patients without gastritis clearly had nervous dyspepsia and should respond to the simplest psychotherapy.

At the end of the war Francis Avery Jones (1910–98) published a survey of dyspepsia among civilians. He had spent the war as Physician in Charge of the Dietetic Department at the Central Middlesex County Hospital. During this time and for many years afterwards he kept meticulous records of his patients and built up a remarkable database of gastro-intestinal diseases long before the introduction of computerised records. The majority of his dyspeptic patients who were all hospital referrals had a peptic ulcer. Even so 40 per cent had "X-ray negative" dyspepsia who in his opinion probably had an ulcer that he was unable to prove, a reasonable assumption in the days before double contrast barium meals and modern endoscopy.[121] Nonetheless he was impressed by the number of non-ulcer patients he was seeing and promised that they would be the subject of a later report. This never materialised but in conjunction with the young Richard Doll (1912–2005) he went on to look at over 6,000 men and women employed in the neighbourhood.

Nearly a third had a history of some dyspepsia in the preceding five years and almost half of these had a peptic ulcer.[122]

So it was peptic ulcer disease that worried people. By 1950 ten per cent of middle-aged men had an ulcer at any one time, an extraordinarily high figure. For the next 35 years with few exceptions everyone's concern was to single out the dyspeptics with ulcers. Even though medical treatment was purely symptomatic, it was unfortunate to overlook an ulcer because it was a disabling disease with serious implications. Gradually new techniques improved diagnostic accuracy.

During the 1960s the Japanese introduced the double contrast barium meal which was popularised in this country by William Scott-Harden, a radiologist in Belfast.[123] This technique could pick up small gastric lesions easily missed by conventional barium meal.

The Japanese also developed a gastrocamera, which caught the imagination of George Hadley (1908–84), physician to the Middlesex Hospital. In his early career Hadley had worked with Izod Bennett (1887–1946) at the Middlesex where he learnt to use the semi-flexible Wolf-Schindler gastroscope. As medical specialist in the army he was captured at Dunkirk and despite several escapes spent five years as a prisoner-of-war. Tall and austere, his imprisonment made him reticent and reserved but his kindness and intellectual honesty inspired devotion from a series of brilliant trainees. In 1963 he was the first Briton to fly to Japan to learn to use and service the gastrocamera.[124] His skills as a fly fisherman, bookbinder and cellist were an advantage as the camera needed fine manipulation and a gentle touch. It was a safe diagnostic tool that theoretically obtained photographs anywhere in the stomach but in practice the technique was tricky and the failure rate twenty per cent.[125]

It was still hoped that chronic gastritis might explain dyspepsia in some cases but this was difficult to prove. Semi-flexible gastroscopy was unsatisfactory because the view was limited and biopsies could not be taken, but in 1955 Nelson Coghill (1912–2002), physician to the West Middlesex Hospital, Isleworth, devised a method of obtaining gastric biopsies. With the help of a pathologist, Professor Wynn Williams, he modified a suction biopsy tube invented by Ian Wood a few years earlier.[126] The tube was placed in the stomach under X-ray control so the technique was relatively blind, but multiple samples of mucosa could be obtained, which were thought sufficient to allow for the patchy nature of gastritis. With the help of Felicity Edwards (born 1927) fresh from Tom

McKeown's social medicine department in Birmingham he studied 200 patients with non-ulcer dyspepsia. Twenty per cent of the patients had gastritis but this was mainly chronic atrophic gastritis and they felt unable to say that it was causing their dyspepsia.[127] Over the next decade they continued to look at the clinical manifestations of dyspepsia but were still unable to differentiate them from ulcers with sufficient accuracy to be useful diagnostically. Coghill, a modest and unassuming man, built one of the earliest gastroenterology units in the country and showed what could be achieved in a district general hospital in the early days of the National Health Service. He was elected president of the British Society of Gastroenterology in 1969.

Gastroenterology changed dramatically with the development of the fully flexible fibrescope in the late 1960s. Many specialties have been born on the back of a special instrument or technique and gastroenterology was no exception. Once it was possible for anyone with average technical ability to examine the upper gastrointestinal tract the specialty blossomed. Duodenal ulcers could be diagnosed with certainty and multiple biopsies obtained from suspicious lesions in the stomach under direct vision. Within a few years upper gastrointestinal endoscopy had almost replaced radiology.[128/129] Shortly afterwards the first really effective treatment for peptic ulcer, the histamine H2 antagonists, became available. This led to a remarkable change in attitude. Doctors now almost hoped they would find an ulcer because they could treat it. It was almost too good to be true and wonderful for the long-suffering ulcer patient.

But what became of the dyspeptics without an ulcer? Previously these people had been considered lucky not to have the disease but now almost the opposite applied. They were not always satisfied with simple reassurance and wanted effective treatment too. Previous surveys of peptic ulcer had already indicated that non-ulcer dyspepsia was common. In 1968 Deans Weir (born 1926) and Maurice Backett (1916–2009), two distinguished epidemiologists in Aberdeen, studied a population in semi-rural north-east Scotland and confirmed Doll's findings that nearly one man in every four suffered from dyspepsia, half of whom had an ulcer. The study was meticulous and brought home just how common both ulcer and non-ulcer dyspepsia were.

b) Definition of functional dyspepsia

It was clear that functional dyspepsia was difficult to define, hard to explain and awkward to treat. It was intangible, frustrating and a huge problem for everybody, patients, doctors and health economists alike; indeed along with irritable bowel syndrome it was becoming the new scourge. For several years the diagnosis was made by excluding significant pathology with an endoscopy. This was a conclusive test, provided excellent training opportunities for fledgling endoscopists and, I dare say, a useful source of income for those engaged in private practice.

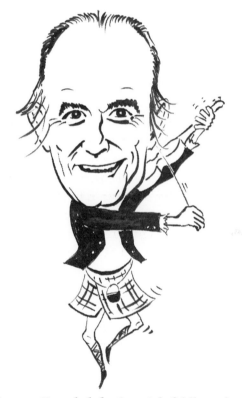

72 Crean – Founded the Scottish fiddle orchestra.

Peptic ulcers were in decline and most endoscopies were normal. This naturally led people to question whether so many tests were necessary. Could the discomfort of an endoscopy, medical workload and financial cost be justified? Surely doctors could be more selective in their requests for endoscopy? Several groups tried to tackle the problem but there were difficulties. The definition of dyspepsia was one; what did people mean by dyspepsia and what did doctors understand by it? Throughout the 1980s several groups pondered this, none more than Gerald Crean and his colleagues in Glasgow.

Gerry Crean (1927–97) qualified in Dublin and worked in Edinburgh for several years studying the effect of hormones on the growth of gastric mucosa. While there he came under the influence of Wilfrid Card (1908–85) and followed him to Glasgow in 1967. Card had formed a diagnostic methodology research unit and on his retirement in 1974 Crean took over as its director. Over the next thirteen years together with his colleague Robin Knill-Jones (born 1940) he measured and analysed the evidence provided by symptoms of dyspepsia and developed a computer program that interrogated patients, elicited evidence from them and calculated the likely diagnosis. By the end of an enormous, prospective study of more than 1,500 patients he was able to make a confident diagnosis of functional dyspepsia in only half the patients who actually had it. He admitted that functional dyspepsia was incapable of explicit definition.[130] Diagnosis still rested on symptomatic evidence supported to a greater or lesser extent by exclusion of organic disease by investigation. The amount of investigation required depended on the confidence with which the diagnosis could be made; generally doctors were more comfortable with a diagnosis of organic disease than a functional disorder that depends on a greater readiness to accept clinical evidence. In his spare time Crean was passionate about Irish and Scottish traditional fiddle music and formed a large and enthusiastic fiddle orchestra. He was a lovable man, and few presidents of the British Society of Gastroenterology have had more charm, wit, and native cunning.[131]

The enigma of dyspepsia also attracted Timothy de Dombal (1935–97), another inspirational character who was also a keen musician, this time a jazz pianist. After qualifying in Cambridge, de Dombal went to Leeds and became senior lecturer in surgery on John Goligher's unit. From the start he was fascinated by the process of clinical diagnosis and was one of the first to use a computer to collect and retrieve data. In 1981 he became director of the clinical information unit at Leeds University and later was awarded a personal chair in this specialty. For many years he worked with Jane Horrocks, a computer programmer in the department of surgery, hoping to show that a computer was at least as effective as a clinician in reaching a diagnosis. Unfortunately in the case of dyspepsia though the computer made an accurate diagnosis of organic disease it struggled with functional dyspepsia, predicting that half the patients with X-ray negative dyspepsia would have organic lesions.[132] There were simply not enough positive features to make the diagnosis.

The size of the problem was emphasised by Richard Harvey (born 1940) and Alan Read (1926–93) in Bristol. Concerned by the apparent frequency of functional disease seen in their outpatient clinics, they looked at 2,000 patients between 1976 and 1979 and found that almost half had a functional disorder.[133] Most had some form of irritable bowel syndrome and one in ten had dyspepsia. In fact the figure for dyspepsia would have been larger had they included patients referred directly by their general practitioner for gastroscopy. They highlighted the problem of definition suggesting that it was somewhat illogical to separate dyspepsia from the irritable bowel group as the two conditions often overlapped. They too were worried by the extensive investigation of these patients and hoped a solution or compromise could be found.

Stimulated by these concerns, a group of ten gastroenterologists from Europe, America and Australia met at the time of the AGA meeting in Chicago in 1987 to suggest a practical approach to the management of dyspepsia.[134] The chairman was Duncan Colin-Jones (born 1938) from Portsmouth who was interested in classifying dyspepsia into clinical subgroups for treatment purposes. The group that included Gerry Crean defined dyspepsia in the broadest terms covering the whole range of symptomatic upper gastrointestinal disease. Non-ulcer dyspepsia was defined as the presence of these symptoms lasting for more than four weeks without a detectable cause, which of course implied that investigation was always needed to exclude focal disease. This was certainly the case in older patients but not necessarily so in the young in whom organic disease was much less likely. In highlighting that younger dyspeptics without alarm symptoms did not require investigation, the working party did a great service to those trying to reduce the workload of endoscopy. In effect the report was the first of many guidelines soon to be so popular with the British Society of Gastroenterology. The committee subdivided non-ulcer dyspepsia into various subgroups according to symptoms including reflux-like, dysmotility-like, ulcer-like and idiopathic (non-specific) dyspepsia, but admitted that the causes of dyspepsia were poorly understood. They reviewed what was known about the pathophysiology and, apart from the old chestnuts of gastritis, acidity and psychological factors, emphasised the overlap with irritable bowel syndrome and the fact that at least half the patients with unexplained dyspepsia have some delay in gastric emptying with antral hypomotility. There was a natural tendency for non-ulcer dyspepsia to improve and patients should be given general advice and firm reassurance. The large placebo response made specific treatments difficult to evaluate or to recommend. Nonetheless, individual subgroups sometimes seemed to benefit from drug therapy, for example H2-receptor antagonists in ulcer-like dyspepsia.

CHAPTER FIFTY-SIX

IRRITABLE COLON SYNDROME IN THE MID-TWENTIETH CENTURY

a) Clinical aspects

It was not until the 1980s that the profession as a whole began to take functional dyspepsia seriously, by which time the irritable bowel syndrome had been the subject of attention for three decades. Precisely who coined the term I do not know but Sir Edmund Spriggs (1871–1949), physician in charge of a clinic for metabolic disease in Ruthin Castle in North Wales, may have been the first to mention it. He had always been interested in gastroenterology but his career at St. George's Hospital was cut short by a tuberculous pleural effusion and he was advised to leave London. In 1931 he reviewed 242 cases of functional disorders of the colon; two thirds had mucous colitis and a third had irritable colon, spasm and nervous diarrhoea.[135] This was an impressive personal series for the time but unfortunately his analysis of the clinical features took no account of his own subdivisions, so the result is somewhat confused. Nonetheless he did emphasise that purgatives, infective dysentery and psychological factors were common predisposing causes. Spriggs was a founder member of the Gastro-Enterological Club in 1937 and President of the British Society of Gastroenterologists in 1947, as the BSG was then known.

The expression "The Irritable Bowel Syndrome" was the title of a review by Arnold Bargen (1894–1976) at the Mayo Clinic in 1942[136] and it was the Americans, notably Thomas Almy (born 1920) and Maurice Tulin in New York, who were the first to show that the colon in these patients seemed unduly susceptible to stress.[137] Their methods would raise the eyebrows of an ethical committee today. For example, a fourth-year medical student was asked to take part in an experiment that would only require a sigmoidoscopy. After ten minutes of observation, it was implied that carcinoma of the rectum had been discovered. Horrified, the poor fellow's rectum went into spasm and became engorged until the hoax was explained. They also studied the effect of physical stress and this was fairly brutal too, producing a similar response; in one series of experiments the subjects had their heads compressed by a head screw for 30 minutes.

In 1957 Walter Palmer (1896–1993) and Joseph Kirsner (1909-2012) presented a remarkably perceptive review of the problem to a postgraduate course in gastroenterology in Denver, Colorado.[138] Palmer himself suffered from an irritable colon which he gave as his reason for specialising in gastroenterology. He became Professor of Medicine in Chicago and was succeeded on his retirement by his colleague Kirsner. Both lived to a great age and were legendary figures in American gastroenterology. In their review, published the following year, they suggested that the irritable bowel was often part of a functional disorder of the entire digestive tract, reflecting an autonomic imbalance that was psychogenic. It was very common, masquerading as a variety of digestive complaints, and often began in childhood. Dysentery could initiate it as could emotional factors, by which they meant the usual problems and frustrations of life rather than serious psychiatric disease. The digestive complaints were frequently accompanied by symptoms such as fatigue, headache, palpitation, dysmenorrhoea and urinary frequency, all in their view physiological concomitants of systemic vasomotor instability. As usual the most important part of treatment was firm but sympathetic reassurance, which had to be repeated again and again. Much of what Palmer and Kirsner had to say in their paper has been rediscovered and regurgitated many times, reflecting how little of note has been added since.

In Britain meanwhile the spastic colon was attracting little attention. Gastroenterology was still practised by general physicians who found other diseases more interesting. For example cardiac surgery had given cardiology a new impetus, metabolic and endocrine diseases were stimulated by advances in biochemistry, and haemodialysis was an exciting new venture. As far as the gut was concerned, interest in peptic ulcer still reigned supreme, though ulcerative colitis was catching up thanks to effective new treatment. People with abdominal pain and an irregular bowel habit were referred to a surgeon in case they had cancer. Once this was excluded they were reassured and sent back to plague their hapless general practitioner. There were exceptions of course and Sidney Truelove (1913–2002) in Oxford was one.

Truelove worked in the Nuffield Department of Clinical Medicine at the Radcliffe Infirmary and was well known for his famous trial showing that cortisone was effective in severe ulcerative colitis. His forte was clinical research and he excelled at identifying a clinical problem and devising an experiment to solve it. He was also interested in the natural history of disease and a keen epidemiologist and was well aware that functional bowel disease was common. In 1962 he published a seminal paper on the irritable colon syndrome with Nazir Chaudhary, his research assistant who later became professor of medicine in Karachi. Their study was an analysis of 130 patients and most of their findings were in agreement with Palmer and Kirsner's observations, but it was an important paper as it drew attention to the irritable colon syndrome in this country for the first time.[139]

Chaudhary and Truelove found that many more patients had a painful spastic colon than painless diarrhoea and they were impressed by the number who had had an unnecessary appendicectomy. Dysentery and psychological factors were important predisposing causes but the regular use of laxatives was not as common as people thought. Treatment centred on reassurance, anticholinergics, phenobarbitone and a bland bulk provider such as isogel. In a few patients who responded poorly to treatment, relaxation under light hypnosis appeared to help. They found that patients with painless diarrhoea as well as those who had had dysentery fared best. Not surprisingly people with insoluble psychological problems did worst.

b) Manometry

Truelove assumed that the symptoms were caused by colonic spasm and attempted to measure this. At the time the study of gastrointestinal motility occupied a small niche in academic gastroenterology and was dominated by physiologists and pharmacologists exploring the function of smooth muscle. The few clinicians showing any interest in the field confined themselves to the oesophagus and stomach.

Truelove confirmed the opinion of Thomas Almy in New York that the colon was unusually active in these people. The Americans had used large balloons inserted into the lower colon and coupled to manometers to measure colonic pressure whereas Truelove used open-ended water-filled tubes inserted through a sigmoidoscope. In fact it is frequently impossible to insert a rigid sigmoidoscope as far as the sigmoid colon, particularly without the use of insufflation, and many recordings were probably taken from the rectum. Nonetheless, the Oxford group believed that in the majority of patients they had managed to show that the colon was highly sensitive to the same psychological events that had originally brought on the symptoms.[140]

Truelove employed an ex-Royal Navy doctor, James Ritchie (1920–90) to continue this research. Ritchie settled down in Oxford as an honorary senior registrar in the Nuffield Department of Clinical Medicine where he became an expert in colonic measurement, indeed his sole medical interest was the colon. Working with Gordon Ardran (1917–94), a distinguished radiologist, he filmed the passage of barium in normal subjects and was able to show how the colon mixed, stored and propelled its contents.[141] Transit was achieved by interhaustral shuttling, propulsion, retropulsion and to-and-fro movements. Ritchie's careful observations were especially valuable because even though he reduced the amount of irradiation by using a time-lapse cine technique, the exposure was considerable and his studies cannot now be repeated. He also measured pressure generated in the sigmoid colon but found no consistent correlation between any form of pressure wave and any type of colonic contraction seen radiologically.[142] "Pressure tracings," wrote Ritchie, "show almost every imaginable form of pressure change." He realised that he was unlikely to find a motor abnormality that was typical of irritable colon syndrome. This was disappointing but he found the cinefluorography technique useful for studying the pain felt by patients with irritable bowel disease, work for which he is best remembered. Using large balloons inserted into the sigmoid colon, he showed that patients were unusually sensitive to distension.[143]

At the same time another group at the Central Middlesex Hospital were carrying out almost identical experiments. The hospital had become the Mecca for young gastroenterologists after the Second World War, thanks to the inspiration of Francis Avery Jones. With funds from the Nuffield Foundation, Medical Research Council and the Regional Hospital

Board he built and equipped a new unit, which was opened in 1957. Eirwyn Rowlands (1912–2003), a clinical physiologist, was in charge of the laboratories at the hospital on a part-time basis. "Tom" Rowlands was also deputy director of the Medical Research Council's department of clinical research at University College Hospital under the leadership of Sir Eric Pochin. Soon after the new gastroenterology unit at the Central Middlesex Hospital opened Avery Jones managed to persuade the Medical Research Council to establish an MRC gastroenterology research unit there, even though it was not a teaching hospital, on the grounds that it was full of gastrointestinal patients suitable for physiological research. Tom Rowlands was appointed its director in 1960.

Avery Jones had told the Medical Research Council that one of his projects was the study of functional gastrointestinal disorders. It was partly with this in mind that he had originally encouraged Rowlands to join his team. Rowlands had long been interested in gut mobility and in the late 1950s teamed up with Heinz Wolff, an electronic wizard at the bioengineering laboratory of the National Institute for Medical Research, Mill Hill. Wolff managed to construct a pressure-sensitive radio pill that could be swallowed and traced in the gut by an aerial.[144] Rowlands hoped that it would be possible to record on a smoke drum both its progress through the intestine and the pressure waves associated with its propulsion. There were many technical problems in the early days, for example, background interference had to be suppressed and he was obliged to screen a room completely with copper foil and install a choke filter in the electricity supply. But they got it to work.

While the radio pill was being developed, the focus of motility studies at the Central Middlesex Hospital had been the oesophagus and stomach, especially the nature of the lower oesophageal sphincter and the mechanism of gastric emptying. Working with David Edwards (1920–2001), A. J. Honour and Michael Atkinson, Rowlands used fine open-ended tubes attached to a manometer to measure the pressure differences across the lower oesophageal sphincter. Unfortunately these were technically unsuitable for measurements in the pylorus so he replaced the open tip with a chain of small balloons. These gave identical recordings as the open tubes did not get blocked with debris and could be positioned with greater accuracy.[145] Their work has been described in the chapter on oesophageal disease, but is mentioned here because Avery Jones and Rowlands realised that the miniature balloons were tailor-made for the measurement of pressures within the rectum and distal colon. Indeed they should complement the work with the radio pill in the proximal colon.

The goal, indeed the Holy Grail, was to elucidate the cause of the irritable bowel syndrome and establish logical and effective treatment for it. For nearly twenty years a series of research fellows at the Central Middlesex Hospital studied the problem. It was tedious and frustrating work, and though interest in motility steadily increased, it was never popular with the majority of gastroenterologists because the measurements were difficult to obtain and interpret and clinically unhelpful.

The first research fellow was Alastair Connell (born 1931) who studied the motility of the sigmoid colon in several hundred patients by recording pressures with these tiny balloons. He devised an index of colonic activity that was a product of the duration of activity and the mean amplitude of the pressure waves. The colon was a surprisingly active organ but as Ritchie had found, its activity varied widely from person to person and from day to day in the same subject.[146] This made it impossible to establish a normal pattern but fortunately the organ was nearly always stimulated by a meal, which was a useful provocation test. Most of the pressure waves were non-propulsive and slowed colonic movement, so people with an overactive colon were often constipated. Conversely colonic movements were reduced in diarrhoeal states.[147] On one occasion Connell visited Cairo to confirm this observation in patients with diarrhoea following amoebic dysentery.[148]

But it was abdominal pain that generated most interest. Generally speaking patients with unexplained abdominal pain (after full investigation) were found to have exceptionally high pressures in the sigmoid colon, especially after the stimulus of a meal. Avery Jones thought the pain was due to local distension of the colon by air trapped in the colon by exaggerated segmentation.[149] Thus many patients with abdominal pain probably had a spastic colon.

Soon after his appointment Connell was joined by George Misiewicz (born 1930). Misiewicz arrived from Poland in 1947 and qualified at St. Bartholemew's Hospital. He had aspirations to a career in clinical haematology but while waiting for a job took a locum post with Avery Jones at the Central Middlesex and never looked back. He quickly became involved in the motility programme, which was just as well because Connell decided that a career in research in Britain was incompatible with a reasonable standard of living and left in 1964 to seek his fortune in America (after a brief stint in Belfast working with Thomas Parks (born 1935) in the department of surgery). Misiewicz became a permanent member of the staff and collaborated with a series of research fellows who went on to have distinguished careers in gastroenterology. Among the first were Douglas Holdstock (born 1935) and Sheila Waller, a pharmacologist. In a study on the mechanism of obscure abdominal pain they demonstrated that the small intestine was involved as well as the colon and speculated that this could be due to the effect of 5-hydroxytryptamine, a well-known gut stimulant. On the other hand not all the patients with hyperactive colons had pain and there were some people with pain whose colons were not hypercontactile, implying that raised intraluminal pressure was not always painful. They could only suggest, like others before them, that people vary in their sensitivity to visceral stimuli,[150] and that stress has a considerable role.[151] Holdstock was later appointed physician to Ashford Hospital, Middlesex and became well known for his vigorous opposition to nuclear power and weapons and was appointed secretary to the campaigning group Medical Action for Global Security.

The work done in Oxford and at the Central Middlesex Hospital during the 1960s was unusual because interest in motility was confined to a small international group of physiologists. So though cyclical fasting motor activity of the gut had been recognised as hunger contractions for many years, few clinicians noticed when Jo Szurszewski, a physiologist working at the Mayo Clinic, made the key observation that this cyclic fasting activity was migratory.[152] Undaunted, the physiologists formed an international motility club and in 1969 held the first biennial international symposium in Erlangen, Germany.

CHAPTER FIFTY-SEVEN

FUNCTIONAL GI DISEASE IN THE 1970S: THE RISE OF FIBRE

During the 1970s three events combined to stimulate interest in functional bowel disease.

Firstly though Truelove and Avery Jones had drawn attention to the irritable bowel syndrome it was a humble substance, wheat bran, that caught the imagination of patients and turned those three words, irritable bowel syndrome, into a household phrase. It was exceedingly common and doctors could no longer ignore it but they found it hard to define, difficult to explain and frustrating to treat.

Secondly new ways to measure gut motility were being developed and research was galvanised by support from the pharmaceutical industry especially Janssen Pharmaceutica. This Belgian company founded by Dr. Paul Janssen, a brilliant pharmaceutical chemist, had recently launched a highly successful product, loperamide, unequalled to this day in the management of diarrhoea. Later in the early 1980s the company discovered another drug for which they needed a clinical role. This was cisapride, which in vitro improved antroduodenal coordination in the isolated guinea pig stomach and duodenum. Undeterred by the fact that impaired antroduodenal coordination was not a recognised clinical disorder, the chemists reasoned that the drug might be helpful in treating the "functional gastrointestinal disorders", especially dyspepsia. Given the worldwide market for such a product the company decided to invest heavily in supporting research across the whole field of gastrointestinal motility.

The third exciting development was the discovery of the "gut hormones". For a time doctors thought that these peptides controlled or at least modulated gut motility and it was hoped that they would provide the key to unlock the mysteries of functional disorders.

In 1967 three surgeons, Peter Cleave, Neil Painter and Denis Burkitt began an extraordinary collaboration. They could not have been more different in background, temperament or careers, but they had one thing in common, a belief in the value of dietary fibre. Thanks to their missionary zeal and utter conviction, by the mid-1970s the citizens of Britain and the United States were either munching bran or knew someone who was, and as a topic of conversation it seemed to be second only to the state of the weather.

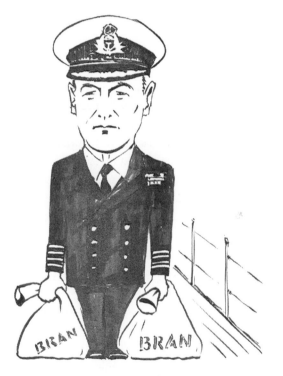

73 Cleave – The bran man.

Surgical Captain T. L. (Peter) Cleave (1906–83) was Director of Medical Research to the Royal Navy with a bee in his bonnet. He had spent his life gathering evidence (he wrote over 20,000 letters in longhand to doctors all over the world) to support his view that the human body was maladapted to the artificial foods of civilisation, in particular the refined carbohydrates, sugar and white flour. If man avoided unnatural foods he would surely avoid unnatural diseases, that is, diseases that did not occur in primitive peoples. These included diabetes, coronary heart disease, peptic ulcer, gall stones, appendicitis, constipation, haemorrhoids and diverticular disease.

Cleave believed that a refined diet led to small stools, straining and high pressures in the colon causing diverticulosis. He was aware that cereals encouraged a regular bowel habit and many years before, in 1941, he had been one of the first to advocate bran in medical practice while serving on the battleship HMS *King George V*. Constipation was endemic on board ship and fresh fruit and vegetables unobtainable so Cleave took raw, unprocessed bran himself for several days and found that it cured his constipation. Subsequently he ordered sacks of bran to be brought on board and given to the sailors.[153] This was so effective that Cleave became known in the navy as "the bran man".

He published several books on the dangers of eating a refined diet, all at his own expense, but they were ignored. These included *Diabetes,Coronary Thrombosis and the Saccharine Disease* written in 1966 with Duncan Campbell, a diabetologist, despite a supportive forward from Richard Doll.[154] The problem was that Cleave had no time for statistical analysis or controlled trials; he was recording big differences in disease patterns worldwide over decades, long before the epidemiology of chronic disease was a recognised discipline. He felt isolated but hated criticism and upset people who dared to disagree with him. But his luck was about to change.

In May 1967 Richard Doll (1912–2005), director of the Medical Research Council's statistical unit, introduced Cleave to Denis Burkitt in what turned out to be a key meeting between the two men. Burkitt (1911–93), a charming Irishman, was by this time famous for his discovery of Burkitt's lymphoma in 1963; a triumph of epidemiological research in Africa undertaken when he was working for the Colonial Office. He had recently returned to London to take up a post with the Medical Research Council.

Cleave told him all about his theory that many Western diseases, including diverticulosis, resulted from the overconsumption of refined sugar. He added that the medical profession had ignored him and that his ideas were unacceptable to conventional medical thought. However, Burkitt agreed to read the first edition of *Diabetes, Coronary Thrombosis*

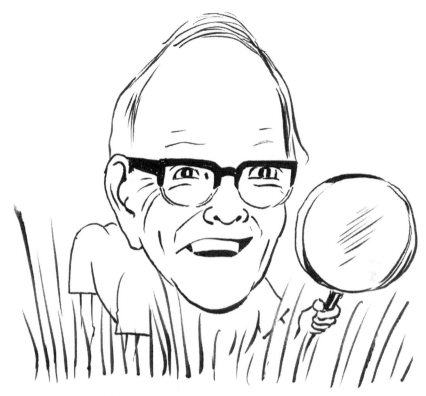

74 Burkitt – Big – stool hunter.

and the Saccharine Disease, which had just been published. He recognised a similarity with his own work on lymphoma – the possibility that several seemingly unrelated diseases could have a common cause. He was also aware from his own experience that several of the Western diseases mentioned by Cleave were virtually unknown in Africa. But he thought that a lack of fibre in the diet was a more likely reason for the problem than an excess of refined sugar. Cleave did not agree, though he accepted that fibre helped constipation.

Both men knew that they needed scientific support for the fibre theory but Cleave was now retired and Burkitt did not have access to patients in Britain. Possibly at Doll's suggestion they arranged to meet a surgeon working at the Manor House Hospital, a small trade union hospital in Golders Green. The surgeon, Neil Painter (1923–89), had been senior registrar at the Radcliffe Infirmary where under the supervision of Sydney Truelove he had studied the pathogenesis of diverticular disease using open-ended tubes inserted up the rectum to measure pressure. By correlating changes in pressure with what he saw using cineradiography he had shown that the sigmoid colon could generate very high pressures by segmenting itself into pockets or "little bladders". Diverticula developed at weak spots in the colonic wall. Painter had noted that these high pressures occurred after certain stimuli such as food and were more likely if the colon had a narrow bore.[155] This seminal work was the subject of his Hunterian lecture in 1963.

Cleave's hypothesis appealed to Painter who was already thinking along the same lines[156] and he agreed to undertake a trial of bran in patients with diverticular disease. He recruited 70 patients over three years and the vast majority were satisfied with the outcome. Their bowels improved and they no longer required laxatives. Furthermore those with colic became almost pain-free.[157] During the study Painter wrote a chapter on diverticular disease in the second edition of Diabetes, Coronary Thrombosis and the Saccharine Disease, which was published in 1969 with Painter as co-editor.[158] This time the book was well received and sold well. Painter had given scientific credibility to Cleave's theory and Cleave had helped to publicise Painter's work. Both men deserved this encouragement, Cleave after years in the wilderness and Painter after his disappointment at not securing a consultant post in a recognised NHS hospital.

Burkitt and Painter next looked into the history of diverticular disease in Britain and found that it was first recognised as a significant problem in 1920. Further research revealed that the amount of fibre consumed in Britain fell dramatically in 1880 when stone-ground flour was replaced by a new milling process that extracted more fibre. Burkitt argued that diverticular disease only became common a generation later in people whose colons had been unable to adapt to this new low-residue diet.[159] Painter agreed and thought that fibre produced a bulky stool, kept the lumen of the colon open and prevented excessive segmentation. Hitherto a low-residue diet had been the standard treatment of diverticular disease in the mistaken belief that "roughage" irritated the colon.

Burkitt also used his influence abroad. At the time he was receiving monthly cancer figures from more than 150 Third World hospitals. He sent his colonial colleagues a questionnaire enquiring about the incidence of diverticular disease in rural Africans. They reported back that they had scarcely, if ever, seen a case. The condition was almost unknown as Cleave had maintained.

Encouraged by this information, Burkitt visited a village in Africa and weighed the stools of fifteen villagers living on a high-fibre diet. Their average daily faecal output was more than four times that of a group of senior boys at an English public school.[160]

He and Painter then teamed up with Alec Walker (1913–2007) to compare gut transit times between Africans and Englishmen. They used a technique to measure transit devised by John Lennard-Jones at St. Mark's Hospital, who had a special interest in constipation.[161] Walker, who worked in Johannesburg, was an old friend of Burkitt and had recently shown that most food residue passed through the African's gut within 48 hours whereas in Englishmen this took twice as long.[162] The swiftly-passed stool required little effort and did not favour the development of diverticula.[163] Walker commented that the South African Bantu passes large moist stools without straining on demand. They must have been a joy to study.

When Burkitt first became enthused with the subject of fibre he was already in demand, giving lectures about his lymphoma. Yet within six months he was extolling the virtues of fibre instead. At a major lymphoma conference in Ann Arbor, Michigan, he surprised his audience by lecturing not on Burkitt's lymphoma as expected but on Cleave's hypothesis. Thereafter in a series of spell-binding lectures, he alerted doctors all over the world to the idea that fibre-depleted diets were harmful.

After one of these lectures Burkitt was approached by a retired clergyman, Hugh Trowell, who had met him years before in Uganda. The Rev Hubert Trowell (1904–89) had been physician/paediatrician at Mulago Hospital, Kampala. In 1957 he referred a five-year-old boy to Burkitt with a tumour in his neck and this turned out to be the first case of Burkitt's lymphoma. Over the years Trowell's main interest had been in nutrition and he was one of the first to identify kwashiorkor as a nutritional disease in the 1930s. He retired in 1959 to enter theological training and published his chief work *Non-infective Disease in Africa* in 1960.[164] In the book he listed 30 diseases that were rare in Africa such as coronary artery disease, diabetes and bowel cancer, but though he believed that nutrition played a key role he had been unable to find a coherent hypothesis to explain their rarity. After hearing Burkitt expounding Cleave's theory in 1970, Trowell realised that it would explain many of the facts he had accumulated. By this time he had retired from the ministry and at Burkitt's suggestion met Cleave for an exchange of views. The meeting was not a success. Cleave was developing Alzheimer's disease and was suspicious of Trowell's motives. Trowell, a sensitive man, felt slighted and never got over it. But he believed in Cleave's theory and worked productively with his old friend, Burkitt, who was a model of diplomacy. With his support Trowell turned the emphasis away from the harmful nature of fibre-depleted foods towards the protective nature of fibre itself. In this sense he can be regarded as the author of the bran hypothesis, though he also stressed the dangers of fat and sugar, especially in regard to coronary artery disease. His chief contribution to the fibre story was a definition. In the early 1970s fibre was accepted as synonymous with plant cell walls that were indigestible, but terms like "crude fibre" and "unavailable carbohydrate" confused the issue.[165] Trowell formally proposed the term "dietary fibre" and defined it as "that part of the plant material taken in our diet which is resistant to digestion by the secretions of the human gastrointestinal tract".[166] Unfortunately he was something of a cyclops intellectually and would turn a conversation about, say, Ming vases back to his beloved fibre at every opportunity.

Burkitt and Trowell were both committed Christians and to a large extent missionaries. They adopted Cleave's hypothesis with considerable fervour and ensured that no one could be in doubt about the importance of fibre. Burkitt wrote a bestseller in 1979, *Don't Forget Fibre in Your Diet,*[167] that was translated into nine languages, Cleave wrote a third and final edition of *The Saccharine Disease*[168] in 1974, which sold thousands of copies, Trowell edited *Western Diseases: Their Emergence and Prevention*[169] with 34 other authors in 1981 at the age of 77 and even Painter came up with *Diverticular Disease of the Colon: A Deficiency Disease of Western Civilisation.*[170]

When Burkitt first met Cleave in 1967 he had been unable to find any articles under the title "Fibre" in the *Cumulative Index Medicus*. He himself soon changed this with his publications but physicians showed little interest. Diverticular disease was not really a disease at all and though diverticula were very common in older people the majority did not have symptoms. The minority who suffered pain or constipation could take bran and if diverticulitis supervened then it was a surgical problem anyway and not all that common.

But suppose irritable bowel was included with diverticular disease, what then? All at once the commonest gastrointestinal disorder in Britain would be a candidate for bran. The argument was seductive. The so-called pre-diverticular state appeared to resemble the irritable colon closely.[171] Truelove wrote, "It appears likely that in both conditions the underlying mechanism is a functional disorder of the colonic musculature."[172] A few years later Painter went further when he suggested that the bowel was not irritable but irritated; irritated by the lack of fibre in its lumen.[173]

When the Nutrition Society decided it was time to hold an international meeting on dietary fibre in 1972 their choice of chairman was limited. Very few physicians knew anything about fibre. In fact the choice was fairly simple, Martin Eastwood, a physician in Edinburgh, and David Southgate, a biochemist in Cambridge.

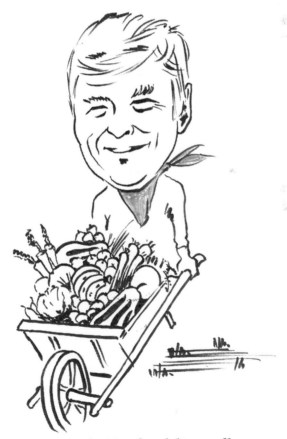

75 *Eastwood – Moral and dietary fibre.*

Eastwood (born 1935) was a gastroenterologist at the Western Infirmary, Edinburgh with the ability to cram two days' work into one. For some years he had been interested in the effect of bile salts on fat absorption and was aware that fibre could reduce this effect by absorbing them in the gut. With this in mind he had fed cereal fibre (bran) to a community of monks in the hope that it would lower their blood cholesterol.[174] It hadn't but in the process of his research Eastwood had become intrigued by the role of dietary fibre.

Southgate (1930–2008) was a biochemist at the Medical Research Council Nutrition Unit, Dunn Nutritional Laboratory in Cambridge. He had studied fibre and other "unavailable" carbohydrates to see if they had any energy value in man. A modest and unassuming man, he knew a great deal about the chemical and physical properties of fibre[175] and later became editor of the *British Journal of Nutrition*.

Eastwood spoke on the physical properties of vegetable fibre at the meeting[176] and subsequently investigated their effect on colonic function in patients with diverticular disease and the irritable bowel syndrome, working for several years alongside Adam Smith, Reader (and later Professor) in Clinical Surgery in Edinburgh.

Among those at the Edinburgh meeting was the highly influential Francis Avery Jones (1910–98). "Avery" (as he was known to his friends and colleagues) had his fingers in so many gastroenterological pies that it would be easy to overlook his interest in dietary fibre. His mother had been a firm believer in the benefits of brown bread thanks to the preaching of the Victorian physician Thomas Allinson (1858–1918), who held that it was the true staff of life, "not a luxury, a necessity".[177] So Avery Jones grew up imbued with the importance of good nutrition and in 1940 was appointed to the staff of the Central Middlesex Hospital as physician to the dietetic department (the nearest thing to a gastroenterology department in those days). After the war he was appointed consultant to the Royal Navy and got to know Cleave, so he was familiar with his views on the dangers of eating refined sugar at a time when most people knew nothing about them or thought they were nonsense. About the time of the Edinburgh meeting Avery edited a book *Management of Constipation* and in the preface credited Painter, Burkitt, Cleave, Walker and others with "a recent advance of outstanding importance" in showing that fibre accelerates bowel transit. In his own chapter on management Avery leant heavily on diet as the first line, including bran, and included a sample high-fibre diet sheet.[178]

Avery knew that Cleave believed in Berkeley Moynihan's old idea that gall stones were the direct result of infection from the gut. "Every gall stone is a tombstone erected to the evil memory of the germs that lie dead within it."[179] According to Cleave a refined diet caused intestinal stasis, which increased the risk of biliary infection and stones. Most people no longer believed this theory but Avery was shrewd enough not to argue the point. Instead he put Cleave in touch with a young gastroenterologist in Bristol, Kenneth Heaton.

Heaton (1936–2013), a gentle thoughtful man, had worked as a clinical clerk for Avery Jones during his training. He moved to Bristol as medical registrar to Professor Alan Read in 1965, where he stayed for the rest of his career becoming Reader in Medicine at Bristol University in 1979. For some years he studied bile salt metabolism and the aetiology of gallstones. In 1969 he was asked by the editor of *Gut*, then Avery Jones, to write a review on the role of bile salts.[180] In the final paragraph Heaton quoted Cleave's book *The Saccharine Disease* with approval, having idly picked it up in the Bristol Medical Library earlier that year. He had been impressed with how Cleave's indictment of refined carbohydrates chimed with his knowledge of bile salt metabolism and the manipulation of bile salts by diet in laboratory animals. When Avery read the review he showed it to Cleave, who wrote to Heaton in August 1969. This was the first of many broadsides, as Heaton called them, from Cleave, who was delighted that Heaton thought excess sugar could cause gall stones but upset that he did not believe in the infection theory. After a lengthy correspondence, Heaton managed to convert Cleave to the view that intestinal stasis caused gallstones by encouraging the formation of lithogenic bile rather than infection. The following year the two men met and became good friends. Later Cleave acknowledged Heaton's work in the third edition of *The Saccharine Disease* and meanwhile Heaton decided he would re-examine the claim that fibre in the form of bran accelerated intestinal transit.

The prospect was appealing; bran was cheap and harmless, patients with irritable bowel syndrome were plentiful and willing to try anything new, the measurement of transit time was simple, and he had the enthusiastic support of Richard Harvey (born 1940) who was interested in functional gastrointestinal disorders. Harvey, a genial man, had been

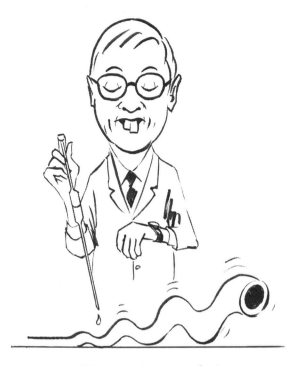

76 Harvey – Gut stimulation.

appointed Lecturer in Medicine at the University of Bristol by Alan Read after holding a research fellowship at the Central Middlesex Hospital where he had gained experience in the measurement of colonic motility. He was particularly interested in the hormonal control of gastro-intestinal motility and with Read had recently shown that an infusion of cholecystokinin given to patients with the "food-related pain" variant of the irritable bowel syndrome produced symptoms identical to those experienced after meals.[181]

Harvey and Heaton found that fibre certainly speeded up gut transit in people with colonic stasis but it also seemed to slow transit in people with diarrhoea.[182] They suggested that bran in some way "normalised" colonic behaviour and was therefore ideal for patients with irritable bowel syndrome. They repeated the study in a group of schoolboys obtaining similar results[183] and sales of bran increased.

In fact these two studies were flawed as they were not placebo controlled and the statistical testing was not rigorous. Harvey and Heaton were observing the phenomenon of data regressing towards the mean with repeated measurement. But the trials were crucial in stimulating an interest in fibre and functional bowel disease that was to remain with them for the rest of their careers. A further controlled trial[184] in a small group of patients showed that bran improved bowel habit and abdominal pain and dampened colonic motor activity but there was indeed a placebo effect.

During the course of this study it became clear to Heaton and his new registrar, Adrian Manning (born 1948), that the term irritable bowel syndrome was imprecise to say the least. An experienced clinician might

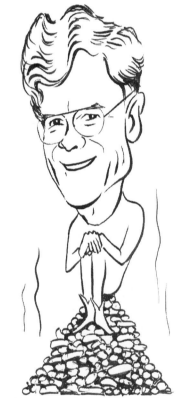

77 Heaton – A – stool – collector.

make a confident diagnosis but find it difficult to cite objective evidence for his conclusion. In the absence of objective signs the defining criteria had to be in terms of symptoms. Symptoms are subjective and Heaton knew that these could later be ignored, forgotten or denied by the patient. A patient's recall could also be unreliable, for example he found that constipated people often exaggerated their problem.[185] What did people mean when they said they were constipated or had diarrhoea? Indeed what was a normal bowel habit by which a patient's constipation or diarrhoea could be compared? People's gut transit time, frequency of defaecation and faecal weight varied enormously.[186] It was not surprising that many clinicians had been satisfied to define the irritable bowel syndrome simply by what it wasn't, that is, it wasn't an organic disease.

Heaton realised that if research into the condition was to continue a clear definition with emphasis on the positive features of the condition was needed. In 1976 he was joined by an enthusiastic Canadian research fellow, Grant Thompson, from Ottawa, who was also interested in defining the irritable bowel syndrome. Together Manning, Thompson and Heaton compared the symptoms of 32 patients with irritable bowel syndrome with 33 patients with organic abdominal disease such as peptic ulcer and colitis. They found that, of the many symptoms thought to be characteristic of irritable bowel syndrome, only distension, relief of pain with a bowel movement and more frequent and looser stools were more common in the people with irritable bowel syndrome. The more of these four symptoms that were present the more likely was the diagnosis to be irritable bowel syndrome. If a patient also passed mucus and had a feeling of incomplete evacuation he almost certainly had the syndrome.[187]

The Manning criteria, as they became widely known to the mild embarrassment of Adrian Manning, who was Heaton's research fellow at the time, were soon adopted by gastroenterologists in Europe and America and stood the test of time.[188] Critics argued that the criteria only discriminated between colonic and non-colonic pain and did not exclude colitis and other colonic diseases, but Heaton insisted that he was simply stressing the positive features of the irritable bowel syndrome,which could indeed be similar to other colonic disorders. He was not providing a definition of irritable bowel syndrome and was well aware that there were several subgroups of the condition that fell outside his criteria, notably unexplained abdominal pain and painless diarrhoea. His criteria were weighted towards patients with pain and distal colonic dysfunction, who were the commonest group.

CHAPTER FIFTY-EIGHT

MOTILITY STUDIES IN THE 1970S

a) Oesophagus

Motility research gathered pace during the 1970s spurred on by financial support from the pharmaceutical industry, improved technology and the need to define the underlying cause of functional disorders. Physiologists felt that a complex clinical classification would not help to elucidate the cause and was a distraction.

People knew more about the motility of the oesophagus than any other part of the gastrointestinal tract, because it was a relatively simple and accessible organ to investigate. Hurst had studied it with X-rays and balloons at the turn of the century. Later two physicians continued the fine tradition for clinical research at Guy's Hospital. Wilfred Payne (1894–1978) and Edward Poulton (1883–1939) working in the Medical Investigation Department in the 1920s suggested that visceral pain resulted from stretching the pain endings in the oesophageal wall. This could be burning or gripping in character and could be referred precordially.[189] After the Second World War, workers both in Britain and America used manometric techniques to study the lower oesophageal sphincter mechanism so that by the mid-1950s normal oesophageal peristalsis had been well defined.

Though cardiologists were well aware that oesophageal pain could have the same quality and distribution as angina pectoris, few physicians took much interest in the subject unless the pain was accompanied by dysphagia or typical reflux in which case it was a surgical problem anyway. The first gastroenterologists to study oesophageal pain were John Bennett (born 1934), then Sheldon research fellow at Birmingham

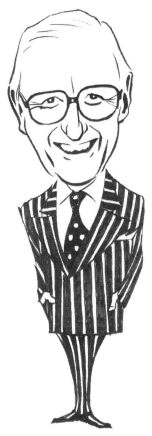

78 Bennett – Sartorial elegance.

and Michael Atkinson (born 1925) then physician at Worcester Royal Infirmary with a longstanding interest in motility. Both were experienced endoscopists, which was unusual among physicians at the time and they found that oesophagitis accounted for precordial pain alone in tweny per cent of their patients.[190] They may have overlooked some people with ischaemic heart disease because they did not have access to coronary angiography nor did they carry out exercise electrocardiography. On the other hand they were confident about the endoscopic diagnosis of oesophagitis and supplemented this by perfusing hydrochloric acid into the oesophagus in doubtful cases.[191] Bennett and Atkinson not only highlighted the importance of oesophageal disease as a cause of chest pain but went on to show that acid could cause oesophageal spasm as well as heartburn, explaining why the pain mimicked angina.[192]

Motility workers in Europe, notably Gaston Vantrappen in Leuven, Belgium identified a variety of oesophageal disorders during the 1970s, the commonest being diffuse oesophageal spasm.[193] By this time coronary angiography had become available, especially in America, and many patients with angina were found to have normal coronary arteries. Unlike Britain every large city in the United States had several gastroenterologists in private practice and soon large numbers of patients with chest pain were being referred to oesophageal manometry laboratories. It was an expanding and lucrative field as Charles Pope II (born 1928) and his colleagues in Seattle found; in a study of 43 patients with normal coronary arteries no fewer than half had oesophageal spasm.[194]

The situation in Britain was different. Patients were carefully selected for coronary angiography because resources were limited and if the investigation was normal the patient was firmly reassured and discharged back to the general practitioner. Access to oesophageal manometry was almost non-existent and gastroenterologists were neither interested nor trained in the technique. Full credit then to the cardiology department in Cardiff who were the first in Britain to use it. Andrew Henderson (born 1932), professor of cardiology, and his registrar Tony Dart (born 1951), were wondering if some of their patients with angina and normal coronary arteries might have coronary artery spasm which was a fashionable diagnosis at the time. They gave them ergometrine which is known to cause coronary spasm, and it certainly reproduced the pain, but this was not due to myocardial ischaemia.[195] Dart then suggested that oesophageal spasm might be responsible and showed this to be the case in half the patients who agreed to undergo oesophageal manometry. Ergometrine caused simultaneous pain and oesophageal spasm.[196] Clearly anginal pain due to oesophageal spasm was easy to overlook and commoner than people realised. About this time a doctor with both angina and oesophageal spasm wrote an amusing letter to the *Brit. Med. J.* explaining how he differentiated between the two by taking a hard swallow of saliva. If the pain was oesophageal, peristalsis overcame the spasm instantly, much to his relief and peace of mind.[197]

b) Stomach

Doctors had long believed that dysmotility was also a common cause of dyspepsia, but the stomach was a much more complicated organ to study than the oesophagus. From a clinical standpoint delayed gastric emptying was the most significant consequence of gastric dysmotility. Unfortunately for many years the only way to measure this in man was by X-rays or serial aspiration of a liquid meal.[198] A simple less invasive method was badly needed and came with the application of radionucleides in 1966 by Gwilym Griffith (born 1933) and Robert Shields, later Sir Robert (1930–2008), from the department of surgery at the Welsh National School of Medicine in Cardiff.[199] Not long afterwards the scanning process was greatly simplified by the arrival of the gamma camera.[200] At the time Robert Heading (born 1941) was a junior lecturer in Edinburgh working with David Shearman, then Senior Lecturer in Medicine, who was interested in how duodenal ulcer affected gastric emptying. Shearman handed Shields' paper to Heading and told him to develop the technique with the physics department. In due course Heading was able to measure the ability of the stomach to empty solid as well as liquid meals, which had been impossible with the older techniques.[201] He also worked with his colleagues in the therapeutics field to show how gastric emptying limited the absorption of drugs by controlling delivery into the small intestine. His research career accelerated and when Shearman unexpectedly left Edinburgh for Adelaide in 1975, Heading took his place as senior lecturer at the early age of 34.

Measurement of gastric emptying proved a valuable research tool and researchers confirmed previous X-ray studies that patients with dyspepsia often had slow or occasionally very rapid emptying. But few research centres in Britain made use of it because it required sophisticated and expensive gamma cameras and the results of emptying studies were difficult to interpret. The relationship between gastric emptying and upper gastrointestinal symptoms was still far from clear.

c) Small intestine

During the 1970s physiologists also began to understand the pattern of small bowel activity. For many years they had known that the jejunum responded to a meal with clusters of small contractions to mix the food thoroughly (so-called minute rhythm) interspersed by much larger contractions to move the contents down the lumen to the colon. An excess of minute rhythm for whatever reason was often associated with diarrhoea. However, Szurszewski's discovery of the migrating myoelectric complex in fasting dogs was important because it ultimately led to a completely new concept of gut innervation. Charles Code (1910–97), the eminent physiologist at the Mayo Clinic, next noticed that the migrating myoelectric complex (MMC) was completely abolished by feeding.[202] He suggested that this background motor activity acted as an intestinal housekeeper necessary to maintain an empty gut and prevent bacterial overgrowth. Subsequently the Leuven group, led by Gaston Vantrappen, demonstrated a similar motor complex in man manometrically using multi-lumen perfused tubes.[203] The MMC was abolished not only by food but by other influences, such as stress, so it was invaluable for study purposes. (Not only is the MMC easily identified but it is much simpler to study the intestine in the fasting state.) In fact the first person to record the cyclical nature of the fasting migratory motor complex in a human being was a Roumanian, Carel Stanciu, who was a research fellow with John Bennett at the Royal Infirmary, Hull. In 1975 he was studying gastro-oesophageal reflux using perfused gastrointestinal tubes and happened to leave a tube in the duodenum recording pressures overnight. He was unaware of Code's work and Bennett admits that neither of them could make much sense of the recordings at the time. Nonetheless, Stanciu published the findings in a little known journal on his return to Iasi in Roumania.[204] The article attracted little attention and would have been forgotten had it not been plucked from obscurity by David Wingate at the London Hospital, himself a pioneer in the motility field.

The study of gastrointestinal motility was also helped by the introduction of two simple tests to measure the speed of intestinal transit. The first measured the time taken for food to pass from one end of the gut to the other using radio-opaque markers and was devised by John Hinton and John Lennard-Jones at St. Mark's Hospital, who were interested in constipation.[205] The second known as the Exhaled Breath Hydrogen Test indicated the speed of transport of a test meal as far as the caecum.[206] This was devised by two Americans, John Bond and Michael Levitt in Minneapolis and proved a useful research tool, though it did not find a place in routine clinical practice. Nonetheless the two tests taken in conjunction with the gastric emptying time made it possible to calculate the individual transit times of the small intestine and the colon.

The early experiments of colonic manometry in Oxford and London were complimented by Herbert Duthie, another pioneer of motility.

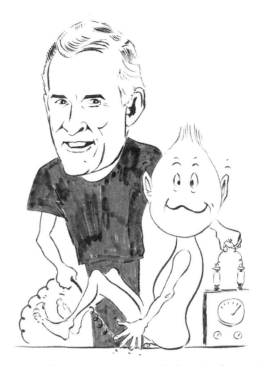

79 Duthie – Testing rectal electrical activity.

Bert Duthie (born 1930) had been appointed professor of surgery in Sheffield in 1966 and was interested in the problem of gastric emptying. He had a great facility for getting the best out of people and built up a fine research department at the university, working with physicists and electrical control engineers to study the effect of vagotomy and various drugs on gastric motility. Together with his colleagues Brian Catchpole (born 1927) and Christopher Stoddard (born 1947) he was one of the first to record migratory myoelectrical activity in post-operative patients using implanted electrodes[207] or mucosal electrodes placed within the stomach with a nasogastric tube.[208]

d) Colon

Later Duthie and his registrar, Irving Taylor (born 1946), used the same technique to study the colon and began to measure electrical activity in the recto-sigmoid region using electrodes implanted through a sigmoidoscope. They identified slow waves in the colon that were similar but far less organised than those in the upper gut.[209] Taylor continued this work when he moved to Liverpool as senior lecturer in 1977 and thought he had managed to identify an abnormal frequency in patients with irritable bowel syndrome,[210] even though he needed a computer to analyse it.[211] This was exciting and others in America found it too but unfortunately the abnormality was later shown to be non-specific.[212] Both Taylor and Duthie enjoyed distinguished careers; the former became Professor of Surgery at Southampton in 1981 and the latter Provost at the Welsh National School of Medicine, work for which he was honoured with a knighthood.

e) Discovery of gut hormones

The discovery of the gut hormones during the 1970s caused great excitement. At the beginning of the decade, gut innervation was defined as cholinergic, adrenergic, or NANC (non-adrenergic, non-cholinergic). By the end of the decade a host of circulating peptides had been identified in the gut and were being postulated as putative NANC neurotransmitters. Two, gastrin and cholecystokinin, were already well known and Richard Harvey in Bristol had shown that an infusion of cholecystokinin increased colonic activity and exacerbated the pain of irritable bowel syndrome.[213] But no one really suspected that the gut also secreted a number of other active peptides. As so often happens their discovery was partly serendipitous. David Wingate recalls that in 1970 he was studying intestinal water absorption at the research institute of the Middlesex Hospital. He was using fresh tissue obtained from urologists who regularly resected small intestine to construct ileal bladders. In the same institute, a young research worker called Stephen Bloom was trying to develop a radioimmunoassay for glucagon, a peptide with hyperglycaemic effects secreted by the pancreas. One day Bloom asked Wingate if he could give him some surplus fresh bowel tissue to use as a control for his assay. To Bloom's surprise the radioimmunoassay consistently identified glucagon-like immunoreactivity from the specimens of intestine he was using as a control. He had stumbled on enteroglucagon, a new peptide arising from the gut, and this was followed by the discovery of a number of other intestinal peptides.[214] People speculated that these peptides might be the unknown NANC neurotransmitters.

One of these peptides, called motilin, seemed to stimulate the activity front of the migrating motor complex.[215] So during the 1970s it was generally believed that the "clock" that controlled the biorhythm of the intestine lay outside the gut and that the different patterns of gut motility were the products of humeral or hormonal control.[216] Perhaps these peptides were the key to the irritable bowel syndrome.

CHAPTER FIFTY-NINE

1980S: THE NEUROTIC BOWEL

a) Localisation of pain

There was an air of expectancy among doctors and physiologists treating functional bowel disease during the 1980s. Meetings were held, symposia attended, articles written and monographs published. Financial support from the pharmaceutical industry flowed into research. The first meeting of the European Motility Society was held in Bologna, Italy in 1981 sponsored by Janssen Pharmaceutica. A new *Journal of Gastrointestinal Motility* appeared in 1987. New names appeared alongside the old such as David Thompson, Nick Read, Peter Whorwell and Robin Spiller, and cooperation with workers in Europe and America increased. Yet the cause of the disease remained elusive.

Ken Heaton in Bristol hoped that the Manning criteria would help gastroenterologists to agree among themselves on what exactly was meant by irritable bowel syndrome.

As with the classification of dyspepsia, the criteria drew attention to the most important symptoms but did not attempt to explain them. Treatment had to be based on symptoms and the effects of different treatments could only be compared if the symptoms themselves were comparable. Some, such as Truelove, preferred a broader brush. He compared the benefit of lorazepam, hyoscine and isphagula husk in patients with irritable bowel syndrome but made no attempt to analyse particular symptoms.[217] He argued that these varied so much and patients' reactions to them were so different that the aim of treatment was simply to obtain an overall symptomatic improvement and not necessarily to eliminate individual symptoms. Though he claimed that all three treatments helped, many thought the benefit was a placebo effect. One difficulty as Heaton had shown was that the colon behaved quite unpredictably in so many healthy people.[218] He and Grant Thompson surveyed 300 healthy people in the Bristol area and found that at least twenty per cent fulfilled their criteria for irritable bowel syndrome, though the individuals themselves felt fine.[219] So why did patients consult their doctor? Were they simply neurotic or was their gut unduly sensitive to certain stimuli?

The Manning criteria did not include patients with unexplained abdominal pain and normal bowel habit. This was a contentious issue as many felt that people with pain alone often had an irritable bowel. Indeed back in 1969 Sheila Waller and George Misiewicz at the Central Middlesex Hospital had found that many patients classified as having the irritable bowel syndrome might have pain in any part of the abdomen.[220] Later in his classic experiments in Oxford James Ritchie frequently saw a peristaltic wave starting up near the splenic flexure about five minutes after inflating a balloon in the sigmoid colon. He also noted that pain could occur anywhere in the abdomen after contraction of the sigmoid colon.[221]

The challenge to correlate isolated abdominal pain with the irritable bowel syndrome was taken up by Anthony Dawson (1928–97), later Sir Anthony, physician to St. Bartholemew's Hospital and to the Queen. Dawson was an outstanding general physician and a formidable academic gastroenterologist. He developed his interest in the absorption of peptides from the small intestine as a research fellow at Harvard Medical School in Boston and returned to a position at the Royal Free Hospital before his appointment at St. Bartholemew's Hospital in 1965. At St. Bartholemew's he built up a gastroenterology department from scratch that enjoyed an enviable reputation.

Dawson took advantage of the technique of colonoscopy with the help of Christopher Williams (born 1938) and Edwin Swarbrick (born 1945), both experts in this new skill. A balloon was inflated in various parts of the colon from the caecum to the sigmoid colon in 48 patients with a long history of severe and often baffling abdominal pain. This reproduced the pain in over half the patients but not all of them.[222] Dawson then studied a further group of patients with a swallowed balloon placed in various parts of the small intestine and lower oesophagus.[223/224] Again the pain could be reproduced in over half

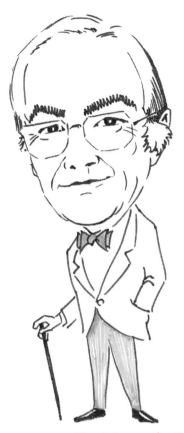

80 Dawson – Physician to the Queen.

the patients and most of the non-responders subsequently responded to colonic balloon distension like the first group. So he had managed to reproduce their pain in the great majority of patients. His most surprising observation was that distension of the distal oesophagus not only caused retrosternal pain as one would expect but also pain in other parts of the abdomen. Furthermore pain from the gut was often referred to various extra-abdominal sites such as the back, ribs and breasts. Dawson concluded that the whole of the alimentary tract was potentially a source of pain in patients with the irritable bowel syndrome and that this pain could be felt anywhere in the abdomen and also in some misleading extra-abdominal sites.

Chest pain that mimicked angina was also attracting more attention. In Cardiff John Rhodes repeated Henderson's work showing that oesophageal spasm caused angina,[225] though Henderson did not agree with the term "oesophageal angina" favoured by Rhodes. Meanwhile in Edinburgh Bob Heading had capitalised on his experience with scintigraphy to measure oesophageal transit, and claimed that this was as good as manometry in detecting motility disorders.[226] He began this work with his registrar, John Blackwell, who spent some time working with Don Castell, the guru of oesophageal motility, in Winston-Salem, North Carolina.[227] While Blackwell was in America, his place was taken by John de Caestecker, who also became interested in the problem of non-cardiac chest pain. Unfortunately this proved much more complicated than Henderson and Rhodes had thought.[228] Like workers elsewhere, the Edinburgh group found it difficult to be sure that oesophageal spasm was actually the cause of chest pain in many patients. Some had spasm without pain and provocation tests were often inconclusive. De Caestecker and Heading found that acid perfusion was more provocative than the use of cholinergic drugs but this technique was also far from foolproof.[229] Even 24-hour ambulatory manometry could miss an attack of pain if it was infrequent. In America Castell revived the use of oesophageal balloons as a provocative test[230] though some thought this had limited use as patients with ischaemic heart disease could not differentiate their angina from the pain of a distended balloon.[231]

Oesophageal dysmotility was common and Dawson's suggestion that it was often a manifestation of the irritable bowel syndrome was supported by a study from Southampton. In 1981 a young Peter Whorwell working with Colin Smith on the professorial medical unit found that patients with irritable bowel syndrome also had a variety of oesophageal motility disturbances even though they had no oesophageal symptoms.

Similarly a group at the Mayo Clinic showed that functional dyspepsia was frequently associated with gastric dysmotility. Many of this group were young men from Italy and Spain anxious to work with Sidney Phillips who was renowned for his work on gut physiology. Subsequently they became household names in the motility field such as Juan Malagelada (Barcelona), Fernando Azpiroz (Barcelona), Vincenzo Stanghellini (Bologna) and Michael Camilleri, who remained at the Mayo Clinic and succeeded Phillips.

b) The enteric nervous system

David Wingate was the first to study the small intestine in patients with the irritable bowel syndrome. Wingate (born 1935) was a physiologist at heart and spent his early years studying water absorption, first with Dennis Parsons in Oxford and later with Sidney Phillips at the Mayo Clinic. On his return to England in 1972 he obtained a clinical senior lectureship in the physiology department at the London Hospital while looking for a senior registrar post. There he came under the influence of David Ritchie (1920–93), an energetic professor of surgery, who had established an academic department of surgical gastroenterology and who also knew several workers from the Mayo Clinic, including Charles Code. Within two or three years Wingate had abandoned his work on absorption, thrown in his lot with the surgeons and switched to motility. Because of his work on absorption he was particularly interested in the small intestine and decided to study its motor activity. At first he used intubation techniques but realised that these were cumbersome and uncomfortable, limiting the periods of observation to a few hours. He then hit on the idea of tethering Tom Rowlands' radio pill in the upper jejunum with a long thread. He could now record the motor activity in one segment of the small intestine for at least 24 hours, including mealtimes and periods of sleep with minimal inconvenience to the subject.

Opposite the surgical unit lay the department of medicine. Here a young lecturer in medicine, David Thompson (born 1948), was looking for a clinical research project. He met Wingate who was keen to start his longterm recordings with the radiotelemetry capsule and they teamed up. One of their first studies was in a patient with severe irritable bowel syndrome who had undergone extensive investigation, including seven barium enemas, three barium meals, three jejunal biopsies, a colonoscopy, various scans and innumerable biochemical tests, all of which had been normal. They recorded the motor activity in his jejunum for 48 hours and found normal migrating motor complexes when he was asleep. On one occasion he was woken by his pain and they saw a period of irregular contractions. During the day he had several episodes of pain associated with irregular contractions, and even though he was fasting there were very few migrating complexes. Whatever this meant it was the first time anyone had recorded an abnormality in this unfortunate man.[232]

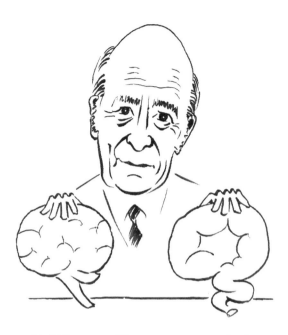

81 Wingate – Neurogastroenterologist.

Wingate and Thompson went on to show that the cycle of the migrating motor complex was much more variable than people thought[233] and that migrating complexes were only slightly less frequent during the waking state than during sleep.[234] In fact a normal range was difficult to pin down and Wingate realised that measurement of small bowel motility would be meaningless unless it was defined.[235] Nonetheless, the biorhythm of the intestine did fit with the concept that it was controlled by neural and not by humoral mechanisms after all. The gut literally seemed to have a mind of its own that resided within the enteric nervous system in its muscle coats (the myenteric plexus).[236] The enteric nervous system contained a profusion of neurotransmitters and became known as the "gut-brain" because it had much in common with the brain. Though largely autonomous its activity could be modulated by the central nervous system. For example, the migrating motor complex cycled more frequently during sleep when the brain was relatively inactive and the gut was left to itself.[237] Stress on the other hand inhibited it as Wingate and Thompson showed in further experiments. They subjected medical students to the psychic stress of dichotic listening and found this inhibited the normal fasting motor activity of the jejunum.[238]

The radiotelemetric capsule was not sufficiently robust to allow subjects to go home during an experiment and was superseded by small-calibre nasoenteric probes with in-built sensors that could be wired to a recorder.[239] Working with John Kellow, an Australian fresh from the Mayo Clinic, Wingate showed that all irregular gut activity disappeared during a good night's sleep at home.[240] So he reasoned that the biorhythm of the intestine was programmed within the enteric nervous system, but modulated by the central nervous system, principally under the opposing influences of sleep and mental stress. Later he found that the sleep pattern was usually normal in patients with irritable bowel but highly abnormal when the patient was awake with a mass of clustered contractions all day, particularly under stressful conditions.[241] The enteric nervous system of patients with irritable bowel syndrome was being bombarded by information from the central nervous system, as might occur for example, during stress.[242] The function of the enteric nervous system might be appropriate, but the demands on it were inappropriate.

David Thompson was fascinated by the effect of stress on the gut. Apart from the obvious clinical implications he hoped that the study of stress would help to clarify how the central nervous system mediated disturbances of gut function. In 1981 he visited Sid Phillips' department at the Mayo Clinic. Here, working with Juan Malagelada, he showed that stress delayed gastric emptying and inhibited gastric secretion.[243] The stress, whether physical or mental, appeared to exert its effect through the sympathetic nervous system.[244] On his return to the London Hospital Thompson obtained a Wellcome senior lectureship and continued this work in collaboration with Rodney Burnham, a gastroenterologist at Oldchurch Hospital in Romford with close ties to the London Hospital. Many of the tests of gut function were invasive and in themselves stressful so he relied as much as possible on transit studies using the hydrogen breath test to measure orocaecal transit.[245] Though he used well tried and tested ways of inducing experimental stress he was concerned that these short-term, artificial techniques did not necessarily reflect the worries of daily life. Indeed the very word stress concerned him as people varied so much in their response to it. Nonetheless, he was able to show that catecholamines were essential for the modulation of the enteric nervous system by the brain.[246]

Academically minded clinicians hoped that the new techniques for studying motility would at least provide a diagnostic test for irritable bowel syndrome, even if they did not explain it. In Britain no one tried harder to define the syndrome physiologically than Nicholas Read in Sheffield.

c) *The hypersensitive gut*

Nick Read (born 1945) qualified at the London Hospital and originally planned to follow a career in tropical medicine, having led an expedition to Ethiopia when he was a medical student. His mentor, Professor Edward Spooner (1904–95) at the London School of Hygiene and Tropical Medicine, advised him to obtain a specialty first and he chose the gut. In 1975 he became registrar to Derek Holdsworth (born 1933) at the Royal Hallamshire Hospital in Sheffield, with whom he studied the absorption of amino acids. In 1977 he spent fifteen months working with John Fordtran, an eminent gastroenterologist in Dallas, who was attempting to elucidate the mechanism of chronic unexplained diarrhoea. Here Read gained experience in the technique of total gut perfusion devised by Fordtran to evaluate patients with secretory diarrhoea.[247] Despite intensive study Fordtran only managed to reach a reasonably satisfactory diagnosis in half his patients. The most common diagnoses were surreptitious abuse of laxatives and anal sphincter defects with incontinence masquerading as diarrhoea.[248]

On his return to Sheffield, Read continued to study the mechanisms of diarrhoea and in particular the influence of motor activity on intestinal absorption[249] and joined the department of physiology in full-time research, becoming an honorary consultant in gastroenterology in 1981 and later Professor of Gastrointestinal Physiology and Nutrition. His research was productive and he harnessed the help of several physiology students for his projects and was generously supported by Janssen Pharmaceuticals. In 1984 he was one of the first to describe the so-called ileal brake when he noticed that an infusion of fat into the ileum caused a prolonged delay in small bowel transit time.[250] This was found to be due to an inhibition of contractile activity in the duodenum and jejunum mediated by the enteric nervous system. Many people were involved in this study and there were no less than thirteen authors on the paper. Read speculated that the phenomenon could influence satiety in some way quite apart from any effect it might have on absorption by the small intestine.[251]

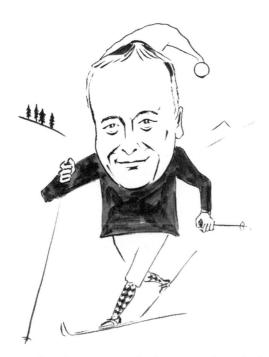

82 Read – Gastroenterologist turned psychologist.

Read's work with diarrhoea inevitably stirred his interest in the irritable bowel syndrome. Many patients with the syndrome had diarrhoea as their predominant symptom so he decided to compare IBS patients with diarrhoea with a group with constipation and a third group with abdominal pain and distension. Aware that many thought of irritable bowel syndrome as a disease of the whole gut he was keen to study the behaviour of the stomach as well as the small intestine and colon. Furthermore because most patients with irritable bowel syndrome reported that food makes them worse he decided to follow the transit of a solid meal as it passed down the gastrointestinal tract. He tried to avoid intraluminal pressure studies as the methods were invasive and the pressures varied so much in normal subjects that it was difficult to decide what was abnormal.

Read and Holdsworth and their research fellow, Paul Cann (born 1953), later appointed physician to Middlesborough General Hospital, found that the transit of food through the small intestine and the colon was faster than normal in patients with irritable bowel syndrome who had diarrhoea, but slower than normal in patients who presented with constipation.[252] Unfortunately, though this supported Wingate and Thompson's view that the small intestine had a role in the irritable bowel syndrome, most of the patients had transit times well within the normal range (admittedly large), even though they continued to have abdominal symptoms and an abnormal bowel habit. Clearly the alteration in transit times could not be the only problem so they speculated that the colon in irritable bowel syndrome was unable to tolerate the usual variations in small bowel transit, noting that many patients complained of pain in the right iliac fossa coinciding with the entry of food into the caecum. This sensitivity of the colon was in keeping with the earlier reports from James Ritchie in Oxford[253] and Irving Taylor in Liverpool[254] of unusually sensitive sigmoid colons in these patients.

The concept that the fundamental problem in IBS was an abnormal motor response to a hypersensitive bowel rather than a primary motor disorder was not new but rather appealing. In 1980 William Whitehead and Marvin Schuster at the Johns Hopkins University School of Medicine had shown that the rectum of IBS patients was more sensitive to distension by a balloon than normal.[255] This was taken up by Ken Heaton in Bristol and his research fellow, Julian Oettle, later professor of surgery in Johannesburg. They compared various parameters of rectal function in fifteen patients with irritable bowel, nine of whom had what they called rectal dissatisfaction. In fact they found no difference between the two groups.[256] They went on to study four patients in detail for a month. Each patient kept a careful record of symptoms and frequency of defaecation. Their stools were weighed and graded by appearance from watery to hard lumps.[257] Again they found no relationship between symptoms and stool weight, form, frequency or transit time. In other words the patients' description of urgency, looseness and frequency of defaecation gave little guide to intestinal events, suggesting that symptoms came from an altered perception of large bowel function rather than alterations in bowel function itself.[258] Heaton, an experienced gastroenterologist, knew that these patients often complained of diarrhoea because they felt the need to defaecate frequently, though the stools were formed or even hard. They had pseudo-diarrhoea as he put it.[259]

Whitehead and Shuster's study of rectal sensitivity was repeated by Peter Whorwell (born 1946) who had moved from Southampton in 1981 to take up an appointment as physician and senior lecturer in the Department of Medicine at the University Hospital of South

Manchester. On arrival he found that all the patients with interesting conditions such as inflammatory bowel disease were attending another hospital whereas he was inundated with patients with irritable bowels desperate for his attention. No one was interested in these people and they were hard to treat. Undaunted he accepted the challenge. During the 1980s money followed the patient so funds were plentiful, and full of optimism Whorwell built up a fine department and did some highly productive research. I shall discuss his treatment of refractory cases by hypnosis for which he is best known later. He knew that the irritable bowel syndrome could affect other parts of the gut and he also noticed that many patients had symptoms that had nothing to do with the gut. At first he had difficulty getting his views published but clearly showed that dyspareunia, urinary symptoms, lassitude, back pain and bad breath were all common and misleading symptoms.[260] Moreover they were just as likely to occur in patients who had no evidence of psychiatric disease. He wondered if a diffuse disorder of smooth muscle might explain the diversity of symptoms.[261]

Whorwell was supported by two research registrars, David Maxton (born 1954) and Alison Prior (born 1958), who were subsequently appointed gastroenterologists to Shrewsbury and Norwich respectively. Aware that patients with irritable colon suffered urgency of defaecation, frequent stools and a sensation of incomplete evacuation, he decided to study their anorectal function and found that a sensitive rectum was common, especially among those with diarrhoea.[262] Perhaps, he speculated, these people had visceral hypersensitivity throughout the gut.

The concept of rectal dissatisfaction also appealed to Read in Sheffield who now felt that patients with irritable bowel syndrome should not be segregated on the basis of their predominant bowel habit, especially as many patients had alternating diarrhoea and constipation. The very terms diarrhoea and constipation were subjective and meant different things to different people, as Heaton had shown. He still believed the best way to categorise patients with irritable bowel syndrome was by the use of a physiological test, if one could be found. He was worried by the trend towards complicated clinical classifications, which he felt were leading nowhere. He was impressed by Whitehead and Schuster's work in Baltimore and believed that measurement of rectal sensitivity to balloon distension was the most useful approach on the grounds that most irritable bowel symptoms were based on rectal sensations.

Alison Prior spent a year with Read in Sheffield in 1990 when they confirmed that over half their patients with irritable bowel syndrome had abnormally sensitive rectums.[263] These people had a frequent desire to defaecate and though a sensitive rectum was common in patients with diarrhoea, many constipated patients also had a sensitive rectum feeling a constant urge to strain. They were much the same as Heaton's patients with rectal dissatisfaction. Earlier Read had shown that normal subjects found it much more difficult to evacuate small objects from the rectum than larger ones.[264] So he speculated that some patients with an irritable bowel who complained of constipation had a rectum that was so sensitive that they were acutely aware of faecal pellets that would not worry a normal subject. This produced a frequent desire to defaecate, but because the pellets were so small, they could not be expelled without a great deal of effort.

Warming to his theme Read went on to suggest that the phenomenon of rectal sensitisation was part of a neurotic bowel.[265] Perhaps the whole of the gut was hypersensitive and hyper-reactive to a variety of stimuli reminiscent of other diseases such as asthma. Echoing the thoughts of Arthur Hurst as far back as 1910 Read wondered if this type of irritable bowel syndrome represented a response to a number of sensitising factors; chemical, physical, inflammatory or psychogenic. If a way could be found to desensitise the rectum and perhaps the rest of the gut to any of these factors, effective treatment might be possible.

Despite the misgivings of those who felt that a classification of functional bowel disease based on clinical groupings was flawed, a small team of experts from Europe and America met to produce guidelines for the diagnosis and study of irritable bowel syndrome. They argued that until the cause was known precise clinical entities had to be established before trials of treatment and research into the cause could be carried out. The team, under the chairmanship of Grant Thompson and with the strong support of Douglas Drossman in North Carolina, was set up after the Twelfth International Congress of Gastroenterology held in Lisbon in 1984. After much discussion the so-called first Rome criteria were presented at the Thirteenth Congress in Rome in 1988.[266] Most of the Manning criteria were adopted but the committee stressed the chronicity of the syndrome. They also highlighted one conundrum: "It is still unclear to what extent irritable bowel syndrome is normal perception of abnormal events or abnormal perception of normal events."

To try to answer this Ken Heaton and his research fellow, Subrata Ghosh (born 1959), now Professor of Gastroenterology at Imperial College School of Medicine, London, studied the defaecatory symptoms, stool consistency and shape, and abdominal pain/bloating of women with irritable bowel syndrome compared with a group of healthy women and a third group who had symptoms but did not complain of them. The study was carried out prospectively and showed that some variation in bowel function, pain and bloating was common in all three groups. But the symptoms were much worse in the patient group who thus had every reason to complain.[267] In effect they had the neurotic bowel described by Read.

CHAPTER SIXTY

TREATMENT IN THE 1980S

a) Bran discredited

Cann, Read and Holdsworth in Sheffield took advantage of their gut transit studies to re-examine the benefit, if any, of treatment with drugs for irritable bowel syndrome. The first compound they looked at was domperidone, a dopaminergic antagonist, which they found had no effect at all on symptoms or gastrointestinal transit.[268] The second, loperamide, an opiate-like antidiarrhoeal agent, at least helped those patients with diarrhoea.[269] Holdsworth reviewed the literature and was appalled by the widespread use of drugs with so little evidence to justify their use.[270] He criticised the majority of drug trials on several counts. It was essential to study patients with consistent and fairly frequent symptoms otherwise a trial would have to continue for months or even years to show anything at all. In many trials the only assessment had been subjective improvement; very few had assessed separately the improvement of individual symptoms, and hardly any had attempted to identify individual therapeutic goals for patients and tailored treatment to these (for example, relief of pain). Few had an adequate run-in period and many did not include a placebo, which made them valueless. The placebo response in irritable bowel syndrome was high and furthermore it varied for different symptoms. People with pain, for example, had a higher placebo response rate than those with, say, diarrhoea. So far more patients were needed in a trial looking at pain relief as opposed to diarrhoea to demonstrate a real therapeutic benefit.

Despite any evidence that they did much good, a large number of drugs were marketed for irritable bowel syndrome, chiefly

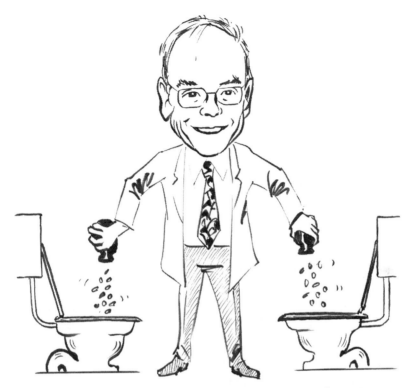

83 Holdsworth – Unimpressed by medication for IBS.

antispasmodics often in combination with antacids and psychotropic drugs. In 1983 Richard Harvey and Alan Read in Bristol published a survey of 2,000 gastroenterology outpatients seen over five years and found that almost one half had functional bowel disease.[271] So the market was huge and in the absence of any better treatment, drugs were being widely prescribed at enormous cost. Good evidence that they worked was needed and Holdsworth called for well-controlled trials to justify their use.

The Sheffield team also took the opportunity to evaluate the place of wheat bran as a preliminary to their drug trial. Fibre had come a long way since Painter's original work in 1972 suggesting that it helped people with diverticular disease. It was certainly a popular remedy. A postal survey of members of the British Society of Gastroenterology in 1975 revealed that they nearly all recommended fibre to patients with spastic colon including those with diarrhoea.[272] There was still no good evidence that fibre actually helped patients but scientists were intrigued and wondered what it did and how it worked. By 1980 more than 300 papers were being published annually on dietary fibre compared with fewer than five per year a decade earlier. There were regular workshops and symposia and even a report from the Royal College of Physicians on *Medical Aspects of Dietary Fibre* (edited anonymously by Ken Heaton).[273]

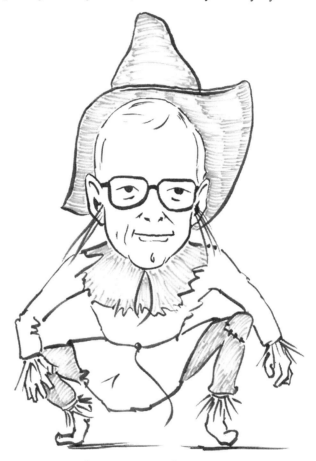

84 Cummings – Fibreman – too.

Much of the credit for what we know about fibre today belongs to John Cummings (born 1942). Cummings' interest in fibre began when he was a senior registrar with the Medical Research Council's gastroenterology unit at the Central Middlesex Hospital. One day in 1973 he was asked by Professor Sheila Sherlock (1918–2001), then editor of *Gut*, to write an editorial on dietary fibre after he had presented a short review about it at a journal club meeting.[274] Thrown in at the deep end, he soon familiarised himself with the subject and this became his chief research interest for many years. He transferred to the Dunn Clinical Nutrition Centre in Cambridge in 1975 where he headed a group of MRC scientists known as the *Gut* Group. At the time fibre in its various forms was thought to increase the bulk of faeces by its ability to absorb water like a sponge.[275] Eastwood believed that plant cell walls exerted a physical effect on intestinal bulk by retaining water within their cellular structure. This would explain why Heaton found that the laxative effect of wheat bran was reduced by cooking. But it seemed unlikely that this was the only explanation, especially as Godfrey Milton-Thompson (1930–2012), working at St. Mark's Hospital, had found that man manages to metabolise over half the cellulose that he ingests[276] and David Southgate, director of the Dunn Nutrition Laboratory, had shown that up to 75 per cent fibre is degraded in the gut by colonic microflora.[277] In due course Cummings and his research fellow in biochemistry, Alison Stephen, demonstrated that the ability of a given type of fibre to hold water in vitro bore little relation to its stool bulking effect.[278] For example, wheat bran, which holds relatively little water, had pronounced faecal bulking properties. So something else was happening. They were aware that bacteria are 80 per cent water and were therefore a potentially important water-holding component of stools. So they wondered if the bulking effect of fibre was at least partly due to its metabolism by micro-organisms in the colon. This would lead to a massive increase in their numbers and Stephen proved it by fractionating the stool and weighing its bacterial mass.[279] This increased significantly after the addition of fibre. In the case of wheat bran, which is only partly fermented, the increase in stool weight was caused by a combination of bran's physical sponge-like property and an increase in faecal microbial mass.[280]

Cummings continued his research, identifying the colon as an important digestive organ. He looked at other properties of fibre (a non-starch polysaccharide of the plant cell wall) and went on to study other carbohydrates, notably starch itself and the so-called prebiotic oligosaccharides, which stimulate the growth of lactobacilli (a probiotic bacterium) in the colon.[281]

Though bran was widely used, the Sheffield trial was the first placebo-controlled evaluation of its benefit in patients with irritable bowel syndrome since Heaton's trial in Bristol in 1977. This may seem odd particularly as the Bristol trial was quite small, no attempt had been made to separate patents according to their bowel habit and only four patients out of twelve obtained complete relief of pain. But it was difficult to organise a trial in patients whose symptoms were so variable and impossible to run a double blind study with bran because patients knew that they are taking it; even if they did not recognise its appearance, they could recognise its chewiness. In fact there were two trials in Britain of bran in patients with diverticular disease though many felt that "symptomatic diverticular disease" was not the same as irritable bowel syndrome.

The first trial was organised by John Brodribb (born 1942), senior registrar in surgery at the Radcliffe Infirmary in Oxford.[282] Eighteen patients were given crispbread biscuits for three months, nine had biscuits with bran and nine without. Nearly all the bran group lost their abdominal pain (which was quite severe) whereas the control group did not. There was an initial placebo response, which settled after a month. The results were so impressive that the trial was stopped as it was considered unethical to deprive further patients of fibre. Brodribb subsequently spent some time in Wisconsin studying the effect of fibre in the colon of monkeys. Fibre had no effect on myoelectrical activity but lowered intraluminal pressure by increasing stool bulk and the diameter of the lumen, confirming Painter's original studies.[283] Later he was appointed surgeon to Plymouth General Hospital.

Despite Brodribb's findings the Medical Research Council were still unconvinced that bran really helped people with diverticular disease so they sponsored a large trial run by Marcus Ornstein (born 1945), senior registrar in surgery at Northwick Park Hospital, Harrow, and Ian McLean Baird (born 1915), physician to the West Middlesex Hospital.[284] Surprisingly this trial appeared to show that fibre had no effect on abdominal pain or bowel symptoms apart from helping constipation. This flatly contradicted the Oxford study but the trial was flawed and heavily criticised. Firstly the patients had very little pain so a positive response was always going to be unlikely. Secondly their colonic function was practically normal to start with so any benefit in transit time or stool weight would be difficult to show. Thirdly there was very little difference between the fibre intake of the treatment group and placebo group. Indeed this criticism from, among others, Avery Jones[285] and Heaton,[286] emphasised their view that the dose of fibre should be increased, provided it was tolerated, until a response was obtained.

The authors of the Sheffield trial of bran for irritable bowel syndrome (as opposed to diverticular disease) were the first to admit that their trial was imperfect; in particular that it was an open one.[287] The patients had never received bran before, knew they were taking bran and were told to increase the dose at weekly intervals for four weeks. Symptoms were analysed separately and the response to bran was no better than to placebo. However, those with constipation did improve their gut transit time and stool weight. But, out of 38 patients, only 18 said they were better for taking bran, and only 5 of these were willing to be discharged from the clinic.

As the Sheffield trial was rather short, Anthony Dawson and Michael Clark at St. Bartholemew's Hospital ran another study of bran lasting three months.[288] Twenty-eight patients responded equally well to bran and placebo as judged by the Manning criteria. There was little difference in stool weight between the two groups, though very few patients were constipated in the first place. Significantly ten additional patients who had been recruited withdrew from the trial for social reasons, including the inconvenience of eating bran-rich biscuits.

Another similar trial of 65 patients was conducted by Hugh Shepherd (born 1950), physician at the Royal Hampshire County Hospital, Winchester, and Jonathan Snook (born 1959), his senior registrar and later gastroenterologist at Poole General Hospital. The trial was well planned and again showed that bran was no better than placebo.[289] By the middle 1990s, bran was finally losing favour with the majority of physicians.

b) Food intolerance

It was disenchantment with bran that led John Hunter in Cambridge to try the opposite, a low-fibre diet. This was quite restrictive but some of his patients responded to it surprisingly well, which made him wonder if they could be intolerant to certain foods. He knew that so-called food allergy was a contentious subject and that he was entering a conceptual minefield strewn with discredited ideas and fanciful fallacies, but he was fortunate to have the support of an experienced dietician, Elizabeth Workman, and an enthusiastic senior house officer, Victoria Alun

Jones. To begin with, the team studied a small group of patients with diarrhoea-type irritable bowel most of whom were female and highly motivated.[290] Two thirds of them responded well to elimination diets and proved to be intolerant of specific foods. They later expanded the study, though the detection of food intolerance required considerable dedication from the staff and determination by the patient. The rewards were well worthwhile. Over 90 per cent of the patients were still well on their diets two years later.[291] Hunter (born 1940) worked hard to make the concept of food intolerance acceptable to a sceptical medical profession and tried to explain its mechanism. He worked closely with the Dunn Clinical Nutrition Centre in Cambridge and had the support of Robin Coombs (1921–2006), the distinguished immunologist, who was unable to find any evidence for an allergy in these patients. Hunter put forward another explanation. He noted that some patients developed irritable bowel symptoms after a course of antibiotics, which altered the gut flora.[292] This would cause abnormal fermentation of certain foods, notably carbohydrates, in the colon, leading in turn to a range of abnormal metabolites. In susceptible individuals these chemicals could pass into the circulation to produce symptoms. In line with this hypothesis he suggested that food allergy should be renamed an "enterometabolic disorder".

Hunter claimed that food intolerance was a major factor in the pathogenesis of IBS but exclusion diets, however effective, only helped patients with diarrhoea-type IBS, the least common group that carried the best prognosis. Furthermore, his theory did not explain why IBS was so much commoner in women.

Another careful study of 49 patients with diarrhoea-type IBS was carried out by John Mackenzie (born 1946), a gastroenterologist in Glasgow.[293] In contrast to the Cambridge study his rigorous, placebo-controlled food challenges revealed only three patients with specific food intolerance and confirmed the general impression that most forms of food reactions were largely psychogenic.

Encouraged by Hunter's work, Derek Jewell (born 1941) in Oxford ran a large open study in which half the patients responded to an exclusion diet.[294] The patients then challenged themselves with a series of foods in succession noting relapses as they occurred, and were subsequently advised to remove them from the diet. As they knew which foods upset them the benefit could have been psychological. Whatever the mechanism a year later the majority were well and had lost their abdominal pain, flatus, distension or diarrhoea. Jewell concluded that the dietary approach was frequently welcomed by patients and was a possible therapeutic approach, noting that those who failed to respond were usually non-compliant.

Most gastroenterologists felt that true food intolerance was rare and not worth investigating. But in the clinical setting it made sense to concur with patients convinced that certain foods disagreed with them whatever the mechanism.

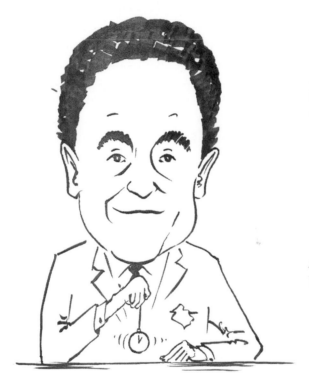

85 Whorwell – Hypnosis helps.

c) Hypnosis

Like everyone else Peter Whorwell in Manchester was well aware that most patients responded to a combination of spasmolytics, bulking agents and a sympathetic explanation of their symptoms. But equally he knew that a significant number failed to respond to anything. So in the early 1980s he decided to try hypnosis. This had been used with some success in patients with asthma and he thought that hypnotic relaxation would help colonic spasm too. Initially he was careful not to mention his ideas to his colleagues because he realised that the profession was highly sceptical of hypnosis. To his delight his patients, all of whom had severe refractory irritable bowel syndrome, responded well to treatment.[295] Furthermore they remained in remission[296] and besides relieving their abdominal symptoms they felt much better and were able to go back to work.[297] Whorwell knew his colleagues would want to know how hypnosis worked and he suggested various mechanisms to explain it. The obvious one was that it helped anxious people to cope with their symptoms but, as he showed, hypnotherapy also modified visceral hypersensitivity in some way.[298] Despite this he had difficulty in convincing doctors and they were reluctant to use the technique. Many thought it was time-consuming and remained sceptical. But patients had no such qualms and were falling over themselves for treatment.

CHAPTER SIXTY-ONE

1990S VISCERAL HYPERSENSITIVITY

For students of functional bowel disease the final decade of the twentieth century was a curious mix of optimism and disillusion. Physiologists welcomed new technology that enabled them to study the autonomic nervous system in a way that was unthinkable a few years earlier. The term "gastrointestinal motility" was inadequate and no longer reflected the work of several disciplines that included neuroscience, psychiatry, immunology, endocrinology and epidemiology. Indeed gastrointestinal motility implied a sterile academic subject to most clinicians whereas the neural control of the gut seemed clinically relevant. The Americans called it "Nerve-Gut Interaction" but David Wingate at the London Hospital and others did not relish being known as "nerve-gut interactivists". He preferred the term "neurogastroenterology" and after canvassing support from his colleagues managed to have it adopted despite initial resistance from America. He did this by forming a temporary "Society for Neurogastroenterology". The society was unorthodox with no officers, meetings or subscription. It was simply a vehicle by which Wingate could get his term "neurogastroenterology" into regular use. In due course the word was accepted and the society was abolished. Finally, in 1997, the *Journal of Gastrointestinal Motility* became the *Journal of Neurogastroenterology and Motility* representing both the European and American Motility Societies.

Physiologists from America and Europe now knew more about the interaction between the gut and the central nervous system, though most of their information came from animal studies. Much of the gut's activity was controlled by the enteric nervous system, a vast array of neurones and peptides responding to the need to absorb food and reject toxins from the lumen. In turn the enteric nervous system was modulated by the autonomic nervous system, which operated a two-way system of messages sent to and from the central nervous system via the sympathetic nerves and the vagus. During the 1990s people realised that thoughts and emotions from the brain could directly influence the gut through the autonomic nervous system. Indeed there was a circular relationship between the gut and the brain with each capable of stimulating the other. Visceral hypersensitivity resulted if this interrelationship was disturbed in some way either at the level of the gut or the autonomic nerves or indeed the brain. This was difficult to study as animal experiments cannot always be extrapolated to human beings, especially those involving stress.

The simplest way to study visceral sensitivity was by distending the gut with a balloon. James Ritchie had used balloons in the distal colon in the early 1970s and several groups had subsequently done the same.[299] Similarly Malagelada in Barcelona had devised a balloon or gastric barostat to show that the stomach was unusually sensitive to distension in people with functional dyspepsia.[300] In Britain Bob Heading, who was interested in the mechanism of non-cardiac chest pain confirmed the suggestion from Donald Castell in North Carolina that the sensory perception of these patients was abnormal.[301] Heading found that patients with minimal oesophageal reflux had a low threshold for pain induced by oesophageal distension. Minimal amounts of acid, it seemed, sensitised the oesophagus to stimuli that would not normally be painful. David Thompson, now in Manchester, thought he would look into this further.

For some time Thompson had been interested in the control of gastrointestinal function by the central nervous system. Many thought that he would stay at the London Hospital but when John Lennard-Jones and John Ledingham retired in 1987 the department of medicine faced an uncertain future and Thompson moved to Manchester as senior lecturer (and later professor of gastroenterology). Here he studied the effects of feeding on gastric motility and gradually built a fine research unit.[302] In the late 1990s he collaborated with Clifford Woolf (born 1952), a South African, who was Professor of Neurobiology at University College, London and later at Harvard. With the help of Sanchoy Sarkar (born 1971), now a gastroenterologist at Aintree Hospital, Liverpool and Qasim Aziz (born 1965), now Professor of Gastroenterology at St. Bartholemew's and the London Hospital, Thompson showed that when acid was instilled into the lower oesophagus of healthy volunteers, it

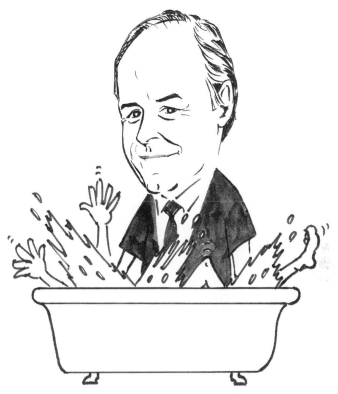

86 Thompson – Experimental stress.

lowered the threshold for pain in the upper oesophagus and on the chest wall. The effect was even greater in patients with non-cardiac chest pain.[303] This hypersensitivity to pain well away from the area of acid exposure implied that there must be a change in sensory processing within the central nervous system. Whatever the initiating cause (acid, for example), changes occurring in the autonomic nerves stimulated central sensitisation and this would explain the visceral hypersensitivity of patients with chest pain.

Could the trigger for visceral hypersensitivity be infection?

a) Post infective irritable bowel syndrome

For many years gastroenterologists had been aware that irritable bowel syndrome sometimes followed a bout of gastroenteritis. In 1931 Spriggs had noted its occurrence after infective dysentery[304] and Chaudhary and

Truelove also described it in their classic paper in 1962. Nick Read in Sheffield realised that this would be an attractive group of patients to study as they represented a natural experiment with a clearly defined start date. Accordingly, in the early 1990s, he approached his colleague, Michael McKendrick (born 1947), on the infectious disease ward who was enthusiastic and able to provide any number of patients with gastroenteritis. A preliminary study supported his hypothesis that an attack of gastroenteritis could cause irritable bowel symptoms and this was always associated with anxiety and rectal hypersensitivity.[305] By this time Read was becoming increasingly convinced that the irritable bowel syndrome and indeed functional bowel disease as a whole were psychological disorders. Though most people agreed that functional disease was characterised by dysregulation of brain-gut function with motor and visceral hypersensitivity to stress, Read after years spent in gastrointestinal research felt that no one had managed to prove that any of these physiological disturbances were actually responsible for the symptoms that patients experienced. Indeed he believed this strongly enough to undertake retraining as a clinical psychologist.

For a while he kept a foot in both camps and his later study on post-infective irritable bowel syndrome reflects this because it was published twice; the first paper stressed the psychological factors but the second emphasised the biological changes. The study was conducted by Kokan Gwee, a PhD student who is now Professor of Gastroenterology in Singapore.[306] A large group of patients with acute gastroenteritis underwent careful psychological assessment as well as the usual studies of rectal function including rectal biopsies. Only a minority developed symptoms of an irritable bowel, though all the patients had persisting rectal hypersensitivity and rapid colonic transit. The difference lay in the personality of the symptomatic patients who were neurotic and prone to somatisation. They had suffered some tragedy in their lives and were hypochondriacal. Read concluded that post-infectious irritable bowel syndrome occurred in psychologically predisposed individuals whose bowel had been sensitised by infection.

Most of the patients had acute inflammatory changes during their infection but only those with subsequent irritable bowels showed evidence of persisting minor chronic inflammation. These changes were not sufficient to be called microscopic colitis. Read sent the rectal biopsies to an old friend of his, Stephen Collins (born 1946), a pathologist at McMaster University, Hamilton, Ontario. Collins had qualified in England but moved to Canada in 1981 where he developed an interest in the immune modulation of the enteric nervous system. Using immunohistochemical techniques in an animal model he had recently shown that stress could reactivate experimental colitis.[307] Collins examined the biopsies sent by Read and found clear evidence of excessive cytokine activity in the rectal mucosa.[308] So the second publication of the paper emphasised the enhanced inflammatory response in these patients, though the authors agreed that the inflammatory aetiology and the psychological factors were not mutually exclusive. The two converged to influence disease expression and underscored the importance of both in the development of irritable bowel syndrome following infection.

By the time the second paper was published Read had resigned from his position in Sheffield and left the National Health Service. Convinced that a psychological approach was the only way to help people with functional bowel disease he completed his training and became a psychotherapist in private practice. He became medical advisor to the Gut Trust, a charity set up in 1986 to help people cope with the irritable bowel syndrome, and in 2004 he wrote a popular book entitled *Sick and Tired, How Modern Life is Affecting our Health*. Like much of his writing this is a stimulating **R**ead.

The baton of post-infectious diarrhoea was taken up in Britain by Robin Spiller (born 1950) in Nottingham. He knew Read well and academically their paths had already crossed with the discovery of the ileal brake. Soon after qualifying Spiller joined the MRC gastrointestinal research unit at the Central Middlesex Hospital working in the field of nutrition with David Silk (born 1944). He also came under the influence of George Misiewicz with his interest in motility. Aware that steatorrhoea was associated with small bowel hypomotility Silk postulated that if unabsorbed fat reached the ileum it would inhibit jejunal motility. The group managed to prove this by using segmental perfusion techniques in human volunteers to show that infusion of fatty acids into the ileum suppressed contractile activity and prolonged transit time along a 30-centimetre length of jejunum. It was Spiller who coined the term "ileal brake".[309] Shortly after he spent a year with Sidney Phillips at the Mayo Clinic where using radio-opaque markers he showed that fat accelerated colonic transit and motility thus explaining why people with coeliac disease had diarrhoea.[310]

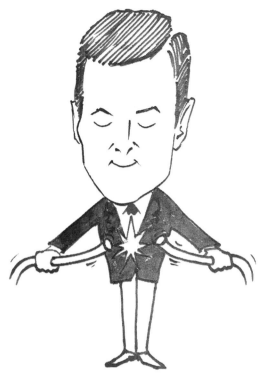

87 Spiller – The ileal break.

Spiller was appointed Gastroenterologist in Nottingham in 1988 where he rekindled his interest in post-infective irritable bowel syndrome acquired at the Central Middlesex Hospital, where he seen several such patients. In 1993 he met Keith Neal (born 1958) who had recently been appointed senior lecturer in the Public Health Department. Neal was interested in food poisoning and the department was routinely informed of all cases of bacterial gastroenteritis. Spiller and Neal decided to look at the fate of 400 patients with gastroenteritis and found that a quarter of them still had loose stools six months later and a quarter of these had full-blown irritable bowel syndrome (one in fourteen).[311] The risk was greater in women and those with severe gastroenteritis. Later they looked at the same group again and found that less than half of them had recovered after six years.[312] As Truelove had observed, diarrhoea was the dominant feature in these patients and recovery was much less likely in those with anxiety or depression.

Spiller went on to show that these people had inflammatory

changes in their gut that were identical to a group of patients recovering from acute bacterial enterocolitis, which supported his theory that infection could sometimes cause an irritable bowel.[313] The changes were subtle because the rectal mucosa looked normal using conventional microscopic techniques. But David Jenkins (born 1946), his pathologist, used immunohistological techniques to show an excess of enteroendocrine cells and T-lymphocytes in the mucosa. Furthermore both groups of patients had increased gut permeability consistent with inflammation. None of these changes were seen in controls. Spiller speculated that peptides released by enteroendocrine cells, notably 5-hydroxytrytamine, were responsible for the diarrhoea in these patients, and the T-lymphocytes were presumably part of a continuing cell mediated or humoral defensive response to the infecting organism. If so the response was being sustained for many years.

Spiller repeated this study on a larger scale and discovered that patients who had had bacterial enteritis and become asymptomatic still had evidence of continuing inflammation (T cells) but normal enteroendocrine cell counts.[314] However, the post-dysenteric irritable bowel patients were much more likely to have been depressed or anxious. A multivariate analysis suggested that an inflammatory process and depression were equally important in predicting post-infective irritable bowel, a conclusion very much in agreement with the Sheffield group.

Robin Spiller was appointed Professor of Gastroenterology at the Wolfson Digestive Diseases Centre in Nottingham in 2000 and has been chairman of the neurogastroenterology and motility section of the BSG. He became editor of *Gut* in 2003 in succession to Michael Farthing and edited the BSG guidelines for the management of irritable bowel syndrome published in 2007.[315]

b) Helicobacter gastritis and functional dyspepsia

When Barry Marshall and John Armstrong discovered Helicobacter pylori in 1984, they initially had difficulty proving that the bacterium caused duodenal ulcers. It certainly caused gastritis and was associated with ulcers but people only became convinced that it was ulcerogenic when its successful eradication cured them. Similarly clinicians hoped that healing the gastritis would also help patients with non-ulcer dyspepsia but this was much more difficult to show. Unlike peptic ulcer, which was a precise pathological entity, non-ulcer dyspepsia was an ill-defined group of symptoms that were hard to define and highly subjective. But if Helicobacter did cause dyspepsia, treatment would be simple and highly rewarding. Non-ulcer dyspepsia was extremely common as recent surveys had again shown.

In 1990 Roger Jones (born 1949), then senior lecturer in primary care at the University of Southampton, carried out a postal survey of nearly 7,500 people from six cities in England and Scotland and found that 41 per cent had suffered from dyspepsia in the previous six months.[316] Fortunately most of them had treated themselves and not bothered to visit a doctor. A few years later Roy Pounder (born 1945), professor of medicine at the Royal Free Hospital, surveyed over 2,000 adults across Britain using the Gallup organisation and found a similar prevalence of 40 per cent.[317] Only a fifth of these had visited their GP and only two per cent had been absent from work.

About the time of Jones' survey a simple screening test (the urea breath test) was introduced making it possible to screen people for Helicobacter pylori non-invasively, and it was apparent that the infection was indeed common, especially in people with dyspepsia. Soon there were several trials suggesting that its eradication helped people with dyspepsia, with one of the best early studies by Colm O'Morain's group in Dublin.[318]

In fact most of the early trials were short and flawed for one reason or another, so Kenneth McColl (born 1950), Professor of Gastroenterology in Glasgow, decided to undertake a much larger study. McColl had spent several years studying Helicobacter pylori in a city renowned for its high prevalence of peptic ulcer, so he had plenty of experience with the organism and its eradication. Many of his patients did not have ulcers of course, but simple dyspepsia, so he was ideally placed to run such a trial. Working with his research fellow, Emad El-Omar (born 1964), he first designed a score for assessing the severity of dyspepsia that was simple but reliable.[319] In the absence of a more objective endpoint this questionnaire was crucial to the study. With backing from the Medical Research Council, McColl treated over 150 dyspeptic patients infected with H. pylori and showed that 21 per cent of them no longer had dyspepsia a year later.[320] By comparison only seven per cent treated with omeprazole on its own were symptom-free a year later. The result was significantly in favour of the treated group and McColl suggested that all patients with H. pylori infection and non-ulcer dyspepsia should be treated. Though only a minority would be cured he believed the potential benefit – curing a chronic disorder with a single course of antibiotics – justified this approach.

Others disagreed, notably Nicholas Talley, an energetic globe-trotting Australian gastroenterologist/epidemiologist, and Andre Blum, professor of gastroenterology in Lausanne, Switzerland. Supported by Astra (the makers of omeprazole) Talley simultaneously supervised two large studies similar in size to the Glasgow trial. The first (the OCAY study) compared omeprazole, clarithromycin and amoxicillin with omeprazole alone and recruited patients from several centres in Europe, Canada and South Africa.[321] One year after treatment there was little difference between the two groups. The second (the ORCHID study – optimal regimen cures H. pylori-induced dyspepsia) compared omeprazole and the same antibiotics with a placebo, recruiting patients from Australia, New Zealand and several countries in Europe.[322] Again there was little evidence that the eradication of H. pylori relieved the symptoms of functional dyspepsia. McColl criticised the ORCHID study on the grounds that follow-up of some of the patients was inadequate and that patients with the motility type of dyspepsia (the group least likely to benefit from treatment) were overrepresented.[323] He also suggested that there results did in fact slightly favour eradication therapy, a view that was rebuffed by Talley.[324]

So far trials had been carried out on patients attending gastroenterology clinics. However, most patients with dyspepsia needing medical help were managed by their family doctor and never went near a hospital. With this in mind Tony Axon in Leeds and his research fellow, Paul Moayyedi (born 1965) devised a simple questionnaire for measuring the presence and severity of dyspepsia that could be used in general practice surveys.[325] In association with the Epidemiology and Primary Care Unit at the university, the Clinical Trials Unit and the Centre for Health Economics at York they set up the Leeds HELP study group (Helicobacter Eradication in General Practice); acronyms were becoming as popular in gastroenterology as they were in cardiology by this time. Using the questionnaire, Moayyedi interviewed over 8,000 people between the ages of 40 and 49 years randomly selected from 36 primary care centres.[326] He also used the urea breath test to determine their H. pylori status. This was an impressive undertaking and as expected

38 per cent had dyspepsia and this was more likely in people who were infected with H. pylori. He calculated that the organism caused nearly six per cent of all dyspepsia in the community.

The Leeds group went on to treat half the infected patients and found a small improvement in dyspepsia compared to the untreated group, though this did not improve their quality of life.[327] The benefit was long lasting and cost effective when reviewed eight years later.[328]

Moayyedi also reviewed twelve studies up to the year 2000 and concluded that eradicating H. pylori seemed to be cost-effective even though the effect on dyspepsia was marginal.[329] This was the first of several reviews that he carried out as a Cochrane editor for the Upper Gastrointestinal Disease Group and he served on various guideline groups including the NICE evaluation of dyspepsia in 2004 before moving to McMaster University, Ontario, to continue his interest in gastrointestinal epidemiology.

Meanwhile the case for treating H. pylori in patients with functional dyspepsia continued to be debated. McColl was convinced that it was worthwhile[330] and went on to show that dyspeptic patients with a positive breath test could be treated effectively without recourse to an endoscopy in selected cases.[331] Patients under the age of 45 were thus spared an invasive procedure and the strategy was considerably cheaper. This "test and treat" policy became widespread. A recent evaluation conducted in Leeds, Birmingham and Nottingham by Brendan Delaney, Professor of Primary Care in Birmingham and an old colleague of Moayyedi, confirmed its value.[332] This was the Medical Research Council's CUBE trial (Carbon Urea Breath test and Eradication), another jolly acronym.

In view of the controversy about treating H. pylori in the community at large, Richard Harvey, gastroenterologist in Bristol, set up the Bristol helicobacter project in 1996. It was an ambitious study in which more than 10,000 patients aged 20 to 59 were selected at random from seven general practices in southwest England.[333] They were all tested for H. pylori infection and fifteen per cent were positive. Half of this group (nearly 800 patients) had their infection eradicated and the other half were given a placebo. After two years Harvey found that the treated group had significantly less dyspepsia, with 30 per cent fewer visits to their doctor. He felt that the benefits and costs were worthwhile even though the prevalence of infection was only fifteen per cent in the Bristol area. The reward would be greater in areas of high H. pylori prevalence, as fewer people would have to be tested for one to gain benefit.

Even if helicobacter infection is a cause of functional dyspepsia, it can only account for a minority of cases as its prevalence in the community is small and falling. It has been difficult to prove that its eradication helps dyspepsia, again suggesting that its role is probably small. Doubtless the debate will continue.

CHAPTER SIXTY-TWO

PSYCHOLOGICAL ASPECTS OF FUNCTIONAL BOWEL DISEASE

The terms nervous dyspepsia and irritable colon reflect how doctors have always thought of these patients – neurotic, anxious or depressed. In 1960 Francis Avery Jones wrote that the commonest cause of functional disturbances was anxiety and nervous tension with depression not far behind.[334] He added that treatment remained within the art of medicine and that a personal approach to the patient by the physician was essential. Men like Watson, Brinton, Osler and Ryle would have agreed with him. The psychological aspects were so self-evident that they were taken for granted. Psychiatrists were not interested in gut problems and gastroenterologists were more attracted by organic diseases and the practice of endoscopy. Pharmaceutical companies promoted antidepressants and tranquillisers on slender scientific evidence, which many physicians thought were unjustified for these chronic, harmless complaints.

At the same time interest in gastrointestinal motility was steadily increasing, inspired by the work of Avery Jones in London and Truelove in Oxford. This distracted people from looking at psychosomatic factors and to hunt for specific abnormalities within the gut itself. So for thirty years after the Second World War little research into the psychological aspects of functional bowel disease took place.

The most demanding problem was unexplained abdominal pain. If a cause could not be found doctors tried reassurance but this often failed, particularly with children. Physicians interested in childhood disorders had been aware of the problem for years. At the turn of the century in his book *Diseases of Children* James Goodhart (1845–1916) of Guy's Hospital commented on the subject of mucous disease, a childhood form of mucous colitis with striking abdominal pain.[335] He had no great liking for the term as he had never seen much mucus but he believed it occurred in nervous children of nervous families. They were "an odd lot and the abdominal pain was compatible with enfeebled nervous control". He recommended small doses of Dover's powders for the pain. The subject attracted little further attention for 50 years until after the formation of the National Health Service when paediatrics (an American term) began to flourish. In 1959 John Apley (1908–80), a paediatrician in Bristol and a prolific author and speaker, wrote an acclaimed book *The Child With Abdominal Pains* in which he showed that children with obscure abdominal pain often had mothers with abdominal pain and continued to be subject to it into adult life.[336] Another paediatrician, John Dodge, Senior Lecturer in Child Health in Cardiff, agreed, emphasising that abdominal pain in childhood was 90 to 95 per cent psychosomatic.

One of the first psychiatrists to take an interest in the evaluation of "non-organic" abdominal pain was Oscar Hill (born 1931) at the Middlesex Hospital who carried out a thoughtful study with Laurence Blendis, a visiting Canadian who was to make his mark in hepatology.[337] Hill confirmed that many of these people were neurotic and came from parents who had themselves suffered from abdominal pain. The symptoms often began in the setting of a bereavement or some other clear upheaval in their lives. At least a quarter of them were considerably depressed and their pain improved when the depression was treated. Hill and Blendis were describing what came to be known as the bio-psycho-social model of functional bowel disease that is fashionable today. Hill anticipated current thought in suggesting that these patients may be aware of pain in the higher centres, unaccompanied by any phenomena in the gut. Alternatively pain might result from an awareness of disordered activity in the gut, the activity having been induced by the subject's psychological state. The two possibilities probably operated simultaneously and potentiated each other.

Ten years later in 1977 Peter Dally (1923–2005), a psychiatrist at the Westminster Hospital, suggested that all patients presenting to a gastroenterology clinic who did not have an organic cause for their pain had a psychiatric illness.[338] This somewhat startling revelation certainly drew attention to the problem but his study was flawed. He did not include a control group and diagnosed tension and hysterical states purely on the basis of the abdominal pain without any evidence of psychological disturbance at all.

A better study by Alasdair MacDonald. a lecturer in psychiatry in Dundee, and Ian Bouchier, a professor of medicine at the university, found a definite association between functional abdominal pain and psychiatric illness but emphasised that many patients with functional disease did not necessarily have a psychiatric illness and conversely some patients with organic disease had treatable anxiety or depression.[339] This seemed more in accord with clinical practice.

In the late 1960s George Misiewicz had shown that obscure abdominal pain correlated with pressure changes in the colon and small intestine[340] and a few years later Anthony Dawson confirmed his observation using inflatable balloons in various parts of the gut.[341] Dawson found that two thirds of his patients, mostly women, were depressed, but this figure was probably because they had suffered severe symptoms. His 22 patients had been seen by a total of 79 consultants and undergone 38 operations to no avail. Work on gut motility and later gut hypersensitivity gradually led people back to the psychosomatic aspects of irritable bowel syndrome as the importance of the brain-gut axis was appreciated. In their original study Chaudhary and Truelove identified psychological factors as a cause or influence in over 80 per cent of their 130 patients. Some were depressed, many were neurotic and several had family or business worries. Women were more often affected than men. Their astute observations required rigorous testing if clinicians were to accept that irritable bowel syndrome and indeed non-ulcer dyspepsia were truly psychosomatic disorders. Towards the end of the century psychiatrists both here and abroad applied themselves to the problem. In Britain Thomas Craig in London, Arthur Crisp at St. George's Hospital, and Francis Creed in Manchester led the way.

Though everyone agreed that approximately one in three patients with irritable bowel syndrome was clinically depressed, early studies to prove that psychiatric illness actually caused IBS were flawed and therefore inconclusive. The first convincing evidence came from a study in 1984 by Thomas Craig, a psychiatrist in South London working with a sociologist, George Brown.[342] They used a sophisticated interview technique – the Life Events and Difficulties Schedule (LEDS) to show that patients with functional bowel disease, especially IBS, were indeed more likely to have psychiatric disease than patients with organic gastrointestinal illness. Their report was convincing because they used a reliable measure of psychiatric illness in a typical group of patients and included a control group.

Similarly most clinicians thought that their patients with irritable bowel syndrome were neurotic but was this more frequent than normal? Arthur Crisp (1933–2005), Professor of Psychiatry at St. George's Hospital, thought it was. In conjunction with Misiewicz at the Central Middlesex Hospital he assessed the personality of 41 patients and found them to be significantly more neurotic than usual but less so than the average psychiatric patient.[343] He thought that neuroticism rather than bowel symptoms took them to the doctor, though obviously this would not account for those who were not neurotic.

Likewise patients and doctors often ascribed their illness to a recent tragedy, marital difficulty or business worry, in which case it was clearly essential to establish that the stressful life event had occurred before the onset of symptoms. As it can be difficult to date the onset of irritable bowel syndrome, Francis Creed (born 1948), senior lecturer in psychiatry in Manchester, studied life events before appendicectomy, which of course could be accurately dated.[344] He found that people who turned out to have a normal appendix were much more likely to have had a recent stressful event than those with appendicitis. This was similar to patients with depression and many of them were depressed. They were not helped by the operation and turned out to have irritable bowel syndrome.

Martin Eastwood and his wife Jenny in Edinburgh came to a similar conclusion, working with Michael Ford, a physician in Leith, and the MRC Unit for Epidemiological Studies in Psychiatry.[345] They found a history of anxiety or depression in a half of their patients with IBS or functional dyspepsia compared with only ten per cent of patients with organic disease. However, the frequency of a stressful event was similar in both groups and in healthy controls. It was only when a stressful life situation caused an anxiety disorder that functional disease ensued.

In a further effort to establish that psychological factors caused functional bowel disease, Creed teamed up with Craig to compare their earlier studies with a group of overdose patients.[346] All three groups, that is Creed's patients who had had a normal appendicectomy, Craig's patients attending a clinic with functional abdominal pain and the overdose group, were far more likely to have had a severe problem such as separation or divorce before their illness, and the majority were extremely anxious or depressed. They could only speculate on the mechanism. Was it emotional stress altering colonic motility, or anxiety leading to a lowered pain threshold, or was a severe life event causing treatment seeking behaviour? Notably, long standing relationship difficulties were more common in gastroenterological clinics than in overdose patients, perhaps explaining why functional abdominal pain often became chronic.

In 1987 Creed and his research fellow Elspeth Guthrie (born 1958), later awarded an honorary chair in psychological medicine in Manchester, reviewed the psychological aspects of the irritable bowel syndrome[347] and followed this with a current review of psychological treatments.[348] Psychotropic drugs were helpful but people were still unsure how much this was due to their antidepressant effect as opposed to their analgesic and anti-diarrhoeal properties. Psychotherapy was little used and still unproved. Hypnotherapy has already been mentioned and seemed effective, and behaviour therapy had yet to find a place.

During the 1990s interest in the psychological approach to functional bowel disease increased as research into control of the enteric nervous system led inexorably to central control mechanisms and emotional factors. Many people had dyspepsia or symptoms of an irritable bowel but ignored them. Their gut might be unduly sensitive or prone to spasm but they put up with it. Others with similar problems did not. What differentiated those who complained from those who did not? Psychological differences seemed likely and two studies from America published simultaneously in 1988 had shown that people who were psychologically distressed were much more likely to consult a doctor about their irritable bowel symptoms.[349/350]

In Britain, when Roger Jones carried out his survey of dyspepsia in the community, he found that the minority who felt the need to consult a doctor were worried about the possible sinister nature of their symptoms.[351] They tended to exaggerate them and were also afraid they might have cancer or heart disease. Jones found the same in a survey of people with irritable bowel symptoms.[352] Only a third of them sought medical advice and again it was fear of serious disease rather than the severity of their symptoms that took them to the doctor. The non-consulters tended to trivialise their symptoms.

About the same time Ken Heaton in Bristol sent a questionnaire to over 1,800 people in the city asking about intestinal symptoms. Nine per cent had diagnosable irritable bowel syndrome but only half had consulted a physician about it.[353] He found that people with multiple symptoms were the most likely to consult their doctor.

This accorded with earlier work by Peter Whorwell, showing that patients with functional gastrointestinal disease frequently complained of other symptoms such as lethargy, urinary frequency, insomnia and backache. He had also found that patients with IBS and lower abdominal pain were over-represented in gynaecology clinics.[354] Indeed he went on to suggest that non-colonic features were helpful in the diagnosis of irritable bowel syndrome.[355]

These were key observations and became the focus of intense study by psychologists, helping to refashion the whole approach to functional disease, not only of the gastrointestinal tract, but other areas as well such as the musculoskeletal system. Gastroenterologists began to collaborate with psychiatrists and psychologists in a manner that was new to them, and equally psychiatrists had to break away from their traditional field of serious psychiatric illness. It was no longer appropriate to separate psychological illness from physical disease; they were intimately linked.

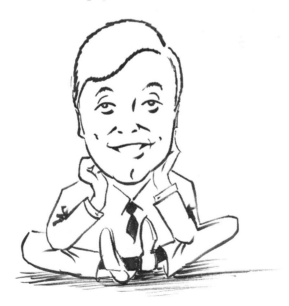

88 Farthing – Unhappy people = unhappy guts.

The Department of Gastroenterology at St. Bartholemew's Hospital, led by Professor Michael Farthing, was one of the first to embrace this approach. Farthing (born 1948) had been appointed senior lecturer at the hospital in 1983 becoming head of the Digestive Diseases Research Centre with a personal chair in 1990. His early research focussed on the pathogenesis of intestinal infection and the mechanisms of intestinal secretion, but his interests were wide and he became fascinated by the relationship between brain and gut and what drove people to seek medical help. Working with two psychiatrists, Gerald Libby and Paul Dewsnap, and a clinical psychologist, Jennifer Gomborone, Farthing organised a community study and showed as expected that consulters with the irritable bowel syndrome had higher anxiety and depression scores than non-consulters.[356] The consulters judged their pain to be more severe, frequent, prolonged and disruptive to daily life than the others. But when the investigator blindly assessed the severity of the symptoms in consulters and non-consulters he found no significant difference between them. So the individual's perception of his or her symptoms seemed to determine whether he or she consulted a doctor. Consulters with the irritable bowel syndrome were more concerned about illness generally, tending to be hypochondriacal and preoccupied with their physical health.[357] Their attitude to illness was worse than that of people with organic disease or even people with depression.

Farthing and his colleagues found that though many patients with IBS were often depressed this could easily be overlooked because they did not have the classic symptoms of an affective disorder. But when he carried out a simple cognitive memory test he found that IBS patients were similar to people with depression.[358] Both groups memorised gloomy words from a list of adjectives in preference to cheerful ones. However, unlike the depressed group, the IBS patients also recalled gloomy words that were not on the list. Farthing thought this was consistent with their negative interpretation of innocent IBS symptoms. They expressed their feelings in terms of physical illness (somatisation) instead of appearing emotionally distressed.

It was now evident that the symptoms of functional bowel disease resulted from abnormal sensitivity and motility within the gut, often strongly influenced by psychological factors. This surprised no one but for the first time clinical impressions were supported by solid scientific evidence, well conducted epidemiology and carefully controlled trials.

The problems did not originate solely in the gut or the brain but in both. Apart from emotional factors and abnormal illness behaviour affecting consultation rates and interpretation of symptoms, there was physiological evidence that emotion could influence the gut directly. This was apparent from Robin Spiller's work on post-infective irritable bowel syndrome in which he showed that persisting inflammation and psychological factors combined to cause continuing symptoms. Another example was the effect of mood on intestinal motor function. Farthing's group showed that patients with anxiety states had fast transit times whereas patients with depression had slow transit times.[359]

Further evidence that emotion affected gut motility and visceral sensation came from Peter Whorwell's studies with hypnosis in Manchester. He induced specific emotions in a specific and reliable way and confirmed the well known fact that anger and excitement increases colonic motility whereas happiness had the opposite effect.[360] Later he showed that altering the emotional state of a patient with irritable bowel syndrome affected their response to rectal discomfort.[361] He speculated that this was due to an alteration in pain processing in the cerebral cortex or changes in cognitive functioning. Some patients with IBS were hypervigilant to expected visceral stimuli and this was increased by emotions such as anger and decreased during relaxation or happiness.

Thus by the early 1990s people, especially in America, were beginning to appreciate the interaction between physiological and psychological factors in functional gut disorders.[362] Biological, psychological and social aspects all had a role to play rather than one of these in isolation. In America clinical psychology was popular and well accepted whereas in Britain it was little used or understood. The attraction of the bio-psycho-social model lay in the opportunities for treatment of a condition that had so far been singularly unsuccessful. Admittedly this approach was time consuming but fortunately the vast majority of patients did not need it. Most responded to simple measures such as reassurance and sympathetic explanation of their problem, sometimes supplemented by an antispasmodic or prokinetic agent and simple dietary advice. Only those with a serious anxiety state, depression or a reaction to their symptoms that was highly abnormal needed specialist psychological help. Broadly speaking the options were antidepressants if the patient was depressed or anxious and some form of psychotherapy if he or she was psychologically disturbed.

Unfortunately few psychiatrists felt inclined to tackle functional gastrointestinal disorders possibly because they did not have the back-up of clinical psychologists. There were of course exceptions such as Farthing's unit at St. Bartholemew's Hospital. Another was in Oxford where Richard Mayou, Professor of Psychiatry at the university, and his colleague, Christopher Bass, consultant liaison psychiatrist at the John Radcliffe Infirmary, were especially interested in psychosomatic disease (liaison psychiatry is the recognition and management of psychiatric problems in general medicine). They spent several years treating non-cardiac chest pain. The vogue for investigating this with oesophageal manometry had never caught on in this country and the relevance of oesophageal disorders to the perception of chest pain was uncertain.[363] The pain might well arise from the oesophagus but demonstrating a motility disturbance rarely helped the management. Mayou and Bass took referrals straight from the cardiologists and showed that cognitive behaviour therapy benefited patients with persistent and disabling chest pain.[364]

The best known centre for the psychological management of functional gut disease was Manchester, curiously enough in two departments working independently. One was Peter Whorwell's unit at Wythenshawe Hospital. Whorwell was of course a gastroenterologist but he had pioneered hypnotherapy for functional disorders, beginning with the irritable bowel syndrome and extending this to functional dyspepsia[365] and non-cardiac chest pain.[366] He was able to claim excellent results but dug his own furrow and received little support from the NHS. He funded most of his research team himself including Dr. Lesley Houghton, Senior Lecturer in Medicine and Physiology, and six hypnotherapists. Unfortunately this proved expensive and by 2008 there were only two therapists working in the department and a disappointing two-year wait for treatment.

The organisation of the other department in Manchester was more conventional. Francis Creed was well established as senior lecturer in psychiatry at Manchester Royal Infirmary when he was appointed Professor of the Department of Psychological Medicine in 1997. He was a prolific author and in 1999 became Editor of the *Journal of Psychosomatic Research*. In 2001 he was elected President of the European Association of Consultation-Liaison Psychiatry and Psychosomatics. As far as the functional gastrointestinal disorders were concerned his chief interest

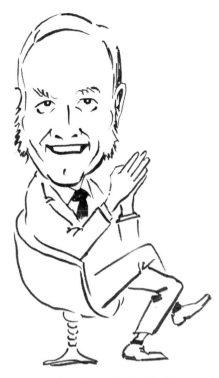

89 Creed – Put simply, the problem is bio-psycho-social.

lay with the irritable bowel syndrome. In the early 1990s, working with Elspeth Guthrie, lecturer in psychiatry and later to be Professor of Psychological Medicine at the University, he showed that psychotherapy was unequivocably superior to standard medical treatment in patients with IBS.[367] About this time Creed and David Thompson, Professor of Gastroenterology, set up the North of England IBS study group as a vehicle for clinical trials. This was a loose association of psychiatrists and psychologists from Manchester and Sheffield, together with Karna Bardham from Rotheram, Nick Read from Sheffield and a health economist from York. For a decade or so, with support from the Medical Research Council, the group published a series of papers on the effect of psychological interventions on quality of life in the irritable bowel syndrome[368] and the cost effectiveness of psychological treatment.[369] In particular they showed that though somatisation was common in patients with IBS not all of them had an excess of bodily symptoms. Those that did had a concurrent psychiatric disorder and/or a history of sexual abuse and it was this group that responded particularly well to psychotherapy.[370] Research from Belgium and America suggested that functional dyspepsia benefited from a similar approach.[371]

Psychologists were making their mark. Creed was a member of the Rome II sub-committee's report on psychosocial factors in functional gastrointestinal disorders in 1999[372] and again when the Rome III sub-committee reported in 2006.[373] When the British Society of Gastroenterology published its guidelines on the management of the irritable bowel syndrome in 2000, four of the editors represented the psychological aspects of treatment;[374] Jennifer Gomborone and Gerald Libby, Nicholas Read (about to retrain as a psychotherapist and leave the National Health Service) and Peter Whorwell. An updated and comprehensive set of guidelines appeared in 2007 in which both Creed and Whorwell were involved.[375] Yet, despite the impressive evidence for psychological intervention, psychiatrists were slow to embrace the challenge of somatisation and hypochondriasis[376] that typified severe functional bowel disease.[377] Creed appealed for a greater involvement of psychiatrists in both the evaluation and treatment of patients with these disorders as well as education and training of practitioners caring for these patients.[378] Unfortunately very few hospitals in Britain employed clinical psychologists, seen as a luxury that the NHS could not afford. Most specialist bowel psychotherapists are in private practice and it seems unlikely that this will change in the foreseeable future.

CHAPTER SIXTY-THREE

5-HYDROXYTRYPTAMINE

Patients with mild to moderate functional dyspepsia or irritable bowel syndrome visited their doctor hoping that reassurance and simple medication would help them, which they usually did. Unfortunately, this approach was ineffective in more severe cases and psychotherapy, which could be useful was rarely available. So the discovery of new drugs affecting 5-hydroxytrytamine metabolism was exciting especially when people realised they might be beneficial in functional gastrointestinal disorders.

Serotonin, or 5-hydroxytryptamine, was identified soon after the Second World War and though most of it came from the gut a small but significant amount was present in the brain, and this was the focus of attention for several years. However, the amine was known to affect gut motility and in 1966 George Misiewicz and Sheila Waller at the Central Middlesex Hospital showed this to be the case in humans when infusions of 5-HT increased small bowel motility.[379] However, apart from its role in the rare carcinoid syndrome 5-HT excited little interest among gastroenterologists until the early 1980s, when the importance of the enteric nervous system in regulating motility and visceral perception was accepted and it was realised that 5-hydroxytryptamine was a key enteric neurotransmitter. By this time several receptor subtypes for 5-HT were being discovered and in the gut the 5-HT3 and 5-HT4 receptors were the most important. It was a distinguished British pharmacologist, John Fozard (born 1942), working for Merrell Dow, who discovered the first potent selective antagonist at the 5-HT3 receptor. Research now took off with enthusiastic support from the pharmaceutical companies.

Glaxo introduced their 5-HT3 receptor antagonist, ondansetron, in 1987 as an antiemetic for patients receiving chemotherapy.[380] Shortly after

Tony Morris in Liverpool, a future president of the BSG, Ian Gilmore (born 1947), a future president of the Royal College of Physicians and their research registrar, Steve Gore, studied the effect of ondansetron on intestinal transit in healthy volunteers and found that it slowed colonic transit.[381]

Meanwhile researchers at Beecham had developed another 5-HT3 receptor antagonist, granisetron, and in 1993 Alison Prior and Nick Read in Sheffield showed that this compound reduced rectal sensitivity and post-prandial colonic activity in patients with IBS.[382] This generated considerable interest because of its potential to relieve symptoms of functional bowel disorders such as pain, urgency and bowel frequency. Further support for this class of drugs came from Peter Whorwell's group in Manchester who found that ondansetron helped people with both functional dyspepsia and irritable bowel syndrome.[383]

By this time Charles Marsden (born 1943), a neuropharmacologist in Nottingham,had introduced a new technique, that of high performance liquid chromatography, to measure 5-hydroxytryptamine sensitively and quickly[384] which was widely adopted. Michael Farthing at St. Bartholemew's Hospital who had long been interested in the pathogenesis of infective diarrhoea used this method to show that 5-hydroxytryptamine was implicated in the secretory effect of cholera toxin.[385] Farthing was also interested in functional bowel disorders and with his registrar, Charlotte Bearcroft, went on to show that patients with diarrhoea predominant IBS had higher post-prandial plasma 5-HT levels than normal. Here was further evidence that serotonin was responsible for some of the symptoms of IBS[386] and it fitted nicely with Robin Spiller's finding that post-dysenteric IBS was associated with an excess of enterochromaffin cells in the small intestine, the chief source of 5-hydroxytryptamine in the gut. Later in Manchester, Peter Whorwell and Lesley Houghton (born 1960), a physiologist with the honorary title of senior lecturer in medicine and physiological sciences, extended Farthing's work and showed that symptoms after a meal in women with diarrhoea predominant IBS were definitely associated with increased levels of plasma 5-HT.[387/388]

5-HT3 receptor antagonists looked set to be a valuable addition to the few effective remedies for severe diarrhoea predominant irritable bowel syndrome especially after Michael Camilleri at the Mayo Clinic published excellent results for another compound, alosetron.[389] But no sooner had his report appeared than the drug was withdrawn by Glaxo because of side effects of constipation and ischaemic colitis. This was a setback for clinicians and the pharmaceutical industry but to the surprise of many the drug was reintroduced into the American market in 2002 with restrictions for its use. The regulatory case of alosetron was highly debated in the literature[390/391] and to date 5-HT receptor antagonists are unavailable in this country.

The discovery of the 5-HT4 receptor in 1988 occurred shortly after the introduction of cisapride, a prokinetic agent that was subsequently found to have 5-HT4 receptor agonist and 5-HT3 receptor antagonist activity. Cisapride increased oesophageal sphincter pressure and accelerated gastric emptying and was promoted as treatment for gastro-oesophageal reflux and functional dyspepsia. It had little effect on the colon probably because of its 5-HT3 receptor antagonist properties. Unfortunately it interacted with many other drugs causing serious cardiac arrhythmias and was withdrawn in 2001. Meanwhile another 5-HT receptor agonist, tegaserod, was undergoing successful trials in patients with constipation-predominant IBS. Most of this work was done in Europe and America but in Manchester Peter Whorwell's group were enthusiastic about the drug, especially its ability to improve bloating,[392] an under-rated but very troublesome symptom for some people.[393] Unfortunately, despite good initial experience concerning safety, the pharmaceutical company, Novartis, suspended sales of tegaserod in March 2007 after an analysis of its clinical database pointed to a higher incidence of myocardial infarction and stroke among patients (typically young women) taking the drug.

Thus despite considerable interest and enthusiasm for 5-HT3 receptor antagonists and 5-HT4 receptor agonists, none is yet available because of safety concerns. Functional bowel diseases are not lethal disorders so their treatment has to be above suspicion. Fortunately it has been possible to harness the benefit of 5-HT thanks to the selective serotonin reuptake inhibitors, antidepressants that are in common use. Serotonin (5-HT) is avidly taken up by platelets where it is deactivated. Serotonin uptake inhibitors prevent this thus increasing the availability of 5-HT. As about 20 per cent of 5-HT is found in the brain much of the early work on 5-HT concerned its role within the brain and the development of antidepressants affecting 5-HT levels. Both the older tricyclic antidepressants and the newer SSRI compounds were effective antidepressants but were also noted to alter help patients with IBS even if they were not depressed. If this was something to do with 5-HT, the benefit could be at two levels, gut and brain. In 1994 Michael Farthing and his registrar, David Gorard, showed that imipramine (a tricyclic) slowed gut transit despite its inhibitory action on 5-HT re-uptake, presumably because of its antimuscarinic effect. On the other hand, paroxetine (an SSRI) speeded up the gut due to the effect of 5-HT on the small intestine.[394] At the time Farthing was careful not to link these changes with the benefits of the drugs in IBS, which he thought were still more likely to be due to a central effect.

Subsequent work by Francis Creed and his co-workers in Manchester showed that paroxetine helped two groups of patients with IBS, those who were clearly depressed and those with somatisation who report numerous bodily symptoms.[395] Creed speculated on how SSRIs helped these people and concluded that they have an as yet undefined effect on the gut itself but undoubtedly help some of the psychological processes,[396] quite apart from their antidepressant effect.

Functional gastrointestinal disorders remain a challenge. As Sir Christopher Booth once asked, "Does anyone have any idea what produces that extraordinary concatenation of symptoms that go under the general diagnosis of irritable bowel syndrome?"[397] That was in 1995 and some, particularly psychologists, feel they are making progress. We now think the mind can influence the gut and that biology, psychology and social factors are inextricably linked and not to be treated in isolation.

The enteric nervous system and the central nervous system work together for better or worse. The 1990s were heralded as the decade of the brain amid excitement that new imaging techniques would allow neuroscientists to unravel the mysteries of the human brain. Gastroenterologists, frustrated by the lack of objective methods to assess gut sensory dysfunction, hoped that they would finally see cortical representation of visceral sensation, which would lead to appropriate treatment. In Manchester, David Thompson and his senior lecturer, Qasim Aziz (now Professor of Neurogastroenterology at Bart's and the London School of Medicine and Director of the Wingate Institute), demonstrated the central processing of visceral afferents using positron emission tomography and functional magnetic resonance imaging.[398] In particular they showed how central sensitisation might explain the symptoms in patients with non-cardiac chest pain.[399] But so far brain imaging has had little impact on the actual management of functional gastrointestinal disorders.[400]

Thus despite considerable progress in our concept of functional gut disorders, there has been little real advance in their treatment over the last 50 years. Indeed a recent review suggested that the time-honoured use of fibre, antispasmodics and peppermint oil were as effective in the treatment of irritable bowel syndrome as any of the newer drugs.[401] This may be so but there seems little doubt that psychological treatment for more serious cases can be highly effective. The physicians of the eighteenth and nineteenth century would agree and the likes of Abernethy and James Johnson might equate the effects of 5-hydroxytryptamine with their concepts of universal sympathy and morbid sensibility of the stomach and bowels.

REFERENCES

SECTION FIVE

1   Carroll L. 1871 *Through the Looking-Glass and What Alice Found There*. Ch 6

2   Lovell R. 1661 *Panzooruktologia Sive Panzoologicominealogia or A Compleat History of Animals and Minerals* Oxford: Godwin 366

3   Sydenham T. 1683 *A Treatise on Gout and Dropsy*. The Works of Thomas Sydenham vol 2 R. G. Latham Sydenham Society, London 1850 129

4   Sydenham T. 1681–2 *Epistolary Dissertation to Dr. Cole* The Works of Thomas Sydenham vol 2 R. G. Latham Sydenham Society, London 1850 56–118

5   Sydenham T. ibid pp111–2

6   Quoted by J. A. Paris in *Pharmacologia* (1825) p48 and in John Brown, Locke and Sydenham (1866) 87–88

7   Woodward J. 1910–11 *Of the Body of Man; Of Health, of Diseases, and of Remedies; Three Physico-Mechanical Lectures Read in the Theater of the College of Physitians.* Gulstonian Lectures. B. M. MS Sloane 2039, ff115–29

8   Observations on the Dissection of Daniel Coates, who was executed at Tyburn, 1710, B. M. MS. Sloane 2039, ff130–35

9   Friend J. 1717 *Hippocratis de Morbis Popularibus* London

10 Woodward J. 1718 *State of Physick and of Diseases* London

11 Aitken G. A. 1892 *The Life and Works of John Arbuthnot*, Oxford Clarendon Press

12 Cheyne G. 1773 *The English Malady or a Treatise of Nervous Diseases of all Kinds.* G. Strachan in Cornhill, London

13 Helmont I. B. van 1648 *Sextuplex Digestio Alimenti Humani*, Ortus Medicinae, Amsterdam p208

14 Sylvius F. D. *1679 De Alimentorum Fermentatione in Ventriculi Caesa*. Opera Medica Praxeos Medicae Idea Nova, lib. 1, cap. Vii, 166. Amsterdam

15 Borelli A. G. 1680 *De Motu Animalum*, 1 287 Rome

16 Viridet J. 1692 *Tractatus Novus Medico-Physicus de Prima Coctione Praecipuque de Ventriculi Fermento*. Geneva pp90, 93, 95, 224

17 Reaumur R. A. F. de, 1752 *Sur la Digestion des Oiseaux. Memoires de Mathematiques et de Physique*. Premier memoire, 461 Paris

18 Spallanzani L. 1783 *Experiences de Digestion de l'Homme et de Differentes Especes d'Animaux*. Translated by J Senebier. Geneva; Barthélemy Chirol.

19 Beddoes T. 1784 *Dissertations Relative to the Natural History of Animals and Vegetables.* Translated from the Italian of the Abbe Spallanzani. 2 vols. J. Murray, London

20 Von Haller A. 1759–66 *Experimenta Physiologiae Corporis Humani*

21 Whytt R. 1764 *Observations on the Nature, Causes and Cures of Those Disorders Which Have Been Commonly Called Nervous, Hypochondriac or Hysteric;* Edinburgh, Balfour

22 Thomson J. 1854 *An Account of the Life, Lectures and Writings of William Cullen MD* Edinburgh: William Blackwood and Sons Vol Methodicae 1 25

23 Cullen W. 1769 *Synopsis Nosologiae* Edinburgh

24 Kendall R. E. 1993 in *William Cullen and the Eighteenth Century World* ed Doig A., Ferguson J. P. S., Milne I. A. and Passmore R. Edinburgh Univ Press 223–228

25 Parkinson, J. W. K. ed. 1833 *Hunterian Reminiscences, Being the Substance of a Course of Lectures on the Principles and Practice of Surgery, Delivered by the Late Mr. John Hunter in the Year 1785; Taken in Short-Hand and Afterwards Fairly Transcribed by the Late Mr. James Parkinson.* Sherwood, Gilbert and Piper, London

26 Hunter J. 1772 *On Digestion of the Stomach after Death*, Philosoph. Trans. London 62 447

27 Beddoes T. 1784 *Dissertations Relative to the Natural History of Animals and Vegetables. Translated from the Abbe Spallanzani. To which are added an appendix, the first containing a paper written by Mr. Hunter FRS and the Experiments of Dr. Stevens* 2 vols J. Murray, London 365–391

28 Gibbs D. D. 2000 *John Hunter and the Stomach.* Delivered to the Trustees of the Hunterian Collection: The Royal College of Surgeons, unpublished

29 Coe T. 1757 *A Treatise on Biliary Concretions: or, Stones in the Gall-Bladder and Ducts.* Printed for D. Wilson and T. Durham at Plato's Head in the Strand, London

30 Grant W. 1779 *Some Observations on the Origins, Progress, and Method of Treating the Atrabilious Temperament and Gout.* printed for T. Cadell in the Strand, London

31 Andree J. 1788 *Considerations on Bilious Diseases and Some Particular Affections of the Liver and the Gall-Bladder.* Hertford. Printed for the Author and sold by J. Murray, and W. Lowndes, in Fleet St. London; and T. Simson, Hertford

32 Adair J. M. 1790 *Essays on Fashionable Diseases.* Bateman, London

33 Trotter T. 1807 *A View of the Nervous Temperament; Being a Practical Enquiry into the Increasing Prevalence, Prevention, and Treatment of Those Diseases Commonly Called Nervous, Bilious, Stomach, and Liver Complaints; Indigestion; Low Spirits; Gout, etc.* Second edition, printed by Edward Walker, Newcastle for Longman, Hurst, Rees, and Orme, London

34 Rees G. 1810 *Practical Observations on Disorders of the Stomach with Remarks on the Use of Bile in Promoting Digestion,* Allen, London

35 Thornton J. L. 1953 *John Abernethy a Biography.* Distributed by Simpkin Marshall Ltd., London

36 Abernethy J. 1806 *Surgical Observations, Part the Second, Containing an Account of the Disorders of Health in General and of the Digestive Organs in Particular.* Longman, London

37   Abernethy J. 1809 *Surgical Observations on the Constitutional Origin and Treatment of Local Diseases, and on Aneurisms.* Longman, London

38   Power Sir Darcy 1930 My Book by John Abernethy, XI Epoch-making Books in British Surgery. *Brit. J. Surg.*, 17, 369–372

39   Pettigrew T. J. 1838–40 *Medical Portraits Gallery, 4 volumes "John Abernethy FRS"* Fisher and Son, London, II, 10

40   Philip A. P. W. 1824 *A Treatise on Indigestion and its Consequences Called Nervous and Bilious Complaints; With Observations on the Organic Diseases in Which They Sometimes Terminate.* 4th edition Thomas and George Underwood, London

41   Johnson J. 1827 *Essay on Morbid Sensibility of the Stomach and Bowels, as the Proximate Cause, or Characteristic Condition of Indigestion, Nervous Irritability, Mental Despondency, Hypochondriasis, etc. etc.* American edition published by Benjamin & Thomas Kite, Philadelphia

42   Osler W. 1959 *William Beaumont,* Dover Publications Inc. New York pxi

43   Beaumont W. 1833 *Experiments and Observations on the Gastric Juice, and the Physiology of Digestion.* Plattsburgh, printed by F. P. Allen

44   Smith T. S. 1835–37 *The Philosophy of Health, or an Exposition of the Physical and Mental Constitution of Man: With a View to the Promotion of Human Longevity and Happiness.* 2 vols London, Knight II pp642–644

45   Combe A. 1836 *The Physiology of Digestion Considered With Relation to the Principles of Dietetics,* Maclachlan and Stewart, Edinburgh

46   Beaumont W. 1838 *Experiments and Observations on the Gastric Juice and the Physiology of Digestion,* Reprinted From the Plattsburgh Edition, With Notes by Andrew Combe MD. Edinburgh: Maclachan and Stewart.

47   Watson T. 1848 *Lectures on the Principles and Practice of Physic; Delivered at King's College, London.* John W. Parker, London Third edition vol II p437

48   Child G. C. 1847 *On Indigestion and Certain Bilious Disorders Often Conjoined With It. To Which are Added, Short Notes on Diet.* John Churchill, London

49   Watson T. 1848 *Lectures on the Principles and Practice of Physic; Delivered at King's College, London.* John W. Parker, London. Third edition vol II 437–454

50   Budd G. 1856 *On the Organic Diseases and Functional Disorders of the Stomach,* Samuel S. and William Wood, New York. 168–179

51   Boyd Sprott. 1836 On the Structure of the Mucous Membrane of the Stomach. *Edin. Med. and Surg. Journal* xlvi 382

52   Brinton W. 1864 *Lectures on the Diseases of the Stomach With an Introduction on its Anatomy and Physiology.* John Churchill & Sons, London Lectures II and VI

53   Gibbs D. D. 1997 The Demon of Dyspepsia: Some Nineteenth-Century Perceptions of Disordered Digestion. in *Gastroenterology in Britain: Historical Essays* ed W. F. Bynum Wellcome Trust p37

54   *The Complete Correspondence of Charles Darwin.* 1985. ed. F. Burkhardt and S. Smith vol II 47–52

55   Gully J. M. 1846 *The Water Cure in Chronic Disease.* John Churchill, London

56   Darwin F. 1887 *Life and Letters of Charles Darwin.* John Murray, London vol 3 p1.

57 Hubble D. 1943 Charles Darwin and psychotherapy. *Lancet*, 30 Jan 129–33

58 Pickering G. 1974 *Creative Malady,* George Allen and Unwin, London

59 Atkins H. 1974 *Down: The Home of the Darwins.* The Royal College of Surgeons, London

60 Bowlby J. 1990 *Charles Darwin. A New Biography.* Hutchinson, London

61 Gould G. M. 1903 *Biographical Clinics.* Redman, London

62 Huxley L. ed 1900 *Life and Letters of Thomas Henry Huxley* 2 vols. New York, Appleton and Company

63 Gould G. M. 1903 *Biographic Clinics: the Origin of the Ill-health of De Quincy, Carlyle, Darwin, Huxley and Browning.* Rebman, Limited, London

64 Quain R. 1895 letter *Brit. Med. J.* 1147

65 T. Lauder Brunton 1886 *Lettsomian Lectures: In Disorders of Digestion, Their Consequences and Treatment.* Macmillan and Co., London 1–79

66 Kussmaul A. 1869 Ueber die Behandlung der Magenereweiterung durch eine neue Methode mittelst der Magenpumpe. *Dtsch. Arch. Klin. Med.* 6: 455–500 (Dec. 23)

67 Leube W. O. 1883 Beitrage zur Diagnostik der Magenkrankheiten. *Dtsch. Arch. Klin. Med.* 33, 1–21

68 Ewald C. A., Boas J. 1885 Beitrage zur Physiologie und Pathologie der Verdauung. *Arch. F. Path. Anat.,* 101: 325–375

69 Osler W. 1901 *The Principle and Practice of Medicine.* Edinburgh Young J. Pentland 497–505

70 Summers J. E. 1905 Surgical treatment of chronic muco-membranous colitis and ulcerative colitis. *Annals of Surgery* 421 97–109

71 Herodotus 1992 *The Histories* Book Two chap 77 The Folio Society, London

72 Doig A., Ferguson J. P. S., Milne I. A., Passmore R. 1991 *William Cullen and the Eighteenth Century World.* Edinburgh University Press 228–229

73 Abercrombie J. 1830 *Pathological and Practical Researches on Diseases of the Stomach, the Intestinal Canal, the Liver, and Other Viscera of the Abdomen.* Carey and Lea, Philadelphia p194

74 ibid pp308–9

75 Howship J. 1830 *Practical Remarks on the Discrimination and Successful Treatment of Spasmodic Stricture in the Colon Considered as an Occasional Cause of Habitual Confinement of the Bowels.* London

76 Watson T. 1848 *Lectures on the Principles and Practice of Physic.* London Vol 1 p160 and p184

77 Hutchinson T., Wilks S. & Clark A. 1857 Tubular Exudation Casts of the Intestine. *Trans. Pathol. Soc.* Vol 9: 188–194

78 Wilks S. 1859 *Lectures on Pathological Anatomy delivered at Guy's Hospital during the summer sessions 1857–58* Longmans, Brown, Green, Longmans, Roberts, London

79 Wilks S. & Moxon W. 1875 *Lectures on Pathological Anatomy* Second edition J. & A. Churchill, London pp409–410

80 Fitz R. H. 1886 Perforating inflammation of the vermiform appendix; with special reference to its early diagnosis and treatment. *Trans. Assoc. Am. Physicians* I; 107–144

81   Deaver J. B. 1896 *Appendicitis*. Blakiston, Philadelphia p132

82   Shoemaker G. E. 1898 The Importance of Chronic Irritability of the Colon, with Mucous Stools as a Symptom of Appendicitis. *Annals of Surgery* 6; 733–740

83   Glenard F. 1885 Application de la methode naturelle a l'analyse de la dyspepsie nerveuse; determination d'une espece. *Lyon Med.*, 48: 449–464; 492–505; 532–543; 563–583

84   Cannon W. B. 1902 The movements of the intestines studied by means of the roentgen rays. *Amer. J. Physiol.* 6: 251–277

85   Osler W. 1901 *The Principle and Practice of Medicine*. Edinburgh Young J. Pentland 541–543

86   Summers J. E. 1905 The surgical treatment of chronic muco-membranous and ulcerative colitis, with special reference to technique. *Annals of Surgery* July; 42 97–109

87   Hurst A. F. 1910 A clinical lecture on muco-membranous colitis *Clinical Journal* August, 36, 263–267

88   Sand G. 1855 *Histoire de ma Vie*. Vol xviii. p295 Paris

89   Editorial 1902 Chronic Dyspepsia. *Lancet* Aug 23rd

90   Moynihan B. G. 1910 *Duodenal Ulcer* Philadelphia, Saunders, p19

91   Moynihan B. G. 1910 *Brit. Med. J.* Jan

92   Hurst A. F. 1922 Chronic appendicitis and appendicular dyspepsia. *Guy's Hosp. Reports*. 72, 386–399

93   Bastedo W. A. 1911 The dilatation test for chronic appendicitis. *Amer. J. Med. Sci.* 142, 11–14

94   Hurst A. F. 1913 Bastedo's sign: a new symptom of chronic appendicitis. *Lancet*, 1, 816–817

95   Hurst A. F. and Stewart M. J. 1929 Diagnosis from reflex dyspepsias. In: *Gastric and Duodenal Ulcer*. Ox Univ Press Part VI chap 2 pp234–237

96   Hawkins H. P. 1906 The reality of enterospasm and its mimicry of appendicitis. *Brit. Med. J.* i, 65–69

97   Hurst A. F., Morton C. J., Cook F., Cox A. N., Gardiner N., Schlinger E. G., Todd, A. H. 1907 The passage of food along the human alimentary canal. *Guy's Hosp. Reports* 61, 85–110

98   Newton H. A. S., Hurst A. F. 1913 The normal movements of the colon in man. *J. Physiol.* (London) 47, 57–65

99   Hurst A. F. 1919 *Constipation and Allied Intestinal Disorders*. Oxford University Press 2nd edit p101

100   Hurst A. F. 1949 *A Twentieth Century Physician, Being the Reminiscences of Sir Arthur Hurst*. E Arnold and Co., London pp120–1

101   Hurst A. F., Cook F., Schlesinger E. G. 1908 The sensibility of the stomach and intestines in man. *J. Physiol.* (London) 37, 481–490

102   Hurst A. F. 1911 *The Goulstonian Lectures on The Sensibility of the Alimentary Canal*. Oxford University Press, London

103   Hurst A. F. 1910 A clinical lecture on muco-membranous colitis, *Clinical Journal* 36, 263–267

104   Osler W. 1901 *The Principle and Practice of Medicine*. Edinburgh Young J. Pentland 544

105   Hurst A. F. 1910 A clinical lecture on muco-membranous colitis. *Clinical Journal*, 36, 263–267

106   Barclay A. E. 1935 Direct X-ray cinematography with a preliminary note on the nature of the non-propulsive movements of the large intestine. *Brit. J. Radiol.* 8, 652–658

107   Hurst A. F. 1922 An address on the sins and sorrows of the colon. (Delivered before the Harrogate Medical Society, November 26th, 1921.) *Brit. Med. J.*, 1, 941–943

108   Root H. K. 1856 *The People's Medical Lighthouse*. New York: Ranney, p114

109   Lane W. A. 1913 An address on chronic intestinal stasis. *Brit. Med. J.* ii: 1126

110   Morrice A. A. G. 2004 *Sir William Arbuthnot Lane. Oxf. Dict. Nat. Biog.* Article 34394

111   Ogilvie H. 1951 The Large Bowel and Its Functions. *Proceedings of the Royal Society of Medicine* 44, 200–206

112   Wilson T. S. 1922 A physiological explanation of pain due to functional disturbance of the muscles of colon. *Brit. Med. J.* i 944–946

113   Wilson T. S. 1927 *Tonic Hardening of the Colon*. Humphrey Milford, Oxford University Press

114   Ryle J. A. 1928 Chronic Spasmodic Affections of the Colon and the Diseases which They Simulate. *Lancet*, ii, 1115–17

115   Ryle J. A. 1936 *The Natural History of Disease*. Oxford University Press

116   Hurst A. F. 1930 "Mythical maladies." *Clinical Journal* 59: pp277–283

117   Hurst A. F. 1930 "Mythical maladies." *Clinical Journal* 59: p282

118   Ogilvie W. H. 1951 The Large Bowel and Its Functions. *Proceedings of the Royal Society of Medicine* 44, 6–12

119   Tidy H. L. 1941 Discussion of dyspepsia in the forces. *Proceedings of the Royal Society of Medicine* XXXIV 411–426

120   Payne R. T. and Newman C. E. 1940 Interim Report on dyspepsia in the Army *Brit. Med. J.* ii, 819–821

121   Jones F. A. and Pollak H. 1945 Civilian dyspepsia *Brit. Med. J.* I 797– 800

122   Doll R., Jones F. A., Buckatzsch M. M. 1951 Occupational factors in the aetiology of gastric and duodenal ulcers. Special Report Series. No 276 Medical Research Council, HMSO., London

123   Scott Harden W. G. 1960 *Mod Trends in Diagnostic Radiology*. Ed. J. W. McLaren, Butterworths

124   Hadley G. D. 1965 The gastrocamera. *Brit. Med. J.* 1209–12

125   Blendis L. M., Cameron A. J. and Hadley G. D. 1967 Analysis of 400 examinations using the gastrocamera *Gut* 8 83-90

126   Coghill N. F. and Williams A. W. 1955 The technique of gastric biopsy *Brit. Med. J.* ii 1111

127   Williams W. A., Edwards Felicity, Lewis T. H. C. and Coghill N. F. 1957 Investigation of non-ulcer dyspepsia by gastric biopsy. *Brit. Med. J.* I 372–377

128   Gear M. W. L. and Barnes R. J. 1980 Endoscopic studies of dyspepsia in a general practice *Brit. Med. J.* ii 1136–37

129   Holdstock G., Wiseman M., Loehry C. A. 1979 Open-access endoscopy service for general practitioners. *Brit. Med. J.* I 457–459

130   Crean G. P., Holden R. J., Knill-Jones R. P., Beattie A. D., James W. B., Marjoriebanks, F. M. and Spiegelhalter, D. J. 1984 A data base on dyspepsia. *Gut*, 35: 191–202

131   Misiewicz J. J. & Baron J. H. 1987 Gerard Crean, a mini-biography. *Gut*, Jubilee Suppl. p48

132   Horrocks Jane C. & de Dombal F. T. 1975 Computer-aided diagnosis of "dyspepsia". *Dig. Dis. Sci.* 20, Number 5 397–406

133   Harvey R. F., Salih S. Y., Read A. E. 1983 Organic and functional disorders in 2000 outpatients attending a gastroenterology clinic. *Lancet.* I 632–634

134   Management of Dyspepsia: Report of a Working Party. 1988 *Lancet* I 576–579

135   Spriggs E. I. 1931 Functional disorders of the colon. *Quart. J. Med.* 24, 533-541

136   Peters G. A. and Bargen J. A. 1944 The irritable bowel syndrome. *Gastroenterology*, 3, 399–402

137   Almy T. P. and Tulin M. 1947 Alterations in colonic function in man under stress: experimental production of changes simulating the "irritable colon". *Gastroenterology* 8, 616–626

138   Kirsner J. B. and Palmer W. L. 1958 The Irritable Colon, *Gastroenterology*, 34, 3, 491–500

139   Chaudhary N. A. & Truelove S. C. 1962 The irritable colon syndrome. *Quart. J. Med.*, *n.s.* xxxi, No 123, 307–322

140   Chaudhary A. S. & Truelove S. C. 1961 Human colonic motility: a comparative study of normal subjects, patients with ulcerative colitis, and patients with the irritable colon syndrome. *Gastroenterology*, 40, 1–34

141   Ritchie J. A. 1968 Colonic motor activity and bowel function. Part 1. Normal movement of contents. *Gut.* 9, 442–456

142   Ritchie J. A., Ardran G. M. & Truelove S. C. 1962 Motor activity of the sigmoid colon of humans. *Gastroenterology*, 43, 642–668

143   Ritchie J. A. 1973 Pain from distension of the pelvic colon by inflating a balloon in the irritable colon syndrome. *Gut*, 14, 125–132

144   Rowlands E. N. & Wolff H. S. 1960 The radio pill. Telemetering from the digestive tract. *Brit. Commun. Electron.* 7, 598–701

145   Atkinson M., Edwards D. A. W., Honour A. J., & Rowlands E. N. 1957 Comparison of cardiac and pyloric sphincters, a manometric study. *Lancet*, 2, 918–922

146   Connell A. M. 1961 The motility of the pelvic colon. I Motility in normals and in patients with asymptomatic peptic ulcer. *Gut* 2 175–186

147   Connell A. M. 1962 The motility of the pelvic colon. II Paradoxical motility in diarrhoea and constipation. *Gut* 3 342–348

148   Connell A. M., Gaafer M., Hassenan M. A., and Khayal M. A. 1964 The motility of the pelvic colon. III Motility responses in patients with symptoms following amoebic dysentery. *Gut*, 5, 443

149 Connell A. M., Avery Jones F. and Rowlands E. N. 1965 Motility of the pelvic colon IV Abdominal pain associated with colonic hypermotility after meals. *Gut* 6 105–112

150 Holdstock D. J., Misiewicz J. J. and Waller S. L. 1969 Observations on the mechanism of abdominal pain. *Gut* 10 19–31

151 Misiewicz J. J., Waller S. L., Fox R. H., Goldsmith R. and Hunt T. J. 1968 The effect of elevated body temperature and of stress on the motility of the stomach and colon in man. *Clin. Sci.*, 34, 149–159

152 Szurszeski J. H. 1969 A migrating electric complex of the canine small intestine. *Amer. J. Physiol.* 217, 1757–63

153 Cleave T. L. 1941 Natural bran in the treatment of constipation. *Brit. Med. J.* i 461

154 Cleave T. L. and Campbell G. D. 1966 *Diabetes, Coronary Thrombosis and the Saccharine Disease.* Wrights of Bristol

155 Painter N. S., Truelove S. C., Ardran G. M. & Tuckey M. 1965 Segmentation and the localisation of intraluminal pressures in the human colon, with special reference to the pathogenesis of colonic diverticula. *Gastroenterology*, 49, 169–177

156 Painter N. S. 1967 Diverticulosis of the Colon–Fact or Speculation. *Amer. J. Dig. Dis.* 12, 222–227

157 Painter N. S., Almeida A. Z. & Colebourne K. W. 1972 Unprocessed bran in the treatment of diverticular disease of the colon. *Brit. Med. J.* ii, 137–140

158 Cleave T. L., Campbell G. D. & Painter N. S. 1969 *Diabetes, Coronary Thrombosis and the Saccharine Disease.* 2nd edition. John Wright and Sons Ltd, Bristol.

159 Painter N. S. & Burkitt D. P. 1971 Diverticular Disease of the Colon: A Deficiency Disease of Western Civilisation. *Brit. Med. J.* ii 450–454

160 Burkitt D. P. 1971 Epidemiology of cancer of the colon and rectum. *Cancer*, 28, 3–13

161 Hinton J. M., Lennard-Jones J. E. & Young A. C. 1969 A new method for studying gut transit times using radiopaque markers. *Gut*, 10, 842–847

162 Walker A. R. P., Walker B. F. & Richardson B. D. 1970 Bowel transit times in Bantu populations. *Brit. Med. J.* iii 48–49

163 Burkitt D. P., Walker A. R. P. & Painter N. S. 1972 Effect of dietary fibre on stools and transit times, and its role in the causation of disease. *Lancet*, ii, 1408–12

164 Trowell H. C. 1960 *Non-infective Disease in Africa.* Edward Arnold, London

165 Heaton K. W. 1989 The rev Hubert Carey Trowell. *Monk's Roll* vol IX 533–536

166 Trowell H. C. 1972 Crude fibre, dietary fibre and atherosclerosis. *Atherosclerosis*, 16, 138–140

167 Burkitt D. P. 1979 *"Don't Forget Fibre in Your Diet" to Help Avoid Many of Our Commonest Diseases.* The Lotuspond

168 Cleave T. L. 1974 *The Saccharine Disease,* John Wright and Son, Bristol

169 Trowell H. C. 1981 Editor, *Western Diseases: Their Emergence and Prevention* Edward Arnold, London

170 Painter N. S. 1975 *Diverticular Disease of the Colon: A Deficiency Disease of Western Civilisation.* Heinemann, London

171 Lumsden K., Chaudhary N. A. & Truelove S. C. 1963 The irritable colon syndrome. *Clinical Radiology*, 14, 54–63

172 Manousos O. N., Truelove S. C. & Lumsden K. 1967 Transit time of food in patients with diverticulosis or irritable colon syndrome and normal subjects. *Brit. Med. J.* iii 760–762

173 Painter N. S. 1972 Irritable or irritated bowel? *Brit. Med. J.* ii, 46

174 Eastwood M. 1969 Dietary Fibre and serum-lipids. *Lancet*, ii, 1222–24

175 Southgate D. A. T. 1978 The definition, analysis and properties of dietary fibre. In *Dietary Fibre: Current Developments of Importance to Health*. ed K. W. Heaton Newman Publishing, London 9-19

176 Eastwood M. A. 1973 Vegetable fibre: its physical properties. In Symposium on "fibre in human nutrition" Proc. Nutr. Soc. 32, 137–143

177 Allinson T. R. 1889 *The Advantages of Wholemeal Bread*. Allinson Publication, London

178 Jones F. A. & Godding E. W. 1972 *Management of Constipation*. Blackwell, Oxford.

179 Moynihan B. G. 1913 The gifts of surgery to medicine. Annual address to Brit. Med. Assoc. *Brit. Med. J.* 169–175

180 Heaton K. W. 1969 Keeping bile salts in their place. *Gut* 10 857–863

181 Harvey R. F. and Read A. E. 1973 Effect of cholecystokinin on colonic motility and symptoms in patients with the irritable bowel syndrome. *Lancet*, I: 1–3

182 Harvey R. F., Pomare E. W. and Heaton K. W. 1973 Effects of increased dietary fibre on intestinal transit. *Lancet*, I: 1278–80

183 Payler D. K., Pomare E. W., Heaton K. W. and Harvey R. F. 1975 The effect of wheat bran on intestinal transit. *Gut*, 16, 209–213

184 Manning A. P., Heaton K. W., Harvey R. F. and Uglow, p1977 Wheat fibre and irritable bowel syndrome. *Lancet* 2 417–418

185 Manning A. P., Wyman J. B. and Heaton K. W. 1976 How trustworthy are bowel histories? *Brit. Med. J.* iii 213–214

186 Wyman J. B., Heaton K. W., Manning A. P. and Wicks A. C. B. 1978 Variability of colonic function in healthy subjects *Gut* 19, 146–150

187 Manning A. P., Thompson W. G., Heaton K. W. and Morris A. F. 1978 Towards positive diagnosis of the irritable bowel. *Brit. Med. J.* 2 653–654

188 Talley N. J., Phillips S. F., Melton L. J., Wiltgen D., Mulvihill C. and Zinsmeister A. R. 1990 Diagnostic value of the Manning criteria in irritable bowel syndrome. *Gut*, 31: 77–81

189 Payne W. W. and Poulton E. P. 1927 Experiments on visceral sensation: Part 1, The relation of pain to activity in the human oesophagus. *J. Physiol.* Lxiii 217–241

190 Bennett J. R. and Atkinson M. 1966 The differentiation between oesophageal and cardiac pain. *Lancet*, ii 1123–27

191 Bennett J. R. and Atkinson M. 1968 Oesophageal acid perfusion in the diagnosis of precordial pain. *Lancet*, ii 1150–52

192 Atkinson M. and Bennett, J. R. 1968 The relationship between motor changes and pain during esophageal acid perfusion. *Amer. J. Dig. Dis.* 13, 4, 346–350

193 Vantrappen G. and Hellemans J. 1976 Diffuse Muscle Spasm of the Oesophagus

and the Lower Oesophageal Sphincter. *Clinics in Gastroenterology* vol 5, No 1, 59 -72

194 Brand D. L., Martin D. and Pope C. E. 1977 Esophageal manometrics in patients with angina-like chest pain. *Dig. Dis. Sci.*; 22, 300–304

195 Dart A. M., Alban Davies H., Dalal J., Ruttley M. and Henderson A. H. 1980 "Angina" and normal coronary arteriograms: a follow-up study. *Eur. Heart J.*; 1, 97–100

196 Dart A. M., Alban Davies H., Lowndes R. H., Dalal J., Ruttley M. and Henderson A. H. 1980 Oesophageal spasm and angina: diagnostic value of ergometrine (ergonovine) provocation. *Eur. Heart J.* 1, 91–95

197 Ellis R. 1980 The uneasy oesophagus. *Brit. Med. J.* vol 280 334

198 Hunt J. and Spurrell, W. R. 1951 The pattern of emptying of the human stomach. *J. Physiol.* (Lond) 113; 151–168

199 Griffith G. H., Owen G. M., Kirkman S. and Shields R. 1966 Measurement of rate of gastric emptying using chromium-51. *Lancet*, i, 1244–45

200 Harvey R. F., Brown N. J. G., Mackie D. B., Keeling D. H. and Davies W. T. 1970 Measurement of gastric emptying time with a gamma camera. *Lancet*, i, 16–18

201 Heading R. C., Tothill P., McLoughlin G. P. and Shearman D. J. C. 1976 Gastric emptying rate measurement in man. A double isotope scanning technique for simultaneous study of liquid and solid components of a meal. *Gastroenterology*, 71, 45–50

202 Code C. F. and Marlett J. A. 1975 The interdigestive myo-electric complex of the stomach and small bowel of dogs. *J. Physiol.* 246, 289–309

203 Vantrappen G., Janssens J., Hellemans J. and Ghoos Y. 1977 The interdigestive motor complex of normal subjects and patients with bacterial overgrowth. *J. Clin. Invest.* 59; 1158–66

204 Stanciu C. and Bennett, J. R. 1975 The general pattern of gastro-duodenal motility: 24 hour recordings in normal subjects. *Rev. Med. Chir. Soc. Med. Nat.* Iasi; 79, 31–36

205 Hinton J. M., Lennard-Jones, J. L. and Young A. C. 1969 A new method for studying gut transit time using radio-opaque markers. *Gut*, 10, 842–847

206 Bond J. H. and Levitt M. D. 1975 Investigation of small bowel transit time in normal subjects utilising pulmonary hydrogen measurements. *J. Clin. Lab. Med.* 86 546–555

207 Duthie H. L., Kwong N. K., Brown B. H. and Whittaker G. E. 1971 Pacesetter potential of the human gastroduodenal junction. *Gut*, 12, 250–256

208 Kwong N. K., Brown B. H., Whittaker G. E. and Duthie H. L. 1972 Effects of gastrin, secretin, and cholecystokinin-pancreozymin on the electrical activity, motor activity and acid output of the stomach in man. *Scand. J. Gastroenterol.* 7, 161–170

209 Taylor I., Duthie H. L., Smallwood R. and Linkens D. 1975 Large bowel myoelectrical activity in man. *Gut*, 16, 808–814

210 Taylor I., Darby C. F., Hammond P. and Basu P. 1978 Is there a myoelectrical abnormality in the irritable bowel syndrome? *Gut*, 19, 391–395

211   Darby C. F., Hammond P. and Taylor I. 1978 Real time analysis of colonic myoelectrical rhythms in disease. *Gastrointestinal Motility in Health and Disease. Proc. VI Int. Symp. GI Moility.* MTP Press, Lancaster, England 287–294

212   Taylor I. 1984 Colonic motility in the irritable colon syndrome. In Read N. W. ed *Irritable Bowel Syndrome.* pp89–104, Grune & Stratton, London

213   Harvey R. F. and Read A. E. 1973 Effect of cholecystokinin on colonic motility and symptoms in patients with the irritable bowel syndrome. *Lancet,* i, 1–3

214   Wingate D. L. 2008 A 20-year perspective – from *Journal of Gastrointestinal Motility to Neurogastroenterology and Motility. Neurogastroenterol. Motil. 20* (Suppl. 1), 1–7

215   Vantrappen G., Janssens J., Peeters T. L., Bloom S. R. and Christofides N. D. 1979 Motility and the interdigestive migrating motor complex in man. *Dig. Dis. Sci.* 24 497–500

216   Wingate D. L. 1976 The eupeptide system: a general theory of gastrointestinal hormones. *Lancet,* i, 529–532

217   Ritchie J. A. and Truelove S. C. 1980 Comparison of various treatments for irritable bowel syndrome. *Brit. Med. J.* 2: 1317–9

218   See ref. 193

219   Thompson W. G. and Heaton K. G. 1980 Functional bowel disorders in apparently healthy people. *Gastroenterology,* 79: 283–288

220   Waller S. L. and Misiewicz J. J. 1969 Prognosis in the irritable bowel syndrome *Lancet,* ii; 753– 756

221   Ritchie J. 1985 Mechanisms of Pain in the Irritable Bowel Syndrome. 163–171 In: *Irritable Bowel Syndrome* ed Read N. W. Grune and Stratton, London

222   Swarbrick E. T., Bat, L., Hegarty J. E., Williams C. B. and Dawson A. M. 1980 Site of pain from the irritable bowel. *Lancet* ii: 443–446

223   Moriarty K. J. and Dawson A. M. 1982 Functional abdominal pain: further evidence that whole gut affected. *Brit. Med. J.* 284 1670–72

224   Kingham J. G. C. and Dawson A. M. 1985 Origin of chronic right upper quadrant pain. *Gut,* 26, 783–788

225   Alban Davies H., Kaye M. D., Rhodes J., Dart A. M. and Henderson A. H. 1982 Diagnosis of oesophageal spasm by ergometrine provocation. *Gut, 23,* 89–97

226   Blackwell J. N., Hannan W. J., Adam R. D. and Heading R. C. 1983 Radionuclide transit studies in the detection of oesophageal dysmotility. *Gut, 24,* 421–426

227   Blackwell J. N and Castell D. O. 1984 Oesophageal chest pain: a point of view. *Gut, 25,* 1–6

228   De Caestecker J. S., Blackwell J. N., Brown J. and Heading R. C. 1985 The oesophagus as a cause of recurrent chest pain: which patients should be investigated and which tests should be used? *Lancet,* ii, 1143–46

229   De Caestecker J. S., Pryde, A. and Heading R. C. 1988 Comparison of intravenous edrophonium and oesophageal acid perfusion during oesophageal manometry in patients with non-cardiac chest pain. *Gut, 29,* 1029–34

230   Barish C. F., Castell D. O. and Richter J. E. 1986 Graded esophageal balloon distension: a new provocative test for non-cardiac chest pain. *Dig. Dis. Sci.* 31, 1292–98

231　Kramer P. 1989 Diagnostic value of esophageal balloon distension (letter). *Gastroenterology*, 96, 271–272

232　Thompson D. G., Laidlow J. and Wingate D. L. 1979 Abnormal small bowel motility demonstrated by radiotelemetry in a patient with irritable colon. *Lancet* ii 1321–23

233　Thompson D. G., Wingate D. L., Archer L., Benson M. J., Green W. J. and Hardy R. J. 1980 Normal patterns of human upper small bowel motor activity recorded by prolonged radiotelemetry. *Gut*, 21, 500–506

234　Thompson D. G., Archer, L., Green W. G. and Wingate D. L. 1981 Fasting motor activity occurs during a day of normal meals in healthy subjects. *Gut*, 22, 489–492

235　Wingate D. L. 1981 Backwards and forwards with the migrating motor complex. *Dig. Dis. Sci.* 26; 641–666

236　Wingate D. L. 1983 Complex clocks. *Dig. Dis. Sci.* 28, 1133–40

237　Ritchie H. D., Thompson D. G. and Wingate D. L. 1980 *J. Physiol.* 305, 54P

238　McRae S., Younger, K., Thompson D. G. and Wingate D. L. 1982 Sustained mental stress alters human jejunal motor activity. *Gut*, 23, 404–409

239　Gill R. C., Kellow J. E., Browning C. and Wingate D. L. 1990 The use of intraluminal strain-gauges for recording ambulant small bowel motility. *Amer. J. Physiol.* 258; G610–15

240　Kellow J. E., Gill R. C. and Wingate D. L. 1990 Prolonged ambulatory recordings of small bowel motility demonstrate abnormalities in the irritable bowel syndrome. *Gastroenterology* 98, 1208–18

241　Kumar D. And Wingate D. L. 1985 The irritable bowel syndrome: a paroxysmal disorder. *Lancet*, ii, 973–977

242　Wingate D. L. 1991 Small Bowel Motor Activity: A Key to Understanding Functional Disorders of the Bowel. In *Irritable Bowel Syndrome*. ed N. W. Read 24–28 Blackwell Scientific Publications

243　Thompson D. G., Richelsen E. and Malagelada J. R. 1982 Perturbation of gastric emptying and duodenal motility via the central nervous system. *Gastroenterology* 73; 1200–06

244　Thompson D. G., Richelson E. and Malagelada J. R. 1983 Perturbation of upper gastrointestinal function by cold stress. *Gut* 24; 277–283

245　Thompson D. G., Binfield P., De Belder A., O'Brien J., Warren S, and Wilson M. 1985 Extraintestinal influences on exhaled breath hydrogen measurement during the investigation of gastrointestinal disease. *Gut*, 26, 1349–52

246　McIntyre A. S., Thompson D. G., Day S., Burnham W. R. and Walker E. R. 1992 Modulation of human upper intestinal nutrient transit by a beta adrenoreceptor mediated pathway. *Gut*, 33, 1062–70

247　Schiller L. R., Davis D. R., Santa Ana C. A., Morawski S. G. and Fordtran J. S. 1982 Studies of the mechanism of the antidiarrheal effect of codeine. *J. Clin. Invest.* 70: 999–1008

248　Fordtran J. S., Santa Ana C. A., Morawski S. G., Bo-Linn G. W. and Schiller L. R. 1986 Pathophysiology of chronic diarrhoea: insights derived from intestinal perfusion studies in 31 patients. *Clinics in Gastroenterology* 15: 3, 477–490

249   Read N. W. 1986 Diarrhee motrice Clinics in gastroenterology 15: 3, 657–686

250   Read N. W., McFarlane, A., Kinsman R. I., Bates T. E., Blackhall N. W., Farrar G. B. J., Hall J. C., Moss G., Morris A. P., O'Neil B., Welch I. Mcl., Lee Y. and Bloom S. R. 1984 The effect of infusion of nutrient solutions into the ileum on gastrointestinal transit and plasma levels of neurotensin and enteroglucagon. *Gastroenterology*, 86: 274–280

251   Read N. W. and Brown N. J. 1991 The small intestine and the ileal brake. In: *Gastrointestinal Transit: Pathophysiology and Pharmacology*. Ed Kamm M. A. and Lennard-Jones, J. E. Wrightson Biomedical Publishing Ltd. Petersfield

252   Cann P. A., Read N. W., Brown C., Hobson N. and Holdsworth C. D. 1983 Irritable bowel syndrome: relationship of disorders in the transit of a single solid meal to symptom patterns. *Gut* 24, 405–411

253   Ritchie J. 1973 Pain from distension of the pelvic colon by inflating a balloon in the irritable colon syndrome. *Gut*, 14, 125–32

254   Flynn M., Hammond P., Darby C., Hyland J. and Taylor I. 1981 Faecal bile acids and the irritable bowel syndrome. *Digestion*, 22: 144–9

255   Whitehead W. E., Engel B. T. and Schuster M. M. 1980 Irritable bowel syndrome. Physiological and psychological differences between diarrhoea-predominant and constipation-predominant patients. *Dig. Dis. Sci.* 25, 404–413

256   Oettle G. J. and Heaton K. W. 1986 "Rectal dissatisfaction" in the irritable bowel syndrome. A manometric and radiological study. *Int. J. Colorect. Dis.* 1, 183–5

257   Davies G. J., Crowder M., Reid B. and Dickerson J. W. B. 1986 Bowel function measurements of individuals with different eating patterns. *Gut*, 27, 164–9

258   Oettle G. J. and Heaton K. W. 1987 Is there a relationship between symptoms of the irritable bowel syndrome and objective measurements of large bowel function? A longitudinal study. *Gut*, 28, 146–9

259   O'Donnell L. J., Virgee J. and Heaton K. W. 1988 Pseudo-diarrhoea in the irritable bowel syndrome: patients' records of stool form reflect transit time while stool frequency does not. *Gut*, 29, A 1455

260   Whorwell P. J., McCallum M., Creed F. H. and Roberts C. T. 1986 Non-colonic features of irritable bowel syndrome. *Gut*, 27, 37–40

261   Whorwell P. J., Lupton E. W., Erduran D. and Wilson K. 1986 Bladder smooth muscle dysfunction in patients with irritable bowel syndrome. *Gut*, 27, 1014–17

262   Prior A., Maxton D. and Whorwell P. J. 1990 Anorectal manometry in irritable bowel syndrome: differences between diarrhoea and constipation-predominant subjects. *Gut*, 31, 458–462

263   Prior A., Sorial E., Sun W. M., and Read N. W. 1990 Rectal sensitivity – a rational means of categorizing patients in the irritable bowel syndrome. Unpublished?

264   Bannister J. J., Dawson P., Timms J. M., Gibbons C. G. and Read N. W. 1987 Effect of the stool size and consistency on defaecation. *Gut*, 28, 1246–50

265   Read N. W. 1991 The neurotic bowel: a paradigm for the irritable bowel syndrome. In *Irritable Bowel Syndrome, New Ideas and Insights Into Pathophysiology*. ed Read N. W. Blackwell Scientific publications, Oxford

266   Thompson W. G., Dotevall G., Drossman D. A., Heaton K. W. and Kruis W.

1989 Irritable bowel syndrome: guidelines for the diagnosis. *Gastroenterology. Int.* 2, 92–95

267   Heaton K. W., Ghosh S. and Braddon F. E. M. 1991 How bad are the symptoms and bowel dysfunction of patients with the irritable bowel syndrome? A prospective, controlled study with emphasis on stool form. *Gut,* 32, 73–79

268   Cann P. A., Read N. W. and Holdsworth C. D. 1983 Oral domperidone: double blind comparison with placebo in irritable bowel syndrome. *Gut,* 24, 1135–40

269   Cann P. A., Read N. W., Holdsworth C. D. and Barends D. 1984 The role of loperamide and placebo in the management of the irritable bowel syndrome. *Dig. Dis. Sci.* 29, 239–247

270   Holdsworth C. D. 1985 Drug treatment of irritable bowel syndrome. in *Irritable Bowel Syndrome.* ed Read N. W. Grune and Stratton 223–232

271   Harvey R. F., Salih S. Y. and Read A. E. 1983 Organic and functional disorders in 2000 gastroenterological outpatients. *Lancet,* I, 632–634

272   Manning A. P. and Heaton K. W. 1976 Bran and the irritable bowel. *Lancet,* I; 588

273   A report of the Royal College of Physicians 1980 *Medical Aspects of Dietary Fibre* Pitman Medical Limited, Tunbridge Wells.

274   Cummings J. H. 1973 Dietary fibre. *Gut,* 14: 69–81

275   McConnell A. A., Eastwood M. A. and Mitchell W. D. 1974 Physical characteristics of vegetable food stuffs that could influence bowel function. *J. Sci. Food Agric.* 25, 1457–64

276   Milton-Thompson G. J. and Lewis B. 1971 The breakdown of dietary cellulose in man. *Gut,* 12, 853–4

277   Southgate D. A. T. and Durnin J. V. G. A. 1970 Colonic conversion factors. An experimental reassessment of the factors used in the calculation of the energy value of human diets. *Br. J. Nut.* 24, 517–535

278   Stephen A. M. and Cummings J. H. 1979 Water holding by dietary fibre and its relationship to faecal output in man. *Gut,* 20, 722–729

279   Stephen A. M. and Cummings J. H. 1980 The microbial contribution to the human faecal mass. *J. Med. Microbiol.* 13, 45–52

280   Cummings J. H. 1984 Constipation, dietary fibre and the control of large bowel function. *Postgrad. Med. J.* 60, 811–819

281   Cummings J. H., Edmond L. M. and Magee E. A. 2004 Dietary carbohydrates and health: do we still need the fibre concept? *Clin. Nutr. Suppl.* 1, 5–17

282   Brodribb A. J. M. 1977 Treatment of symptomatic diverticular disease with dietary fibre. *Lancet.* i. 664–666

283   Brodribb A. J. M., Condon R. E., Cowles V. and De Cosse J. J. 1979 Effect of dietary fibre on intraluminal pressure and myoelectrical activity of left colon in monkeys. *Gastroenterology.* 77, 70–74

284   Ornstein M. H., Littlewood E. R., Baird I. M., Fowler J., North W. R. S. and Cox A. G. 1981 Are fibre supplements really necessary in diverticular disease of the colon? A controlled clinical trial. *Brit. Med. J.* 282: 1353–56

285   Avery Jones F. A. 1981 Are fibre supplements really necessary in diverticular disease of the colon? A controlled clinical trial. *Brit. Med. J.* 282: 1629

286 Heaton K. W. 1981 Is bran useful in diverticular disease? *Brit. Med. J.* 283. 1523–24

287 Cann P. A., Read N. W. and Holdsworth C. D. 1984 What is the benefit of coarse wheat bran in patients with irritable bowel syndrome? *Gut*, 25, 168–173

288 Lucey M. R., Clark M. L., Lowndes Jo, and Dawson A. M. 1987 Is bran efficacious in irritable bowel syndrome? A double blind placebo controlled cross over study. *Gut*, 28, 221–225

289 Snook J. A. and Shepherd H. A. 1994 Bran supplementation in the treatment of irritable bowel syndrome. *Alimentary Pharmacology and Therapeutics* 8, 511–514

290 Alun Jones V., McLaughlan P., Shorthouse M., Workman E. and Hunter J. O. 1982 Food intolerance: a major factor in the pathogenesis of irritable bowel syndrome. *Lancet*, ii, 1115–17

291 Hunter J. O. 1985 Irritable bowel syndrome. *Proc. Nutr. Soc.* 44, 141–3

292 Hunter J. O. 1991 Food allergy – or enterometabolic disorder? *Lancet*, ii, 495–496

293 Farah D. A., Calder I., Benson L. and Mackenzie J. F. 1985 Specific food intolerance: its place as a cause of gastrointestinal symptoms. *Gut*, 26, 164–8

294 Nanda R., James R., Smith H., Dudley C. R. K. and Jewell D. P. 1989 Food intolerance and the irritable bowel syndrome. *Gut*, 30, 1099–1104

295 Whorwell P. J., Prior, A, and Faragher E. B. 1984 Controlled trial of hypnotherapy in the treatment of severe refractory irritable-bowel syndrome. *Lancet*, ii 1232–34

296 Whorwell P. J., Prior A. and Colgan S. M. 1987 Hypnotherapy in severe irritable bowel syndrome: further experience. *Gut*, 28, 423–425

297 Houghton L. A., Heyman D. J. and Whorwell P. J. 1996 Symptomatology, quality of life and economic features of irritable bowel syndrome – the effect of hypnotherapy. *Alimentary Pharmacology and Therapeutics* 10, 91–95

298 Prior A., Colgan S. M. and Whorwell P. J. 1990 Changes in rectal sensitivity after hypnotherapy in patients with irritable bowel syndrome. *Gut*, 31, 896–898

299 Whitehead W. E., Holtcotter B., Enck P., Hoelzl R., Holmes K. D., Anthony J., Shabsin H. S. and Shuster M. M. 1990 Tolerance for recto-sigmoid distension in irritable bowel syndrome. *Gastroenterology*, 98, 1187–92

300 Mearin F., Cucala M., Azpiroz F. and Malagelada J. R. 1991 The origin of symptoms on the brain-gut axis in functional dyspepsia. *Gastroenterology*, 101, 999–1006

301 Trimble K. C., Pryde A. and Heading R. C. 1995 Lowered oesophageal sensory thresholds in patients with symptomatic but not excess gastro-oesophageal reflux: evidence for a spectrum of visceral hypersensitivity in GORD. *Gut*, 37, 7–12

302 Ahluwalia N. K., Thompson D. G. and Barlow J. 1996 Effect of distension and feeding on phasic changes in human proximal gastric tone. *Gut*, 39, 757–761

303 Sarkar S., Aziz Q., Woolf C. J., Hobson A. R. and Thompson D. G. 2000 Contribution of central sensitisation to the development of non-cardiac chest pain. *Lancet*, ii, 1154–9

304 Spriggs E. I. 1931 Functional disorders of the colon. *Quart. J. Med.* 24, 533–541

305 Bergin A. J., Donelly T. C., McKendrick M. W. and Read N. W. 1993 Changes in ano-rectal function in persistent bowel disturbance following salmonella gastroenteritis. *Eur. J. Gastroenterol. & Hepatol.* 5, 617–620

306　Gwee K. A., Leong Y. L., Graham C., McKendrick M. W., Collins S. M., Walters S. J., Underwood J. E. and Read N. W. 1999 The role of psychological and biological factors in postinfective gut dysfunction. *Gut*, 44, 400–406

307　Collins S. M., McHugh K., Jacobson K., Khan I., Riddell R., Murase K. and Weingarten H. P. 1996 Previous inflammation alters the response of the rat colon to stress. *Gastroenterology*, 111, 1509–15

308　Gwee K. A., Collins S. M., Read N. W., Rajnakova A., Deng Y., Graham J. C., McKendrick M. W. and Moochhala S. M. 2003 Increased rectal mucosal expression of interleukin 1B in recently acquired post-infectious irritable bowel syndrome. *Gut*, 52, 523–526

309　Spiller R. C., Trotman I. F., Higgins B. E., Ghatel M. A., Grimble G. K., Lee Y. C., Bloom S. R., Misiewicz J. J. and Silk D. B. A. 1984 The ileal brake–inhibition of jejunal motility after ileal fat infusion in man. *Gut*, 25, 365–374

310　Spiller R. C., Brown M. L. and Phillips S. F. 1986 Decreased fluid tolerance, accelerated transit, and abnormal motility of the human colon induced by oleic acid. *Gastroenterology*, 91, 100–7

311　Neal K. R., Hebden J. and Spiller R. C. 1997 Prevalence of gastrointestinal symptoms six months after bacterial gastroenteritis and risk factors for development of the irritable bowel syndrome: postal survey of patients. *Brit. Med. J.* 314: 779–782

312　Neal K. R., Barker L. and Spiller R. C. 2002 Prognosis in post-infective irritable bowel syndrome: a six year follow up study. *Gut*, 51: 410–413

313　Spiller R. C., Jenkins D., Thornley J. P., Hebden J. M., Wright T., Skinner M. and Neal K. R. 2000 Increased rectal mucosal enteroendocrine cells, T lymphocytes, and increased gut permeability following acute Campylobacter enteritis and in post-dysenteric irritable bowel syndrome. *Gut*, 47, 804–811

314　Dunlop S. P., Jenkins D., Neal K. R. and Spiller R. C. 2000 Relative importance of enterochromaffin cell hyperplasia, anxiety, and depression in postinfectious IBS. Gastroentrology, 125: 1651–59

315　Spiller R., Aziz, Q., Creed F., Emmanuel A., Houghton L., Hungin P., Jones R., Kumar D., Rubin G., Trudgill N. and Whorwell P. 2007 Guidelines on the irritable bowel syndrome: mechanisms and practical management. *Gut*, 1770–98

316　Jones R. H., Lydeard S. E., Hobbs F. D. R., Kenkre J. E., Williams E. I., Jones S. J., Repper J. A., Caldow J. L., Dunwoodie W. M. B. and Bottomley J. M. 1990 Dyspepsia in England and Scotland. *Gut*, 31, 401–405

317　Penston J. G. and Pounder R. E. 1996 A survey of dyspepsia in Great Britain. *Alimentary Pharmacology and Therapeutics* 10, 83–89

318　Gilvarry J., Buckley M. J. M., Hamilton H. and O'Morain C. A. 1997 Eradication of Helicobacter pylori affects symptoms in non-ulcer dyspepsia. *Scand. J. Gastroenterol.* 32: 535–540

319　El-Omar E., Banerjee S., Wirz A. and McColl K. E. L. 1996 The Glasgow Dyspepsia Severity Score–a tool for the global measurement of dyspepsia. *Eur. J. Gastroenterol. & Hepatol.* 8, 967–971

320　McColl K., Murray L., El-Omar E., Dickson A., El-Nujumi A., Wirz A., Kelman

A., Penny C., Knill-Jones R. and Hilditch T. 1998 Symptomatic benefit from eradicating Helicobacter pylori infection in patients with non-ulcer dyspepsia. *New England Journal of Medicine* 339 1869–74

321   Blum A. L., Talley N. J., O'Morain C., Veldhuyzen van Zanten S., Labenz J., Stolte M., Louw J. A., Stubberod A., Theodors A., Sundin M., Bolling-Sternevald E. and Junghard O. 1998 Lack of effect of treating Helicobacter pylori infection in patients with non-ulcer dyspepsia. *New England Journal of Medicine* 339, 1875–81

322   Talley N. J., Janssens J., Lauritsen K., Racz I, and Bolling-Sternevald E. 1999 Eradication of Helicobacter pylori in functional dyspepsia: randomised double blind placebo controlled trial with 12 months' follow up. *Brit. Med. J.* i 833–837

323   McColl K. E. L., Gillen D. and Dickson A. S. 1999 Eradication of Helicobacter pylori in functional dyspepsia *Brit. Med. J.* ii, 451[L]

324   Talley N. J., Lauritsen K. and Bolling-Sterneveld E. Eradication of Helicobacter pylori in functional dyspepsia. *Brit. Med. J.* ii 451[L]

325   Moayyedi P., Duffett S., Braunholtz D., Mason S., Richards I. D, G., Dowell A. C. and Axon A. T. R. 1998 The Leeds Dyspepsia Questionnaire: a valid tool for measuring the presence and severity of dyspepsia. *Alimentary Pharmacology and Therapeutics.* 12, 1257–62

326   Moayyedi P., Braunholtz D., Duffett S., Mason S., Richards I. D. G., Dowell A. C. and Axon A. T. R. 1998 What proportion of dyspepsia in the general population is attributable to Helicobacter pylori? *Gut*, 42 (Suppl. 1) A75

327   Moayyedi P., Feltbower R., Brown J., Mason S., Mason J., Nathan J., Richards I. D. G., Dowell A. C. and Axon A. T. R. 2000 The effect of population H. pylori screening and treatment on dyspepsia and quality of life in the community: results of a randomised controlled trial. *Lancet*, 355, 1665–69

328   Ford A. C., Forman D., Bailey A. G., Axon A. T. R. and Moayyedi P. 2005 A community screening program for Helicobacter pylori saves money: 10 year follow up of a randomised controlled trial. *Gastroenterology* 129, 1910–17

329   Moayyedi P., Soo S., Deeks J., Forman D., Mason J., Innes M. and Delaney B. 2000 Systematic review and economic evaluation of Helicobacter pylori eradication treatment for non-ulcer dyspepsia. *Brit. Med. J.* ii 659–664

330   McColl K. E. L. 2001 Protagonist: Should we eradicate Helicobacter pylori in non-ulcer dyspepsia? *Gut* 48, 759

331   McColl K. E. L., Murray L. S., Gillen D., Walker A., Wirz A., Fletcher J., Mowat C., Henry E., Kelman A. and Dickson A. 2002 Randomised trial of endoscopy with testing for Helicobacter pylori compared with non-invasive H. pylori testing alone in the management of dyspepsia. *Brit. Med. J.* i 999–1002

332   Delaney B., Qume M., Moayyedi P., Logan R. F. A., Ford A. C., Elliott C., McNulty C., Wilson S. and Hobbs F. D. R. 2008 Helicobacter pylori test and treat versus proton pump inhibitor in initial management of dyspepsia in primary care: multicentre randomised controlled trial (MRC-CUBE trial) *Brit. Med. J.* ii, 651–654

333   Lane J. A., Murray L. J., Noble S., Egger M., Harvey I. M., Donovan J. L., Nair P. and Harvey R. F. 2006 Impact of Helicobacter pylori eradication on

dyspepsia, health resource use, and quality of life in the Bristol helicobacter project: randomised controlled trial *Brit. Med. J.* i 199–204

334   Jones F. A. and Gummer J. W. P. 1960 *Clinical Gastroenterology.* Blackwell Sci. Pub. Oxf. 54–64

335   Goodhart J. F. 1905 *The Diseases of Children.* ed by G. F. Still 8th edition J & A Churchill, London 111–2

336   Apley J. 1959 *The Child With Abdominal Pains.* Blackwell, Oxford

337   Hill O. W. and Blendis L. M. Physical and psychological evaluation of "non-organic" abdominal pain. *Gut*, 8, 221–229

338   Gomez J. and Dally P. 1977 Psychologically mediated abdominal pain in surgical and medical outpatient clinics. *Brit. Med. J.* i 1451–53

339   MacDonald A. J. and Bouchier I. A. D. 1980 Non-organic gastrointestinal illness: a medical and psychiatric study. *Br. J. Psychiatry.* 136, 276–283

340   Holdstock D. J., Misiewicz J. J. and Waller S. L. 1969 Observations on the mechanism of abdominal pain. *Gut*, 10, 19–31

341   Kingham J. C. G. and Dawson A. M. 1985 Origin of chronic right upper quadrant pain. *Gut*, 26, 783–788

342   Craig T. K. and Brown G. W. 1984 Goal frustrating aspects of life event stress in the aetiology of gastrointestinal disorder. *J. Psychosom. Res.* 28, 411–421

343   Palmer R. L., Stonehill E., Crisp A. H., Waller S. L. and Misiewicz J. J. 1974 Psychological characteristics of patients with the irritable bowel syndrome. *Postgrad. Med. J.* 50, 416–419

344   Creed F. H. 1981 Life events and appendicectomy. *Lancet*, i, 1381–85

345   Ford M. J., McMiller P., Eastwood J. and Eastwood M. A. 1987 Life events, psychiatric illness and the irritable bowel syndrome. *Gut*, 28, 160–5

346   Creed F., Craig T. and Farmer R. 1988 Functional abdominal pain, psychiatric illness, and life events. *Gut*, 29, 235–242

347   Creed F. H. and Guthrie E. 1987 Psychological factors in the irritable bowel syndrome. *Gut* 28, 1307–18

348   Creed F. H. and Guthrie E. 1989 Psychological treatments of the irritable bowel syndrome. *Gut* 30, 1601–09

349   Drossman D. A., McKee D. C., Sandler R. S., Mitchell C. M., Cramer E. M., Lowman B. C. and Burger A. L. 1988 Psychosocial factors in the irritable bowel syndrome. A multivariate study of patients and nonpatients with irritable bowel syndrome. *Gastroenterology*, 95, 701–708

350   Whitehead W. E., Bosmajian L., Zonderman A. B., Costa P. T. Jr. and Shuster M. M. 1988 Symptoms of psychological distress associated with irritable bowel syndrome. Comparison of community and medical clinic samples. *Gastroenterology*, 95, 709–714

351   Lydeard S. and Jones R. 1989 Factors affecting the decision to consult with dyspepsia: comparison of consulters and non-consulters. *J. R. Coll. Gen. Pract.* 39, 495–498

352   Kettell J., Jones R. H. and Lydiard S. 1992 Reasons for consultation in irritable bowel syndrome. *Br. J. Gen. Pract.* 42, 459–461

353   Heaton K. W., O'Donnell L. J., Braddon F. E., Mountford R. A., Hughes A. O. and Cripps P. J. 1992 Symptoms of irritable bowel syndrome in a British urban community: Consulters and non-consulters. *Gastroenterology*, 102, 1962–67

354   Prior A., Wilson K., Whorwell P. J. and Faragher E. B. 1989 Irritable bowel syndrome in the gynaecological clinic. Survey of 798 new referrals. *Dig. Dis. Sci.* 34, 1820–24

355   Maxton D. G., Morris J. and Whorwell P. J. 1991 More accurate diagnosis of irritable bowel syndrome by the use of "non-colonic" symptomatology. *Gut*, 32, 784–786

356   Gomborone J. E., Dewsnap P. A., Libby G. W. and Farthing M. J. G. 1993 Community study reveals that dysfunctional illness attitudes in irritable bowel syndrome are not wholly a reflection of patient status. *Gastroenterology*, 104, A:153

357   Gomborone J. E., Dewsnap P. A., Libby G. W. and Farthing M. J. G. 1995 Abnormal illness attitudes in irritable bowel syndrome. *J. Psychosom. Res.* 39, 227–230

358   Gomborone J. E., Dewsnap P. A., Libby G. W. and Farthing M. J. G. 1993 Selective affective biasing in recognition memory in the irritable bowel syndrome. *Gut*, 34, 1230–33

359   Gorard D. A., Gomborone J. E., Libby G. W. and Farthing M. J. G. 1996 Intestinal transit in anxiety and depression. *Gut*, 39, 551–555

360   Whorwell P. J., Houghton L. A., Taylor, E. E. et al. 1992 Physiological effects of emotion: assessment via hypnosis. *Lancet*, 340, 69–72

361   Houghton L. A., Calvert E. L., Jackson N. A., Cooper P. and Whorwell P. J. 2002 Visceral sensation and emotion: a study using hypnosis. *Gut*, 51, 701–704

362   Drossman D. A. 1993 Psychosocial and psychologic mechanisms in GI disease. In: Kirsner, J. B. ed. *The Growth of Gastroenterologic Knowledge in the 20th Century.* Lea and Febiger, Philadelphia 419–432

363   De Caestecker J. 1998 Oesophageal chest pain: an update. In: Kaski J. ed. *Chest Pain With Normal Coronary Angiograms; Pathogenesis, Diagnosis and Management.* Philadelphia. Kluwer Academic

364   Mayou R., Bryant B., Sanders D., Bass C., Klimes I. and Forfar C. 1997 A controlled trial of cognitive behaviour therapy for non-cardiac chest pain. *Psychol. Med.*, 27, 1021–31

365   Calvert E., Houghton L. A., Cooper P., Morris J. and Whorwell P. J. 2002 Long term improvement in functional dyspepsia using hypnotherapy. *Gastroenterology*, 123, 1778–85

366   Jones H., Cooper P., Miller V., Brooks N. and Whorwell P. J. 2006 Treatment of non-cardiac chest pain: a controlled trial of hypnotherapy. *Gut*, 55, 1403–08

367   Guthrie E., Creed F. H., Dawson D. and Tomenson B. 1993 A controlled trial of psychological treatment for the irritable bowel syndrome. *Br. J. Psychiatry*, 163, 315–321

368   Creed F., Ratcliffe J., Fernandes L., Palmer S., Rigby C., Tomenson B., Guthrie E., Read N. and Thompson D. G. 2005 Outcome in severe irritable bowel

syndrome with and without accompanying depressive, panic and neurasthenic disorders. *Br. J. Psychiatry* 186, 507–515

369   Creed F., Ratcliffe J., Fernandes L., Tomenson B., Palmer S., Rigby C., Guthrie, E., Read, N. and Thompson, D. G. 2001 Health-related quality of life and health care costs in severe, refractory irritable bowel syndrome. *Ann. Intern. Med.* 134, 860–868

370   Creed F., Guthrie E., Ratcliffe J., Fernandes L., Rigby C., Tomenson B., Read N. and Thompson, D. 2005 Reported sexual abuse predicts impaired functioning but a good response to psychological treatments in patients with severe irritable bowel syndrome. *Psychosom. Med.* 67, 490–9

371   Creed F. 2008 Somatisation in functional dyspepsia: integrating gastric physiology with psychological state. *Gut*, 57, 1642–43

372   Drossman D. A., Creed F. H., Olden K. W., Svedlund J., Toner B. B. and Whitehead W. E. 1999 Psychosocial aspects of the functional gastrointestinal disorders. *Gut*, 45 (Suppl. II): II25–II30

373   Levy R. L., Olden K. W., Naliboff B. D., Bradley L. A., Francisconi C., Drossman D. A. and Creed F. H. 2006 Psychological aspects of the functional gastrointestinal disorders. *Gastroenterology*, 130, 1447–58

374   Jones J., Cann P., Gomborone J., Forbes A., Heaton K., Hungin P., Kumar D., Libby G., Spiller R., Read N., Silk D. and Whorwell P. 2000 Guidelines for the management of the irritable bowel syndrome. *Gut* 47 (Suppl. II): ii1–ii19

375   Spiller R., Aziz Q., Creed F., Emmanuel A., Houghton L., Hungin P., Jones R., Kumar D., Rubin G., Trudgill N. and Whorwell P. 2007 Guidelines on the irritable bowel syndrome: mechanisms and practical management. *Gut*, 56, 1770–98

376   Creed F. H. 2006 Should general psychiatry ignore somatisation and hypochondriasis? *World Psychiatry.* 5, 146–150

377   Creed F. H., Tomenson B., Guthrie E., Ratcliffe J., Fernandes L., Read N., Palmer S. and Thompson D. G. 2008 The relationship between somatisation and outcome in patients with severe irritable bowel syndrome. *J. Psychosom. Res.* 64, 613–620

378   Jones M., Crowell M., Olden K. and Creed F. H. 2007 Functional gastrointestinal disorders: an update for the psychiatrist. *Psychosomatics*, 48, 93–102

379   Misiewicz J. J., Waller S. L. and Eisner M. 1966 Motor responses of human gastrointestinal tract to 5-hydroxytryptamine in vivo and in vitro. *Gut*, 7, 208–216

380   Cunningham D., Hawthorn J., Pople A., Gazet J. C., Ford H. C., Challoner T. and Coombes R. C. 1987 Prevention of emesis in patients receiving cytotoxic drugs by GR38032F, a selective 5-HT3 antagonist. *Lancet*, i, 1461–63

381   Gore S., Gilmore I. T., Haigh C. G., Brownless S. M., Stockdale H. and Morris A. I. 1990 Colonic transit in man is slowed by ondansetron (GR38032F), a selective 5-hydroxytryptamine receptor (type 3) antagonist *Alimentary Pharmacology and Therapeutics* 4, 139–144

382   Prior A. and Read N. 1993 Reduction of rectal sensitivity and post-prandial motility by granisetron, a 5 HT3–receptor antagonist, in patients with irritable bowel syndrome. *Alimentary Pharmacology and Therapeutics* 7, 175–180

383   Maxton D. G., Morris J. and Whorwell P. J. 1996 Selective 5-hydroxytryptamine antagonism: a role in irritable bowel syndrome and functional dyspepsia? *Alimentary Pharmacology and Therapeutics* 10, 595–599

384   Marsden C. A. 1981 Effect of L-tryptofan on mouse brain 5-hydroxytryptamine: comparison of values obtained using a fluorimetric assay and liquid chromatographic assay with electrochemical detection. *J. Neurochem.* 36, 1621–26

385   Bearcroft C. P., Perrett D. and Farthing M. J. G. 1996 5–Hydroxytryptamine release into human jejunum by cholera toxin. *Gut*, 39, 528–531

386   Bearcroft C. P., Perrett D. and Farthing M. J. G. 1998 Postprandial plasma 5-hydroxytryptamine in diarrhoea predominant irritable bowel syndrome: a pilot study. *Gut*, 42, 42–46

387   Houghton L. A., Atkinson W., Whitaker R. P., Whorwell P. J. and Rimmer M. J. 2003 Increased platelet depleted plasma 5-hydroxytryptamine concentration following meal ingestion in symptomatic female subjects with diarrhoea predominant irritable bowel syndrome. *Gut*, 52, 663–670

388   Houghton L. A., Brown H., Atkinson W., Morris J., Fell C., Whorwell P. J., Lockhart S. and Keevil B. 2009 5-hydroxytryptamine signalling in irritable bowel syndrome with diarrhoea: effects of gender and menstrual status. *Alimentary Pharmacology and Therapeutics* 30, 919-929

389   Camilleri M. D., Northcutt A. R., Kong S., Dukes G. E., McSorley D. and Mangel A. W. 2000 Efficacy and safety of alosetron in women with irritable bowel syndrome: a randomised, placebo-controlled trial. *Lancet*, 355, 1035–40

390   Horton R. 2001 Lotronex and the FDA: a fatal erosion of integrity. *Lancet*, 357, 1544–45

391   Moynihan R. 2002 Alosetron: a case study in regulatory capture, or a victory for patient's rights? *Brit. Med. J.* 325, 592–595

392   Whorwell P. J., Ruegg P., Earnest D., Dunger-Baldauf C. 2004 Tegaserod significantly improves bloating in female irritable bowel syndrome patients with constipation. *Gastroenterology* 126, A-643. W1470

393   Houghton L. A. and Whorwell P. J. 2005 Towards a better understanding of abdominal bloating and distension in functional bowel disorders. *Neurogastroenterol. Motil.* 17, 500–511

394   Gorard D. A., Libby G. W. and Farthing M. J. G. 1994 Influence of antidepressants on whole gut and orocaecal transit times in health and irritable bowel syndrome. *Alimentary Pharmacology and Therapeutics* 8. 159 -166

395   Creed F., Fernandes L., Guthrie E., Rigby C., Tomenson B., Read N. and Thompson D. 2003 The cost-effectiveness of psychotherapy and paroxetine for severe irritable bowel syndrome. *Gastroenterology*, 124, 303–317

396   Creed F. 2006 How do SSRIs help patients with irritable bowel syndrome? *Gut*, 55, 1065–67

397   Booth C. 1997 Factors influencing the development of gastroenterology in Britain. In: *Gastroenterology in Britain: Historical Essays*. Ed: W. F. Bynum. Wellcome Institute for the History of Medicine Occasional Publications, No. 3

398   Aziz Q., Thompson D. G., Ng V. W. K., Hamdy S., Sarkar S., Brammer M. J., Bullmore E. T., Hobson A. R., Tracey I., Suckling K., Simmons A. and Williams S. C. R. 2000 Cortical processing of human somatic and visceral sensation. *J. Neurosci.* 20, 2657–2663

399   Sarkar S., Aziz Q., Woolf C. J., Hobson A. R. and Thompson D. G. 2000 Contribution of central sensitisation to the development of non-cardiac chest pain. *Lancet*, 356, 1154–59

400   Hobson A. R. and Aziz Q. 2004 Brain imaging and functional gastrointestinal disorders: has it helped our understanding? *Gut*, 53, 1198–1206

401   Ford A. C., Talley N. J., Spiegel B. M. R., Foxx-Orenstein A. E., Schiller L., Quigley E. M. M. and Moayyedi P. 2008 Effect of fibre, antispasmodics, and peppermint oil in the treatment of irritable bowel syndrome: systematic review and meta-analysis. *Brit. Med. J.* 337, 1388–92

SECTION SIX

GASTROINTESTINAL ENDOSCOPY

Despite their enthusiasm for endoscopy from the start, one has to admit that the British contribution to the manufacture and design of endoscopes has been small. The Germans led the way with a variety of rigid gastroscopes at the turn of the twentieth century and followed this up with a semi-flexible instrument in 1932. The best known exponent of gastroscopy at the time was Rudolf Schindler and much has been written about him and his colleagues over the years.[1/2] Subsequently, in 1958, Basil Hirschowitz, a South African working in America, introduced the fully flexible fiberscope. This was taken up by the Japanese who revolutionised endoscopy making it the safe and simple investigation that it is today. Yet at each stage of its development, from rigid to fully flexible instruments, the British have played their part.

CHAPTER SIXTY-FOUR

RIGID ENDOSCOPY

A handful of Victorian physicians described illuminated tubes that they grandiosely called gastroscopes. They must have been optimists because their only source of light was a candle reflected by mirrors and the instruments they produced were well-nigh impossible to swallow. They took their inspiration from professional sword swallowers who were well trained in their art but scarcely represented the average patient. The endoscopes were simple tubes made of wood or metal. The chief incentive for endoscopy apart from a natural inclination to peer down any orifice was the need to remove foreign bodies from the oesophagus. In addition, bearing in mind that this was well before the discovery of X-rays people hoped it would be possible to see a gastric ulcer or cancer, both of which were well recognised by the nineteenth century.

One of the first instruments was made by a surgeon at Charing Cross Hospital called John Avery (1807–55), who was one of the original 300 Fellows of the college. He was well known for his ingenious gadgets and put together a lamp, a tube and reflectors through which "he was able to examine the ear, urethra, bladder, oesophagus, and larynx, as probably no surgeon had ever examined them before him". It certainly sounded an impressive instrument and for his invention he received two medals, one from Prince Albert, as President of the Society of Arts, and the other from the adjudicators of the Great Exhibition in 1851. A modest man he did not publish his results on the grounds that he had yet to perfect his technique.[3] Unfortunately he died aged 48 and it is largely from his obituary that we learn about his gastroscope.[4] His obituary incidentally gave full details of his terminal illness, which was marked by repeated vomiting and profound cachexia that had defied diagnosis. His friends and indeed Avery himself thought he had malignant intestinal obstruction but in fact he had unsuspected pulmonary tuberculosis.

About the same time another enthusiast, Dr. David Campbell (died 1848), a surgeon in Glasgow, invented a gastroscope, which he presented at a meeting of his brethren in the Southern Medical Society of that city. Unsurprisingly, none of the brethren would allow him to examine them but "as luck would have it the Glasgow Fair was taking place at the time and among the wonderful feats to be seen was the swallowing of a sword by one of the performers. Dr. Campbell naturally concluded that if the man could swallow a sharp, rigid, flat sword, he would have no difficulty in getting him to swallow his smooth, flexible, round gastroscope. Accordingly he called at the sword swallower's booth and, producing his gastroscope, tackled him by explaining its intended use, and requesting liberty to experiment on him with it. The showman looked askance at the gastroscope and gently declined. Dr. Campbell insisted that the experiment would be simple, and added that if one could swallow a sword without danger, he could surely swallow Dr. Campbell's comparatively harmless instrument. But the showman was inflexible, and put a damper on Dr. Campbell's ardent hopes about the future of his gastroscope by abruptly exclaiming, "I know I can swallow a sword, but I'll be – – if I can swallow a trumpet."[5] History does not record if anyone subsequently swallowed the instrument but it is unlikely that the stomach would have been visible even if they had.

Another instrument was described by a surgeon at Guy's Hospital, John Bevan, in 1868. It was lit by reflected candle light and was only four inches long. In a brief article entitled "Oesophagoscope" he claimed that he could see the precise position and nature of foreign bodies, strictures, morbid growths etc., obviating the need for oesophagotomy and facilitating extraction with forceps by mouth.[6] He added that visibility was improved by a magnesium lamp made for him by a Mr. Mayor of Great Portland Street to such an extent that any part of the oesophagus and the stomach were demonstrable. This would have been a remarkable achievement but we have no idea if he actually used it. A decade or so later Morrell Mackenzie (1837–92) had his doubts; "a perusal of Bevan's paper will convince any reader that the experiments were the result of work in the laboratory rather than in the wards of a hospital; and, in fact, that the instrument is of no practical value".[7] Morrell Mackenzie, physician to the Hospital for Diseases of the Throat and to the Royal Society of Musicians, was the leading laryngologist of his day. In 1880 he himself invented a slick device consisting of an expandable tube of rods through which he managed to remove a piece of impacted meat and bone from a woman's mid-oesophagus. He called it a "skeleton tube" but it had no potential as a gastroscope and fell into disuse with his death.

The end of the nineteenth century was notable for the introduction of antiseptic and aseptic surgery. For the first time surgeons could contemplate gastric surgery and German doctors led the way. This was a golden age for German medicine and it was supported by the quality of their instruments and their expertise with optics. The most notable was a surgical instrument maker from Vienna called Joseph Leiter (1830–92) who collaborated with a surgeon, Max Nitze (1848–1906) from Dresden, to develop the first effective cystoscopes. Before long their instruments were improved considerably by the invention of the electric light bulb in 1879 by Thomas Edison (1847–1931).

But examining the bladder was a far cry from looking at the stomach. As far back as 1868 the great German physician in Freiburg, Adolf Kussmaul (1822–1902), attempted to look directly into the stomach and ordered two special tubes to be made, 47 centimetres in length with a diameter of 13 millimetres. He managed to find a more cooperative sword swallower than Campbell and gave a demonstration to the medical section of the Society of Naturalists in Freiburg.[8] Unfortunately he had insufficient light to see anything at the lower end but he did at least prove that a straight tube could be passed into the stomach with the aid of an obturator.

Eleven years later Nitze, now working in Vienna, used a longer version of his cystoscope to examine the stomach but the instrument was angulated at the level of the throat, which interfered with its manipulation in the stomach.[9] Nitze moved to Berlin and lost interest in gastroscopy but Leiter now cooperated with the Austrian surgeon, Johann von Mikulicz (1850–1905), to produce an optical gastroscope angulated this time at the lower end. Though he was able to discern sufficient detail to be diagnostically helpful, he used a platinum-loop lamp rather than an Edison bulb at the distal end, which required water-cooling, and the technical difficulties made him abandon the project. For two decades interest in gastroscopy waned and only a handful of enthusiasts on the continent persevered with it. The rewards were small, the risk of perforation great and the technique was shunned in Britain and America. This led James Sherren (1872–1945), a distinguished surgeon at the London Hospital, in an address on the early recognition of carcinoma of the stomach to say, "You may be surprised that I have not mentioned the gastroscope as a diagnostic instrument. In its present form its use is probably more dangerous than exploratory laparotomy in the hands of a competent surgeon."[10] By this time (1910) surgical exploration of the abdomen was feasible and X-rays had revolutionised gastric imaging.

By a curious coincidence, two colleagues of Sherren at the London Hospital had just resuscitated Mikulicz's original technique. One, Theodore Thompson (1878–1935), known as "Turtle" owing to his rotund build and waddling gait, was a fine diagnostician. The other, Henry Souttar (1875–1964), was still only a house surgeon when he used his considerable technical ability to design an angulated gastroscope. In fact he produced several prototypes based on the Mikulicz gastroscope, which he tested on himself, refining each in the light of his experience. The final model was made in Berlin and was very expensive (£60) but he managed to obtain a grant from the British Research Council to develop it. Souttar and Thompson obtained good views of the stomach, including the pylorus, and observed cancer, atrophic gastritis and a case with petechial haemorrhages.[11] The instrument was inserted blindly and unfortunately Souttar felt obliged to discard it after sharp criticism from an influential throat, nose and ear surgeon at St. Mary's Hospital, William Hill (1858–1928), who thought it was dangerous.[12] Hill published a short monograph in 1912 extolling the virtues of his own method of oesophago-gastroscopy using direct vision down a straight tube.[13] He claimed that Arthur Hurst among others had adopted his technique but there is no evidence that Hurst used it. In fact Hill's procedure was also extremely difficult and dangerous and consequently gastroscopy in Britain lay dormant for several more years. Hurst made no mention of it in his well known book on gastric and duodenal ulcer published in 1929.

Despite the problems physicians in Germany continued to devise all manner of rigid gastroscopes, none of which were satisfactory until 1920 when Rudolf Schindler (1888–1968) first became interested in gastroscopy. After World War One he had noticed that half the patients in hospital were young women with stomach troubles, which seemed to be functional. There was no way of proving this and he was worried that he might be overlooking some undiscovered organic change, particularly as many of these girls were malnourished because of the war. He then recalled that, before the war, his compatriots had attempted to examine the stomach endoscopically. He found an old gastroscope that had lain in a cupboard unused for ten years and soon became remarkably proficient with it. Within two years he presented the results of 120 gastroscopies to the Medical Society of Munich, at which he described various types of gastritis, carcinoma and the action of the pylorus.[14] The same year, 1922, he married his wife, Gabriele Winkler, who became indispensable as his assistant. Her ability to help a patient relax while simultaneously supporting the head in an iron grip was crucial to Schindler's success. A year later he published the first important textbook and atlas on gastric pathology illustrated by colour drawings.[15] According to his biographer, Audrey Davis, it was "a monument to the fortitude of Schindler and the cooperation of his patients". By this time he had carried out 400 gastroscopies and claimed that patients were demanding the examination. He was able to reach the stomach in 97 per cent of his patients, though he considered the examination to be successful in only 55 per cent and expected to see the pylorus in only 20 per cent.

CHAPTER SIXTY-FIVE

SEMI-FLEXIBLE GASTROSCOPY

Even Schindler found the rigid instrument difficult to use and when he had a fatal perforation he became determined to improve the technique. In 1928 he approached Georg Wolf (1873–1938), an optical physicist from Berlin who had made many gastroscopes, to see if he could devise a flexible instrument. After two years Wolf came up with a fully flexible gastroscope that incorporated a series of thick convex lenses enabling him to see through a curved tube. Unfortunately this was too floppy and unmanageable and the images were distorted. At Schindler's suggestion he altered the instrument so that only the distal six inches were flexible, making it easier to use and optically more efficient. The famous Wolf-Schindler gastroscope was introduced in 1932 at a meeting of the Physician's Association in Munich,[16] and was given the immediate backing of Norbert Henning (1896–1985), an influential and experienced endoscopist in Leipzig who had been given one to try.[17] The semiflexible instrument proved to be far superior to the rigid gastroscope and physicians from all over the world began to visit Schindler to learn gastroscopy. Wolf made his fortune from sales of the instrument. But with the rise of Nazism Schindler, being Jewish, was obliged to flee Germany in 1934. He emigrated to America where he was welcomed by Walter Palmer in Chicago and given the title of visiting professor at the university in order to introduce gastroscopy. In 1937 he published the first edition of his classic book on gastric pathology, which included detailed instruction on the art of endoscopy based on his personal experience of 6,000 cases.[18]

The British were quick to recognise the value of Schindler's gastroscope. One of the first was a newly qualified young surgeon from St. Bartholemew's Hospital called Hermon Taylor (1905–2001). He was on a visit to Leipzig in 1932 where he happened to meet Schindler (who was presumably there to see Henning) and as a result bought a gastroscope from Wolf in Berlin. Export of such items from Germany was forbidden, so he slipped it down his trouser leg and limped through customs with it. Subsequently he mastered the skill of using the instrument and later modified it as we shall see.

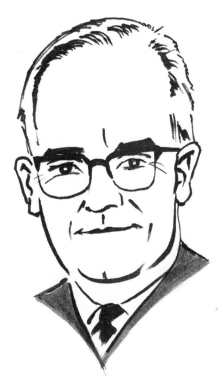

90 Edwards – First editor of **Gut.**

In 1933 an editorial appeared in the *Lancet* extolling the virtues of the flexible gastroscope, which caught the eye of another surgeon, Harold Edwards (1899–1989).[19] Edwards had won several prizes during his meteoric career and had been appointed surgeon at King's College Hospital only five years after qualification. In 1934 he went to Henning in Leipzig who taught him how to use the new gastroscope, after which he also bought one from Wolf, which he also smuggled through customs. Fifty years later he wrote an amusing confession about his visit to Germany in the *British Medical Journal.*[20] Apparently he was able to afford the instrument only because Hitler, in order to lure students to the Reich, had recently doubled the number of reichsmarks that could be exchanged for a pound sterling. Despite this Edwards still had insufficient funds to pay the excise duty. Fortunately he managed to convince the customs officer in Harwich that his gastroscope was an old instrument that he had taken to Germany for repair so he escaped the duty. Edwards was one of the earliest surgical members of the Gastro-Enterological Club and was elected President of the British Society of Gastroenterology in 1959. A prodigious writer he was also the first editor of *Gut* when it finally appeared in 1960.

In the same year,1934, yet another surgeon, Harold Rodgers (1907–2001) then chief assistant at St. Bartholemew's Hospital, travelled to Leipzig to learn gastroscopy with Henning. He bought an instrument at his own expense and began to use it at St. Bartholemew's Hospital a month after Harold Edwards. He was assisted by a house physician, Francis Avery Jones (1910–98), who made himself available to hold the patient's head. In no time Avery was using the gastroscope himself and became one of the few physicians practising endoscopy on a regular basis. Rodgers admired the work of the department in Leipzig and personally translated a copy of Henning's book on gastroscopy into English in 1937.[21] In the preface he made the point that Henning was a physician who had retained his interest in general medicine and had not let the gastroscope lead him "from erudition to a narrow peeping specialty"; a warning that is relevant today.

Though Edwards, Rodgers and Hermon Taylor are rightly credited for introducing semi-flexible gastroscopy to Britain, Schindler also mentioned one other person who visited him from the "Anglo-Saxon country" by the name of Arafa. In fact Mohamed Arafa was an Egyptian who had come from Cairo to work as medical assistant at Guy's Hospital in 1932. He worshipped Arthur Hurst (1879–1944) and wrote a book on modern aspects of gastroenterology that was slated by the press; according to one disgruntled reviewer there was nothing new in it and the book would have been better called "Recent Expressions in Gastroenterology by Sir Arthur Hurst" because it contained so many of Hurst's favourite sayings.[22] Probably at Hurst's instigation, Arafa took himself off to Germany in 1933 where he learnt the technique of gastroscopy from Schindler himself. Soon after in January 1935 he presented the results of 78 gastroscopies he had performed in Cairo at a discussion on diagnosis of diseases of the stomach at the Royal Society of Medicine.[23] This was just as Edwards and company were starting to do gastroscopies in Britain.

Inspired perhaps by Rodgers, another physician to travel to Germany in 1934 was Percy Thompson Hancock (1904–2004), who visited Schindler in Munich. Hancock was chief assistant to Lord Horder at St. Bartholemew's Hospital but fortunately was not put off by the great man's pronouncement that "gastroscopy was repugnant to the English character". Unfortunately he had to leave Munich after only two attempts at using the new gastroscope because Schindler was about to be betrayed to the Gestapo. Undaunted he returned to St. Bartholemew's Hospital and introduced gastroscopy alongside Rodgers.[24] Years later Thompson met Schindler again in Chicago and was made an honorary member of the American Gastroscopy Society.

Schindler's original interest in gastroscopy had been driven by his anxiety to study unexplained dyspepsia and gastritis. In Britain and America people were concerned with the link between atrophic gastritis and gastric cancer. In 1937 during his Harveian oration Sir Arthur Hurst, recently knighted in the Coronation Honours, stressed the usefulness of gastroscopy in the study of gastritis.[25] He also prophesied that for some purposes, such as the investigation of post-operative gastric disorders and of the healing of gastric ulcers under treatment, gastroscopy would in future take the place of radiology; this was somewhat optimistic in 1937 but time would eventually prove him right. He added that several younger physicians were using the gastroscope and he was glad that it was not regarded as a purely surgical instrument.

A month later in November 1937 the *Lancet* published a leading article on gastroscopy advocating that "every large hospital should possess a gastroscope and an experienced gastroscopist".[26] The same weekend Hurst chaired the inaugural meeting of the British Gastroenterological Club which opened with a discussion on the technique and value of gastroscopy led by Stanley Hartfall (1899–1982), then medical assistant to Hurst at Guy's Hospital and later Professor of Medicine in Leeds.[27]

So it seemed that gastroscopy was about to take off with several physicians and surgeons keen to use it. In fact it did not because it was a difficult technique requiring considerable skill on the part of the gastroscopist and his accomplice. Furthermore the instrument was expensive. Gastroenterology was regarded as part of general medicine and few physicians felt that gastroscopy contributed enough to the diagnostic process to justify the discomfort and cost involved. There was no National Health Service and most provincial hospitals were run by general practitioners with reasonable radiological facilities. So it was only in the larger cities that there were sufficient specialists prepared to take on gastroscopy. In fact the majority of gastroscopists worked in London with a few scattered among cities such as Birmingham, Liverpool and Newcastle numbering perhaps two dozen in all.

Nonetheless it was thanks to the gastroscope that Arthur Douthwaite (1896–1974) at Guy's Hospital was able to prove that aspirin caused gastric bleeding. Working with another gastroscopist, Gordon Lintott (1908–40), he collected thirteen cases and presented them to the second meeting of the British Gastroenterological Club in 1938.[28] In each case radiology had been normal. Not long afterwards the Second World War began to disrupt medical research and prevented the import of gastroscopes from Germany for several years.

One of the frustrations of the Wolf–Schindler instrument was the inability to control the distal end while inspecting the stomach so that there were many blind areas particularly on the posterior wall. This particularly irked Hermon Taylor at the London Hospital so he sought the help of Sir Henry Souttar who was now approaching retirement but was renowned for his technical wizardry. Souttar lent him his engineering workshop and after three years experimenting with various designs he produced a gastroscope with a flexible tip that could be curled up or down by the operator using a pair of wires attached to a handle.[29] This made it possible to see most of the stomach quite easily and the principle has been used in flexible endoscopes to this day. Furthermore, the Hermon Taylor gastroscope, as it became known, could be bought from the Genito–Urinary Manufacturing company in London whereas, during the Second World War, the Schindler gastroscope was impossible to obtain.

After the war, practice slowly returned to normal and the National Health Service was introduced in 1948. An interesting survey looking at the risks of gastroscopy was carried out by Avery Jones and Harold Rodgers (with the help of Richard Doll and Charles Fletcher) in 1951.[30] They sent a letter to 40 gastroscopists in Britain, which was in effect everyone who was undertaking gastroscopy. Altogether 49,000 gastroscopies had been done during the preceding fifteen years. Of these nearly one half had been carried out by just eight gastroscopists

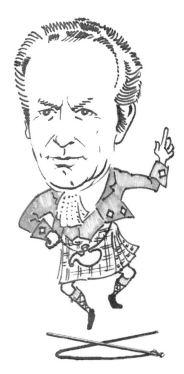

91 Sircus – Caledonian Society of Gastroenterology.

suggesting that in many parts of the country the service was unavailable. London had the lion's share including St. Bartholemew's Hospital (Harold Rodgers), the London Hospital (Hermon Taylor), King's College Hospital (Harold Edwards), Central Middlesex Hospital (Avery Jones), Guy's Hospital (Arthur Douthwaite), The Queen Mary's Hospital, Roehampton (Percy Hancock), the Middlesex Hospital (George Hadley), St. Mary's Hospital, Paddington (John Goligher) and St. James Hospital, Balham (Norman Tanner). Notable by its absence was St. Thomas's Hospital where Wilfred Card was not allowed to open a specialised department. Card was an experienced gastroscopist and was lured to Edinburgh by Sir Stanley Davidson in 1948 where Bill Sircus was using the Hermon-Taylor instrument. Sircus carried out many thousands of endoscopies without mishap.[31] Others in those postwar days included Ernest Bulmer (Birmingham), Thomas Boon (Newcastle), Stanley Hartfall (Leeds), and Howell Hughes (Liverpool). Bulmer reported that he performed about three gastroscopies per week.

The survey showed that there had been 35 deaths as a result of gastroscopy, mostly from perforation of the oesophagus, a rate of 0.3 per cent. Nearly all the perforations occurred with the Hermon Taylor instrument, which was slightly larger and less flexible than the Schindler gastroscope. However, most endoscopists preferred to use the Hermon Taylor instrument because it provided a better view of the stomach. (The authors added that Hermon Taylor had personally made several thousand examinations without a single fatal perforation of the oesophagus.)

However, the fact remained that, despite the enthusiasm of the experts, semiflexible gastroscopy was never widely practised in Britain. Many clinicians recall how uncomfortable it was for the patient and inconclusive for the gastroscopist. An added drawback was the inability to obtain biopsies reliably if at all. An attempt was made by Percy Hancock and Margot Shiner to combine gastroscopy with biopsy using a tube attached to the gastroscope, but though they had some success it did not catch on.[32] Gastroscopy was regarded as a specialised technique that most clinicians did not consider an option in the management of their gastric patients. For example, as far as I am aware, no one along the south coast of England ever used a semi-flexible gastroscope.

CHAPTER SIXTY-FIVE

INVENTION OF FIBREOPTIC (FULLY FLEXIBLE) ENDOSCOPY

In 1951 Hugh Gainsborough, a physician at St. George's Hospital, London, happened to meet the distinguished physicist, Harold Hopkins, at a dinner party. Gainsborough (1893–1980) was an academic type who cared little for the affectations sometimes thought necessary for successful private practice. But besides his commitment to science

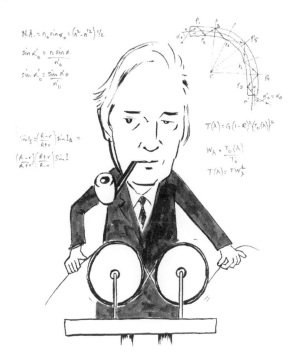

92 Hopkins – Winding his first glass fibres.

he was a highly competent and compassionate doctor. Like many he appreciated the potential of gastroscopy but abhorred its use because of the discomfort and difficulties of intubation. He knew that Hopkins (1918–1994) specialised in optics and had already designed the zoom lens so he asked him if it would not be possible to invent a more flexible gastroscope that would be easier to use and make the procedure less of an ordeal for the patient.[33]

Hopkins gave the matter some thought and knew that light could be made to travel in a curve if trapped in a column of water or a bent glass tube. For example the fountains in several major cities had been illuminated for years using this principle with spectacular results. In the mid-nineteenth century, Jacques Babinet (1794–1872), professor of optical physics in Paris, showed that light could also be transmitted through thin glass rods[34] and by the end of the century several people had shown that glass could be drawn into fibres that were flexible and robust. One of the first to recognise the potential of light transmission through glass fibres was John Logie Baird (1888–1946), the pioneer of television. In 1927 he filed a patent for the manufacture of bundles of rigid glass tubes, five centimetres long, heaped in parallel rows that transmitted light from one end to the other.[35] But he became preoccupied with television and never made use of his patent.

In his book on gastric pathology, Schindler mentions the case of a foreign body in the stomach that was extracted under fluoroscopic control using a hook. The case was reported by a young doctor in Munich called Heinrich Lamm (1908–73).[36] What Schindler does not mention is that Lamm, when he was a third-year medical student, published a paper in which he showed that a bundle of bent glass filaments could transmit light from one end to the other.[37] He also suggested that fibres could transmit images as well as light provided that they were properly aligned. But his bundle only contained about 400 fibres and suffered from leakage of light where adjacent fibres touched, so the image was poor. In his paper he wrote, "I hope that some optical instrument firm with more means and experience than I have, will succeed, thanks to my work, in making a clinically useful flexible gastroscope." Unfortunately, Schindler was too tied up with his own experiments to take Lamm seriously. Lamm tried to obtain a patent for his discovery but found that an American, Clarence Hansell (1899–1967) had beaten him to it with a patent based on the transmission of light through cables, though he had no plans to develop his ideas.

Hopkins was probably unaware of Lamm's work but after his chat with Gainsborough he will have soon familiarised himself with what was known about glass fibres. He realised that to produce a useful image he would need to assemble tens of thousands of fibres in a coherent, carefully aligned, bundle. In July 1952 he managed to obtain a grant from the Royal Society, the amount being £750 for each of two years, and took on a young research assistant, Narinder Kapany.[38] Together they wound a single long fibre in a figure-of-eight around a pair of drums. When sufficient turns had been added, they sealed a short section in resin, cut through it and straightened it out to produce the coherent bundle. Hopkins used his experience with optics to add an objective to one end of the bundle and an eyepiece to the other. Finally they added a flexible jacket to protect the bundle and the fibrescope was born.[39]

They published details of their invention in *Nature* in January 1954.[40] The instrument was nine inches long and transmitted an image with enough definition to read large print. But the loss of light from the bare fibres was so great that a bundle long enough to reach the stomach would have been useless. As it happened there was another article in the same issue of *Nature* that complemented Hopkins' work.[41] A distinguished Dutch physicist Abram Van Heel (1899–1966), professor of optics at Delft University, produced a coherent bundle of only 400 fibres but they were each coated with dark varnish to prevent loss of light and image. Van Heel suggested his invention might have a medical application but it was Hopkins' article with the words "flexible fibrescope" in the title that attracted attention.

Unfortunately Hopkins was unable to obtain a patent for his fibrescope because of the earlier patents granted to Logie Baird and Hansell. He tried to persuade one of the British optical manufacturers to develop an instrument but failed. He also tried to interest the industry on the continent, including Siemens, and was again unsuccessful. He was a modest and unassuming man, which may have partly explained his inability to convince people of the significance of his work. With hindsight it is a pity that Hopkins and Van Heel did not join forces, in fact Heel's application for a patent for his discovery went to an American, Brian O'Brien, professor of optics at Rochester University.

According to Booth, one physician who showed considerable interest in Hopkins' discovery was Francis Avery Jones who, unusually for a gastroenterologist, was a subscriber to *Nature* and had read Hopkins' article. He immediately realised that fibreoptics offered the possibility of a greatly improved gastroscope".[42] It happened that he had recently trained a young South African doctor, Basil Hirschowitz, in the technique of semi-flexible gastroscopy in his clinic at the Central Middlesex Hospital. By this time Hirschowitz (1925–2013) had taken up a fellowship arranged for him by Avery with Professor Marvin Pollard at the University of Michigan but fortunately he was alerted to the articles in *Nature* by a young research worker, Keith Henley (1925–2013), who had recently arrived in Michigan to work with Pollard. Henley in turn had had his attention drawn to Hopkins' work by Tim Counihan, a registrar at the Hammersmith Hospital, who had worked alongside Henley when he was a research fellow in Sheila Sherlock's department.[43]

Hirschowitz was quick to see the potential of the fibrescope and hurried back to England to meet Hopkins whom he described as warm and friendly and one of the "most modest of men". Despite the limitations of the prototype he returned to Michigan determined to produce a workable instrument. In this he was strongly supported by Pollard who found the funds needed to support his work. At first he had hoped that Kapany would join him but the latter decided to join a large American optical company instead. However, Pollard introduced him to Wilbur Peters, an assistant professor in physics at Ann Arbor who in turn recommended a brilliant young physics student, Larry Curtiss, to join them. The following year (1955) they bought £3-worth of glass fibre from Fibreglass Ltd. in England, the same material used by Hopkins and Kapany, and started work. The fibreglass from England was unfortunately too green and opaque to be useful but they collaborated with Dow Corning who managed to provide clear material. Eventually they devised a method of making one-metre-long bundles containing up to 200,000 coherent fibres. Later still Larry Curtiss discovered a way of insulating each fibre with more refractive glass to prevent loss of light. His invention of the glass-coated glass fibre was the key to their success and in February 1957 Hirschowitz used the first prototype on a patient.[44]

Hirschowitz was unable to find a backer to develop his gastroscope in America and came to England in 1957 hoping to interest Genito-Urinary Manufacturing Ltd. in London but found that they were also unwilling to support him. Returning to the United States, he finally convinced the giant American Cystoscope Makers Inc (ACMI) to help him and the first commercial gastroscope eventually appeared in 1960. Hirschowitz reported his clinical experience with it in the *Lancet* in 1961 and it was a revelation.[45] Apart from easy intubation of the patient, he was able to see all of the stomach and to enter the duodenum for the first time. He described duodenal ulcers and duodenitis and also took photographs with his simple camera (the *Lancet* published the first colour plates to appear in that journal for many years). The gastroscope was a side-viewing instrument so it was unsuitable for examination of the oesophagus. Hirschowitz wrote, "It may be stated unequivocably that the fiberscope has already reached the stage where it should replace the conventional gastroscope." This was encouraging but slightly overoptimistic and not an opinion shared by the first British endoscopists to use it.

CHAPTER SIXTY-SEVEN

FLEXIBLE ENDOSCOPY IN BRITAIN

a) Gastroscopy

The first people in Britain to try their hand with the fiberscope were, naturally enough, the doctors already familiar with the semi-flexible endoscope, and within a year of the *Lancet* publication about twenty clinicians had tried their hand with the new instrument. They all agreed that it was much easier and safer to insert than the old gastroscope but, unlike Hirschowitz, who claimed that he could always examine the duodenum, the British and others found it almost impossible to negotiate the pylorus. The tip of the gastroscope was large (half an inch in diameter) and there was no mechanism for manipulating it, which was a serious drawback. On the other hand the views of the antrum were excellent and good photographs could be obtained, so people felt confident that with modifications the fiberscope had a bright future.

Bright indeed was the future if the light could be improved. William Burnett (1921–81), a senior lecturer in surgery with Charles Illingworth in Glasgow, actually suggested in 1962 that "if part of the fibre bundle were to be used for light transmission in a distal direction, the tungsten bulb and its connections could be eliminated thus effecting a considerable reduction in the size of the distal head".[46] Unfortunately, he did not pursue this prescient observation and left Glasgow the following year to take up a chair in surgery in Brisbane.

The light source for the early gastroscopes was a miniature incandescent bulb built into the tip of the instrument similar to Schindler's gastroscope. This was not particularly bright but a more powerful lamp was risky because it was liable to burn the gastric mucosa.

The same dilemma arose with rigid instruments such as cystoscopes and laparoscopes.

The problem was solved by the founder of a small medical instrument company in Germany called Karl Storz (1910–96), who realised that glass fibres could be used to convey light from a powerful external lamp to an endoscope. As he was only interested in light conduction he was able to use non-coherent fibre bundles, which were cheaper to manufacture than the coherent bundles needed to transmit an image. In 1960 he produced the first cystoscopes and laparoscopes to be illuminated in this way and coined the term "cold light". For a short time he also manufactured a semi-flexible gastroscope designed by Henning, using cold light transmitted down the instrument through fibreoptic bundles. Subsequently all fiberscopes were illuminated by cold light, which was much brighter than the old system and eliminated the risks of heat and electrical harm in the process.

While on the subject of Storz it is worth mentioning his successful partnership with Harold Hopkins. In the late 1950s Hopkins was approached by a frustrated urologist working in Liverpool called James Gow (1917–2001), asking if he could develop a better cystoscope.[47] Hopkins responded with his brilliant invention of the rod-lens system. This consisted of a flexible tube containing a series of cylindrical glass rods separated by short convex air spaces or "lenses". The system was much more robust than the glass lenses then in use and improved the optical efficiency of the cystoscope at least nine fold. A prototype cystoscope using rod lenses was made at Imperial College in 1961 but, almost inevitably it seems, manufacturers in Britain and America were not interested in it. It was not until 1965 after a lecture in Dusseldorf that he met Karl Storz who quickly obtained a patent to combine the use of the rod-lens system with fibreoptic illumination.[48] Thus were born the Storz-Hopkins cystoscopes and laparoscopes, which were highly successful and transformed Storz from a small local company into a huge multinational one. Once again a British invention was lost to a foreign competitor. Hopkins was elected a fellow of the Royal Society in 1973 and a fellow of both Royal Colleges (Physicians and Surgeons). The British Society of Gastroenterology commemorates him with their Hopkins endoscopy prize. He also received many honorary doctorates and several tempting offers to work abroad, but he was a modest and unpretentious man and preferred to remain at

Reading University. Inexplicably he did not receive a knighthood for his remarkable inventions.

In 1963 ACMI introduced their first fibreoptic oesophagoscope lit by cold light. It was a forward-viewing instrument and included a biopsy channel.[49] But there was still no mechanism for guiding the tip of the fibrescope and it was this together with lack of biopsy facilities that was preventing the widespread adoption of flexible gastroscopes. Radiology of the stomach was widely available and vastly improved by the use of air contrast techniques so clinicians saw little need for gastroscopy. Endoscopes were expensive, fiddly, fragile and time consuming. Furthermore there was no infrastructure in most hospitals for the care and maintenance they required.

It was now, in the middle 1960s, that the Japanese stepped in and stole a march on the Americans. The incidence of stomach cancer in Japan was very high and a matter of national concern. In 1950 the Olympus optical company had developed a gastric camera, or gastrocamera, to screen for early gastric cancer, and it was being used on a massive scale. The instrument consisted of a miniature camera attached to a flexible tube resembling a thin gastroscope. Nurses learnt to use it and literally millions of asymptomatic Japanese citizens had their stomachs photographed during the 1950s and 1960s. In London, George Hadley (1908–84), a physician at the Middlesex Hospital, was an enthusiast and visited Japan in 1963 to learn and service the gastrocamera, though he admitted that pictures of the entire stomach could not be guaranteed. The technique was never popular in Britain. The film had to be processed in Japan, gastric cancer was not the scourge here that it was in that country and crucially the camera could not provide tissue for histology. But thanks to its use, the Japanese developed considerable expertise in gastric instrumentation.

The fully flexible gastroscope must have seemed the answer to a prayer to the Japanese. They soon acquired a gastroscope from ACMI and by 1963 the Machida corporation had manufactured an instrument of their own using high quality glass fibres that were far superior to anything in America. The following year Olympus brought out a gastrocamera fibrescope with a controllable tip and by 1966 both companies had developed gastroscopes with a mechanism for controlling the tip of the instrument similar to the Hermon Taylor device. A channel for biopsy, cytology, water and air soon followed. The ingenuity of the Japanese instrument makers was matched by the remarkable dexterity and inventiveness of their clinicians. By 1970 several groups were reporting success with duodenoscopy using forward and side viewing instruments, colonoscopy and the first attempts at endoscopic retrograde cholangio-pancreatography (ERCP).

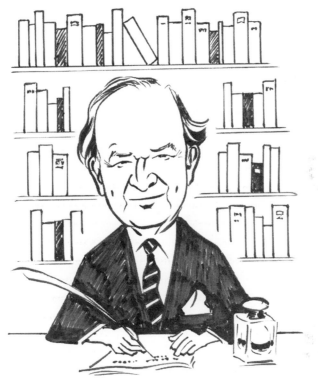

93 Gibbs – Medical historian.

In Britain Denis Gibbs was one of the first to acquire a combined fibrescope and gastrocamera (GTF). Gibbs (born 1927), a physician working at the Good Hope General Hospital, Sutton Coldfield, was interested in the diagnosis of gastric cancer using saline washings to look for malignant cells.[50] He had had some experience with George Hadley using "blind" gastric photography[51] and in 1966 the Birmingham Regional Hospital Board bought him a GTF fibrescope / gastrocamera. The instrument was easy to handle (he taught himself) and he soon appreciated the advantage of direct inspection over blind photography.[52] Another to use it was Geoffrey Chandler (born 1923), a physician at St.

James's Hospital, Leeds, who had been senior registrar to Avery Jones at the Central Middlesex Hospital.

Olympus next introduced an angulating mechanism that permitted better views of the proximal stomach. By this time, 1968, they were actively promoting their endoscopes in Britain with the help of Albert Reddihough, who ran a small business called Air Shields in Southend, later to become highly successful as the Key Med company. Reddihough sold one of the modified gastroscope/gastrocameras (GTF-A) to Clifford Hawkins, a physician at Queen Elizabeth Hospital, Birmingham in March 1968 for about £1,000 donated by Merck, Sharp and Dohme Limited. Hawkins paid one visit to Gibbs to learn the technique and, within eighteen months, together with his young colleague, Roy Cockel (born 1937), who was also self-taught, he had examined 100 patients.[53] They concluded that the examination was particularly rewarding in patients with gastric haemorrhage or when radiology was equivocal.

But biopsies with this instrument were not possible and it was not until Sidney Truelove in Oxford, with a grant from the Nuffield Foundation, bought an Olympus gastroscope through which biopsies could be taken that people began to take a serious interest in gastroscopy. In 1968 working with Michael Gear (born 1933), then senior surgical registrar at the Radcliffe Infirmary, he used the new side-viewing instrument (GFB) to examine and take biopsies from lesions anywhere in the stomach.[54] They obtained excellent views of the pylorus but did not intubate the duodenum or if they did the view was unsatisfactory. However, their ability to obtain biopsies completely changed people's perspective on endoscopy and suddenly a group of young enthusiasts sprang up as if from nowhere.

Among the first were two research fellows working with Brian Creamer at St. Thomas's Hospital. Peter Cotton (born 1939) was investigating lipid absorption in the small intestine and Mervyn Rosenberg (born 1934) was studying the effect of carbenoloxone on gastric ulcers in rats. Both were clinicians at heart and in 1968 Cotton had asked Creamer about the Schindler gastroscope gathering dust in a cupboard. Creamer's response was that it was a fiendish instrument, nobody believed what was seen and until it was possible to obtain biopsies gastroscopy was a waste of time. Shortly afterwards Truelove's article appeared and the two researchers persuaded the hospital, with Creamer's blessing, to buy them a flexible endoscope (GFB). The pair made one visit to watch Klaus Schiller (1927–2010) at St. Peter's Hospital, Chertsey, who had learnt endoscopy in Oxford with Truelove, and never looked back. Cotton, a master craftsman, took to endoscopy like a ferret to a trouser leg and Rosenberg used his endoscopy expertise throughout his surgical career. Incidentally neither have taken responsibility for their attempt to biopsy a strange black object (the inverted endoscope) the first time they saw it.

At the same time Professor Alan Read in Bristol asked his new lecturer in medicine, Paul Salmon (born 1939), to develop endoscopy in his department. Salmon took himself up to Oxford to see Mike Gear at work and was enthralled. For him endoscopy was the discovery of a wonderland and he relished the new technology. In the same year, 1968, John Lennard-Jones at University College Hospital, who already had experience of the Hermon Taylor semi-flexible instrument, obtained a GFB gastroscope and arranged a demonstration from a visiting Japanese endoscopist with experience of 5,000 cases. Ironically the first case was a failure because the patient had an unsuspected pharyngeal pouch. Not long afterwards, Lennard-Jones took sabbatical leave and Duncan Colin-Jones (born 1938), his senior registrar, took over endoscopy, teaching himself the technique and picking up tips from colleagues. Colin-Jones moved to Southampton in 1970 where John Bamforth (born 1930) was using a GFB instrument and soon became one of the leading upper GI endoscopists in Britain.

These men were young, enthusiastic and blessed with considerable dexterity. They were largely, if not entirely, self-taught and fed off one another, exchanging ideas and experience regularly. The instrument companies, notably Olympus and ACMI as far as Britain was concerned, developed a series of modifications and improvements to their endoscopes with such regularity that some instruments seemed almost obsolete by the time they were marketed. Olympus in particular soon dominated the field partly due to the marketing skills of Reddihough. Paul Salmon who first met him in 1968 recalls visiting him in Southend when his company was just an office block with two tables and chairs and a filing cabinet. Reddihough had managed to secure the marketing agency from Olympus Photo-Optical for the United Kingdom and realised that a highly efficient repair and replacement service would be crucial to the success of endoscopy. He made his fortune but helped the fledgling industry in return, sponsoring endoscopy meetings and supporting training courses for doctors, technicians and nurses.

Longer side-viewing endoscopes could be used to examine the second part of the duodenum[55] but it was not until forward-viewing duodenoscopes were developed in 1968 that the duodenal bulb could be examined directly. In Britain Paul Salmon and Paul Brown (1945–96), later appointed gastroenterologist in Shrewsbury, examined 150 patients using the first panendoscope made by ACMI (7089–A).[56] This was the first series of complete "oesophago-gastro-duodenoscopies" to be published in Britain and demonstrated the value of the procedure in X-ray negative dyspepsia, the follow-up of ulcer therapy and acute upper gastro-intestinal haemorrhage in a manner that was well beyond anything seen hitherto. Salmon extended this series to 1,000 cases using a new Olympus panendoscope (GIF-D2) with facilities for angulation of the tip in four directions that was to become very popular with endoscopists in Britain. Paul Brown was later appointed secretary to the endoscopy committee of the British Society of Gastroenterology but died at the early age of 51 from a small cell carcinoma.

b) Colonoscopy

Early attempts to peer up the gut paralleled those to peep down it and were similarly bedevilled by the lack of good illumination. The few enthusiasts had to rely on candlelight or simple sunlight. The first person in the British Isles (as they then were) to use an effective light was an Irish urologist from Dublin, Sir Francis Cruise (1834–1912). Cruise came from an old and distinguished family and was himself a literary man and a fine musician. He had an illustrious career for which he received a knighthood and towards the end of his life he was appointed Honorary Physician to King Edward VII in Ireland. In 1865 he designed a cystoscope that was similar to one that had recently been invented by the great Parisian surgeon, Antonin Jean Desormeaux (1815–94).[57] It consisted of a simple tube lit by a lamp burning a mixture of paraffin and camphor. The light was reflected down the tube by an angulated mirror but became so hot that it had to be encased in a wooden box, which made it rather cumbersome. Like Desormeaux, Cruise used different sized tubes, which allowed him to examine other orifices including the vagina and the rectum. His endoscopes were quite popular until superseded by those of Nitze and Leiter in the 1880s.

The real advance came with Edison's discovery of the electric light bulb in 1879. Several instruments were soon available in Europe and America incorporating an electric lamp but it was Hermann Strauss (1868–1944) in Berlin in 1903 who introduced the first successful sigmoidoscope that we would recognise today with a handle, an insufflation balloon and an obturator as well as a light carrier with a distal lamp.[58] Strauss was an eminent physician among the Jewish community who years later in his eighth decade was to die at the hands of the Nazis in a concentration camp. In England his instrument was quickly adopted by one of the pioneers of colonic surgery, Percy Lockhart-Mummery (1875–1957), as I have described in the chapter on inflammatory bowel disease. Clearly excited by the instrument he surely spoke for all endoscopists when he wrote: "The human mind is so constituted that we always experience a certain pleasure when we have succeeded in obtaining access to some spot hitherto difficult or impossible to explore."[59] Lockhart-Mummery extolled the virtues of the new sigmoidocope at a symposium on ulcerative colitis held at the Royal Society of Medicine in 1909.[60]

For nearly half a century the sigmoidoscope was used almost entirely by surgeons, though there were a few exceptions, notably Arthur Hurst who did his best to champion its use by physicians. "Nobody," he said, "would think of treating a case of tonsillitis without looking at the tonsils; it is even less justified to treat a case of colitis without looking at the colon."[61] But his words were ignored by the majority. It was not until after the Second World War that physicians (there were still very few gastroenterologists) took an interest when O. W. "Ossie" Lloyd-Davies (1905–87), a meticulous colo-rectal surgeon at St. Mark's Hospital, developed a small-bore proximally-lit sigmoidoscope. This was much more comfortable for the patient and did not require an anaesthetic, so it could be used in outpatients. It was quickly adopted by Francis Avery Jones who did his best to encourage its use by other physicians; indeed he would produce it from a specially designed poacher's pocket in his jacket at every opportunity. The growing interest of physicians in colitis and Crohn's Disease and the fact that many radiologists rightly insisted on endoscopic examination of the rectum before undertaking a barium enema, gradually made sigmoidoscopy and rectal biopsy a routine procedure. As Basil Morson (1918–2007), the leading colonic pathologist, put it, "where surgeons 'bit', physicians 'nibbled' and they were more prepared to use the smaller sigmoidoscope".[62]

During the early 1960s Professor Fujio Matsunaga[63] and Professor Hiruhomi Niwa,[64] working independently, attempted to examine the colon with a camera though they never enjoyed the success of the gastrocamera because the pictures were poor and unreliable. When fibre-optic instruments became available they abandoned the camera and experimented with various prototypes of colonoscope and soon realised that colonoscopy was a much more difficult procedure than gastroscopy. While they were struggling to master the technique, a young American intern in the Department of Medicine at the University of Michigan at Ann Arbor, called Bergein Overholt, constructed a series of life-like models of the sigmoid colon from casts of silastic foam enemas. With the help of the Eder company who manufactured rigid and semi-flexible endoscopes Overholt designed a flexible sigmoidoscope that proved to be far superior to the rigid instrument and fairly easy to use. He expected to be able to examine the entire sigmoid colon in at least 80 per cent of his cases.[65] I should emphasise that at this time (late 1960s) most people apart from the Japanese were thinking in terms of extended sigmoidoscopy rather than colonoscopy. Admittedly there were one or two enthusiasts on the continent who attempted to feed a colonoscope over a guide wire that had previously been swallowed a day or two before (so-called transintestinal intubation) but this was time consuming and never popular.[66]

Meanwhile in Britain while most clinicians were happily using the rigid sigmoidoscope to take biopsies, a senior surgical registrar at the Royal Free Hospital, John Fox (born 1933), attempted to obtain what he described as high colonic biopsies using a soft polyvinyl tube 120 centimetres long inserted through a Lloyd-Davies sigmoidoscope under X-ray screening. He called his technique "retrograde colonic intubation" and managed to secure biopsies from the upper sigmoid and descending colon in most patients.[67] In the process he was gaining valuable experience at intubation and ACMI provided him with a microbore fibreoptic colonoscope (7.5 millimetre diameter), which could be inserted through the polyvinyl tube to obtain views as high as the transverse colon.[68] Fox demonstrated the colonoscope to the consultant staff at St. Mark's Hospital but they were not interested. The technique was cumbersome and soon overtaken by larger colonoscopes through which biopsies could be obtained under direct vision. Later he used one of the first colonoscopes designed by Overholt for ACMI but the instrument had limitations and he had difficulty negotiating the sigmoid and rarely reached the caecum.[69]

The redoubtable entrepreneur, Albert Reddihough, began to promote the first colonoscope made by Olympus in the late 1960s. His first customer was Alan Dean (born 1932), a gastrointestinal surgeon in Edinburgh who had become interested in endoscopy while working at King's College Hospital as senior registrar to Harold Edwards. Dean teamed up with David Shearman, a gastroenterologist who later moved to Australia, and they managed to raise the funds to buy an instrument from Reddihough. The colonoscope (model CF-SB) could only be passed to a maximum of 70 centimetres so it was in effect a flexible sigmoidoscope and Dean and Shearman saw it simply as an improvement on the rigid sigmoidoscope. They always managed to enter the sigmoid colon but had difficulty getting through it and rarely reached the descending colon.[70] At the first sign of patient discomfort, or difficulty with a sharp bend, they abandoned the procedure but they were impressed by its potential.

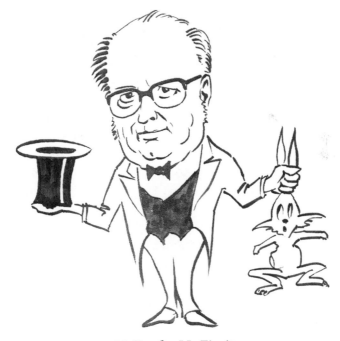

94 Read – Mr Fix-it.

About the time that Dean and Shearman were doing their trial, Sidney Truelove (Oxford) and Paul Salmon (Bristol) were invited to meet Professor Niwa from Japan at the Gordon Hospital in London. Niwa now had extensive experience of flexible sigmoidoscopy and had brought an Olympus colonoscope (CF-SB) with him. They both tried their hand with the instrument with mixed fortune. Truelove had difficulty passing the instrument into the sigmoid colon and was more interested in Niwa's tri-valve rectal speculum, sometimes used to help insert instruments into the rectum. However, Salmon had more success and, in a state of excitement, returned to Bristol where he persuaded Alan Read to buy the very instrument that Niwa had brought with him. When one considers the cost of the colonoscope and the light source and accessories amounted to £5,000, this was a brave decision in 1969 and highlights Read's support for endoscopy from the start.

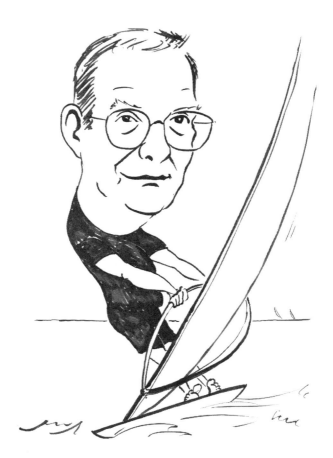

95 Teague – Bristol-Liverpool-Torquay.

Salmon, together with Bob Branch (later an eminent pharmacologist in America) and Robin Teague (born 1944) (later gastroenterologist in Torquay), soon became proficient with the short colonoscope expecting to reach at least as far as the descending colon.[71] As well as experimenting with various sedation techniques and bowel preparations, they recognised the importance of careful photographic recordings for both clinical and teaching purposes and accumulated a fine series of slide tapes and cine film. Enjoying full support from Bristol University, they were among the first to acquire longer colonoscopes from both ACMI and Olympus. The team learnt their trade by trial and error, exchanging ideas with others and even threading the colonoscope through the colon at laparotomy in a few instances.[72] By the end of 1972, Teague and Salmon had experience of 250 cases and were managing to reach the caecum in two-thirds of their patients.[73]

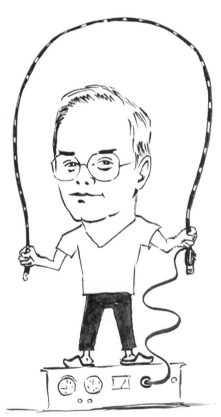

96 Williams – Horshoe is his favourite shape.

However, the man whose name became synonymous with colonoscopy in Britain was Christopher Williams at St. Mark's Hospital, London. Williams (born 1938) qualified at University College Hospital where he did the usual junior posts before moving to St. Mark's Hospital in 1969 as medical registrar to John Lennard-Jones. Not long afterwards, Alan Parks (1920–82), a forward-looking surgeon and later President of the Royal College of Surgeons, returned from a visit to Japan with a short colonoscope. The surgical registrars were too busy to grapple with it so Parks gave it to Williams who used it for the first time in December 1970. He soon realised he was facing a formidable challenge but a combination of skill and perseverance helped him to master the technique. He had a great facility for working in three dimensions. In 1971 Parks acquired a long, improved colonoscope (Olympus model CF-LB) and Williams spent hours with Tetsuichiro Muto, an honorary registrar from Japan, endeavouring to reach the caecum with it. It is a tribute to their tenacity that the pair achieved their goal in 94 per cent of cases.[74] In the early days a single case often took three hours and they would take turns every fifteen minutes, one manipulating the controls and the other advancing or withdrawing the instrument as instructed, but their success rate far exceeded that of anybody else. The first 100 examinations took two years to complete but altered the management of 30 per cent of the patients. Colonoscopy was here to stay.

Further grist was added to the colonoscopist's mill by polypectomy. First pioneered by Professor Demling's department in Erlangen, Germany, in the early 1970s, Williams was quick to undertake polypectomy. He began by experimenting with hot wires on pieces of meat at home in his kitchen, and by the end of 1972 had removed over 150 polyps from 100 patients without complications.[75] Even the most sceptical surgeon now accepted that colonoscopy was desirable.

Alan Parks and Lennard-Jones realised that Williams was indispensable and were determined to keep him at St. Mark's Hospital. At that time there was only one gastroenterologist on the staff (Lennard-Jones) and his registrar. So they created a job for him as a part-time consultant with a special interest in colonoscopy (six sessions at St. Mark's Hospital and three sessions at St. Bartholemew's Hospital) in 1974. The job description stated that the candidate "must have an established international reputation in the performance and teaching of colonoscopy" thus ensuring his appointment. Williams was asked by one interviewer whether he would still be as keen on colonoscopy when he was in his 40s, a fair question. In the event he was, and in retirement still is, thanks to his enthusiasm and also to the tremendous support from his backers. The hospital immediately stumped up £100,000 to convert and equip part of the X-ray department, and subsequently over the years Williams was rewarded with more than £3 million for equipment and facilities from charitable funds raised by well wishers.

c) Endoscopic retrograde cholangio-pancreatography

I can still recall the amazement with which I first saw pictures of the bile ducts in a paper by Peter Cotton and colleagues in the *Lancet* in 1972.[76] At the time scanning was still unheard of and the diagnosis of jaundice relied on palpation, plain radiography and biochemical tests that were frequently misleading. Anyone with prolonged jaundice needed a careful laparotomy sooner or later to exclude biliary tract obstruction.

The British may not have been the first to tackle ERCP (as it became known) but they were not far behind. The first description of endoscopic cannulation of the papilla of Vater appeared in America in 1968. William McCune (1909–98), a surgeon in Washington DC, used an Eder fibrescope and managed to see the papilla in about 50 patients with successful cannulation in half of them. But the X-ray pictures were poor, the Eder fibrescope was awkward to use and McCune's work was overtaken by the Japanese using their own duodenoscopes. In 1970 Itaru Oi and his colleagues from Tokyo presented their first year's experience with ERCP at the Second World Congress of Digestive Endoscopy in Copenhagen. They used a purpose-built duodenoscope made by Machida (FDS-1b) and the pictures caused a sensation.[77]

Early in 1970, Ludwig Demling and Meinhard Classen at Erlangen University, Germany, who had also been trying to cannulate the papilla of Vater finally succeeded with the new Olympus duodenoscope (JFB). At the autumn meeting of the British Society of Gastroenterology in London that year, Meinhard Classen showed an awe-inspiring sixteen-millimetre movie film on endoscopy of the duodenum, which included pictures of chronic pancreatitis and stones in the bile duct. After his presentation Classen was approached by Peter Cotton wishing to visit Erlangen to watch his technique. In the event Cotton went to Japan in May 1971 where he spent three precious weeks with Dr. Kazuei Ogoshi in Niigata and brought the technique of ERCP back to Britain. A new duodenoscope was bought by the Cancer Research Campaign after Cotton promised to stamp out pancreatic cancer with it.

To be the first to establish an ERCP service from scratch required

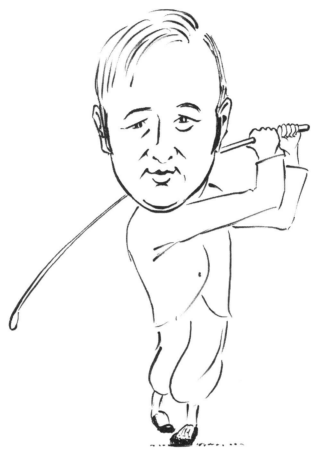

97 Cotton – Stones out of ducts, balls into holes, all in a day's work.

someone with endoscopic experience, considerable skill, confidence in his own ability and persistence. Peter Cotton possessed all these in abundance combined with disarming humility and a laconic sense of humour. He was a tall man with a commanding presence and inspired and taught a generation of ERCPists from Britain and all over the world. The task was daunting as anyone learning ERCP knows only too well. Furthermore the instruments and accessories were still being developed and initially successful cannulation of the papilla was achieved in about 80 per cent of cases.[78] This improved with experience and by the time therapeutic ERCP began in 1975, Cotton was a world leader. By then he had moved to the Middlesex Hospital having inexplicably failed to secure a permanent appointment at St. Thomas's Hospital. Rumour has it that his chief backer, Brian Creamer, left the interview during the discussion of candidates to catch his usual train home at 5.30 p.m.

ERCP required good radiology and Cotton was fortunate to have the enthusiastic cooperation of John Beales (born 1938) who was appointed to St. Thomas's Hospital in 1972. Their early interest was in the pancreas and in those days the contrast medium was ionic and highly irritant. Overfilling of the pancreas was very painful and could precipitate pancreatitis. With poor screening facilities it was difficult to judge how much contrast was required to outline the ducts. The X-ray department in the basement was tiny and poorly equipped. On one occasion when Cotton and Beales made one of the first films of ERCP, they gratefully accepted an offer from the new Greenwich Hospital to use their facilities. Together with a large film crew and long-suffering patient volunteers they sweated through all of a lovely summer Sunday.

Unfortunately St. Thomas's Hospital was not willing to re-equip the X-ray department and Beales moved to Bath in 1974 where he worked with Ken Gough for four years and built up a fine unit. Beales was peripatetic; he spent a short time in New Zealand, then six years as Director of Radiology at Riyadh-Al-Kharj Hospital before returning to the Lister Hospital in 1984. He prided himself on being a general radiologist with an interest in gastroenterology and deliberately avoided sub-specialisation.

About the time that Cotton went to Japan, Alan Read and Paul Salmon from Bristol were invited to spend a week with Professor Demling in Erlangen to observe his team doing ERCP. On their return, Read obtained funds for an Olympus duodenoscope and Salmon, a great enthusiast, soon became proficient at ERCP. They were superbly supported by their radiological colleague, Professor Middlemiss, who provided a university X-ray suite equipped with the latest image-intensifier and floating table. Within a few months Cotton and Salmon were reporting their first 60 patients, with successful cannulation in 73 per cent.[79]

In 1972 a key meeting took place during the European Society of

Gastroenterology meeting in Paris organised by Olympus for about fifteen people in Europe undertaking ERCP. At the time it was widely stated that ERCP was feasible only for Japanese musicians (Ogoshi played the clarinet and Oi also played an instrument). The Europeans soon disabused people of such a notion, though Cotton assumed that their host in Paris must have been a trombone player by the way he used the endoscope. The success of ERCP brought responsibilities and the small European group agreed on the need for proper funding and policies, careful evaluation and research, and teaching. They knew each other and their Japanese counterparts well and later the same year in New York Cotton participated in the first of many international ERCP demonstrations alongside Classen and Itaru Oi.

CHAPTER SIXTY-EIGHT

BRITISH SOCIETY FOR DIGESTIVE ENDOSCOPY

By the early 1970s a few dozen physicians and surgeons throughout Britain were tinkering with endoscopy. With few exceptions they were generalists with an interest in gastroenterology and after watching another endoscopist at work they were learning the technique on the job. Most had one or possibly two instruments for upper gastrointestinal endoscopy and were performing two or three examinations per week, either in a ward side room or the operating theatre, as very few had a purpose designed endoscopy room. As often as not the endoscopes were bought with charitable funds though the NHS generally paid for the high maintenance costs. Not many were tackling colonoscopy because it was a difficult technique and only 250–300 examinations were recorded in 1971 and 1972. Apart from Williams and Salmon most were done by surgeons usually in theatre or the X-ray department.

Many of these clinicians were young consultants or senior registrars and were not members of the British Society of Gastroenterology. They did not fulfil the criteria for election "in recognition of achievement and continuing activity, in any discipline relevant to gastroenterology" though they could apply to be associate members for a limited period. They felt they needed some sort of organisation to represent them and to formalise their training. As there was little enthusiasm or support at the time from the British Society of Gastroenterology a separate group seemed inevitable and it fell to Klaus Schiller (1927–2010), an energetic gastroenterologist at St. Peter's Hospital, Chertsey, to set one up. Schiller had worked with Sidney Truelove at Oxford on a large survey of haematemesis and melaena[80] and taken the opportunity to learn a little of the technique of fibreoptic gastroscopy. After his appointment to St.

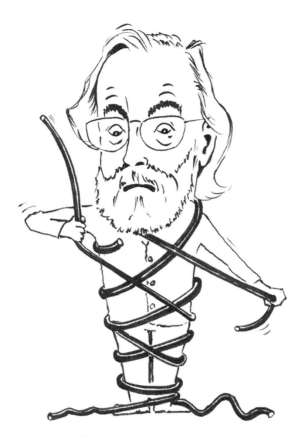

98 Schiller – First to regulate endoscopy.

Peter's Hospital in 1968 he persuaded his health authority to acquire an Olympus gastroscope (GFB) of the type that Truelove had pioneered, and taught himself to use it. He was thus one of the first physicians to be using a gastroscope in routine practice.

In 1971 Schiller organised an informal meeting of like-minded young endoscopists at St. Peter's Hospital, Chertsey, to discuss the possibility of a small specialist society: this was well attended and lively. As their spokesman and ambassador Schiller was deputed to ask Truelove, a senior and highly respected gastroenterologist, to lead such a society if one was formed. Over a beer at the Royal Oak, across the road from the Radcliffe Infirmary, Truelove agreed on condition that Schiller became the honorary secretary and did all the work.[81] In the event, the British Society of Digestive Endoscopy (BSDE) was inaugurated at a private meeting during the 32nd Annual Meeting of the British Society of Gastroenterology held at Newcastle in September 1971. There were more than 60 doctors present and the executive committee practically chose itself, representing the most experienced endoscopists in Britain at the time. Sidney Truelove (Oxford) was duly elected President, Klaus Schiller (Chertsey) Honorary Secretary and Professor Alan Read (Bristol) Honorary Treasurer. The other members were Geoffrey Chandler (Leeds), Peter Cotton (London), Alan Dean (Edinburgh), Denis Gibbs (Sutton Coldfield), John Lennard-Jones (representing the British Society of Gastroenterology), Professor Ian McColl (London), Paul Salmon (Bristol) and Richard Whitehead (an Oxford pathologist). Within a year, McColl and Whitehead stood down to be replaced by Duncan Colin-Jones (Southampton) and Christopher Williams (St. Mark's Hospital). After some correspondence in the press, the name of the new society was changed to the more accurate "for" rather than "of" Endoscopy.

The society flourished. Within six months it had 200 ordinary members and by the end of 1975 there were 370. A few people were given honorary membership for their distinguished contributions to the art of endoscopy, including Harold Hopkins and Basil Hirschowitz. Furthermore corporate membership was offered to companies manufacturing and supplying endoscopes, and to pharmaceutical companies whose drugs were of special value in endoscopy. Foremost among these was Keymed, the instrument company founded by Albert Reddihough and his partner Dr. Tony Hanwell PhD in 1969. Reddihough's intention was to market Olympus endoscopes on a large scale in Britain and he recognised the need to provide a first class repair and replacement service at his workshop in Southend. Endoscopes were delicate instruments that were easily damaged and Keymed became indispensable to everyone doing endoscopy. The success of the company can be measured by the increase in its staff from 5 in 1970 to nearly 600 when Reddihough retired in 1991.

At first Truelove met unexpected criticism when he reported the birth of BSDE to the British Society of Gastroenterology but he was a determined and forthright man and not the sort to be deterred by uninformed and prejudiced opposition.[82]

The success of the society reflected the intense enthusiasm of its committee led by the honorary secretary who was a key figure. Schiller was succeeded by Colin-Jones in 1974 who in turn was replaced by Roy Cockel (Birmingham) in 1977. These three devoted a great deal

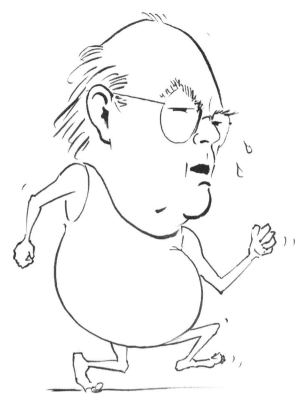

99 Cockel – Endoscopy is fun – so is running.

of time and energy to the society. When BSDE was formed there were probably 150 doctors practising endoscopy (mostly gastroscopy) of whom the majority were physicians with a minority of surgeons and a handful of radiologists. The first priority was to highlight the need for a proper endoscopy service throughout Britain and in 1972 the society produced an influential memorandum on future national needs for fibreoptic endoscopy, ostensibly addressed to Sir George Godber, then Chief Medical Officer, but in reality aimed at a much wider audience.[83] The document, which described in detail the staffing, organisation and financial implications of setting up and running an endoscopy service, was revised in 1973 and distributed to all regional medical officers and other interested parties including the British Society of Gastroenterology and all members of BSDE. No document of this type had previously been written and there was a big demand for it both in Britain and abroad.

The next priority of the society was to ensure that endoscopists were properly taught. Hitherto most had acquired the art of gastroscopy by trial and error. A training subcommittee was formed comprising the secretary (Klaus Schiller), Peter Cotton, Paul Salmon, Duncan Colin-Jones and Christopher Williams, who were to prove indispensable to the society. Initially they concentrated on basic endoscopy for beginners with one-day courses, a series of slide-tape lectures, and stomach models on which to practise. The first workshops for what Cotton called "expert beginners" on ERCP and colonoscopy were held at Imperial College, London in 1973 during the annual meeting of the British Society of Gastroenterology. They were so popular that further successful workshops were arranged at the Middlesex Hospital, St. Mark's Hospital, the Royal Free Hospital, and Bristol Royal Infirmary over the next few years. These centres had state-of-the-art endoscopy units with closed-circuit television and good training facilities.

Endoscopists require skilled assistants and the society promoted the recruitment of nurses as endoscopy assistants despite some initial misgivings from the Joint Board of Clinical Nursing Studies. Nurses were given associate membership of the society but it was many years before their true worth in managing endoscopy units was fully appreciated and funded.

From its inception BSDE was anxious to maintain good relations with the British Society of Gastroenterology (BSG). Several members belonged to both societies and in 1973 the proportion increased as the restriction on ordinary membership of the BSG was relaxed to include people simply with "a special interest or experience in any discipline relevant to gastroenterology". Endoscopists acknowledged that endoscopy was just one facet of gastroenterology. The endoscope was merely one of the tools used by specialists in gastrointestinal disease. There was no wish to foster endoscopy as a specialty in its own right. As early as December 1974 the committee of BSDE realised that their society would be superfluous if the BSG was to relax its membership rules and be prepared to take responsibility for teaching endoscopy. Co-operation between the societies steadily increased, joint registration for meetings began and two presidents of the society (Truelove and Bill Sircus) both became presidents of the BSG after completing their term of office with BSDE. In 1977 negotiations began for a merger and in 1978 a working party chaired by Peter Cotton with representatives from both societies recommended unification. This was accepted by the vast majority of members from both societies at their annual meeting in Guildford in September 1979. On 1st January 1980 the BSDE disappeared as a separate organisation and its ordinary members became full members of the BSG. Associate members, especially nurses, became endoscopy assistant members of the BSG, and corporate membership ceased to exist. From now on the interests of endoscopy would be managed by an endoscopy subcommittee of the British Society of Gastroenterology chaired by the Vice-President (Endoscopy).[84]

CHAPTER SIXTY-NINE

RECOGNITION OF GASTROENTEROLOGY AS A SPECIALTY

At the same time the BSG was pressing for gastroenterology to be recognised as a medical specialty. This was clearly driven by the arrival of endoscopy, which brought meaning to the word specialty in practical terms, and in 1975 the Standing Committee on Gastroenterology of the Royal College of Physicians published a report on the "Organisation of a Gastroenterological Service".[85] This called for hospitals throughout the country to be provided with adequate gastroenterological services. The role of endoscopy was stressed but therapeutic endoscopy was still in its infancy and the need for proper endoscopy units was not spelt out.

During the 1970s the number of physicians with an interest in gastroenterology increased rapidly. Surprisingly no one knew exactly how many physicians were practising gastroenterology because they were categorised as general physicians by the Department of Health. An educated guess suggested that by 1976 there were probably 200 with most practising some upper gastrointestinal endoscopy. But endoscopy was expensive and expansion of the service was coinciding with a time of economic restraint. Clinicians were short of instruments and having to tap private funds for almost half the equipment they needed. As a frustrated Martin Sarner, physician in Portsmouth, wrote in 1974, "It is very noticeable that nephrologists are able to lay claims to departmental monies where I must go cap in hand to local charities etc. Presumably the situation will continue until gastroenterology is a recognised specialty." Sarner resolved his particular problem by transferring to University College Hospital, London in 1975 and Duncan Colin-Jones moved from Southampton and took his place. By this time Colin-Jones was Honorary Secretary to BSDE and two years later he collaborated with Klaus

Schiller and Roy Cockel to review endoscopic practice in the United Kingdom.[86] They confirmed the explosive, unplanned and haphazard growth in gastrointestinal endoscopy in the face of considerable financial difficulties and hoped their report would stimulate a rational forward-looking policy in the future.

To an extent Sarner was correct; many thought that until gastroenterology was recognised as a specialty by the Department of Health (DHSS), a formal policy with an appropriate budget would never occur. Most thought recognition was a long way off and would have been surprised to learn that the DHSS was sympathetic to their cause. For some years various gastroenterological committees had been in dialogue with the department and the man driving the discussions was Nelson Coghill (1912–2002), physician to the West Middlesex Hospital.

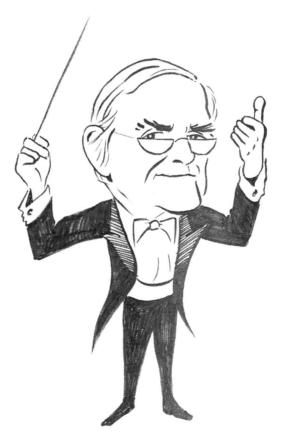

100 Coghill – Liaison officer and negotiator.

Coghill was an influential gastroenterologist; he had been President of the British Society of Gastroenterology in 1970 and was elected Chairman of the Training and Education Committee of the BSG in 1973 which had published a report on training issues in 1974.[87] He was also Chairman of the Specialist Advisory Committee responsible for gastroenterology to the Joint Committee on Higher Medical Training (JCHMT). At the behest of the Standing Committee on Gastroenterology of the Royal College of Physicians, Coghill formed a Liaison Committee on behalf of all these groups to meet representatives of the DHSS at regular intervals, and the first meeting took place in March 1976. It had no executive function but was a forum for free discussion and an opportunity to champion various matters of topical interest, notably endoscopy and recognition of gastroenterology, with the DHSS.

After much deliberation the profession and the DHSS agreed that gastroenterology should remain in the realm of general medicine but that physicians who spent at least half of their time in gastroenterology should be recognised as part-time gastroenterologists. In 1977 they were encouraged to apply for accreditation with the JCHMT. This sensible arrangement suited everyone and allowed considerable flexibility during specialist training and the creation of consultant posts tailored to meet local need. Most clinicians did not wish to relinquish general medicine, but they did want support for their gastroenterological work. The specialty now appeared in the DHSS statistics and was "recognised".

A member of the Department of Health, Dr. Tom Sweeney, also visited more than a dozen gastroenterology units in district general hospitals around the country in 1976 and was able to see for himself what people were doing and how they were coping. He was amazed by what he found. The commonest problem was lack of suitable accommodation in which to run the service. He noted that there had been many ingenious and successful adaptations to existing buildings such as the conversion of a Nightingale ward or a vacated theatre suite or even an old nurses' home, and in one instance, a large unoccupied private house within the hospital compound.

In 1977 Coghill and Sweeney began to put together a joint paper on the provision of a gastroenterological service in the district general hospital. A draft was sent to all members of the British Society of Gastroenterology and the committee of the BSDE for their comments before it appeared in October 1978. The final version was edited by John Lennard-Jones who had by this time succeeded Nelson Coghill as convenor on the liaison committee.[88] The document emphasised the need for a properly funded basic endoscopy service with appropriate instruments, staffing and accommodation and was important because it had the blessing of the DHSS and could be used to put pressure on regional authorities. But it was not a diktat and individual clinicians still had to compete with other specialties for their share of the rather small cake.

CHAPTER SEVENTY

ENDOSCOPY IN THE DISTRICT
GENERAL HOSPITAL IN THE 1970S

Shortly after its implosion the three former secretaries of the BSDE, Cockel, Colin-Jones and Schiller, published an update on the state of endoscopy services in Britain to the end of 1978.[89] All types of endoscopy were increasing but the absolute number of ERCPs and colonoscopies per unit was still small and well behind the activity in Europe. Most units were only managing about 50 ERCPs and 50 colonoscopies annually. Only a third of the hospitals had a designated endoscopy room and far too many procedures were being done in the operating theatre, the X-ray department or an adapted side room. Money to buy endoscopes was hard to get and the British were buying fewer instruments than their colleagues abroad. An unofficial league table prepared by Keymed's Albert Reddihough showed that Britain was seventh out of the eight leading countries of Western Europe in the purchase of endoscopes per doctor and per head of population.

What was actually happening between one hospital and the next varied considerably. Most places had a physician doing one upper gastrointestinal endoscopy list per week but hospitals in a position to make a new appointment were able to improve the service as young consultants with experience in endoscopy filled these posts. Much depended on vacancies arising at the time, the whim of the health authority and, inevitably, cash.

A good example of what could be achieved was seen in Stoke. Charles Swan (born 1937) was appointed to the North Staffordshire Hospitals in 1972 with the brief to develop gastroenterology. He first handled a gastroscope in Birmingham in 1969 and gained further experience as a research fellow in New York. Once settled in Stoke he converted an

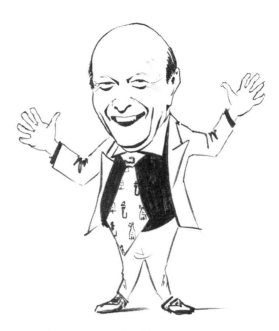

101 Swan – Hands off endoscopy course.

empty ward into one of the most spacious endoscopy units in Britain with two endoscopy rooms, recovery area, waiting room and offices for all. Recognising the value of the "hands-on" approach to teaching, he enlisted the support of Reddihough from Keymed and began a one-week course in 1977 for a maximum of eight trainees in upper GI endoscopy and followed this in 1982 with a similar course in colonoscopy. Delegates practised on routine patients from the waiting list and were overseen by experts (who were under instructions not to commandeer the endoscope from the trainee). The courses proved immensely popular and later in 1987 when radiology improved Jonathan Green (born 1946) added ERCP to the repertoire. Ultimately more than 300 delegates passed through the system and each received a certificate and a specially designed course tie at the end of it.

In stark contrast, the author was appointed to the West Dorset Group Hospitals in 1972 with no gastroenterological experience, in the expectation that he would take on endoscopy. There were three physicians working in two small hospitals eight miles apart. For fifteen years upper GI endoscopy took place in the bowel prep room of the X-ray department with patients waiting and recovering in the corridor. It was rare to have the same nurse for consecutive lists and most GI bleeds had to be endoscoped in the other hospital, which probably shortened the life of the instrument (if not the patient and the endoscopist). Colonoscopy crept in during the late 1970s in an X-ray room when space was available, and ERCP (learnt with a radiologist, Roger Frost, at Salisbury) began in the early 1990s. This was nothing of which to be proud but I suspect many had a similar experience and Yeovil District Hospital, for instance, had no endoscopy at all until the appointment of a surgeon, Robin Kennedy, in 1987.

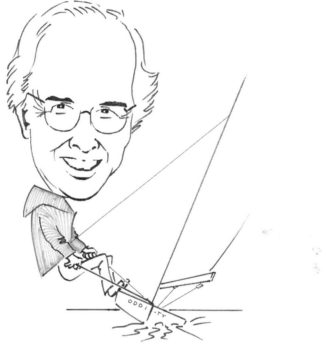

102 Colin-Jones – Time for everyone.

While routine upper gastrointestinal endoscopy became widespread, ERCP and colonoscopy lagged behind. By the end of the 1970s there were only a handful of units undertaking ERCP and even less doing sphincterotomy. Cotton and his team of registrars and trainees from all over the world led the way at the Middlesex Hospital with Paul Salmon in Bristol some way behind. Other physicians included Tony Axon at Leeds who had trained with Cotton at St. Thomas's Hospital, Roy Cockel in Birmingham, Alexander Dellipiani in Middlesbrough and

Duncan Colin-Jones in Portsmouth. Colin-Jones began ERCP at the beginning of 1973 and like most others watched Cotton at work and took the opportunity to visit Meinhard Classen in Erlangen, who ran workshops sponsored by the Keymed company. He recalls how after one of these visits the aircraft carrying the delegates took off for England in thick fog and I shudder to think of the setback to gastroenterology had the plane crashed with the cream of British endoscopists on board.

Funding was always a problem, and apart from the expense of endoscopes, accessories such as sphincterotomy knives, balloons and baskets were costly. As an economy Colin-Jones used to repair the knives at home enabling him to get an extra ten sphincterotomies from each knife.

A few surgeons were also prominent ERCPists. Michael Gear (born 1933) left Oxford in 1970 to take up a consultant post in Gloucester. He already had a reputation in endoscopy after his work with Truelove and built up a flourishing unit in a disused theatre taking on two general practitioners to assist him. Fortunately, a new district hospital in Gloucester was under construction and he was able to incorporate a purpose-built endoscopy suite within it. He learnt ERCP from Peter Cotton at St. Thomas's Hospital soon after the latter's trip to Japan in 1971, and was also one of the first to offer an open access OGD service for general practitioners.[90] His colleague, Hamish Thomson (born 1937), joined him when the new hospital opened in 1975 and took over colonoscopy, leaving him free to concentrate on upper GI endoscopy.

Another surgeon, Christopher Venables (born 1935) in Newcastle was one of the first after Cotton to undertake ERCP. Inspired by Oi's remarkable demonstration at the World Congress of Digestive Endoscopy in Copenhagen in 1970 Venables managed to persuade the Professor of Surgery, Ivan Johnstone, to buy a duodenoscope for the department which he initially used as a gastroscope (he did not have a forward-viewing instrument). At the time a radiological colleague, Ian Lavelle (born 1934), was starting to do double contrast barium meals. To help each other understand what they were seeing they set up a joint clinic together and soon became highly proficient with the side-viewing instrument. From there ERCP was a natural progression, which they began in 1972, taking turns to cannulate the papilla. Both were self-taught and Venables said that he was fortunate that his first attempt was successful, which encouraged him to persevere, and he too visited Classen's unit in Erlangen. On one occasion he was asked to advise on a six year old child who had sustained an abdominal injury and had a raised serum amylase. Using his adult duodenoscope he obtained a pancreatogram and demonstrated a disrupted pancreatic duct. At laparotomy he managed to repair this with a duodenal patch and the child survived. Despite this remarkable event Venables spent years battling for funds and used a side room for routine upper GI endoscopy, where he did more than 3,000 procedures each year.

Naturally radiologists were actively involved in ERCP from the start because X-rays and screening were essential and they helped to interepret pancreatograms, which nobody had seen before. Some were also accomplished ERCPists themselves such as Ian Lavelle. Another was Giles Stevenson (born 1939) who was appointed to Plymouth in 1973. At the time Plymouth had a district hospital on two sites, Devonport and Freedom Fields. There was one gastroenterologist, Michael Grayson (1929–2005), a diligent and gifted clinician who had bought a gastrocamera in 1967 and replaced it with an Olympus GIFD panendoscope in 1971. By 1973 he was doing three or four upper GI endoscopies each week, which was fairly typical of many units around the country. Colonoscopy was virtually non-existent; the surgeons had a short Olympus SF colonoscope and used it in theatre just seven times in 1973.

Stevenson had experience in endoscopy and managed to persuade the regional board in Bristol to buy him two gastroscopes, a duodenoscope and a colonoscope, a Keymed trolley, teaching attachment and cautery equipment before he took up his appointment. Though he was lucky in that a capital project in Plymouth had just fallen through and money was unexpectedly available, he deserved his luck. When he was a senior registrar at King's College Hospital, he was asked by Cotton and Rosenberg to collaborate in a study showing the value of endoscopy in stomachs distorted by previous surgery.[91] He realised that it was frequently impossible for the radiologist to detect lesions in these patients and decided to learn endoscopy himself. On Cotton's advice he arranged to visit Dr. Kasugai in Nagoya but failed to get a Kodak scholarship to fund the project. Undaunted, he worked for a year in Northern Canada and with the proceeds spent six months in 1973 with Kasugai who taught him all aspects of endoscopy. It was while in Japan that he secured his job in Plymouth, starting in 1974 together with all the endoscopes he had requested.

Stevenson galvanised endoscopy in Plymouth and a year later wrote a report outlining his ideas for future developments. This was an ambitious document reflecting everything published in the BSDE memorandum of 1974 and must have given his health authority plenty of food for thought. However, he left Plymouth in 1976 to take up a post at McMaster University, Hamilton, Ontario and his place was taken by another radiologist, David Beckly.

Beckly (born 1940) had worked in Bristol where he learnt the essentials of upper and lower GI endoscopy from Paul Salmon and Robin Teague. He then spent several months in Leeds learning selective visceral angiography with Hans Herlinger (1915–2006), a legendary radiologist and Nazi fugitive.[92] While there he took the opportunity to begin ERCP with Tony Axon (born 1941) who had worked with Peter Cotton at St. Thomas's Hospital and had just been appointed in Leeds. When he came to Plymouth he gave up radiology and became a full-time endoscopist building on the foundation laid by Stevenson. He was probably the only full-time, all-round endoscopist in Britain and prided himself in providing a comprehensive service. His position was unusual and at odds with those who felt that endoscopy should be merely one aspect (admittedly an important one) of gastroenterology.

Despite all this activity, a survey of British experience of duodenoscopic sphincterotomy at the end of the 1970s showed that only 14 centres were active in this field with Cotton's group at the Middlesex Hospital doing far more than anybody else (more than 500 cases[93]). Only six other centres had done more than twenty cases.[94]

Colonoscopy was also slow to catch on and as late as 1979 the vast majority was still done in one or two centres such as St. Mark's Hospital (Christopher Williams) and Bristol (Robin Teague). Elsewhere most places were only managing about one procedure per week and the reasons or excuses were not hard to find. Physicians found it difficult and time consuming and it was expensive. Colonoscopy was still thought of as a diagnostic procedure and surgeons seemed content with rigid sigmoidoscopy and barium enema. In 1979 Christopher Williams made a strong plea for more colonoscopy, arguing that it radically affected the management of colonic disease because it often answered questions that the barium enema could not resolve, and frequently prevented the need for surgery. It was also the investigation of choice in patients with rectal bleeding.[95]

Towards the end of the decade the combined efforts of the BSDE and the joint liaison committee for gastroenterology began to bear fruit. Health authorities realised that therapeutic endoscopy in particular was cost effective and might save them money quite apart from the advantages to the patient.

CHAPTER SEVENTY-ONE

1980S – EXPANSION OF ENDOSCOPY AND OPERATIVE ENDOSCOPY

At the start of the 1980s the number of people doing endoscopy accelerated, driven by the ability to carry out therapeutic procedures. There were now about 270 clinicians devoting three to six weekly sessions to gastroenterology and many were fully trained endoscopists. Nearly all district general hospitals had a physician with a special interest in gastroenterology on their staff but few had purpose-built endoscopy rooms in which to work. Despite this there was a 30 per cent rise in operative upper GI endoscopy between 1980 and 1981 and a 70 per cent rise in colonoscopies.[96]

The oesophagus was particularly amenable to therapeutic attack. Impacted foreign bodies were rare but the use of paediatric endoscopes to remove marbles and coins from the oesophagi of quite small children avoided the need for rigid endoscopy. Benign inflammatory strictures could be treated quite easily and safely by bouginage and malignant strictures by insertion of plastic stents. Michael Atkinson, an experienced endoscopist in Nottingham, developed an introducer that was used to insert a modification of the tube developed earlier by Celestin.[97] This was widely used and known as Atkinson's tube.

Medical endoscopists also found themselves dealing with bleeding oesophageal varices for the first time. Hitherto variceal sclerotherapy had been undertaken by surgeons using a Negus rigid oesophagoscope.[98] In 1979 Kenneth Williams (born 1937) a surgeon at Farnborough Hospital in Kent, and John Dawson (1932-99), surgeon to King's College Hospital showed that varices could be injected safely using a flexible endoscope.[99] They used an overtube to isolate each varix, which also compressed the site of injection and controlled bleeding during the procedure.

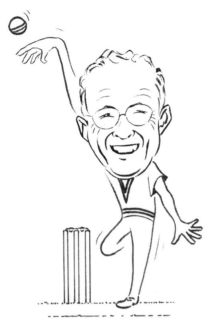

103 Smith – Laughter is the best medicine.

Subsequently Professor Roger Williams and his team on the liver unit at King's followed up more than 100 patients for three years and proved that sclerotherapy was effective.[100] At the same time (early 1980s) Paul Smith, an ebullient gastroenterologist in Llandough Hospital, Cardiff, showed that varices could be obliterated safely without the need for an overtube.[101] His results were impressive and the main complication, stricture formation, was easily overcome by simple dilatation. Generally sclerotherapy was considered to be a safe procedure, though ulceration of the mucosa sometimes led to bleeding and even on one occasion to a broncho-oesophageal fistula.[102]

Straightforward diagnostic gastroscopy was already popular and widely practised and it was particularly valuable in identifying the precise cause of upper gastrointestinal bleeding provided it was done immediately after the bleed.[103/104] Though the ability to treat bleeding peptic ulcers endoscopically had yet to be realised some work with laser photocoagulation was in the pipeline. Peter Cotton sent his registrar, Alan Vallon, to the large Francisco Franco Hospital in Barcelona where the endoscopy unit lay alongside the emergency department, making it an ideal place in which to study gastrointestinal bleeding. In a large trial he found that a group treated with an argon laser did little better than controls.[105] At the same time, Paul Salmon and Steven Bown (born 1944), at University College Hospital, teamed up with Paul Swain at the London Hospital and Tim Northfield and John Kirkham at St. James' Hospital, Balham, and showed that rebleeding could be prevented provided that the ulcer was accessible to laser therapy.[106] While in Bristol Salmon had obtained funds to study the potential of lasers to control bleeding ulcers and had recruited Bown, who had a physics degree, to develop the project. Bown became besotted by lasers and moved to University College Hospital at the same time as Salmon and was later appointed professor of laser medicine at the newly established National Medical Laser Centre at UCH.

Unfortunately lasers were expensive and few units could afford the equipment. Most opted for cheaper but less effective alternatives such as a heater probe or the injection of adrenaline to control bleeding ulcers.[107]

Endoscopic sphincterotomy accelerated during the 1980s as the number of young people trained in the art increased partly as a result of the teaching workshops run by the endoscopy subcommittee of the British Society of Gastroenterology. Clinicians and radiologists began to enjoy removing gallstones from bile ducts. It was exciting and highly satisfying especially in sick, elderly patients unsuitable for surgery. The usual indication was for retained stones or recurrent calculi after a cholecystectomy. However, David Carr-Locke (born 1948), Lecturer in Medicine at Leicester, with extensive ERCP experience, and David Fossard (born 1941), consultant surgeon who had trained under Venables, showed that patients who were unfit for cholecystectomy still did well if their bile ducts were cleared without removing the gall bladder.[108] Peter Cotton reached the same conclusion.[109]

The introduction of prostheses to relieve malignant obstruction of the biliary tract by endoscopists in Germany[110] and Holland[111] in 1980 was another advance quickly taken up by Peter Cotton[112] and others in Britain. To be able to place a small tube through a growth in the head of the pancreas and see bile flowing down the duodenum was miraculous and spared the patient a miserable surgical bypass procedure. But consultants in many hospitals were doing only one or two procedures a week, too few to maintain their skills, and some hospitals still did not have access to ERCP. In 1990 it was estimated that the demand for ERCP in an average district hospital serving 250,000 people was 125 procedures annually. A study by Gear (Gloucester) and Colin-Jones (Portsmouth) on behalf of the British Society of Gastroenterology suggested this was barely sufficient to justify the cost of an ERCP service in every hospital and that adjoining districts should share the service. Not only would this be cost-effective but two consultants could share the work, maintain their experience and cover each other's leave.[113]

Colonoscopy was stimulated by more studies showing that cancers were often missed by radiologists. For example, Paul Farrands, a lecturer in surgery at Nottingham working on Professor Jack Hardcastle's unit, found several neoplastic lesions using a colonoscope in patients who had had a "normal" barium enema. Similarly, Paul Salmon and Charles Clark at University College Hospital noted that colonoscopy frequently picked up a cancer or polyp in patients with diverticular disease that had been overlooked radiologically.[114] This was still the commonest reason for colonoscopy but increasingly clinicians were using the technique to remove polyps and to keep patients with extensive colitis or previous polyps under surveillance.[115] But like the provision of ERCP, colonoscopy services throughout the country were patchy. During 1986 only six units performed more than 400 colonoscopies with ten others managing 250 or more, whereas some did none at all.[116] As usual the common complaints were lack of a specific annual budget to buy new endoscopes and pay for repairs, inadequate accommodation, too few nurses, lack of clinical assistants and the need for more sessions.

CHAPTER SEVENTY-TWO

ENDOSCOPIC RADIOLOGISTS

Ironically, despite the shortcomings of the service, gastroenterology had become such a popular specialty that there were too many trainees. A report prepared by John Lennard-Jones revealed that in 1980 there were almost 100 senior registrars training in gastroenterology with only 30 consultant posts likely to be available during the next decade. The future for many was bleak and the situation was no better two years later, by which time several trainees had become general physicians or switched to radiology, which as we have seen attracted some radiologists from the start. Two further examples illustrate this.

Derrick Martin (born 1948) became interested in gastroenterology after moving to Manchester in 1975 and began upper gastrointestinal endoscopy as a senior house officer. After his appointment as Lecturer in Medicine at South Manchester University Hospital he gained experience in operative endoscopy such as oesophageal intubation and variceal sclerotherapy. In 1976 David Tweedle (born 1940) arrived in South Manchester as Senior Lecturer in Surgery from Chris Venables' unit in Newcastle. Tweedle's interest lay in hepato-biliary surgery and as no one was doing ERCP at the time he started a service in 1977 drawing inspiration from visits to Classen and Cotton. He recalls watching Cotton perform the then incredible feat of completing four sphincterotomies in one day. Initially his biggest difficulty was obtaining radiological support, but demand grew and his problem was solved when Derrick Martin joined him. Martin enjoyed operative endoscopy but as career prospects in gastroenterology were so poor he switched to radiology and in 1986 became Lecturer in Radiology with honorary consultant status. Thereafter he took over the running of the ERCP service and steadily expanded all aspects of upper gastrointestinal endoscopy and radiology making South Manchester one of the leading centres in Britain.

Similarly Roger Frost (born 1949) began training as a gastroenterologist with John Bamforth in Southampton and Duncan Colin-Jones in Portsmouth. In 1980 he joined Peter Cotton at the Middlesex Hospital, becoming accomplished in ERCP, but realised that job opportunities in gastroenterology were poor. So he switched to radiology and spent two years training with David Beckly in Plymouth before retuning to the Middlesex Hospital as a senior registrar in radiology, where he continued to practise endoscopy, including endoscopic ultrasound. He was appointed radiologist to Salisbury Infirmary in 1989 where he has provided an excellent ERCP service.

By this time there were several radiologists doing endoscopy in Britain including Beckly, Frost, Martin, Daniel Nolan (Oxford), Philip Shorvon (Central Middlesex Hospital), John Beales (Bath), Brian Lawrie (Cardiff) and Ian Lavelle (Newcastle), to name but a few. Frost and Beckly thought it would be good to meet regularly and formed the European Society of Gastrointestinal Radiologists in 1989, with Nolan as the first president. The society flourished, holding its annual meeting in a different European capital each year. In 1994 it became the European Society of Gastrointestinal and Abdominal Radiologists (ESGAR) and now has more than 800 members. But the number of radiologists undertaking endoscopy is declining and today few, if any, take it on; gastroenterologists have cornered the market and radiologists have found other imaging and interventional techniques to keep them busy.

CHAPTER SEVENTY-THREE

GASTROENTEROLOGY AS A SERVICE SPECIALTY

Lennard-Jones knew that the solution to the shortage of job opportunities in gastroenterology was to increase the number of consultant posts. The case was overwhelming as several reports showed. For example two senior gastroenterologists, Derek Holdsworth and Michael Atkinson, noted a huge increase in the demand for upper gastrointestinal endoscopy and colonoscopy in the Trent region between 1975 and 1981, which the clinicians were unable to satisfy.[117] Likewise in 1984 the gastroenterology committee of the Royal College of Physicians emphasised the need for more physician-gastroenterologists in order to maintain the service; every hospital, they concluded, required one physician with a special interest and training in gastroenterology and many larger hospitals needed two or more.[118] The biggest demand was for colonoscopy, as very few units were in a position to follow up patients who had had a polypectomy or excision of a carcinoma. The workload of general physicians with an interest in gastroenterology was also highlighted by surveys of hospitals in the North East Thames and East Anglia regions.[119] Seven sessions in endoscopy were necessary to fulfil the demand quite apart from outpatient clinics and acute general medicine. The point was hammered home again by an enquiry into manpower needs in gastroenterology prepared by the BSG in 1990 (written by Paul Smith and chaired by Roger Williams). Remarkably there were still 17 district general hospitals without even a single gastroenterologist. Gastroenterologists had a considerably greater workload than their other physician colleagues and at least another 100 gastroenterologists were needed[120].

In fact the government was supporting extra consultant posts partly to help the service but largely to improve career prospects for trainees. In 1985 it formed a joint planning advisory committee (JPAC) to correct the imbalance between the numbers of trainee and career posts in many specialties. In the case of gastroenterology there was a steady expansion in the number of consultants from 279 in 1980 to 352 in 1988. This was impressive and fast approaching the target suggested by the Royal College of Physicians' Gastroenterological Committee of one physician in the specialty for every 150,000 of the population, a total of 380 posts in Britain.

Apart from the number of endoscopists practising in Britain the BSG was increasingly concerned about their competence. It was no longer acceptable to do an occasional endoscopy nor should they be done without experienced assistants. One of the members of the endoscopy committee of the BSG who had written the report on the future requirements for colonoscopy in 1987, Tony Axon from Leeds, carried out a questionnaire that confirmed the shortfall in staff and administration needed for endoscopy in England and Wales.[121] He then chaired a working party of prominent endoscopists to advise on the number of medical and nursing staff needed to put this right.[122] The working party also recommended that endoscopists, nurses and ancillary staff should receive more formal training, though they stopped short of individual certification. This was the responsibility of the Committee for Higher Specialist Training. But in future, trainees should keep a careful record of their experience and training.

During the 1980s the BSG also concerned themselves with the safety of endoscopy. Though obviously anxious not to harm patients during a procedure, doctors gave the matter of infection little thought and were generally rather cavalier about ensuring that endoscopes were adequately disinfected between cases. As far back as 1973 Tony Axon and Peter Cotton, then at St. Thomas's Hospital, had recommended thorough cleaning followed by soaking in glutaraldehyde.[123] Yet despite many reports of serious infection after endoscopy, a survey of 52 large endoscopy units in 1980 showed that less than half were using effective disinfecting schedules. Axon and Cotton again spelt out precise recommendations for disinfecting endoscopes.[124] Subsequently with the arrival of the human immune deficiency virus a committee of microbiologists and endoscopists met again under the chairmanship of Ian Weller, Senior Lecturer in Infectious Diseases and Genito-Urinary

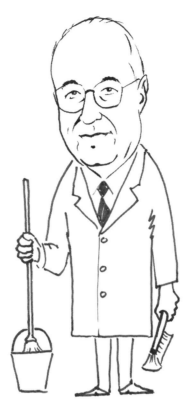

104 Axon – Concern about infection.

Medicine at the Middlesex Hospital. By this time endoscopes were totally immersible and the working party recommended a prolonged protocol for disinfection taking up to fifteen minutes between cases.[125] This implied the need for at least two endoscopes to run a list efficiently, which meant that many units had to buy additional instruments.

Another concern was the use of sedation. The benzodiazepines were introduced in the 1960s just in time for the explosive growth in flexible endoscopy. For many years more than 90 per cent of all upper gastrointestinal endoscopies were conducted using an intravenous benzodiazepine. The early gastroscopes such as the popular Olympus GIF D2 were quite a mouthful and most patients preferred to be sedated. But a survey by Clifford Hawkins in Birmingham and his senior registrar, Antony Hoare, noted the disadvantages.[126] Patients were amnesic afterwards so it was pointless to discuss the result of the investigation with them. They were unable to drive so had to be fetched and carried.

Occasionally young people went beserk during "sedation" and damaged the endoscope. Most worrying was the risk of respiratory depression that necessitated facilities for recovery of semi-conscious patients. Hawkins suggested that older patients should be offered endoscopy without sedation as they tolerated the procedure better and were at greater risk.

In 1982 a new benzodiazepine, midazolam, was introduced. It was twice as potent as diazepam but had a much shorter half life. Many publications comparing the two appeared but the fact was that both caused respiratory depression and hypoxia. Such events were rare and it was easy to be complacent but respiratory depression and occasional deaths were reported. This particularly concerned Duncan Bell, a gastroenterologist working in Ipswich, who showed that these drugs caused significant hypoxia during endoscopy due to their effect on the respiratory centre combined with muscle relaxation and partial blockage of the upper airway by the endoscope.[127] Bell believed that the risk of respiratory depression was under reported and with the blessing of the endoscopy committee conducted a national survey of sedation for upper gastrointestinal endoscopy. With the help of Tawfique Daneshmend and Richard Logan in Nottingham, he found that most endoscopists still used sedation.[128] During the course of two years there were 119 respiratory arrests, 37 cardiac arrests and 52 deaths (about 1 in 10,000 procedures). These startling figures prompted a new set of recommendations for sedation and monitoring during endoscopy including the routine use of pulse oximetry and oxygen in risky patients.[129]

Clearly the safest option was to perform upper gastrointestinal endoscopy without any sedation whatsoever. Indeed this was the normal practice in Germany and Japan. The advantages mentioned by Hoare and Hawkins were obvious, patients could come and go under their own steam, the endoscopist could explain exactly what had been found, often reassure, prescribe and frequently discharge the patient, and nurses were free to get on with other duties and not be detained by semi-conscious patients long after a list was finished. During the early 1990s, attitudes in Britain changed and endoscopy without sedation was widely practised. Apart from the above considerations, the newer endoscopes were slimmer and easier to use, the next generation were properly trained and technically better and quicker at endoscoping, and finally nurse endoscopists were beginning to appear. Though admittedly few in number at first, they were not permitted to administer sedation.

Another matter that concerned the endoscopy committee was record keeping. As far back as 1973 Paul Salmon emphasised that good endoscopy records were essential.[130] For many years various card index systems were tried. Bristol used an automated system using the hospital computer to store information from the card index, which enabled data to be analysed fairly easily. Later, other centres, notably St. Mark's Hospital, the Middlesex Hospital and Wythenshaw Hospital, refined the Bristol system. By 1980 there were any number of record systems in use varying from simple ledgers to complex card indexes, so Peter Cotton, then chairman of the endocopy committee of the BSG, felt the time was ripe to look into the role of computers, which were beginning to make their presence felt. The committee appointed Chris Venables in Newcastle to undertake this with a subcommittee that included Robin Knill-Jones in Glasgow, Tony McCann (Leeds Department of Computer Studies), and Tim de Dombal (Leeds) all of whom were computer literate. Over the next few years they developed a software program for endoscopy records that was cheap and compatible with the then popular BBC-B microcomputer. The endoscopy staff in Newcastle and Leeds found it quick and easy to use and it was well received by delegates to the Newcastle meeting of the BSG in 1985. The particular problem of endoscopic terminology was largely overcome and the computer actually encouraged clinicians to report their findings in greater detail. In fact Venables became the UK representative in Europe when they were thrashing out a new terminology for digestive endoscopy and he helped design the minimal standard terminology (MST) for endoscopy. (Recording of endoscopy was extremely poor at the time.) The endoscopy committee decided that the BBC-B system should be carefully evaluated and Venables appealed to the Department of Health for funds to do this, but was turned down. This was a great disappointment but he and McCann continued to use their system for upper gastrointestinal endoscopy, later changing to Microsoft personal computers when these were introduced. Known as the ULCERS program it was especially helpful when they were developing the minimal standard terminology. Elsewhere his work was not taken up due to lack of support and the first computer program used by most gastroenterologists was probably the Endoscribe system supplied free by Astra in the mid-1990s.

Towards the end of the 1980s a working party was set up by the clinical services committee of the BSG to inform managers of the ever-changing and escalating needs for gastrointestinal endoscopy. The group was chaired by John Lennard-Jones who was also a member of the liaison committee with the DHSS and of the gastroenterology committee of the Royal College of Physicians. It comprised representatives from the endoscopy committee and radiology section of the BSG, the Endoscopy Associates Group and representatives from public health and the Primary Care Society, with observers from the Royal College of Nursing and the DHSS. The report, issued in 1990, incorporated several of the surveys and studies already mentioned and was a comprehensive and authoritative document that clearly stated the current demand for endoscopy, the need for highly trained professional staff at all levels, and the planning, equipment and costs of an endoscopy unit.[131] Its influence was considerable and raised the status of endoscopy, but it took time, almost a decade, before the changes in practice, training and appraisal were implemented.

CHAPTER SEVENTY-FOUR

ACCREDITATION IN ENDOSCOPY

The primary purpose of the British Society for Digestive Endoscopy during its brief existence had been to train people in the art of endoscopy, and by 1980 several hundred clinicians had attended its courses. Thereafter the BSG assumed this responsibility. But formal training was not compulsory and anyone with access to an endoscope could use it if he wished. There were many doctors up and down the country doing endoscopy sporadically. They may have attended one of the many courses organised on an "ad hoc" basis. The best known were those run at St. Mark's and the Middlesex Hospitals and at Stoke on Trent. Meanwhile the endoscopy associates group (mainly but not exclusively nurses) received their training from courses run by the nursing establishment, the BSG (notably at Shrewsbury Hospital and St. Bartholemew's Hospital) or the Keymed Company in Southend. The Keymed course was very popular and always oversubscribed. Delegates were taught about the care and maintenance of endoscopes and received a certificate of attendance. As a result they probably knew more about endoscopes than many of their medically qualified peers. By 1990 there were more than 400 endoscopy associate members of the BSG.

The haphazard practice of some endoscopists worried the endoscopy committee of the BSG who knew that it was bad practice but could do little to stop it. In 1985 David Beckly in Plymouth asked the BSG to produce a certificate that could be given to doctors from America that came to him for training. They needed some sort of official recognition in order to gain privileges back home, perhaps a certificate from the BSG stating the number and type of examinations performed. The endoscopy committee felt this was inappropriate at the time but in their report on staffing of endoscopy units in 1987, chaired by Tony Axon, they recommended a formal training programme and hinted at certification. Graeme Kerr from Shrewsbury pointed out that this had been introduced in Australia and it was a feature of some European countries.

Under the chairmanship of John Bennett (Hull), the endoscopy committee appointed an education officer in 1987 with a remit to formalise the training programme. The first incumbent was Tony Morris, who worked closely with Tony Axon to introduce a basic course in endoscopy for novice endoscopists and endoscopy associates. Its object was to provide a highway code of the do's and don'ts of endoscopy that are easily overlooked during informal apprenticeship in district hospitals. The first course took place at Warwick in 1990 and a certificate of attendance was awarded. A log book of the individual's experience was also encouraged but the whole exercise was still on a voluntary basis. By this time video-endoscopy (originally introduced in 1983) was just becoming available in Britain. The charged couple device or "chip" revolutionised endoscopy; the quality of the picture displayed on a monitor was vastly superior to anything seen before and broken fibres became a thing of the past. Endoscopists no longer needed to crane their necks to the eyepiece of an instrument, everyone in the room could see what was going on, images could be stored on a computer and best of all teaching became infinitely easier.

Meanwhile a working party of the endoscopy committee grasped the nettle and produced proposals for accreditation of endoscopists. Their report in 1989 laid the foundation for the future. The key points were that all endoscopists should be accredited in diagnostic upper digestive endoscopy, preferably including therapeutic endoscopy, and/ or colonoscopy or ERCP. This meant that endoscopy units must be approved for training purposes and experienced endoscopists should be recognised as trainers. Having completed a given number of procedures satisfactorily, the BSG should grant voluntary certification to individual endoscopists.

The proposals were turned down at the annual business meeting of the BSG in Dublin in 1989 mainly because the body responsible for certification was the BSG. Surgeons argued that many endoscopists (including radiologists and general practitioners) were not members of the BSG and could not therefore be certified as trainers. However, everyone agreed that certification was desirable and that the fundamentals of the proposals were sound. Accordingly Miles Irving, later Sir Miles, Professor of Surgery at the University of Manchester, was seconded from the council of the Royal College of Surgeons to find a solution. He formed a small intercollegiate working party that included Christopher Williams, Roger Leicester (St. George's Hospital) and representatives from the colleges of radiologists and general practitioners, and they came up with a procedure for accreditation of trainers. This proved acceptable to all parties; the British Society of Gastroenterology would effectively still be responsible for training individuals (through a new endoscopy training and standards committee), and accreditation would be issued by the specialist advisory committees of the individuals' colleges.

During these negotiations it became clear to the intercollegiate group that there was also an urgent need for formal inspection and accreditation of endoscopy units responsible for training. The British Society of Gastroenterology was unwilling to assume this responsibility as the society was dominated by physicians so the intercollegiate group seized the initiative and formed the joint advisory group (JAG) in 1994. This represented all endoscopists (physicians, surgeons, radiologists, general practitioners and others) and the first chairman, Miles Irving, soon handed the baton on to Charles Swan. In future endoscopy units would be inspected by JAG to insure that they were suitable to supervise training and in due course regular inspection would be compulsory.[132]

Accreditation could not come too soon. A prospective audit of upper gastrointestinal audit by the British Society of Gastroenterology in 1991 found that there were many clinicians performing fewer than twenty endoscopies per year.[133] There were even a few inexperienced doctors with minimal training doing unsupervised endoscopies. The audit also revealed an alarming number of deaths, mainly from cardio-respiratory complications associated with sedation in whom monitoring had been inadequate.

1990s Further expansion

The determination to improve standards and training by the BSG and royal colleges coincided with another surge in demand for endoscopy. This was driven by two developments, open access upper digestive endoscopy and surveillance colonoscopy. Though the concept of an open access service was not new, a survey by Michael Bramble (born 1950) showed that it had suddenly, in 1990, become widely available.[134] This was in response to long outpatient waiting lists and people assumed that open access would reduce the load and shorten the wait. Many hospitals offered a censored service whereby consultants decided if an endoscopy should be done before seeing the patient in clinic. The following year Bramble himself set up a true open access service in Middlesbrough whereby general practitioners referred their patients directly for an endoscopy rather than a consultant opinion and managed the patient themselves.[135] This increased the workload of the endoscopy unit but certainly reduced the wait for an outpatient appointment. Some of the extra work was absorbed by existing endoscopists in Middlesbrough but a new consultant, Paul Cann, was also appointed in the wake of government policy at the time, as well as a GP clinical assistant. The service undertook 100 extra gastroscopies per month, equivalent to three extra sessions a week.

Open access gastroscopy was expensive, though probably cost-effective, but many, including Christopher Booth, thought there was a danger of gastroenterologists becoming mere technicians.[136] The endoscopy tail was threatening to wag the gastroenterology dog. Michael Clark at St. Bartholemew's Hospital thought there were far too many unnecessary endoscopies being undertaken, open access or not.[137] One of the first tasks undertaken by the new joint committee of royal colleges (JAG) and the British Society of Gastroenterology was to issue guidelines on appropriate indications for upper gastrointestinal endoscopy.[138] Prominent among the committee members representing the BSG were Tony Axon, Graham Bell, Peter Fairclough and Rory McCloy. As well as outlining the well-known indications for gastroscopy, the panel emphasised that a clear history of irritable bowel syndrome without features of ulcer disease was a common but wholly inappropriate reason to perform gastroscopy.

Nurse endoscopists

Though clinical assistants were invaluable they were not easy to find. In many places general practitioners were unwilling or unable to take up endoscopy. Yet the demand for endoscopy was inexorable and approaching one per cent of the population. More endoscopists had to be conjured up from somewhere and one solution was the nurse endoscopist. By the early 1990s nurses in America were performing screening flexible sigmoidoscopy. The concept of nurses performing endoscopy was particularly appealing to single-handed physicians with an interest in gastroenterology working in small district hospitals. In Dorchester for example the author obtained support from the hospital authorities to train an endoscopy staff nurse, Pauline Matthews, in upper digestive endoscopy in 1995. Having done 200 endoscopies under supervision in unsedated patients, Matthews (born 1952) was assessed by an external endoscopist and given a certificate of competence in 1996. Subsequently she attended an ENB course for nurse endoscopists when it became available in order to obtain official recognition. Matthews left school at fifteen and became a nurse after raising her family. She typified the best features of apprenticeship learning[139] and combined her endoscopy skills with overall management of the unit. She was awarded an MBE for her services in 2001 and is now lead nurse for the Strategic Health Authority's bowel cancer screening program in the south-west region.

Traditionally diagnosis had been a doctor's business and nurses were afraid to take responsibility for it. This was the problem encountered by Malcolm Bateson (born 1945), a gastroenterologist in Bishop Auckland, who was anxious to train his nurses to endoscope. The nurses were worried that the Royal College of Nursing would not accept that nurses could diagnose peptic ulcers for example. Accordingly Bateson wrote to the endoscopy committee for guidance and support. As a result a working party of the BSG was set up under the chairmanship of Michael Hellier and issued its report in 1994.[140] The committee fully supported the role of the nurse endoscopist and crucially the UK Central Council for Nursing did too. The report spelt out the need for the service and laid down sensible stipulations for those wishing to undertake endoscopy. By 1996–7 courses for nurse endoscopists were available in Hull and Southampton and others soon followed. By 2001 approximately 75 nurses were receiving accreditation in endoscopy per year and several studies confirmed that they were as proficient as their medical colleagues and highly cost-effective.[141/142] Yet in 2002 a survey by Michael Bramble identified only 149 nurse endoscopists working in 96 units registered with the JAG.

If open access endoscopy was fuelling demand for upper digestive endoscopy, surveillance of patients at risk of colorectal cancer was driving the demand for colonoscopy. As if this was not enough, there was a groundswell in favour of screening an entire section of the population for colorectal cancer. The prospect was daunting as there were far too few trained colonoscopists. Graeme Duthie (born 1959), a surgeon in Hull, showed that nurses could help to fill the shortfall by undertaking flexible sigmoidoscopy.[143] But a survey at the end of 1991 revealed that there were still 17 health districts without a single gastroenterologist and 34 large districts serving more than 250,000 people with only one gastroenterologist.[144] Clearly more endoscopists were needed and they had to be properly trained. The newly formed training committee of the British Society of Gastroenterology took advantage of the initiative taken by the Chief Medical Officer, Kenneth Calman, to implement the unified training grade of specialist registrar in gastroenterology.[145] All specialist registrars would receive five years' training and be awarded a certificate of specialist training (CCST) entitling them to apply for consultant posts. The first trainees were appointed in 1996 and by 2001 a steady stream of fully fledged gastroenterologists was emerging throughout Britain. They could not come quickly enough. A survey in 1999 by Bruce Macfarlane at Mount Vernon Hospital showed that only a half of the units in Britain were reaching their colonoscopy targets for lack of endoscopists.[146] As a result of the Calman expansion the number of gastroenterologists rose from 466 in 1998 to 677 in 2003.

But it was not just a numbers game. Colonoscopy was a much more difficult technique than gastroscopy. A competent colonoscopist expected to reach the caecum in 90 per cent of his patients and many endoscopists fell far short of this figure. This was worrying because an incomplete colonoscopy could miss a treatable cancer. The main difficulty was caused by looping of the instrument during the procedure and Brian Saunders and Christopher Williams at St. Mark's Hospital, both expert colonoscopists, devised a non-radiological imaging system to help inexperienced practitioners to untangle loops as they formed.[147] This was an ingenious aid that became indispensable for teaching purposes. Experienced endoscopists also found it useful on occasion but it was expensive and few units were able to afford it.

The real problem was that most trainees served a patchy apprenticeship augmented by occasional demonstrations by world experts beamed across the globe by satellite. Assessment was in-house and informal and was based on the number of colonoscopies undertaken rather than the ability of the endoscopist. A prospective study carried out in the late 1990s by the JAG of Royal Colleges in conjunction with the BSG and the Association of Coloproctology found that training in colonoscopy was often inadequate.[148] Trainees were not supervised and the majority had not attended a formal training course. Good training was utterly dependent on the quality of the trainers and their units. In 1999 JAG published a document entitled *Recommendations for training in gastrointestinal endoscopy.*[149] This was based on a programme for both trainers and trainees being developed by the Raven Department of Education at the Royal College of Surgeons. Trainers would now be taught how to teach endoscopy, trainees would have to attend courses held in approved units, and their subsequent progress at their own hospital would be carefully monitored.

CHAPTER SEVENTY-FIVE

NATIONAL ENDOSCOPY PROGRAMME

The case for nationwide screening for colorectal cancer was compelling. It was the second most common cancer in Britain and the risk of developing it after the age of 54 was about one in 20. The mortality was more than 50 per cent but if the cancer was caught early it was curable. The problem was who and how to screen and the government wanted answers before investing in a national screening programme. Most agreed that people between the ages of 50 and 70 years were most likely to benefit but opinion was divided on the best method. The options were repeated faecal occult blood (FOB) testing followed by colonoscopy if positive, or a one-off flexible sigmoidoscopy. Either would stretch the endoscopy services.

A trial in the Nottingham area during the 1980s led by Jack Hardcastle and Tom Balfour from the Department of Surgery at the University Hospital showed that screening patients by faecal occult blood testing every two years reduced mortality from colorectal cancer by fifteen per cent.[150] This was an impressive study of 152,000 people, half of whom were screened, and the trial took fifteen years. As a result, in the year 2000, the Departments of Health in England and Scotland commissioned a large pilot study in Coventry and Warwickshire (population 800,000) and Grampian, Tayside and Fife (population 1.2 million). The English arm was led by Ronald Parker and the Scottish arm by Professor Robert Steele. Their first report in 2002 confirmed the benefits of screening a healthy population.[151]

The alternative approach was to offer everyone at about the age of 60 a single flexible sigmoidoscopy. This was championed by Professor Wendy Atkin at the UK Colorectal Cancer Unit, St. Mark's Hospital, who argued that this was a more reliable way to detect polyps, the precursors of cancer, and would prevent colorectal cancer rather than simply detecting it. Two-thirds of adenomas and cancers were located in the rectum and sigmoid colon, which was within reach of the flexible sigmoidoscope and the procedure took only five minutes. Fourteen centres throughout Britain took part and over 40,000 patients were recruited between 1996 and 1999.[152] The results of the trial were finally published in 2010 and the results were impressive. First, to people's surprise, more than 70 per cent of the 55- to 64-year-olds offered the examination accepted. Screening seemed to make people happier. Secondly the test cut the incidence of cancer by a third and the death rate by 43 per cent over a decade.

Though Atkin made a good case for screening by single flexible sigmoidoscopy, people were concerned that cancers in the proximal colon would remain undetected.[153] Furthermore, the government was keen to get screening underway but wanted evidence from trials before committing to a national project. It would be several years before Atkin's trial was completed so the government plumped for the faecal occult blood screening programme. This would generate a staggering extra 60,000 colonoscopies per year and the provision of colonoscopy was woefully inadequate.[154]

As part of the NHS cancer plan published in 2000 the government agreed to invest heavily in the prevention, screening and treatment of cancer. This included diagnostic services such as endoscopy and a National Endoscopy Programme was introduced that would address both training and the service. In 2001 the Modernisation Agency (previously the National Patient Access Team), led by Liz Allan, was set up to ensure that the government's investment was matched by results. This was great news for the colonoscopy service and the agency soon threw its weight (and cash) behind JAG to support colonoscopy training. With the help of £2.4 million from the National Cancer Project, the agency selected three centres to run full-time "hands on" training courses along the lines developed by the Raven Department at the Royal College of Surgeons. The chosen units were the Royal Liverpool Hospital led by Professor Anthony Morris, St. George's Hospital (Roger Leicester) and St. Mark's Hospital (Brian Saunders). These men were well known for their commitment to training and had been heavily involved in setting up the programme at the Royal College of Surgeons together with Robin Teague (Torquay) and Ed Swarbrick (Wolverhampton). By the end of 2003 a total of 250 trainees had attended the courses. The results spoke

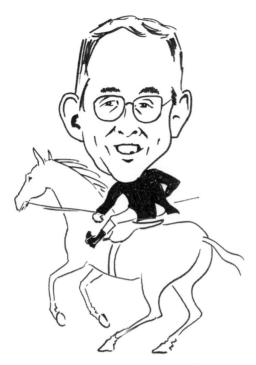

105 Swarbrick – Endoscopist and equestrian.

for themselves as the colonoscopy completion rate of those individuals attending them was well in excess of 90 per cent.

The Modernisation Agency was also concerned about the state of the endoscopy service as a whole, which was still a Cinderella of the health service. So it introduced its plan *Modernising Endoscopy Services* to improve it. The first priority was to collect data with which to argue the case for improvements. Twelve endoscopy units from around the country were selected to examine the deficiencies in their service using a prompt or "tool kit" devised by the agency. The units next took steps to correct their shortcomings with further help from the Agency. Apart from the usual lack of endoscopists the study highlighted the need to examine the service from the patient's perspective and also showed that strong local leadership was essential to make things happen. The successful pilot scheme was expanded in 2002 to include a further 29 units with similar results.

Armed with this powerful evidence the National Endoscopy Programme was rolled out in 2003. First the agency allocated a further

£8.2 million, via the National Cancer Plan, to support nationwide endoscopy training from 2003–2006. In addition to the three national training centres in London and Liverpool, a further seven regional training centres were established in Gloucester (John Anderson), Hull (Graeme Duthie), Norwich (Richard Tighe), Sheffield (Stuart Riley), Middlesbrough (Mike Bramble), Torquay (Robin Teague) and Wolverhampton (Edwin Swarbrick). Each centre was chosen for the excellence of its facilities and the reputation of its endoscopists. Second, all endoscopy units were to be scrutinised and supported in a similar way to those in the pilot studies. JAG and the Modernisation Agency realised that strong local leadership was essential if the endoscopy programme was to succeed and in 2003 took the innovative step of appointing clinical leads in endoscopy for the 28 newly created strategic health authorities in England. These clinicians (mostly gastroenterologists but including two surgeons) were to be responsible for ensuring that the endoscopy units in their area were meeting their targets and that patients were getting a fair deal. The clinical leads would in turn be led by the National Clinical Lead, a key appointment, who would be responsible for driving the whole project. This job was given to Roland Valori, a gastroenterologist in Gloucester.

Valori (born 1954) qualified at the Middlesex Hospital. In 1989 he was appointed consultant gastroenterologist at the recently united Middlesex/University College Hospital but moved to Gloucester in 1993 where he became involved in endoscopy training and joined the BSG endoscopy committee. In 2002 he was appointed National Clinical Lead by the Modernisation Agency and set up his headquarters with the East Midlands Health Authority in Leicester in January 2003.

He faced a daunting task with about 300,000 people waiting up to a year for a colonoscopy. Several endoscopy units were underperforming and staff morale was low. His first job was to establish a small national endoscopy team and he recruited Debbie Johnston, a nurse from Salford, to join Liz Allan. Debbie (born 1964) had extensive management experience and was very good at dealing with disgruntled staff. She was working with the National Booking Team when she was seconded to work with Valori and they clicked immediately. From the start the team made a point of harnessing support from several influential parties such as the Cancer Action Team, JAG, PCTs, the screening programme, the DHSS's waiting-list team, various professional societies and not least patients themselves.

Valori put the patient at the heart of the service and realised that he would have to be able to prove that his innovations were effective. He and Debbie spent a year developing a way of monitoring the performance of endoscopy units and devised the so-called global rating scale (GRS), which measured the experience of patients having an endoscopy and pointed the way to constant improvements. Beginning in April 2005 all units were asked to complete an assessment every six months of the patient's experience of their endoscopy. The data were collected online using simple yes or no answers and a computer automatically calculated each unit's GRS score. Units that were struggling were readily identified and given appropriate support by the National Endoscopy Team. Despite some initial misgivings, clinicians responded positively to GRS and the results were spectacular. Endoscopy was safer and more comfortable, patients were seen quickly and the waiting list fell to 5,000.

Fuelled by nurse endoscopists the number of properly trained endoscopists rose. A survey by the national team in 2008 identified 349 nurse endoscopists, half of whom had been appointed since 2003. In recognition of his effort, Valori won NHS Change Leader of the Year in 2009 for his work with endoscopy services. But his greatest reward has been the success so far of the bowel cancer screening programme, which began in 2007 and is steadily expanding.

However, the remarkable results of the flexible sigmoidoscopy trial organised by Wendy Atkin cannot be ignored. Detection, diagnosis and treatment were delivered all at the same time, in a single five- or ten-minute appointment, with no need for a repeat – ever. By dealing with polyps the treatment was preventative, stopping cancer before it began. There has been no sign of recurrence after eleven years so the incidence of bowel cancer should fall. I suspect that flexible sigmoidoscopy will have to be incorporated into the bowel cancer screening programme if indeed it does not replace it. It is certainly cheaper.

CHAPTER SEVENTY-SIX

ERCP

ERCP quietly ploughed its own furrow. Usually regarded as the most difficult endoscopic procedure, aficionados derived great satisfaction in providing an indispensable service. By the late 1980s there were several competent practitioners of the art, though the NHS did lose three of the best known, Cotton, Salmon and Carr-Locke. Peter Cotton finally managed to persuade the Middlesex Hospital to provide him with a new endoscopy unit in 1982 but the hospital had a fixed budget and Cotton actually received written instructions "to do 25 per cent less procedures next year". As the only gastroenterologist he relied heavily on excellent junior staff and overseas trainees. In 1985 he took unpaid leave to travel and while he was away the authorities decided that they would stop overseas trainees working at the hospital because, though unpaid, they had to be fed and bathed. This was the final straw, Cotton resigned and accepted a post at Duke University, North Carolina in 1987. Next Paul Salmon was seduced by the private sector and left the Middlesex Hospital where he had recently joined Cotton after its amalgamation with University College Hospital. Finally in 1989 David Carr-Locke, gastroenterologist in Leicester and treasurer to the British Society of Gastroenterology, accepted a chair in gastroenterology at Harvard University where he had a distinguished career, becoming in due course President of the American Society of Gastrointestinal Endoscopy.

It was also in 1989 that Alfred Cuchieri (born 1938) in Dundee performed his first laparoscopic cholecystectomy[155] and in no time this became the standard technique for removing gall bladders. As surgeons could not explore the bile ducts laparoscopically, endoscopists were called upon to do the job for them and the demand for endoscopic sphincterotomy increased significantly. Therapeutic ERCP was more difficult and dangerous than simple diagnostic ERCP and many struggled with the technique. A survey in the north of England in 1995 by Andrew Tanner in Stockton-on-Tees confirmed this. Tanner (born 1948) identified wide variations in imaging success, outcomes and serious complication rates.[156]

ERCP training was a problem. The number of budding gastroenterologists increased steadily during the 1990s and they had to be proficient in all areas of endoscopy, including ERCP if they were to secure a consultant appointment. But there were simply not enough people to train them. In 1996 the Conference of Royal Colleges commissioned the recently formed JAG to tackle the whole issue of endoscopy training, especially colonoscopy and ERCP. This was a huge task but eventually under the chairmanship of Charles Swan in Nottingham its recommendations were accepted, published and distributed to all endoscopy units and endoscopists throughout Britain.[157] The key elements for ERCP were that an endoscopy unit had to be doing at least 250 procedures a year to register for training, and the trainee had to carry out at least 100 ERCPs under supervision and achieve cannulation and biliary drainage in more than 90 per cent of cases. This caused quite a stir as the majority of district general hospitals did fewer than 250 procedures a year. Furthermore the average consultant (mainly gastroenterologists but many surgeons and a few radiologists) probably did only two ERCPs a week. This was hardly enough to maintain their own skills, let alone provide the opportunity to train trainees.

JAG's proposals were echoed by a call for structured training and assessment from a group of endoscopists in Leicester who independently came to the same conclusions.[158] Based on their extensive teaching experience, Anthony Wicks, Gavin Robertson and Peter Veitch argued that ERCP and training should be concentrated in large hospitals with specialist pancreatobiliary expertise, serving populations of at least 500,000 people. In fact this was impractical as many patients were too old and frail to tolerate hospital transfers.

At the very time that JAG were putting together their proposals for training, Miles Allison, a gastroenterologist in Newport, South Wales, and a member of the Specialty Committee in Gastroenterology of the Royal College of Physicians, was worried that he was trying to train too many ERCP students and having to compete with colleagues for patients to maintain his own competence. Allison (born 1955) raised his concerns with the committee and secured the influential support of Duncan Colin-Jones who raised the issue with the BSG. As a result the clinical services committee of the BSG delegated Allison and Colin-Jones to review the position of ERCP in Britain as a whole.[159] Several points of interest emerged. Firstly medical gastroenterologists were gradually taking over ERCP from surgeons and radiologists. This was a good thing as it would concentrate expertise and training within one specialty and facilitate appraisal of specialist registrars in training. Secondly there was a handful of units carrying out fewer than 100 ERCPs per year, which was clearly too few for training purposes. On the other hand there were a significant number of centres performing fewer than the recommended 250 ERCPs a year, which could still offer useful training opportunities for an individual trainee. Third, most trainees said that they were reasonably satisfied with their training, though many were given one or less ERCP to do per week. Several were not starting their training until their final year, which was too late for them to achieve independence before completing their training. In fact half the trainees were being awarded their CCST without fulfilling JAG's proposals.

Allison and Colin-Jones reckoned that a typical district general hospital serving a population of 250,000 people were doing 200 ERCPs per annum, no doubt due to the rise in therapeutic procedures especially in the elderly. In fact the need for simple diagnostic ERCP was fast disappearing thanks to the use of magnetic resonance scanning. First developed by Sir Peter Mansfield in Nottingham to scan the brain in the 1970s, MRI was refined during the 1980s to achieve images of moving parts in the chest and abdomen. In 1991 Wallner and his colleagues in Germany managed to obtain MR images of the bile ducts, though at the time they could only demonstrate ducts that were dilated.[160] Further refinements during the 1990s improved the quality of the pictures and it was eventually possible to delineate the normal, undilated biliary tract. MR cholangio-pancreatography (MRCP) was not only comparable with ERCP but the technique was safer and quicker (a few minutes). Conventional MRI systems across the country were updated and by the end of the century non-invasive MRCP was replacing ERCP.

Given the ERCP requirements calculated by Allison and Colin-Jones, if every gastroenterologist were to offer ERCP he would be performing less than two examinations per week – too few to maintain his skills. If fewer gastroenterologists concentrated on ERCP, the results would be better and the complications fewer. The corollary of this was that training should be concentrated on those trainees showing the greatest potential. Though Allison and Colin-Jones found that the majority of trainees were keen to learn ERCP, nearly half said they would be content to give up the procedure on appointment if colleagues were already meeting the requirements.

When Allison presented his conclusions to the BSG in 1999 at the March meeting in Glasgow, many senior gastroenterologists were astonished. The JAG, now under the chairmanship of Tony Morris from Liverpool, wasted no time in persuading the Specialist Advisory Committee (SAC) in Gastroenterology to the Joint Committee for Higher Medical Training (JCHMT) that ERCP should no longer be an essential requirement for CCST. A letter to this effect was sent to all trainees in January 2000. This was a great relief for those with poor hand/eye coordination, especially now that nearly all ERCPs were therapeutic. Trainers also heaved a sigh of relief because they would no longer need to endure long sessions with struggling trainees nor cannulate damaged papillae abandoned by the trainee.

The new millennium began with an air of optimism. There were now competent ERCPists in most district general hospitals working in units keen to be recognised by the JAG for training purposes. Guidelines for good practice were flowing from the BSG covering topics such as informed consent, monitoring and sedation. Specialist registrars were starting to receive regular training in their district and being encouraged to attend special ERCP courses. Several units laid on stimulating programmes, but only two centres offered complete "hands on" ERCP training: Stoke and Liverpool.

Jonathan Green (born 1946) was appointed to North Staffordshire Hospital in 1979 just a year after Charles Swan had started his well known endoscopy course there. While a senior registrar at St. Mary's Hospital, Green had occasionally watched Peter Cotton doing an ERCP with an optical endoscope at the Middlesex Hospital in a darkened room with 30 other aspiring endoscopists, but he did not get his hands on a duodenoscope until his arrival in Stoke. He soon made up for lost time and recalling what he had seen at the Middlesex Hospital he taught himself ERCP. Swan was clearly impressed and in 1987 asked Green to add ERCP teaching to the prestigious Stoke course. Green's initial apprehension only increased when his first case failed as the patient had

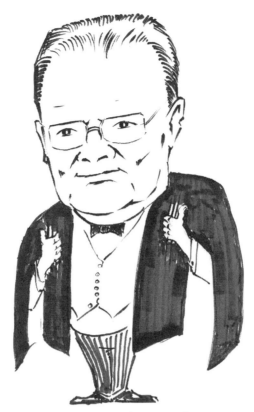

106 Green – Hands on teaching.

an unsuspected carcinoma of the pylorus, but ever since he has run five or six highly successful "hands-on" courses every year for beginners and revalidation purposes.

Liverpool had been at the heart of endoscopy training since Robin Teague's appointment as senior lecturer in 1978. He introduced ERCP and colonoscopy to the city but left in 1980 to take up a post in Torquay. By then Tony Morris had arrived as senior lecturer from Manchester. Morris (born 1946) had watched Tony Axon in Leeds and effectively taught himself ERCP while in Manchester. He was a great enthusiast and steadily built up a superb department at the Royal Liverpool Hospital. A born teacher he was the first education officer to be appointed by the endoscopy committee of the BSG in 1987 and the second chairman of JAG from 1999 to 2004. During this time he developed a "hands-on" ERCP course modelled on the one at Stoke. Later, in 2001, he left clinical

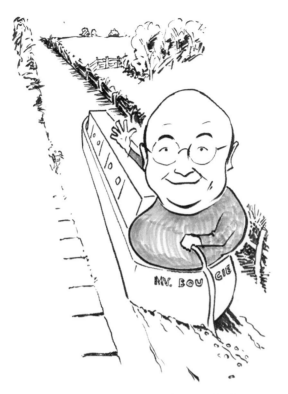

107 Morris – Interventionalist and educator.

medicine to become a full-time endoscopist. He was elected Director of National Endoscopy Training Centre in 2004 and President of the BSG in 2007.

There were, of course, many other excellent practitioners of ERCP besides those in Nottingham and Liverpool, some of whom I have already mentioned. It would be an invidious task to list them all but several were trained by Peter Cotton, including Mark Denyer at Leeds, Mark Wilkinson at Guy's Hospital, and Kelvin Palmer in Edinburgh who was appointed the third chairman of JAG from 2004 to 2006 and President of BSG in 2009.

Despite the surveys in the late 1990s the service needs for ERCP were still unclear. ERCP had spread in a somewhat random and uneven manner. No one knew to what extent magnetic resonance cholangiopancreatography, and for that matter the new technique of endoscopic ultrasound, were affecting the demand for ERCP.

How successful were the British at performing ERCP and how did our complication rates compare with Europe and America? These questions were brought to a head by a startling report from the National Confidential Enquiry into Patient Outcome and Death (NCEPOD) in 2004.[161] Though retrospective and looking at deaths the report suggested that 68 per cent of ERCPs undertaken were futile or inappropriate. It was also critical of sedation practice and monitoring. Stung into action the BSG funded a large prospective audit of ERCP across five metropolitan regions of England in 1994.[162] The study was led by Earl Williams, a lecturer in the Department of Gastroenterology at the Royal Liverpool Hospital. Williams (born 1971) had been taught by two hepatobiliary specialists in the department, Howard Smart and Martin Lombard, and was well aware that patient selection and safety were as important as the technique of ERCP itself. In all 81 hospitals took part in the audit that monitored the procedures of 190 consultants and 74 trainees over six months. The vast majority of ERCPs were therapeutic and appropriate, which was encouraging, and the complication rate was very small. However, there were still too many trainees trying to learn ERCP and unable to gain adequate experience. The authors again called for a reduction in the number of trainees and more specialised training in designated centres. Some units were performing fewer than 100 procedures a year. Only three quarters of our endoscopists managed to cannulate the papilla more than 80 per cent of the time. (This included trainees.) Worse still only 42 per cent of endoscopists managed a successful cannulation more than 90 per cent of the time.

Clearly there was a need to re-think the service and training in ERCP. In 2006 the endoscopy committee of the BSG convened a stakeholders group under the chairmanship of Jonathan Green (Nottingham) to produce a consensus statement about future provision and training in ERCP. The group represented all disciplines and was a miniature Who's Who of top trainers that included Howard Smart and Martin Lombard (Liverpool), Miles Allison (Newport), Kel Palmer and Roger Barton (successive chairmen of JAG), Derrick Martin (Manchester, representing the dying breed of radiologists doing ERCP), Roland Valori (National Endoscopy Team) and Nick Hayes (Tyneside) and Don Menzies (Colchester) representing the Association of Upper Gastro Intestinal Surgeons (AUGIS).

The group met twice and called themselves stakeholders in

recognition of all the disciplines involved in ERCP. They reaffirmed that nearly all ERCP was now therapeutic and approximately 54,000 procedures were done annually. If anything this number was likely to rise as the population became older. To be any good a unit needed to be doing an absolute minimum of 150 procedures per year and individual endoscopists should complete at least 75 cases a year with the prospect of revalidation in some form. Trainee numbers should be reduced as there were too many. Some form of selection was required, ideally by natural selection of those with good hand/eye co-ordination. Trainees should then receive intensive periods of training, perhaps incorporating a "fellowship" in specialised endoscopy.

The stakeholder group submitted their recommendations to JAG who are to take matters forward with the newly formed Postgraduate Medical Education and Training Board. As with other areas of endoscopy Britain has been at the forefront of standards, audit and training and has set the example that is the envy of many.

CONCLUSION

The impact of flexible endoscopy on medicine has been remarkable. Specialties frequently originate and depend on an instrument for their existence and gastroenterology has been no exception. In the last 40 years the specialty has flourished because gastroscopy is relatively simple and hundreds of doctors want to do it. The motives are not new; excitement of the peeping tom, precision of diagnosis, minimally invasive surgery and financial reward. Upper gastrointestinal endoscopy grew rapidly for two decades but this was haphazard and unregulated. Risks were taken that could have been avoided, especially with therapeutic procedures.

Colonoscopy on the other hand was slower to catch on because it was more difficult and experts were few and far between. But it has been the demand for colonoscopy that has driven endoscopy forward in the last two decades. Colonoscopy is almost pointless unless the whole colon is examined and it is here that Britain has led the field in training and audit. Thanks to population screening there are now probably as many colonoscopists as there are gastroscopists.

ERCP is technically the most demanding procedure but the numbers are smaller and thankfully not every endoscopist has to (or should) embrace it. Again the British have grasped the nettle in establishing this.

The demand for gastroscopy has now levelled off and indeed is probably falling. Young people with functional dyspepsia do not need an endoscopy. Investigation should be reserved for older people or those with alarming symptoms. The "test and treat" policy can deal with hidden peptic ulceration. Attention today is focused on operative upper GI endoscopy and surveillance of Barrett's oesophagus and specialist procedures such as endoscopic ultrasound. In his valedictory speech to the annual general meeting of the British Society of Gastroenterology in 2010, Professor Christopher Hawkey suggested that we may have been doing too many gastroscopies in recent years. I think he was right.

REFERENCES

SECTION SIX

1   Davis A. B. 1972 Rudolf Schindler's role in the development of gastroscopy. *Bull. Hist. Med.* 46: 150–170

2   Vilardell F. 2006 Digestive Endoscopy in the Second Millenium. *Grupo Aula Medica*, S. L. chap 4

3   Yearsley. 1862 Introduction to the art of laryngoscopy *Med. Circ.* Vol XX

4   Obituary 1855 The late Mr. Avery *Lancet*, i, 331–332

5   Richmond T. 1909 The gastroscope and its uses. *Brit. Med. J.*, ii, 1195–96

6   Bevan J. A. 1868 Oesophagoscope *Lancet*, i, 470–471

7   Mackenzie M. 1881 On the use of the oesophagoscope in diseases of the gullet. *Med. Times & Gazette*, July 16 1881

8   Kussmaul A. 1868 Uber Magenspiegelung. Berichte uber die Verhandlungen der naturforschenden Gesellschaft Freiberg I. B. 5, 112

9   Walk L. 1966 The history of gastroscopy. *Clio Medica*, 1, 209–222

10 Sherren J. 1912 On the Early recognition of, and Prevention of Carcinoma of the Stomach. Quoted by Hill, in *On Gastroscopy*, John Bale Sons & Danielson, Oxford St., London p1

11 Souttar H. S. and Thompson T. 1909 The gastroscope and its uses. *Brit. Med. J.* ii, 843–846

12 Hill W. 1909 The gastroscope and its uses. *Brit. Med. J.* ii 1096–97

13 Hill W. 1912 *On Gastroscopy*. John Bale, Sons and Danielsson, Ltd. Oxford House, London

14 Schindler R. 1922 Bericht uber 120 Falle von Gastroskopie. Arztl. Verein Munchen 25. Reported in *Deutsche Med. Wehnschr.*, 48, 310

15 Schindler R. 1923 *Lehrbuch und Atlas der Gastroskopie*. Munich, I. F. Lehmann

16 Schindler R. 1932 Ein vollig ungefahrliches, flexible Gastroskop. *München Med. Wsch.* 32, 1268–69

17 Henning N. 1932 Erfahrungen mit dem flexible Gastroskop nach Wolf-Schindler. *München Med. Wsch.* 32, 1269–71

18 Schindler R. 1937 *Gastroscopy: The Endoscopic Study of Gastric Pathology* Univ. of Chicago Press, Chicago, Illinois

19 Leading article 1933 The flexible gastroscope. *Lancet* 2, 813

20   Edwards H. C. 1984 On the acquisition of a gastroscope *Brit. Med. J.* 289 1784–85

21   Rodgers H. W. 1937 *Textbook of Gastroscopy by N. Henning* (trans). Oxford University Press, London

22   Vorhaus M. G. 1934 Modern aspects of gastroenterology: book review *Amer. J. Dig. Dis.* vol 1, p211

23   Arafa M. A. 1935 Discussion on Diagnosis of Diseases of the Stomach. *Proceedings of the Royal Society of Medicine.* 777–782

24   Hudson T. 2004 Obituary. P. E. Thompson Hancock. *Monk's Roll* vol XI p240

25   Hurst A. 1937 Observation and experiment and the physiology of the stomach. *Brit. Med. J.* ii, 785–789

26   Leading article 1937 Gastroscopy as an established method *Lancet* ii, 1200–01

27   Jones F. A. 1987 Gastroenterology in Britain before 1937 and the founding of the Gastro-Enterological Club *Gut*, Jubilee Suppl. p4

28   Douthwaite A. H. and Lintott, G. A. M. 1938 Gastroscopic observation of the effect of aspirin and certain other substances of the stomach. *Lancet* ii, 1222–25

29   Hermon Taylor 1941 A new gastroscope with controllable flexibility. *Lancet* ii 276–277

30   Jones F. A., Doll R., Fletcher C. And Rodgers, H. W. 1951 The risks of gastroscopy. A survey of 49,000 examinations. *Lancet* i, 647–651

31   Sircus W. Milestones in the evolution of endoscopy; a short history. *J. R. Coll Phys Edinb.* 33, 124–134

32   Hancock P. E. T. and Shiner M. 1958 Combined gastroscopy and gastric biopsy under direct vision. *Lancet* i, 1204–05

33   Booth C. C. 1997 Factors influencing the development of gastroenterology in Britain. In *Gastroenterology in Britain: Historical Essays* ed W. F. Bynum, Wellcome Institute Occas Publications, No 3 p100

34   Frankel Eugene. 1970 Babinet, Jacques. *Dict Scientific Biography.* 1, 357–8 Charles Scribners & Sons, N. Y.

35   Baird J. L. 1927 *Brit. Pat. Spec.* No. 20,969/27

36   Schindler R. 1950 *Gastroscopy: The Endoscopic Study of Gastric Pathology.* Univ. of Chicago Press p377

37   Lamm H. 1930 *Biegsame optische Gerate. Ztschr. f. Instrumentenk.*, 50: 579–581

38   Booth, C. C. 1985 What has technology done to gastroenterology? A point of view. *Gut*, 26, 1088–94

39   McCombie C. W., Smith, J. C. 1998 Harold Horace Hopkins 1918–94, *Biograph. Memoirs Fell. R. Soc.* 44, 239–244

40   Hopkins H. H. and Kapany N. 1954 A flexible fibrescope, using static scanning. *Nature*, 173, 39–41

41   Van Heel A. C. S. 1954 A new method of transporting optical images without aberrations. *Nature*, 173, 39

42   Jones F. A. 1976 Foreword to *Modern Topics in Gastrointestinal Endoscopy* eds Schiller K. F. R. and Salmon, P. R. William Heinemann Medical Books Ltd., London vii

43 Vilardell F. 2006 Fibreoptics and the clinician: Basil Hirschowitz. In: *Digestive Endocopy in the Second Millennium*. Georg Thieme Verlag, KG, Stuttgart, Germany Chap 6 115

44 Hirschowitz B. I. 1979 A personal history of the Fiberscope. *Gastroenterology* 76, 864–869

45 Hirschowitz B. I. 1961 Endoscopic examination of the stomach and duodenal cap with the fiberscope. *Lancet*, i, 1074–78

46 Burnett W. 1962 An evaluation of the gastroduodenal fibrescope. *Gut*, 3, 361–365

47 Baron J. H. 2000 *Harold Horace Hopkins Munk's Roll: Lives of the Fellows of the Royal College of Physicians of London* vol X 228

48 Linder T. E., Simmen D. and Stool S. E. 1997 The history of endoscopy. In *Onary Inventions in the 20th Century. Arch. Otolaryngol, Head, Neck Surgery* 123, 1161–63

49 Hirschowitz B. I. 1963 A fibre optic flexible oesophagoscope. *Lancet*, ii, 388

50 Gibbs D. D. 1968 *Exfoliative Cytology of the Stomach*. Butterworths, London

51 Blendis L. M., Beilby J. O. W., Wilson J. P., Cole M. J. and Hadley G. D. 1967 Carcinoma of stomach: evaluation of individual and combined diagnostic accuracy of radiology, cytology, and gastrophotography. *Brit. Med. J.* i 656–659

52 Gibbs D. D. 1967 Gastric endoscopy. *Hosp. Med.* 2, 154–8

53 Cockel R. and Hawkins C. F. 1970 Gastroscopy and gastric photography with the Olympus GTF-A. *Gut*, 11, 176–181

54 Gwyn Williams, D., Truelove S. C., Gear, M. W. L., Massarella G. R. and Fitzgerald N. W. 1968 Gastroscopy with biopsy and cytological sampling under direct vision *Brit. Med. J.* i 535–539

55 Shearman D. J. C., Warwick R. R. G., MacLeod I. B. and Dean A. C. B. 1971 Clinical evaluation of the Olympus duodenoscope. *Lancet*, i, 726–729

56 Salmon P. R., Brown P., Htut, T. and Read A. E. 1972 Endoscopic examination of the duodenal bulb: clinical evaluation of forward- and side-viewing fibreoptic systems in 200 cases. *Gut*, 13, 170–5

57 Cruise F. R. 1865 The endoscope as an aid to the diagnosis and treatment of disease. *Brit. Med. J.* i 345–347

58 Strauss H. 1903 Methodik der Rectoskopie. *Berlin Klin. Wschr.* 48; 1100–04

59 Lockhart-Mummery J. P. 1904 The diagnosis of tumours in the upper rectum and sigmoid flexure by means of the electric sigmoidoscope. *Lancet* i 1781–83

60 Symposium and discussion on ulcerative colitis 1909. *Proceedings of the Royal Society of Medicine vol 2, part 2, medical section* 59–151

61 Hurst A. F. 1926 Diagnosis and treatment of colitis. *Lancet*, ii, 1151–54

62 Morson B. C. 1971 Interpretation of rectal biopsies in IBD. Sir Arthur Hurst Lecture to British Society of Gastroenterology

63 Matsunaga F. 1959 Clinical studies in ulcerative colitis and its related diseases in Japan. Proc First World Congress *Gastroenterology*. Washington 1958 Williams and Wilkins vol 2 Baltimore 955–963

64 Niwa H. 1965 Endoscopy of the colon. *Gastroenterol. Endosc.* (Tokyo) 7, 402–408

65   Overholt B. 1968 Clinical experience with the fibersigmoidocope. *Gastrointest. Endosc.* 15, 27

66   Provenzale I. and Revignas A. 1969 An original method for guided intubation of the colon. *Gastrointest. Endosc.* 16, 73–76

67   Fox J. A. and Kreel L. 1967 Technique of retrograde colonic intubation and its initial application to high colonic biopsy. *Gut*, 8, 77–82

68   Fox J. A. 1969 A fibreoptic colonoscope *Brit. Med. J.* 3, 50

69   Fox J. A. 1971 Fibreoptic colonoscope. *Proceedings of the Royal Society of Medicine* 64, 1191–92

70   Dean A. C. B. and Shearman David J. C. 1970 Clinical evaluation of a new fibreoptic colonoscope. *Lancet*, i, 550–552

71   Salmon P. R., Branch R. A., Collins C., Espiner H. and Read A. E. 1971 Clinical evaluation of fibreoptic sigmoidoscopy employing the Olympus CF-SB colonoscope. *Gut*, 12, 729–735

72   Espiner H. J., Salmon P. R., Teague R. H. and Read A. E. 1973 Operative Colonoscopy. *Brit. Med. J.* i, 453–454

73   Teague R. H., Salmon, P. R. and Read A. E. 1973 Fibreoptic examination of the colon: a review of 255 cases. *Gut*, 14, 139–142

74   Williams C. B. and Muto T. 1972 Examination of the whole colon with the fibreoptic colonoscope. *Brit. Med. J.* iii, 278–281

75   Williams C., Muto T. and Rutter K. R. P. 1973 Removal of polyps with fibreoptic colonoscope: a new approach to colonic polypectomy. *Brit. Med. J.* i, 451–452

76   Cotton P. B., Salmon P. R., Blumgart L. H., Burwood R. J., Davies G. T., Lawrie B. W., Pierce J. W. and Read A. E. 1972 Cannulation of papilla of Vater via fiber-duodenoscope. Assessment of retrograde cholangiopancreatography in 60 patients. *Lancet*, i, 53–58

77   Oi I., Kobayashi, S. and Kondo T. 1970 Endoscopic pancreatocholangiography. *Endoscopy*, 2, 103–6

78   Cotton P. B. 1972 Cannulation of the papilla of Vater by endoscopy and retrograde cholangiopancreatography (ERCP). *Gut*, 13, 1014–25

79   Cotton P. B., Salmon P. R., Blumgart L. H., Burwood R. J., Davies G. T., Lawrie B. W., Pierce J. W. and Read A. E. 1972 Cannulation of the papilla of Vater via fiber-duodenoscope. *Lancet*, i, 53–58

80   Schiller K. F. R., Truelove S. C. and Williams D. G. 1970 Haematemesis and melaena, with special reference to factors influencing the outcome. *Brit. Med. J.* i, 7–14

81   Truelove S. C. 1987 British Society for Digestive Endoscopy. *Gut*. Jubilee Suppl. BSG 1937–87

82   Schiller K. F. R. 2003 Sidney Truelove and gastrointestinal endoscopy. A look at the contributions of Sidney Truelove to gastrointestinal medicine and the history of the endoscope. *Oxford Medical School Gazette* Issue 54, vol 1

83   British Society for Digestive Endoscopy. 1973 Memorandum on Future National Needs for Fibre-Optic Endoscopy of the Gastrointestinal Tract. Samuel Walker Ltd., Hinckley, Leics.

84   Cotton P. B. 1980 Editorial. Merger of BSG and BSDE *Gut*, 21, i, 1–2

85   Standing Committee on Gastroenterology RCP 1975 The organisation of a gastrointestinal service. The College, London

86   Colin-Jones D. G., Cockel R. and Schiller K. F. C. 1978 Current endoscopic practice in the United Kingdom. *Clinics in Gastroenterology*. Vol 7, No 3, 775–786

87   The British Society of Gastroenterology Report 1974 Training in *Gastroenterology* C Nicholls and Company Ltd., Manchester

88   Working Party of the Gastroenterological Liaison Committee with the DHSS. 1978 Provision of a gastroenterological service in the District General Hospital. 1979 HMSO booklet and BSG

89   Cockel R., Colin-Jones, D. G. and Schiller K. F. C. 1982 Gastrointestinal endoscopy services–a review of the 70s with predictions for the 80s. *Health Trends*, 14, 46–49

90   Gear M. W. L., Ormiston M. C., Barnes R. J., Rocyn-Jones J. and Voss G. C. 1980 Endoscopic studies of dyspepsia in the community: an "open-access" service. *Brit. Med. J.* i, 1135.

91   Cotton P. B., Rosenberg M. T., Axon A. T. R., Davis M., Pierce J. W., Price A. B., Stevenson G. W. and Waldram R. L. 1973 Diagnostic yield of fibre-optic endoscopy in the operated stomach. *Brit. J. Surg.*, 60, 111

92   Hans Herlinger with Laurel Marshfield, 2005 *A Dream Surpassing Every Impasse: Becoming a Doctor Against all the Odds: As an Austrian Jew, on the Eve of World War 2, a Memoir*. Blue Horizon Communications

93   Cotton P. B., Frost R. G. and Shorvon P. J. 1982 Computer analysis of a decade of ERCP *Gut*, 23, A432

94   Cotton P. B. and Vallon A. G. 1981 British experience with duodenoscopic sphincterotomy for removal of bile duct stones. *Brit. J. Surg.* 68, 373–375

95   Williams C. 1979 Colonoscopy – a new view. *J. Roy. Soc. Med.* 72, 483–484

96   Design of Gastrointestinal Endoscopy Units. 1983 Brit. Soc. Gastroenterology Report by the Endoscopy Committee

97   Atkinson M., Ferguson R. and Parker G. C. 1978 Tube introducer and modified Celestin tube for use in palliative intubation of oesophago-gastric neoplasms at fibreoptic endoscopy. *Gut*, 19, 669–671

98   Johnston G. W. and Rodgers H. W. 1973 A review of fifteen years experience in the use of sclerotherapy in the control of acute haemorrhage from oesophageal varices. *Brit. J. Surg.*, 60, 797–800

99   Williams K. D. G. and Dawson J. L. 1979 Fibreoptic injection of oesophageal varices. *Brit. Med. J.* ii, 766–7

100   Westaby D., Macdougall B. R. D. and Williams R. 1985 Improved survival following injection sclerotherapy for esophageal varices: final analysis of a controlled trial. *Hepatology*, 5, 827–30

101   Smith P. M., Brian Jones D. and Rose J. D. R. 1982 Simplified fibre endoscopic sclerotherapy for oesophageal varices. *J. Roy. Coll. Phys.* 16, 4, 236–8

102   Carr-Locke D. L. and Sidky K. 1982 Broncho-oesophago fistula: a late complication of endoscopic variceal sclerotherapy. *Gut*, 23, 1005–07

103 Cotton P. B., Rosenberg M. T., Waldram R. P. L. and Axon A. T. R. 1973 Early endoscopy of the oesophagus, stomach and duodenal bulb in patients with haematemesis and melaena. *Brit. Med. J.* ii, 505–509

104 Hoare A. M. 1975 Comparative study between endoscopy and radiology in acute upper gastrointestinal haemorrhage. *Brit. Med. J.* i, 27–30

105 Vallon A. G., Cotton P. B., Laurence B. H., Armengol Miro J. R. and Salord Oses J. C. 1981 Randomised trial of endoscopic argon laser photocoagulation in bleeding peptic ulcers. *Gut*, 22, 228–233

106 Swain C. P., Bown S. G., Storey D. W., Kirkham J. S., Salmon P. R. and Northfield T. C. 1981 Controlled trial of argon laser photocoagulation in bleeding peptic ulcer. *Lancet*, ii, 1313–16

107 Chung S. C. S., Leung J. W. C., Steele R. J. C., Crofts T. J. and Li A. K. C. 1988 Endoscopic injection of adrenaline for actively bleeding ulcers: a randomised trial. *Brit. Med. J.* i, 1631–33

108 Neoptolemos J. P., Carr-Locke D. L. and Fossard D. P. 1984 The management of common bile duct calculi by endoscopic sphincterotomy in patients with gallbladders in situ. *Brit. J. Surg.* 71, 69–71

109 Cotton P. B. and Vallon A. G. 1982 Duodenoscopic sphincterotomy for removal of bile duct stones in patients with gallbladders. *Surgery*, 91, 628–630

110 Soehendra N. and Reynders-Frederix V. 1980 Palliative bile duct drainage–a new endoscopic method of introducing a transpapillary drain. *Endoscopy*, 12, 8–11

111 Huibregtse K., Haverkamp H. J. and Tytgat G. T. 1981 Transpapillary positioning of a large 3.2 mm biliary endoprosthesis. *Endoscopy*, 13, 217–219

112 Laurence B. H. and Cotton P. B. 1980 Decompression of malignant biliary obstruction by duodenoscopic intubation of bile duct *Brit. Med. J.* i, 522–523

113 Gear M. W. L., Dent N. A., Colin-Jones D. G., Lennard-Jones J. L. and Colley J. R. T. 1990 Future needs for ERCP: incidence of conditions leading to bile duct obstruction and requirements for diagnostic and therapeutic biliary procedures. *Gut*, 31, 1150–55

114 Boulos P. B., Karamanolis D. G., Salmon P. R. and Clark C. G. 1984 Is colonoscopy necessary in diverticular disease? *Lancet*, i, 95–96

115 Lennard-Jones J. L. 1986 Compliance, cost, and common sense limit cancer control in colitis. *Gut*, 27, 1403–07

116 Report by the Endoscopy Section Committee of the British Society of Gastroenterology. Future requirements for colonoscopy in Britain. 1987 *Gut*, 28, 772–775

117 Holdsworth C. D. and Atkinson M. 1984 Gastroenterology services: a regional review. *Brit. Med. J.* I, 1245–47

118 College Committee on Gastroenterology 1984 The need for an increased number of consultant physicians with specialist training in gastroenterology. Report for the Royal College of Physicians of London. *Gut*, 25, 99–102

119 Burnham W. R., Lennard-Jones J. E. and Sladen G. E. 1989 Special Report: Staffing of a combined general medical service and gastroenterology unit in a district general hospital. *Gut*, 30, 546–550

120   Smith P. M. and Williams R. 1992 A comparison of workloads of physician-gastroenterologists and other consultant physicians. *J. Roy. Coll. Phys.* 26, 2, 167–8

121   Axon A. T. R., Bottrill P. M. and Campbell D. 1987 Results of a questionnaire concerning the staffing and administration of endoscopy in England and Wales. *Gut*, 28, 1527–30

122   Report of a working party on the staffing of endoscopy units. 1987 *Gut*, 28, 1682–85

123   Axon A. T. R., Cotton P. B., Phillips I. and Avery S. A. 1974 Disinfectant of gastrointestinal fibre endoscopes. *Lancet*, i, 656–658

124   Axon A. T. R. and Cotton P. B. 1983 Endoscopy and infection. *Gut*, 24, 1064–66

125   Cleaning and disinfection of equipment for gastrointestinal flexible endoscopy: interim recommendations of a Working Party of the British Society of gastroenterology. 1988 *Gut*, 29, 1134–51

126   Hoare A. M. and Hawkins C. F. 1976 Upper gastrointestinal endoscopy with and without sedation: patients' opinions. *Brit. Med. J.* ii, 20

127   Bell G. D., Morden, A., Coady T., Lee, J. and Logan R. F. A. 1988 A comparison of diazepam and midazolam as endoscopy premedication assessing changes in ventilation and oxygen saturation. *Br. J. Clin. Pharmacol.* 26, 595–600

128   Daneshmend T. F., Bell G. D. and Logan R. F. A. 1991 Sedation for upper gastrointestinal endoscopy: results of a nationwide survey. *Gut*, 32, 12–15

129   Bell G. D., McCloy R. F., Charlton J. E., Dent N. A., Gear M. W. L., Logan R. F. A. and Swan C. H. J. 1991 Recommendations for standards of sedation and patient monitoring during gastrointestinal endoscopy. *Gut*, 32, 823–827

130   Cotton P. B. and Schiller K. F. R. 1973 Running a gastrointestinal endoscopy service Report of a symposium of the BSDE held at Oxford, 4 April 1973 Held in BSDE files

131   Report of a Working Party of the Clinical Services Committee of the British Society of Gastroenterology. 1991 Provision of gastrointestinal endoscopy and related services for a district general hospital. *Gut*, 32, 95–105

132   Joint Advisory Group. 1999 *Recommendations for Training in Gastrointestinal Endoscopy*. Royal College of Physicians, London

133   Quine M. A., Bell, G. D., McCloy R. F., Charlton J. E., Devlin H. B. and Hopkins A. 1995 Prospective audit of upper gastrointestinal endoscopy in two regions of England: safety, staffing. and sedation methods. *Gut*, 36, 462–467

134   Bramble M. G. 1992 Open access endoscopy–a nationwide survey of current practice. *Gut*, 33, 282–285

135   Bramble M. G., Cooke W. M., Corbett W. A., Cann P. A., Clark D., Contractor, B and Hungin A. S. 1993 Organising unrestricted open access gastroscopy in South Tees. *Gut*, 34, 422–427

136   Booth C. C. 1985 What has technology done to gastroenterology? A point of view. *Gut*, 26, 1088–94

137   Clark M. L. 1985 Upper intestinal endoscopy. *Lancet*, i, 629

138   Axon A. T. R., Bell G. D., Jones R. H., Quine M. A. and McCloy R. F. 1995 Guidelines on appropriate indications for upper gastrointestinal endoscopy. *Brit. Med. J.* i, 853–856

139   Matthews P. M. 2001 Developing the role of the nurse endoscopist. *Nursing Times*, 97, 56–57

140   Report of the British Society of Gastroenterology Working Party. 1994 The nurse endoscopist. BSG

141   Smale S., Bjarnason I., Forgacs I., Prasad P., Mukhood M., Wong M., Ng A. and Mulcahy H. E. 2003 Upper gastrointestinal endoscopy performed by nurses: scope for the future? *Gut*, 52, 1090–94

142   Williams J., Russell R., Durai D., Cheung W. Y., Farrin A., Bloor K., Coulton S. and Richardson G. 2009 Effectiveness of nurse delivered endoscopy: findings from randomised multi-institution nurse endoscopy trial. (MINuET) *Brit. Med. J.* 338, b231

143   Duthie G. S., Drew P. J., Hughes M. A., Farouk R., Hodson R., Wedgewood K. R. and Monson J. R. T. 1998 A UK training programme for nurse practitioner flexible sigmoidoscopy and a prospective evaluation of the practice of the first UK trained nurse flexible sigmoidoscopist. *Gut*, 43, 711–714

144   Farthing M. J. G. et al 1993 Nature and standards of gastrointestinal and liver services in the United Kingdom. Special report of BSG clinical services committee. *Gut*, 34, 1728–39

145   Report of the Working Group on Specialist Medical Training 1993 Hospital Doctors Training for the Future. Calman Implementation Steering Group HMSO

146   MacFarlane B., Leicester R., Romaya C. and Epstein O. 1999 Colonoscopy services in the United Kingdom. *Endoscopy*, 31, 409–412

147   Saunders B. P., Bell G. D., Williams C. B., Bladen J. S. and Anderson A. P. 1995 First clinical results with a real time, electronic imager as an aid to colonoscopy. *Gut*, 36, 913–917

148   Bowles C. J. A., Leicester R., Romaya C., Swarbrick E., Williams C. B. and Epstein O. 2004 A prospective study of colonoscopy practice in the UK today: are we adequately prepared for national colorectal cancer screening tomorrow? *Gut*, 53, 277–283

149   Joint Advisory Group–*Recommendations for Training in Gastrointestinal Endoscopy.* Royal College of Physicians, London April 1999

150   Hardcastle J. D., Chamberlain J. O., Robinson M. H. E., Moss S. M., Amar S. S., Balfour T. W., James P. D. and Mangham C. M. 1996 Randomised controlled trial of faecal-occult-blood screening for colorectal cancer. *Lancet*, 348, 1472–77

151   UK Colorectal Cancer Screening Pilot Group. 2004 Results of the first round of a demonstration pilot of screening for colorectal cancer in the United Kingdom. *Brit. Med. J.* 329, 133–5

152   UK Flexible Sigmoidoscopy Screening Trial Investigators. 2002 Single flexible sigmoidoscopy screening to prevent colorectal cancer: baseline findings of a UK multicentre randomised trial. *Lancet* 359, 1291–1300

153 McCallion K., Mitchell R. M. S., Wilson R. H., Kee, F., Watson R. G. P., Collins J. S. A. and Gardiner K. R. 2001 Flexible sigmoidoscopy and the changing distribution of colorectal cancer: implications for screening. *Gut*, 48, 522–525

154 Rhodes J. M. 2000 Colorectal cancer screening in the UK: Joint Position Statement by the British Society of Gastroenterology, the Royal College of Physicians, and the Association of Coloproctology of Great Britain and Ireland. *Gut*, 46, 746–748

155 Nathanson L. K., Shimi S. and Cuschieri A. 1991 Laparoscopic cholecystectomy: the Dundee Technique. *Brit. J. Surg.*, 78, 155–9

156 Tanner A. R. 1996 ERCP: present practice in a single region. Suggested standards for monitoring performance. *Eur. J. Gastroenterol. & Hepatol.*, 8, 145–8

157 Joint Advisory Group on Gastrointestinal Endoscopy. 1999 *Recommendations for Training in Gastrointestinal Endoscopy*. Brit Soc Gastroenterology, London

158 Wicks A. C. B., Robertson G. S. M. and Veitch P. S. 1999 Structured training and assessment in ERCP has become essential for the Calman era. *Gut*, 45, 154–6

159 Allison M. C., Ramanaden D. N., Fouweather M. G., Knight Davis D. K. and Colin-Jones D. G. 2000 Provision of ERCP Services and Training in the United Kingdom. *Endoscopy*, 32 (9) 693–699

160 Waller B. K., Schumacher K. A., Weidenmaier W. and Friedrich J. M. 1991 Dilated biliary tree: evaluation with MR cholangiography with T-2 weighted contrast-enhanced fast sequence. *Radiology*, 181, 805–808

161 NCEPOD Scoping our practice; The 2004 Report of the National Confidential Enquiry into Patient Outcome and Deaths. London: NCEPOD <www.ncepod. org.uk/ 2004>

162 Williams E. J., Taylor S., Fairclough P., Hamlyn A., Logan R. F., Martin D., Riley S. A., Veitch P., Wilkinson M., Williamson P. R. and Lombard M. 2007 Are we meeting the standards set for endoscopy? Results of a large-scale prospective survey of endoscopic retrograde cholangio-pancreatograph practice. *Gut*, vol 56, 821–829

BIBLIOGRAPHY

Note

Bracketed figures after each entry indicate section followed by reference number.

A Twentieth Century Physician, Being the Reminiscences of Sir Arthur Hurst, 1949, Edward Arnold and Co., London (1,1)

Abercrombie J. 1830 *Pathological and Practical Researches on Diseases of the Stomach, the Intestinal Canal, the Liver, and Other Viscera of the Abdomen.* Philadelphia pp87–88 (1,38)

Abercrombie J. 1830 *Pathological and Practical Researches on Diseases of the Stomach, the Intestinal Canal, the Liver, and Other Viscera of the Abdomen* .Philadelphia pp284–285 (4, 48)

Abercrombie J. 1830 *Pathological and Practical Researches on Diseases of the Stomach, the Intestinal canal, the Liver, and Other Viscera of the Abdomen.* Philadelphia, p119 (2, 12)

Abercrombie J. 1830 *Pathological and Practical Researches on Diseases of the Stomach, the Intestinal Canal, the Liver, and Other Viscera of the Abdomen.* Philadelphia, p194 (5, 73)

Abercrombie J. 1830 *Pathological and Practical Researches on Diseases of the Stomach, the Intestinal Canal, the Liver, and Other Viscera of the Abdomen.* Philadelphia, pp308–309 (5, 74)

Abernethy J. 1806 *Surgical Observations, Part the Second, Containing an Account of the Disorders of Health in General and of the Digestive Organs in Particular.* Longman, London (5, 36)

Abernethy J. 1809 *Surgical Observations on the Constitutional Origin and Treatment of Local Diseases, and on Aneurisms.* Longman, London (5, 37)

Acheson E. D. 1960 An association between ulcerative colitis, regional enteritis and ankylosing spondylitis. *Quart. J. Med.* 29:489–499 (4, 134)

Acheson E. D. 1960 The distribution of ulcerative colitis and regional enteritis in United States veterans with particular reference to the Jewish religion. *Gut* I: 291–293 (4, 114)

Adair J. M. 1790 *Essays on Fashionable Diseases*. Bateman, London (5, 32)

Adams F. 1856 *The Extant Works of Aretaeus, the Cappadocian*. Printed for the Sydenham Society (3, 7)

Adams W. E., Phemister D. B. 1938 Carcinoma of the lower thoracic esophagus: report of a successful resection and esophagogastrostomy.*J. Thorac. Surg.* 7 621–632 (1, 62)

Afzal M. A., Minor P. D., Begley M. L., Armitage E., Ghosh S., Ferguson A. 1998 Absence of measles-virus genome in inflammatory bowel disease. *Lancet* i 646–647 (4, 223)

Ahluwalia N. K., Thompson D. G. and Barlow J. 1996 Effect of distension and feeding on phasic changes in human proximal gastric tone. *Gut*, 39, 757–761 *(5, 302)*

Aitken G. A. 1892 *The Life and Works of John Arbuthnot* Oxford Clarendon Press (5, 11)

Alban Davies, H., Kaye M. D., Rhodes J., Dart A. M. and Henderson A. H. 1982 Diagnosis of oesophageal spasm by ergometrine provocation. *Gut*, 23, 89–97 (5, 225)

Allchin W. H. 1885 Case of acute extensive ulceration of the colon. *Trans. Path. Soc. Lond.* 36: 199–202 (4, 7)

Allchin W. H. 1909 Ulcerative colitis. Symposium and discussion of 314 cases reported by the London Hospitals. *Proceedings of the Royal Society of Medicine II med. sec.* 59 (4, 22)

Allingham W. 1888 Inguinal colotomy. In *Diseases of the Rectum* by W. Allingham. London 5th edition 313–328 (4, 19)

Allinson T. R. 1889 *The Advantages of Wholemeal Bread*. Allinson Publication, London (5, 177)

Allison M. C.,Cornwall S., Poulter L. W., Dhillon A. P., Pounder A. P. 1988 Macrophage heterogeneity in normal colonic mucosa and inflammatory bowel disease. *Gut* 29: 1531–38 (4, 191)

Allison M. C., Ramanasden, D. N., Fouweather, M. G., Knight Davis, D. K. and Colin-Jones, D. G. 2000 Provision of ERCP services and training in the United Kingdom. *Endoscopy* 32, 693–699 (6, 159)

Allison P. R. 1941 Excision of oesophagus via a left thoracotomy *Brit. J. Surg.* 30:132– 141 (1, 67)

Allison P. R. 1948 Peptic ulcer of the oesophagus. *Thorax* 3: 20– 42 (1, 92)

Allison P. R. 1951 Reflux esophagitis, sliding hiatus hernia, and the anatomy of repair. *Surg. Gynae. Obstet.* 92: 419– 431 (1, 93)

Allison P. R. 1973 Hiatus hernia: (A 20 year retrospective survey) *Annals of Surgery.* 178: 273– 276 (1, 94)

Allison P. R., Borrie J. 1949 Bypass oesophagectomy for carcinoma. *Brit. J. Surg.* 37: 1–21 (1, 70)

Allison P. R., Johnstone A. S. 1953 The oesophagus lined with gastric mucous membrane. *Thorax* 8: 87–101

Allison P. R., Johnstone A. S., Royce G. B. 1943 Short oesophagus with simple peptic ulceration. *J. Thorac. Surg.* 12:432– 457 (1, 91)

Allison S. P. 1986 Some psychological and physiological aspects of enteral nutrition. *Gut* 27 Suppl. 118–24 (4, 297)

Allison S. P., Walford S., Todovoric V., Elliott E. T. 1979 Practical aspects of nutrition support. *Research & Clin. Forums.* 149–57 (4, 299)

Almy T. P. and Tulin M. 1947 Alterations in colonic function in man under stress: experimental production of changes simulating the "irritable colon".*Gastroenterology* 8, 616–626 (5, 137)

Alun Jones V., Dickinson R. J., Workman E., Freeman A. H., Hunter J. O. 1984 Controlled trial of diet in the management of Crohn's disease *12th Internat Cong Gastroenterology, abstr.* 943 (4, 313)

Alun Jones V., Dickinson R. J., Workman E., Wilson A. J., Freeman A. H., Hunter J. O. 1985 Crohn's disease: maintenance of remission by diet. *Lancet* ii 177–180 (4, 314)

Alun Jones V., McLaughlan P., Shorthouse M., Workman E., Hunter J. O. 1982 Food intolerance: a major factor in the pathogenesis of irritable bowel syndrome. *Lancet* ii 1115–17 (4, 312; 5, 290)

Alvarez A. S., Summerskill W. H. J. 1958 Gastrointestinal haemorrhage and salicylates. *Lancet* ii 920– 925 (2, 80)

Ament M. E., Ochs H. D. 1973 Gastrointestinal manifestations of chronic granulomatous disease. *New England Journal of Medicine.* 288: 382–387 (4, 177)

Anand B. S., Piris J., Jerrome D. W., Offord R. E., Truelove S. C. 1981 The timing of histological damage following a single challenge with gluten in treated coeliac disease. *Quart. J. Med. n.s.* 1978 3–94 (3, 212)

Anand B. S., Truelove S. C., Offord R. E. 1977 Skin test for celiac disease using a subfraction of gluten. *Lancet* i: 118–120 (3, 213)

Andersen D. H. 1947 Celiac syndrome VI The relationship of celiac disease. starch intolerance, and steatorrhea. *J. Paed.* 30: 564–582 (3, 66)

Anderson C. M., Frazer A. C., French J, M., Gerrard J. W., Sammons H. G., Smellie J, M. 1952 Coeliac disease: gastro-intestinal studies and the effect of dietary wheat flour. *Lancet* i 836–842 (3, 76)

Andree J. 1788 *Considerations on Bilious Diseases and Some Particular Affections of the Liver and the Gall-Bladder*. Hertford. Printed for the Author and sold by J. Murray, and W. Lowndes, in Fleet St. London; and T. Simson, Hertford (5, 31)

Anonymous. 1948 Antihistamine drugs and gastric secretion. *Brit. Med. J.* ii: 1028 (2, 168)

Anonymous. 1990 Gastroenterologists in Sydney. *Lancet* 336: 779–780 (2, 196)

Apley J. 1959 *The Child With Abdominal Pains*. Blackwell, Oxford (5. 336)

Arafa M. A. 1935 Discussion on diagnoses of diseases of the stomach *Proceedings of the Royal Society of Medicine* 777–782 (6, 23)

Arden Jones R. 1969 Immunosuppressive therapy in ulcerative colitis. *Proceedings of the Royal Society of Medicine. Sect. of Proctology.* 499–501 (4, 326)

Armstrong C. P., Blower A. L. 1987 Non-steroidal anti-inflammatory drugs and life threatening complications of peptic ulceration. *Gut* 28 527–532 (2, 88)

Arthur L. J. H., Langman M. J. S. 1981 Prevalence of coeliac disease in Derby. In *The Genetics of Coeliac Disease*, ed R. B. McConnell, M. T. P. Press 15–17 (3,202)

Astley R., French J. M. 1951 The small intestine pattern in normal children and in coeliac disease: its relationship to the nature of the opaque medium. *Brit. J. Radiol.* 24: 321–330 (3, 54)

Atherton J. C., Peek R. M., Tham K. T., Cover T. L., Blaser M. J. 1997 Clinical and pathological importance of heterogeneity in vacA, the vacuolating cytotoxin gene of Helicobacter pylori. *Gastroenterology* 11: 292–299 (2, 114)

Atkins H 1974 *Down: The Home of the Darwins*. The Royal College of Surgeons, London (5, 59)

Atkinson M. 1959 The oesophago-gastric sphincter after cardiomyotomy. *Thorax* 14:125–131 (1, 34)

Atkinson M., Edwards D. A. W., Honour A. J., Rowlands E. N. 1957 The oesophago-gastric sphincter in hiatus hernia. *Lancet* ii 1138–42 (1, 33)

Atkinson M., Ferguson R. 1977 Fibreoptic endoscopic palliative intubation of inoperable oesophago-gastric neoplasms. *Brit. Med. J.* i 266–267 (1, 51)

Atkinson M., Ferguson R., Parker G. C. 1978 Tube introducer and modified Celestin tube for use in palliative intubation of oesophago-gastric neoplasms at fibreoptic endoscopy. *Gut* 19: 669–671 (1, 52 and 6, 97)

Atkinson M and Bennett, J. R. 1968 The relationship between motor changes and pain during esophageal acid perfusion. *Amer. J. Dig. Dis.* 13,4, 346–350 (5, 192)

Atkinson M., Edwards D. A. W., Honour A. J., & Rowlands E. N. 1957 Comparison of cardiac and pyloric sphincters,a manometric study. *Lancet*, ii, 918–922 (5, 145)

Austad W. I., Cornes J. S., Gough K. R., McCarthy C. F., Read A. E. 1967 Steatorrhoea and malignant lymphoma. *Amer. J. Dig. Dis.n.s.*12:475–490 (3, 115)

Axon A. T. R., Bottrill P. M., and Campbell D. 1987 Results of a questionnaire concerning the staffing and administration of endoscopy in England and Wales. *Gut* 28: 1527–30 (6, 121)

Axon A. T. R., Cotton P. B., Phillips, I. and Avery S. A. 1974 Disinfection of gastrointestinal fibre endoscopes. *Lancet* i, 656–658 (6, 123)

Axon A. T. R., and Cotton P. B. 1983 Endoscopy and infection *Gut* 24: 1064–66 (6, 124)

Axon A. T. R., Bell G. D., Jones R. H., Quine M. A. and McCloy R. F. 1995 Guidelines on appropriate indications for upper gastrointestinal endoscopy. *Brit. Med. J.* i: 853–856 (6, 138)

Aylett S 1959 The surgery of diffuse ulcerative colitis including a review of 100 cases of colitis treated by total colectomy and ileo-rectal anastomosis. *Postgrad. Med. J.* 35:67– 74 (4, 339)

Azad Khan A. K., Piris J., Truelove S. C. 1977 An experiment to determine the active therapeutic moiety of sulphasalazine. *Lancet* ii 892–895 (4, 99)

Aziz Q., Thompson D. G., Ng V. W. K., Hamdy S., Sarkar S., Brammer M. J., Bullmore E. T., Hobson A. R., Tracey I., Suckling, K., Simmons A. and Williams S. C. R. 2000 Cortical processing of human somatic and visceral sensation. *J. Neurosci.* 20, 2657–2663 (5, 398)

Badenoch J. 1960 Steatorrhoea in the adult. *Brit. Med. J.* ii: 879 & 963 (3, 96)

Baillie M. 1833 *The Morbid Anatomy of Some of the Most Important Parts of the Human Body.* 8th London pp86–87 (2, 10)

Baillie M. 1833 *The Morbid Anatomy of Some of the Most Important Parts of the Human Body.* 8th edition London p61 (1, 37)

Baird J. L. 1927 *Brit. Pat. Spec.* No 20,969/27

Baker W. N. W., Glass R. E., Ritchie J. K., Aylett S. O. 1978 Cancer of the rectum following colectomy and ileorectal anastomosis for ulcerative colitis. *Brit. J. Surg.* 65: 862– 868 (4, 343)

Baldwin E. 1961 *Gowland Hopkins The discovery of vitamins.* Van Den Bergh (3, 29)

Bannister J. J., Dawson, P., Timms J. M., Gibbons C. G. and Read N. W. 1987 Effect of the stool size and consistency on defaecation. *Gut,* 28, 1246–50 (5, 264)

Barbour R. F., Stokes A. B. 1936 Chronic Cicatrising Enteritis. A phase of benign non-specific granuloma of the small intestine. *Lancet* i 299–303 (4, 54)

Barclay A. E. 1915 *The Radiology of the Alimentary Tract.* Oxford University Press, London (2, 28)

Barclay A. E. 1935 Direct X-ray cinematography. With a preliminary note on the nature of the non-propulsive movements of the large intestine. *Brit. J. Radiol.* 8, 652–658 (5, 106)

Bardhan K. D., Naesdal J., Bianchi Porro G., Petrillo M., Lazzaroni M., Hinchliffe R. F. C., Thompson M., Morris P., Daly M. J., Carroll N. J. H., Walan A., Rikner L. 1991 Treatment of refractory peptic ulcer with omeprazole or continued H2–receptor antagonists: a controlled clinical trial. *Gut* 32:435–438 (2, 199)

Bargen J. A. 1928 Chronic ulcerative colitis associated with malignant disease. *Arch. Surg. Chicago.*17: 561–576 (4, 243)

Bargen J. A. 1949 Treatment of ulcerative colitis with salicylazosulfapyridine (salazopyrine) *Med. Clin. North America* 33: 935 (4, 61)

Bargen J. A. 1956 Report on his experience of ulcerative colitis to the Internat Congress of Gastroenterology. *Lancet* ii 185. (4, 67)

Bargen J. A., Logan A. H. 1925 The etiology of chronic ulcerative colitis: experimental studies with suggestions for a more rational form of treatment. *Arch. Int. Med.* 36: 818–829 (4, 31)

Bargen J. A., Weber 1929 *Collected Papers Mayo Clinic* xxi 209 (4, 30)

Barham C. P., Jones R. L., Biddlestone L. R., Hardwick R. H., Shepherd N. A., Barr H. 1997 Photothermal laser ablation of Barrett's oesophagus: endoscopic and histological evidence of squamous re-epithelialisation. *Gut* 41: 281–284 (1, 117)

Barish, C. F., Castell, D. O. and Richter, J E. 1986 Graded esophageal balloon distension: a new provocative test for non-cardiac chest pain. *Dig. Dis. Sci.* 31: 1292–98 (5, 230)

Baron J. H., Sonnenberg A. 2002 Hospital admissions for peptic ulcer and indigestion in London and New York in the 19th and early 20th centuries. *Gut* 50: 568–570 (2, 14)

Baron J, H., Burrows L., Wildstein W., Kark A. E., Dreiling D. A. 1965 The maximum histamine response of denervated fundic pouches in dogs. *Amer. J. Gastroenterol.* 44:333–344 (2, 44)

Baron H. J. 1969 Timing of peak acid output after pentagastrin. *Gastroenterology* 56:641–643 (2, 50)

Baron J. H., Logan R. P. H. 1994 Infection by Helicobacter pylori is the major cause of duodenal ulcer. *Proc. Roy. Coll. Phys Edin.* 24: 21–36 (2, 112)

Baron J. H., Connell A. M., Lennard-Jones J. E., Jones F. A. 1962 Sulphasalazine and salicyl-azo-sulphadimidine in ulcerative colitis. *Lancet* i 1094–96 (4, 90)

Baron J. H. 2000 Harold Horace Hopkins. *Munk's Roll: Lives of the Royal College of Physicians of London.* Vol 10 228 (6, 47)

Barr H., Shepherd N. A., Dix A., Roberts D. J. H., Tan W. C., Krasner N. 1996 Eradication of high-grade dysplasia in columnar-lined (Barrett's) oesophagus by photodynamic therapy with endogenously generated protoporphyrin 1X. *Lancet* Vol 348 584–585 (1, 116)

Barrett N. R. 1950 Chronic Peptic ulcer of the oesophagus and oesophagitis. *Brit. J. Surg.* 38 175–182 (1, 97)

Barrett N. R. 1956 The oesophagus lined by columnar epithelium. *Gastroenterologia* 86 183–6 (1, 99)

Barrett N. R. 1957 The lower oesophagus lined by columnar epithelium. *Surgery* 416: 881–894 (1, 100)

Barrett N. R., Franklin R. H., 1949 Concerning the unfavourable late results of certain operations performed in the treatment of cardiospasm. *Brit. J. Surg.* 37: 194–202 (1, 24)

Bassett-Smith P. 1919 A case of sprue with associated tetany *Lancet* i 178 (3, 23)

Bastedo W. A. 1911 The dilatation test for chronic appendicitis. *Amer. J. Med. Sci.* 142,11–14 (5, 93)

Bate C. M., Keeling P. W. N., O'Morain C., Wilkinson S. P., Foster, D. N., Mountford, D. A., Temperley, J. M., Harvey, R. F., Thompson, D. G., Davis, M., Forgacs, I. G., Bassett, K. S., Richardson, P. D. I. 1990

Comparison of omeprazole and cimetidine in reflux oesophagitis: symptomatic, endoscopic, and histological evaluations. *Gut* 31: 968–972 (1, 107)

Bean R. H. D. 1966 Treatment of ulcerative colitis with antimetabolites. *Brit. Med. J.* i 1081–84 (4, 322)

Bearcroft C. P., Perrett D. and Farthing M. J. G. 1996 5-Hydroxytryptamine release into human jejunum by cholera toxin. *Gut*, 39: 528–531 (5, 385)

Bearcroft C. P., Perrett D. and Farthing M. J. G. 1998 Postprandial plasma 5-hydroxytryptamine in diarrhoea predominant irritable bowel syndrome: a pilot study. *Gut*, 42: 42–46 (5, 386)

Beaumont W. 1833 *Experiments and Observations on the Gastric Juice, and the Physiology of Digestion.* Plattsburgh, printed by F. P. Allen (5, 43)

Beaumont W. 1838 *Experiments and Observations on the Gastric Juice and the Physiology of Digestion,* Reprinted From the Plattsburgh Edition, With Notes by Andrew Combe MD. Edinburgh: Maclachan and Stewart. (5, 46)

Beddoes T. 1784 *Dissertations Relative to the Natural History of Animals and Vegetables. Translated from the Abbe Spallanzani. To which are added an appendix, the first containing a paper written by Mr. Hunter FRS and the Experiments of Dr. Stevens* 2 vols J. Murray, London 365–391 (5, 19 & 27)

Bell G. D. et al. 1987 14C-urea breath analysis, a non-invasive test for campylobacter pylori in the stomach. *Lancet* i: 1367–68 Letter. (2, 194)

Bell G. D., Morden A., Coady T., Lee J. and Logan R. F. A. 1988 A comparison of diazepam and midazolam as endoscopy premedication assessing changes in ventilation and oxygen saturation. *Br. J. Clin. Pharmacol* 26: 595–600 (6, 127)

Bell G. D., McCloy, R. F., Charlton, J. E., Dent, N. A., Gear, M.W. L., Logan, R. F. A. and Swan, C. H. J. 1991 Recommendations for standards of sedation and patient monitoring during gastrointestinal endoscopy. *Gut* 32: 823–827 (6, 129)

Bell J. R., MacAdam W. 1924 The variations in gastric secretion of the normal individual. *Quart. J. Med.* 17: 215–222 (2, 35)

Belsey R. H. R. 1972 Recent progress in oesophageal surgery. *Acta. Chir. Beg.*71: 230 (1, 82)

Bennett T. I. 1921 Action of atropine and belladonna on gastric secretion *Guy's Hosp. Reports.* lxxi 54– 57 (2, 124)

Bennett T. I., Hardwick C. 1940 Chronic jejuno-ileal insufficiency. *Lancet* ii 381–384 (3, 51)

Bennett T. I., Hunter D., Vaughan J. M. 1932 Idiopathic steatorrhoea (Gee's disease). A nutritional disturbance associated with tetany, osteomalacia and anaemia. *Quart. J. Med. n.s.* 4: 603–667 (3, 45)

Bennett T. I., Ryle J. A. 1921 Studies in gastric secretion. V. A study of normal gastric function based on the investigation of one hundred healthy men by means of the fractional test meal. *Guy's Hosp. Reports.* 71: 268–318 (2, 34)

Bennett J. R. and Atkinson M. 1966 The differentiation between oesophageal and cardiac pain. *Lancet*, ii 1123–27 (5, 190)

Bennett J. R. and Atkinson M. 1968 Oesophageal acid perfusion in the diagnosis of precordial pain. *Lancet*, ii 1150–52 (5, 191)

Bergin A. J., Donelly T. C., McKendrick M. W. and Read, N. W. 1993 Changes in ano-rectal function in persistent bowel disturbance following salmonella gastroenteritis. *Eur. J. Gastroenterol. & Hepatol.* 5, 617–620 (5, 305)

Best C. N., Cook P. B. 1961 Case of Mesenteric Reticulosarcoma Associated with Gluten-sensitive Steatorrhoea. *Brit. Med. J.* ii: 496–498 (3, 112)

Bevan J. A. 1868 Oesophagoscope *Lancet* (6, 6)

Biemond I., Burnham W. R., d'Amaro J., Lanbman M. J. S. 1986 HLA-A and-B antigens in inflammatory bowel disease. *Gut* 27: 934–941 (4, 136)

Bjarnason I., O'Morain C., Levi A. J., Peters T. J. 1983 Absorption of 51 chromium–labelled ethylene diamine tetra acetate in inflammatory bowel disease.*Gastroenterology* 85: 318–322(4, 307)

Bjarnason I., Peters T. J., Veall N. 1983A persistent defect of intestinal permeability in coeliac disease demonstrated by a 51Cr-labelled EDTA absorption test. *Lancet* i 323–5 (4, 306)

Black J. W. 2002 in *Peptic Ulcer: Rise and Fall. Wellcome Witnesses to Twentieth Century Medicine* vol 14. eds. Christie D. A., Tansey E. M. 63–67 (2, 169)

Black J. W., Duncan W. A. M., Durant C. J., Ganellin C. R., Parsons E. M. 1972 Definition and Antagonism of Histamine H2–receptors. *Nature* 236: 385– 390 (2, 170)

Blackburn G., Hadfield G., Hunt A. H. 1939 Regional ileitis. *St. Barts. Hosp. Rep.* 72: 181–224 (4, 168)

Blackwell J. N and Castell D. O. 1984 Oesophageal chest pain: a point of view. *Gut*, 25, 1–6 (5, 227)

Blackwell J. N., Hannan W. J., Adam R. D. and Heading R. C. 1983 Radionuclide transit studies in the detection of oesophageal dysmotility. *Gut*, 24: 421–426 (5, 226)

Blendis L. M., Cameron A. J. and Hadley G. D. 1967 Analysis of 400 examinations using the gastrocamera *Gut* 8: 83 -90 (5, 125)

Blendis L. M., Beilby J. O. W., Wilson J. P., Cole M. J. and Hadley G. D. 1967 Carcinoma of stomach: evaluation of individual and combined diagnostic accuracy of radiology, cytology and gastrophotography. *Brit. Med. J.* i 656–659 (6, 51)

Blum A. L., Talley N. J., O'Morain C., Veldhuyzen van Zanten S., Labenz, J., Stolte M., Louw J. A., Stubberod A., Theodors A., Sundin M., Bolling-Sternevald E. and Junghard O. 1998 Lack of effect of treating Helicobacter pylori infection in patients with non-ulcer dyspepsia. *New England Journal of Medicine* 339, 1875–81 (5, 321)

Bodley Scott R. 1974 *The Royal Hospital of St. Bartholemew* 1123–1973. ed. by Medvei V. C., Thornton J. L. London p188 (3, 9)

Bond J. H. and Levitt M. D. 1975 Investigation of small bowel transit time in normal subjects utilising pulmonary hydrogen measurements. *J. Clin. Lab. Med.* 86: 546–555 (5, 206)

Booth C. C. 1961 The metabolic effects of intestinal resection in man. *Postgrad. Med. J.* 37: 725–739. (3, 101)

Booth C. C. 1985 What has technology done to gastroenterology? A point of view. *Gut* 26, 1088–94 (6, 38 &136)

Booth C. C. 1989 History of coeliac disease. *Brit. Med. J.* I527 (3, 69)

Booth C. C. 1997 Factors influencing the development of gastroenterology in Britain. In: *Gastroenterology in Britain: Historical Essays*. Ed: W. F. Bynum. Wellcome Institute for the History of Medicine Occasional Publications, No. 3 (5, 397; 6, 33)

Booth C. C., Chanarin I., Anderson B. B., Mollin D. L. 1957 The site of absorption and tissue distribution of orally administered 56 Co – labelled vitamin B12 in the rat. *Brit. J. Haematol.* 3: 253–261 (3, 99)

Booth C. C., Dowling R. H. 1970 *Coeliac Disease* Churchill Livingstone, Edinburgh (3, 122)

Booth C. C., Mollin D. L. 1959 The site of absorption of vitamin B12 in man. *Lancet* i: 18 (3, 100)

Borelli A. G. 1680 *De Motu Animalum*,1287 Rome (5, 15)

Boulos P. B., Karamanolis D. G., Salmon P. R. and Clark C. G. 1984 Is colonoscopy necessary in diverticular disease? *Lancet*, i, 95–96 (6,114)

Bowen G. E., Irons G. U., Rhodes J., Kirsner J. B. 1965 Precautionary early experiences with immunosuppressive medication (Azathioprine) in ulcerative colitis. *Gastroenterology* 48: 807–808. (4, 323)

Bowlby J. 1990 *Charles Darwin. A New Biography*. Hutchinson, London (5, 60)

Bowles C. J. A., Leicester R., Romaya C., Swarbrick E., Williams C. B. and Epstein, O. 2004 A prospective study of colonoscopy practice in the UK today: are we adequately prepared for national colorectal cancer screening tomorrow? *Gut*, 53, 277–283 (6, 148)

Boyd E., Johnston D., Penston J. G., Wormsley K. G. 1988 Does maintenance therapy keep duodenal ulcer healed? *Lancet* i: 1324–28 (2, 181)

Boyd Sprott. 1836 On the Structure of the Mucous Membrane of the Stomach. *Edin. Med. and Surg. Journal* xlvi 382 (5, 51)

Bramble M. G. 1992 Open access endoscopy – a nationwide survey of current practice *Gut*, 33, 282–285 (6, 134)

Bramble M. G., Cooke W. M., Corbett W. A., Cann P. A., Clark D., Contractor B. and Hungin A. S. 1993 Organising unrestricted open access gastroscopy in South Tees. *Gut*, 34, 422–427 (6,135)

Brand D. L., Martin D. And Pope C. E. 1977 Esophageal manometrics in patients with angina-like chest pain. *Dig. Dis. Sci.* 22, 300–304 (5, 194)

Brewerton D. A., Hart F. D., Nicholls A., Caffrey M., James R. C. O., Sturrock R. D. 1973 Ankylosing spondylitis and HL-A27. *Lancet* i 904–907 (4, 135)

Bridger S., Lee J. C. W., Bjarnason I., Lennard-Jones J. E., MacPherson A. J. 2002 In siblings with similar genetic susceptibility for inflammatory bowel disease, smokers tend to develop Crohn's disease and non-smokers develop ulcerative colitis. *Gut* 51: 21–25 (4, 156)

Briggs P. J., Dick R. C. S., Hurst Sir A. 1939 Simple ulcer of the oesophagus and short oesophagus. *Proceedings of the Royal Society of Medicine* XXXII 11 1423–45 (1, 87)

Brinton W. 1857 *On the Pathology, Symptoms, and Treatment of Ulcer of the Stomach*. John Churchill, New Burlington Street, London (2, 2)

Brinton W. 1858 *Lectures on the Diseases of the Stomach*. First edition John Churchill & Sons, London (2, 1)

Brinton W. 1864 *Lectures on Diseases of the Stomach*. 2nd edition Churchill & Son. p115 (2, 66)

Brinton W. 1864 *Lectures on Diseases of the Stomach*. London: 2nd edition p174–5 (1, 40)

Brinton W. 1864 *Lectures on the Diseases of the Stomach With an Introduction on its Anatomy and Physiology*. John Churchill & Sons, London Lectures II and VI (5, 52)

Brock R. C. 1942 Cardio-oesophageal resection for tumour of the cardia. *Brit. J. Surg.* 30: 146–160. (1, 64)

Brodribb A. J. M. 1977 Treatment of symptomatic diverticular disease with dietary fibre. *Lancet*, i. 664–666 (5, 282)

Brodribb A. J. M., Condon R. E., Cowles V. and De Cosse J. J. 1979 Effect of dietary fibre on intraluminal pressure and myoelectrical activity of left colon in monkeys. *Gastroenterology*. 77, 70–74 (5, 283)

Brooke B. N. 1952 The management of an ileostomy including its complications. *Lancet* ii 102–4. (4, 75)

Brooke B. N. 1954 *Ulcerative Colitis and its Surgical Treatment*. Livingstone Edin & Lond (4, 77)

Brooke B. N. 1956 Outcome of surgery for ulcerative colitis. *Lancet* ii 532–536 (4, 83)

Brooke B. N., Hoffmann D. C., Swarbrick E. T. 1969 Azathioprine for Crohn's disease. *Lancet* ii 612–614 (4, 327)

Brooke B. N., Javett S. L., Davison O. W. 1970 Further experience with azathioprine for Crohn's disease. *Lancet* ii 1050–53 (4, 328)

Brown R. C., Langman M. J. S., Lambert P. M. 1976 Hospital admissions for peptic ulcer during 1958–72 *Brit. Med. J.* i: 35–37 (2, 63)

Budd G. 1856 *On the Organic Diseases and Functional Disorders of the Stomach* Samuel S. and William Wood, New York. 168–179 (5, 50)

Burge H., Stedeford R. D., Hollanders D. 1970 Recurrent ulceration after vagotomy and drainage with electrical stimulation test, 1957–69. *Br. Med. J.* ii: 372–375 (2, 164)

Burge H., Vane J. R. 1958 Method of testing for complete nerve section during vagotomy. *Brit. Med. J.* i: 615–618 (2, 163)

Burkitt D. P. 1971 Epidemiology of cancer of the colon and rectum. *Cancer*, 28, 3–13 (5, 160)

Burkitt D. P. 1979 *"Don't Forget Fibre in Your Diet" to Help Avoid Many of Our Commonest Diseases*. The Lotuspond. (5, 167)

Burkitt D. P., Walker A. R. P. & Painter N. S. 1972 Effect of dietary fibre on stools and transit times, and its role in the causation of disease. *Lancet*, ii, 1408–12 (5, 163)

Burland W. L., Duncan W. A. M., Hesselbro T., Mills J. G., Sharpe P. C., Haggie S. J., Wyllie J. H. 1975 Pharmacological evaluation of cimetidine, a new histamine H2–receptor antagonist, in healthy man. *Br. J. Clin. Phar.* 2 481–486 (2, 179)

Burland W. L., Sharpe P. C., Colin-Jones D. G., Turnbull P. R. G., Bowskill P. 1975 Reversal of metiamide-induced agranulocytosis during treatment with cimetidine. *Lancet* ii: 1085 (2, 178)

Burnett W. 1962 An evaluation of the gastroduodenal fibrescope. *Gut*, 3, 361–365 (6, 46)

Burnham W. R., Lennard-Jones J. E. and Sladen G. E. 1989 Special Report: staffing of a combined general medical service and gastroenterology unit in a district general hospital. *Gut*, 30, 546–550. (6, 119)

Calman K. C. 1995 Measles vaccination as a risk factor for inflammatory bowel disease. *Lancet* i 1362 (4, 222)

Calvert E., Houghton L. A., Cooper P., Morris J. and Whorwell P. J. 2002 Long term improvement in functional dyspepsia using hypnotherapy. *Gastroenterology*, 123, 1778–85 (5, 365)

Cameron A. H., Astley R., Hallowell M., Rawson A. B., Miller C. G., French J. M., Hubble D. V. 1962 Duodenal-jejunal biopsy in the investigation of children with coeliac disease. *Quart J. Med. n.s.* 31: 125–140 (3, 92)

Camilleri M. D., Northcutt A. R., Kong S., Dukes G. E., McSorley D. and Mangel, A. W 2000 Efficacy and safety of alosetron in women with irritable bowel syndrome: a randomised, placebo-controlled trial. *Lancet*, 355, 1035–40 (5, 389)

Campbell J. M. H., Coneybeare J. J. 1924 Comparison of the test meal and X-ray examination of the stomach in health. *Guy's Hosp. Reports.* 74: 354–366 (2,30)

Campieri M. et al. 1981 Treatment of ulcerative colitis with high dose 5–aminosalicylic acid enemas. *Lancet* ii 270–271 (4, 100)

Cann P. A., Read N. W. and Holdsworth C. D. 1983 Oral domperidone: double blind comparison with placebo in irritable bowel syndrome. *Gut*, 24, 1135–40 (5,268)

Cann P. A., Read N. W. and Holdsworth C. D. 1984 What is the benefit of coarse wheat bran in patients with irritable bowel syndrome? *Gut*, 25, 168–173 (5, 287)

Cann P. A., Read N. W., Brown C., Hobson N. and Holdsworth C. D. 1983 Irritable bowel syndrome: relationship of disorders in the transit of a single solid meal to symptom patterns. *Gut* 24, 405–411 (5, 252)

Cann P. A., Read N. W., Holdsworth C. D. and Barends D. 1984 The role of loperamide and placebo in the management of the irritable bowel syndrome. *Dig. Dis. Sci.* 29, 239–247 (5, 269)

Cannon W. B. 1902 The movements of the intestines studied by means of the roentgen rays. *Amer. J. Physiol.* 6: 251–277 (5, 84)

Cantlie J. 1913 Some recent observations on sprue. *Brit. Med. J.* ii 1296–97 (3, 22)

Card W. I. 1952 *Peptic ulcer: Aetiology.* In Avery Jones. F. (ed) Modern Trends in Gastroenterology, Butterworths, London 380–388 (2, 41)

Card W. I., Marks I. N. 1960 The relationship between the acid output of the stomach following "maximal" histamine stimulation and the parietal cell mass. *Clin. Sci.* 19:147–163 (2, 43)

Carrie A. 1950 Adenocarcinoma of the upper end of the oesophagus arising from ectopic gastric epithelium. *Brit. J. Surg.* 37: 474. (1,101)

Carr-Locke D. L. and Sidky K. 1982 Broncho-oesophageal fistula: a late complication of endoscopic variceal sclerotherapy. *Gut*, 23, 1005–07 (6, 102)

Carroll L. 1871 *Through the Looking-Glass and What Alice Found There.* Ch 6 (5, 1)

Carter C., Sheldon W., Walker C. 1959 The inheritance of coeliac disease. *Ann. Hum. Genet.* 23 266–278 (3, 125)

Carter D. C., Forrest J. A. H., Werner M., Heading R. C., Park J., Shearman D. J. C. 1974 Effect of histamine H2–receptor blockade on vagally induced gastric secretion in man. *Br. Med. J.* iii: 554–556 (2, 175)

Carter M. J., Willcocks M. M., Mitchison H. C., Record C. O., Madely C. R. 1989 Is a persistent adenovirus infection involved in celiac disease? *Gut* 30: 1563–67 ((3,181)

Catassi C., Ratsch I. M., Fabiani E., Rossini M., Bordicchia F., Candela et al. 1994 Coeliac disease in the year 2000: exploring the iceberg. *Lancet* 343: 200–203 (3, 228)

Celestin L. R. 1959 Permanent intubation in inoperable cancer of the oesophagus and cardia. A new tube. *Ann. Roy. Coll. Surg. (Eng.)* 25: 165–170 (1, 48)

Celestin L. R., Campbell W. B. 1981 A new and safe system for oesophageal dilatation. *Lancet* i 74– 75 (1, 49)

Celestin L. R., Harvey V., Saunders J. H. B.,Wormsley K. G., Forrest J. A. H., Logan R. F. A., Shearman D. J. C., Fermont D., Haggie S. J., Wyllie J. H., Albinus M., Thompson M.H., Venables C. W., Burland W. L. 1975 Treatment of duodenal ulcer by metiamide. A multicentre trial. *Lancet* ii: 779–781 (2, 177)

Challacombe D. N., Bayliss J. M. 1980 Childhood coeliac disease is disappearing. *Lancet* ii 1360–61 (3, 204)

Chambers T. 1856 *Digestion and its Derangements* Churchill, London p402 (2, 5)

Chan R. A., Pope D. J., Gilbert A. P., Sacra P. J., Baron J. H., Lennard-Jones J. E. 1983 Studies of two novel sulfasalazine analogs, Ipsalazide and Balsalazide. *Dig. Dis. Sci. n.s.* 28 609–615 (4, 105)

Charles Darwin, the Complete Correspondence of 1985. ed. F. Burkhardt and S. Smith vol II 47–52 (5, 54)

Chaudhary A. S. & Truelove S. C. 1961 Human colonic motility: a comparative study of normal subjects, patients with ulcerative colitis, and patients with the irritable colon syndrome. *Gastroenterology*, 40, 1–34 (5, 140)

Chaudhary N. A. & Truelove S. C. 1962 The irritable colon syndrome. *Quart. J. Med., n.s.* xxxi, No 123, 307–322 (5, 139)

Cheadle W. B. 1903 A clinical lecture on Acholia. *Lancet* i: 1497–1500 (3, 12)

Cheyne G. 1773 *The English Malady or a Treatise of Nervous Diseases of All Kinds.* G. Strachan in Cornhill, London (5, 12)

Child G. C. 1847 *On Indigestion and Certain Bilious Disorders Often Conjoined With It. To Which are Added, Short Notes on Diet.* John Churchill, London (5, 48)

Chorzelski T. P., Beutner E. H., Sulej J., Chorzewska H., Jablonska S., Kumar V. et al.1984 IgA anti-endomysium antibody. A new immunological marker of dermatitis herpetiformis and coeliac disease. *Brit. J. Dermatol.* 111 395–402 (3, 223)

Chung S. C. S., Leung J. W. C., Steele R. J. C., Crofts T. J. and Li A. K. C. 1988 Endoscopic injection of adrenaline for actively bleeding ulcers: a randomised trial. *Brit. Med. J.* i, 1631–33 (6, 107)

Ciclitera P. J., Hunter J. O. and Lennox E. S. 1980 Clinical testing of bread made from millisonic 6A wheats in celiac patients. *Lancet*, ii 234–236 (3, 183)

Clamp J. R., Fraser G., Read A. E. 1981 Study of the carbohydrate content of mucus glycoproteins from normal and diseased colons. *Clin. Sci.* 61: 229–234 (4, 232)

Clark M. L. 1985 Upper intestinal endoscopy. *Lancet* i, 629 (6, 137)

Clarke C. A. 1981 Clinical genetics: the wider horizon. In *The Genetics of Coeliac Disease*. Ed R. B. McConnell MTP Press Ltd, Lancaster pxxiii (3, 149)

Clarke C. A., Edwards J. W., Haddock D. R. W., Howel Evans A. W., McConnell R. B., Sheppard P. M. 1956 ABO blood groups and secretor character in duodenal ulcer. *Br. Med. J.* ii 725–731 (2, 115)

Clarke C. A., McConnell R. B. 1954 Six cases of carcinoma of the oesophagus occurring in one family. *Brit. Med. J.* ii 1137–38 (1, 78)

Clarke J. 1815 *Commentaries on Some of the Most Important Diseases of Children*. Longman, Herst, Rees, Orme & Brown, London p86–90 (3, 18)

Cleaning and disinfection of equipment for gastrointestinal flexible endoscopy: interim recommendations of a Working Party of the British Society of Gastroenterology. 1988 *Gut*, 29, 1134–51 (6, 125)

Cleave T. L. 1941 Natural bran in the treatment of constipation. *Brit. Med. J.* i 461 (L) (5, 153)

Cleave T. L. 1974 *The Saccharine Disease* John Wright and Son, Bristol (5, 168)

Cleave T. L. and Campbell G. D. 1966 *Diabetes, Coronary Thrombosis and the Saccharine Disease*. Wrights of Bristol (5, 154)

Cleave T. L., Campbell, G. D. & Painter, N. S. 1969 *Diabetes, Coronary Thrombosis and the Saccharine Disease*. 2nd edition. Bristol: John Wright and Sons Ltd. (5, 158)

Clinch D., Banerjee A. K., Ostick G., Levy D. W. 1983 Non-steroidal anti-inflammatory drugs and gastrointestinal adverse effects. *J. R. Coll. Gen. Pract.* 17 228–230 (2, 86)

Cockel R. and Hawkins C. F. 1970 Gastroscopy and gastric photography with the Olympus GTF-A *Gut* 11, 176–181 (6, 53)

Cockel R., Colin-Jones D. G. and Schiller K. F. C. 1982 Gastrointestinal endoscopy services–a review of the 70s with predictions for the 80s. *Health Trends* 14, 46–49 (6, 89)

Code C. F. and Marlett J. A. 1975 The interdigestive myo-electric complex of the stomach and small bowel of dogs. *J. Physiol.* 246, 289–309 (5, 202)

Coe T. 1757 *A Treatise on Biliary Concretions: or, Stones in the Gall-Bladder and Ducts*.London. Printed for D. Wilson and T. Durhamat Plato's Head in the Strand. (5, 29)

Coggon D., Lambert P., Langman M. J. S. 1981 20 years of hospital admissions for peptic ulcer in England and Wales. *Lancet* i:1302–04 (2, 64)

Coghill N. F. and Williams A. W. 1955 The technique of gastric biopsy *Brit. Med. J.* ii 1111 (5,126)

Colin-Jones D. G., Langman M. J. S., Lawson D. H., Logan R. F. A., Paterson K. R., Vessey M. P. 1992 Postmarketing surveillance of the safety of cimetidine: 10 years mortality report. *Gut* 33:1280–84 (2, 182)

Colin-Jones D. G., Cockel R. and Schiller K. F. C. 1978 Current endoscopic practice in the United Kingdom. *Clinics in Gastroenterology* Vol 7, No 3, 775–786 (6, 86)

College Committee on Gastroenterology 1984 The need for an increased number of consultant physicians with specialist training in gastroenterology. Report for the Royal College of Physicians of London. *Gut,* 25, 99–102 (6, 118)

Collier D. St. J., Pain J. A. 1985 Non-steroidal anti-inflammatory drugs and peptic ulcer perforation. *Gut* 26, 359–363 (2, 87)

Collier H. Personal communication (2, 91)

Collins S. M., McHugh K., Jacobson, K., Khan I., Riddell, R., Murase, K. and Weingarten, H. P. 1996 Previous inflammation alters the response of the rat colon to stress. *Gastroenterology*,111, 1509–15 (5, 307)

Collis J. L. 1957 Carcinoma of the oesophagus; the case for surgical excision *Lancet* ii 613–616 (1, 72)

Collis J. L. 1971 Surgical treatment of carcinoma of the oesophagus and cardia *Brit. J. Surg.* 58, 801–804 (1, 50)

Combe C., Saunders W. 1813 A singular case of Stricture and Thickening of the Ileum, read at the College July 4th 1806. *Med. Trans. Coll. Phys. London.* 4:16–21 (4, 47)

Combe A. 1836 *The Physiology of Digestion Considered With Relation to the Principles of Dietetics* Maclachlan and Stewart, Edinburgh (5, 45)

Connell A, M., Kamm M. A., Dickson M., Balkwill A. M., Ritchie J. K., Lennard-Jones J. E. 1994 Long-term neoplasia risk after azathioprine treatment in inflammatory bowel disease. *Lancet* 343:1249–52 (4, 333)

Connell W. R., Sheffield J. P., Kamm M. A., Ritchie J. K., Hawley P. R., Lennard-Jones J. E. 1994 Lower gastrointestinal malignancy in Crohn's disease. *Gut,* 35: 347–352 (4, 288)

Connell A. M. 1961 The motility of the pelvic colon. I Motility in normals and in patients with asymptomatic peptic ulcer. *Gut,* 2 175–186 (5, 146)

Connell A. M. 1962 The motility of the pelvic colon. II Paradoxical motility in diarrhoea and constipation. *Gut 3*, 342–348 (5, 147)

Connell A. M., Avery Jones F. and Rowlands E. N. 1965 Motility of the pelvic colon IV Abdominal pain associated with colonic hypermotility after meals. *Gut 6*, 105–2 (5, 149)

Connell A. M., Gaafer M., Hassenan M. A. and Khayal M. A. 1964 The motility of the pelvic colon. III Motility responses in patients with symptoms following amoebic dysentery. *Gut, 5*, 443 (5, 148)

Cook M. G., Goligher J. C. 1975 Carcinoma and epithelial dysplasia complicating ulcerative colitis. *Gastroenterology 68*: 1127–36 (4, 261)

Cooke W. T. 1970 Azathioprine in Crohn's disease. *Lancet* ii 1195–96 (4,329)

Cooke W. T., Brooke B. N. 1955 Non-specific enterocolitis. *Quart. J Med. n.s.* 24: 1–22 (4,123)

Cooke W. T., Peeney A. L. P., Hawkins C. F. 1953 Symptoms, signs, and diagnostic features of idiopathic steatorrhoea. *Quart. J. Med. n.s.* 22: 59–77 (3, 80)

Cooper B. T., Barbezat G. O. 1987 Barrett's oesophagus: a clinical study of 52 patients. *Quart. J. Med. n.s.* 62, 238 97–108 (1, 106)

Cooper B. T., Neumann C. S., Cox M. A., Iqbal T. H. 1998 Continuous treatment with omeprazole 20mg daily up to 6 years in Barrett's oesophagus. *Aliment. Pharmacol. Ther* 12 893–897 (1, 112)

Cooper E. C., Shaw L. E. 1893 On diseases of the duodenum. *Guy's Hosp. Reports* 50:171–308 (2, 13)

Corfield A. P., Myersclough N., Longman R., Sylvester P., Arul S., Pignatelli M. 2000 Mucins and mucosal protection in the gastrointestinal tract: new prospects for mucins in the pathology of gastrointestinal disease. *Gut 47*: 589–594 (4, 238)

Cornes J. S., Stecher M. 1961 Primary Crohn's disease of the colon and rectum. *Gut 2*: 189–201 (4, 126)

Cotton P. B. 1972 Cannulation of the papilla of Vater by endoscopy and retrograde cholangiopancreatography (ERCP) *Gut 13*, 1014–25) (6, 78)

Cotton P. B. 1980 Editorial. Merger of BSG and BSDE. *Gut 21*, i, 1–2 (6, 84)

Cotton P. B., Salmon P. R., Blumgart L. H., Burwood R. J., Davies G. T., Lawrie B. W., Pierce J. W. and Read A. E. 1972 Cannulation of papilla of Vater via fibre-duodenoscope. Assessment of retrograde cholangiopancreatography in 60 patients. *Lancet*, i, 53–58 (6, 76 & 79)

Cotton P. B., Rosenberg M. T., Axon A. T. R., Davis M., Pierce J. W., Price A. B., Stevenson, G. W. and Waldram, R. L. 1973 Diagnostic yield of fibre-optic endoscopy in the operated stomach. *Brit. J. Surg.* 60, 111 (6, 91)

Cotton P. B., Rosenberg M. T., Waldram R. L. and Axon A. T. R. 1973 Early endoscopy of the oesophagus, stomach and duodenal bulb in patients with haematemesis and melaena. *Brit. Med. J.* ii, 505–509 (6, 103)

Cotton P. B. and Schiller K. F. R. 1973 *Running a gastrointestinal endoscopy service*. Report of a symposium of the BSDE held at Oxford, 4 April 1973. Held in BSDE Files. (6, 130)

Cotton P. B. and Vallon A. G. 1981 British experience with duodenoscopic sphincterotomy for removal of bile duct stones. *Brit. J. Surg.* 68, 373–375 (6, 94)

Cotton P. B. and Vallon A. G. 1982 Duodenoscopic sphincterotomy for removal of bile duct stones in patients with gall bladders. *Surgery* 81, 628–630 (6, 109)

Cotton P. B., Frost R. G. and Shorvon P. J. 1982 Computer analysis of a decade of ERCP. *Gut*, 23, A432 (6, 93)

Cottone M., Bunce M., Taylor C. J., Ting A., Jewell D. P. 1985 Ulcerative colitis and HLA phenotype. *Gut* 26: 952–954 (4, 142)

Counsell P. B., Dukes C. E. 1952 The association of chronic ulcerative colitis and carcinoma of the rectum and colon. *Brit. J. Surg.* 39: 485–495 (4, 248)

Crabbe P. A., Heremans J. F. 1966 Distribution of immunoglobulin-containing cells along the gastrointestinal tract. *Gastroenterology* 51: 305–316 (3, 142)

Crabtree J. E., Taylor J. D., Wyatt J. I., Heatley R. V. et al. 1991 Mucosal IgA recognition of Helicobacter pylori 120 KDa protein, peptic ulceration, and gastric pathology. *Lancet*, 338 332–335 (2, 113)

Craig T. K. and Brown, G. W. 1984 Goal frustrating aspects of life event stress in the aetiology of gastrointestinal disorder. *J. Psychosom. Res.* 28, 411–421 (5, 342)

Creamer B. 1962 Dynamics of the mucosa of the small intestine in idiopathic steatorrhoea. *Gut*, 3: 295–300 (3, 104)

Creamer B. 1964 Variations in small-intestinal villous shape and mucosal dynamics. *Brit. Med. J.* ii: 1371–73 (3, 105)

Creamer B. 1964 Malignancy and the small intestinal mucosa. *Brit. Med. J.* ii: 1435–36 (3, 114)

Creamer B., 1966 Coeliac thoughts. *Gut*, 7, 569–571 (3, 109)

Creamer B., Olsen A. M., Code C. F. 1957 The esophageal sphincter in achalasia of the cardia (cardiospasm) *Gastroenterology*, 33, 293–301 (1, 31)

Creamer B., Pierce J. W. 1957 Observations on the gastro-oesophageal junction during swallowing and drinking *Lancet* ii 1309–12 (1, 32)

Crean G. P., Holden R. J., Knill-Jones R. P., Beattie A. D., James W. B., Marjoriebanks F. M. and Spiegelhalter D. J. 1984 A data base on dyspepsia. *Gut*, 35:191–202 (5, 130)

Creed F. H. 1981 Life events and appendicectomy. *Lancet*, i,1381–85 (5, 344)

Creed F. H. 2006 Should general psychiatry ignore somatisation and hypochondriasis? *World Psychiatry*, 5, 146–150 (5, 376)

Creed F. H. 2006 How do SSRIs help patients with irritable bowel syndrome? *Gut*, 55, 1065–10. (5, 396)

Creed F. H. 2008 Somatisation in functional dyspepsia: integrating gastric physiology with psychological state. *Gut*, 57, 1642–43 (5, 371)

Creed F., Craig T. and Farmer R. 1988 Functional abdominal pain, psychiatric illness, and life events. *Gut*, 29, 235–242 (5, 346)

Creed F., Fernandes L., Guthrie E., Rigby C., Tomenson B., Read N. and Thompson D. 2003 The cost-effectiveness of psychotherapy and paroxetine for severe irritable bowel syndrome. *Gastroenterology*, 124, 303–317 (5, 395)

Creed F. H. and Guthrie E. 1987 Psychological factors in the irritable bowel syndrome. *Gut* 28, 1307–18 (5, 347)

Creed F. H. and Guthrie E. 1989 Psychological treatments of the irritable bowel syndrome. *Gut* 30, 1601–09 (5, 348)

Creed F., Guthrie E., Ratcliffe J., Fernandes L., Rigby C., Tomenson B., Read N. and Thompson D. 2005 Reported sexual abuse predicts impaired functioning but a good response to psychological treatments in patients with severe irritable bowel syndrome. *Psychosom. Med.* 67, 490–9 (5, 370)

Creed F., Ratcliffe J., Fernandes L., Tomenson B., Palmer S., Rigby C., Guthrie E., Read N. and Thompson D. G. 2001 Health-related quality of life and health care costs in severe, refractory irritable bowel syndrome. *Ann. Intern. Med.* 134, 860–868 (5, 369)

Creed F., Ratcliffe J., Fernandes L., Palmer S., Rigby C., Tomenson B., Guthrie E., Read N. and Thompson D. G. 2005 Outcome in severe irritable bowel syndrome with and without accompanying depressive, panic and neurasthenic disorders. *Br. J. Psychiatry* 186, 507–515 (5, 368)

Creed F. H., Tomenson B., Guthrie E., Ratcliffe J., Fernandes L., Read, N., Palmer S. and Thompson D. G. 2008 The relationship between somatisation and outcome in patients with severe irritable bowel syndrome. *J. Psychosom. Res.* 64, 613–620 (5, 377)

Crisp E. 1842–43 Cases of perforation of the stomach from simple ulceration. *Lancet* ii 639 (2, 11)

Croft D. N., Loehry C. A., Creamer B. 1968 Small bowel cell- loss and weight-loss in the coeliac syndrome. *Lancet* ii: 68–70 (3, 106)

Croft D. N., Loehry C. A., Taylor J. F. N., Cole J. 1968 D. N. A. and cell loss from normal small-intestinal mucosa. *Lancet* ii: 70–73 (3, 107)

Croft J. 1882 Relief of oesophageal malignancy by endotubation. Report of a case. *St. Thos. Hosp. Reports* 12: 45–53 (1, 43)

Crohn B. B. 1934 Broadening conception of regional ileitis. *Amer. J. Dig. Dis. & Nutr.* I, 97 (4, 44)

Crohn B. B., Ginzberg L., Oppenheimer G. D. 1932 Regional ileitis: a pathologic and clinical entity. *J. Amer. Med. Assoc.* 99: 1323–29 (4, 42)

Crohn B. B., Rosenberg H. 1925 The sigmoidoscopic picture of chronic ulcerative colitis (non-specific). *Amer. J. Med.* 170: p226 (4, 242)

Crosby W. H., Kugler H. W. 1957 Intraluminal biopsy of the small intestine. The intestinal biopsy capsule. *Amer. J. Dig. Dis. n.s.* 2, 236–241 (3, 88)

Crude annual mortality rate from ulcerative colitis (I. S. C. 572.2) for England and Wales, 1940–62 Quoted by J. G. Evans and E. D. Acheson *Gut* 1965, 6: p322 (4, 111)

Cruise F. R. 1865 The endoscope as an aid to the diagnosis and treatment of disease. *Brit. Med. J.* i, 345–347 (6, 57)

Cullen W. 1769 Synopsis Nosologiae Edinburgh. (5, 23)

Cullinan E. R., Price R. K. 1932 Haematemesis following peptic ulceration; prognosis and treatment. *St. Barts. Hosp. Rep.* 65 185 (2, 142)

Cummings J, H., Edmond L. M. and Magee E. A. 2004 Dietary carbohydrates and health: do we still need the fibre concept? *Clin. Nutr. Suppl.* 1, 5–17 (5, 281)

Cummings J. H. 1973 Dietary fibre. *Gut*, 14: 69–81 (5, 274)

Cummings J. H. 1984 Constipation, dietary fibre and the control of large bowel function. *Postgrad. Med. J.* 60, 811–819 (5, 280)

Cunningham D., Hawthorn J., Pople A., Gazet J. C., Ford H. C., Challoner, T. And Coombes, R. C. 1987 Prevention of emesis in patients receiving cytotoxic drugs by GR38032F, a selective 5-HT3 antagonist. *Lancet*, i, 1461–63 (5, 380)

Curling T. B. 1842 On acute ulceration in the duodenum in cases of burn. *Med. Chir. Transact.* London 25 260 (2, 70)

Cuschieri A. 1980 Laparoscopy in general surgery and gastroenterology. *Brit. J. Hosp. Med.* 24: 252–258 (4, 346)

Dale H. H., Laidlaw P. P. 1910 The physiological action of B-iminazolylethylamine *J. Physiol.* 41:318–344 (2, 32)

Dalziel T. K. 1913 Chronic interstitial enteritis. *Brit. Med. J.* ii 1068–70 (4, 45)

Daneshmend T. F., Bell G. D. and Logan R. F. A. 1991 Sedation for upper gastrointestinal endoscopy: results of a nationwide survey. *Gut*, 32, 12–15 (6, 128)

Darby C. F., Hammond P. and Taylor I. 1978 Real time analysis of colonic myoelectrical rhythms in disease. Gastrointestinal Motility in Health and Disease. *Proc. V1 Int. Symp. GI Moility.* MTP Press, Lancaster, England 287–294 (5, 211)

Darke S. G., Parks A. G., Grogono J. L., Pollock D. J. 1973 Adenocarcinoma and Crohn's disease: a report of 2 cases and analysis of the literature. *Brit. J. Surg.* 60: 169–175 (4, 283)

Dart A. M., Alban Davies H., Dalal J., Ruttley M. and Henderson A. H. 1980 "Angina" and normal coronary arteriograms: a follow-up study. *Eur. Heart J.*; 1, 97–100 (5, 195)

Dart A. M., Alban Davies H., Lowndes R. H., Dalal J, Ruttley M. and Henderson A. H. 1980 Oesophageal spasm and angina: diagnostic value of ergometrine (ergonovine) provocation. *Eur. Heart J.* 1, 91–95 (5, 196)

Darwin F. 1887 *Life and Letters of Charles Darwin.* John Murray, London vol 3 p1 (5, 56)

Darzi A., Lewis C., Menzies Gow N. et al 1993 Laparoscopic assisted surgery of the colon: operative technique. *Endosc. Surg. Allied Technol.* 1: 13–15 (4, 352)

Das K. M., Eastwood M. A., McManus J. P. A., Sircus W. 1974 The role of the colon in the metabolism of salicyl-azo-sulphapyridine. *Scand. J. Gastroenterol.* 9: 137–141 (4, 96)

Das K. M., Eastwood M. A., McManus J. P. A., Sircus W. 1973 Adverse reactions during salicyl-azo-sulfapyridine therapy and the relation with drug metabolism and acetylator phenotype. *New England Journal of Medicine*. 289: 491–495 (4, 97)

Davidson L. S. P., Fountain J. R. 1950 Incidence of sprue syndrome with some observations on the natural history. *Brit. Med. J.* i: 1157–61 (3, 79)

Davidson L. S. P., Girdwood R. H., Innes E. M. 1947 Folic acid in the treatment of the sprue syndrome. *Lancet*, i, 511–515 (3, 97)

Davidson S. 1931 Vitamin B in anaemia. *Lancet* ii 1395–98 (3, 43)

Davies D. T. 1935 Some observations on peptic ulcer. Bradshaw Lecture *Lancet* i 521 & 585 (2, 68)

Davies G. J., Crowder, M., Reid, B. and Dickerson, J. W. B. 1986 Bowel function measurements of individuals with different eating patterns. *Gut*, 27, 164–9 (5, 297)

Davis A. B. 1972 Rudolf Schindler's role in the development of gastroscopy. *Bull. Hist. Med.* 46: 150–170 (6, 1)

Dawson I. M. P., Pryse-Davies J. 1959 The development of carcinoma of the large intestine in ulcerative colitis. *Brit. J. Surg.* 47: 113–128 (4, 249)

"Days like these 11 April 1817" compiled by Ian Irvine for *the Independent* 17 April 2005 (4, 355)

De Caestecker, J. S., Blackwell, J. N., Brown, J. and Heading, 1985 The oesophagus as a cause of recurrent chest pain: which patients should be investigated and which tests should be used? *Lancet*, ii, 1143–46 (5, 228)

De Caestecker, J. 1998 Oesophageal chest pain: an update. In: Kaski, J. ed. *Chest Pain With Normal Coronary Angiograms; Pathogenesis, Diagnosis and Management*. Kluwer Academic, Philadelphia (5, 363)

De Caestecker, J. S., Pryde, A. and Heading, R. C. 1988 Comparison of intravenous edrophonium and oesophageal acid perfusion during oesophageal manometry in patients with non-cardiac chest pain. *Gut*, 29, 1029–34 (5, 229)

De Dombal F. T., Watts J. McK., Watkinson G., Goligher J. C. 1966 Local complications of ulcerative colitis: stricture, pseudopolyposis and carcinoma of colon and rectum. *Brit. Med. J.* i 1442–47 (4, 253)

Dean A. C. B. and Shearman, D. J. C. 1970 Clinical evaluation of a new fibreoptic colonoscope. *Lancet*, i 550–552 (6, 70)

Dearing W. H., Brown P. W. 1950 Experience with cortisone and ACTH in chronic ulcerative colitis. *Proc. Staff Meet. Mayo Clin.* 25: 486–488 (4, 63)

Deaver J. B. 1896 *Appendicitis*. Blakiston, Philadelphia, p132 (5, 81)

Deer B. 2011 How the case against the MMR vaccine was fixed. *Brit. Med. J.* 342 77–82 and 136–142 (4, 229)

Delaney B., Qume M., Moayyedi P., Logan R. F. A., Ford A. C., Elliott C., McNulty C., Wilson S. and Hobbs F. D. R. 2008 Helicobacter pylori test and treat versus proton pump inhibitor in initial management of dyspepsia in primary care: multicentre randomised controlled trial (MRC-CUBE trial) *Brit. Med. J.* ii, 651–654 (5, 332)

Dennis C. 1945 Ileostomy and colectomy in chronic ulcerative colitis. *Surgery* 18: 435–452 (4, 73)

Design of Gastrointestinal Endoscopy Units. 1983 Brit Soc Gastroenterology. Report by the Endoscopy Committee (6, 96)

Devlin H. B., Datta D., Dellipiani A. W. 1980 The incidence and prevalence of inflammatory bowel disease in North Tees District. *World J. Surg.* 4: 183–193 (4, 116)

Dew M. J., Harries A. D., Evans B. K., Rhodes J. 1983 Treatment of ulcerative colitis with oral 5–aminosalicylic acid in patients unable to take sulphasalazine. *Lancet* ii 801–803 (4, 110)

Dew M. J., Hughes P. J., Harries A. D., Williams G., Evans B. K., Rhodes J. 1982 Maintenance of remission in ulcerative colitis with oral preparation of 5–aminosalicylic acid. *Brit. Med. J.* ii 1012. (4, 109)

Dew M. J., Hughes P. J., Lee M. G., Evans B. K., Rhodes J. 1982 An oral preparation to release drugs in the human colon. *Br. J. Clin. Phar.* 14: 405–408 (4, 108)

Dick R. C. S., Hurst A. 1942 Chronic peptic ulcer of the oesophagus and its association with congenitally short oesophagus and diaphragmatic hernia. *Quart. J. Med.* 11 105–120 (1, 88)

Dicke W. K. 1941 Simple dietary treatment for the syndrome of Gee-Herter. *Ned. Tijdschr. Geneeskd.* 85 1715 (in Dutch) (3, 70)

Dicke W. K. 1950 *Coeliac disease. Investigation of the harmful effects of certain types of cereal on patients with coeliac disease*. Thesis. Univ. of Utrecht, The Netherlands (in Dutch). (3, 73)

Dicke W. K., Van de Kamer J. H., Weijers H. A. 1953 Coeliac disease II The presence in wheat of a factor having a deleterious effect in cases of coeliac disease. *Acta. Paediatr.* 42:34 (3, 72)

Dickinson R. J., Ashton M. G., Axon A. T. R., Smith R. C., Yeung C. K., Hill G. L. 1980 Controlled trial of intravenous hyperalimentation and total bowel rest as an adjunct to the routine therapy of acute colitis. *Gastroenterology* 79: 1199–1204 (4, 292)

Dickinson R. J., Dixon M. F., Axon A. T. R. 1980 Colonoscopy and the detection of dysplasia in patients with longstanding ulcerative colitis. *Lancet* ii 620–622 (4, 262)

Dieterich W., Elmis T., Bauer M., Donner P., Volta U., Riecken E. O. 1997 Identification of tissue transglutaminase as the auto-antigen of celiac disease. *Nat. Med.* 3, 797–801 (3, 224)

Dissanayake A. S., Jerrome D. W., Offord R. E., Truelove S. C., Whitehead R. 1974 Identifying toxic fractions of wheat gluten and their effect on the jejuna mucosa in celiac disease. *Gut* 15: 931–946 (3, 182)

Dissanayake A. S., Truelove S. C. 1973 A controlled therapeutic trial of long-term maintenance treatment of ulcerative colitis with sulphasalazine (salazopyrin). *Gut* 14: 923–926 (4, 92)

Dixon J. S., Pipkin G. A., Mills J. G., Wood J. R. 1997 Ranitidine bismuth citrate plus clarithromycin for the eradication of H. pylori. *J. Physiol. Pharmacol.* 48: 47–58 (2, 202)

Doe W. F., Henry K., Booth C. C. 1974 Complement in celiac disease In *Coeliac Disease: Proceedings of the 2nd Internat. Coeliac Symposium, Leyden* Ed. W. Th. J. M. Hekkens, A. S. Pena Stenfert Kroese, Leyden (3, 211)

Doe W. F., Henry K., Booth C. C. 1975 Complement in coeliac disease. In *Coeliac Disease*. Ed. W. Th. J. M. Thekkens and A. S. Pena, pp189–194, Stenfert Kroese, Leiden (3, 144)

Doig A., Ferguson, J. P. S., Milne I. A., Passmore R. 1991 *William Cullen and the Eighteenth Century World*. Edinburgh University Press 228–229 (5, 72)

Doll R., Peto R. 1976 Mortality in relation to smoking; 20 years observations on male British doctors. *Brit. Med. J.* ii:1525–36 (2, 72)

Doll R. 2002 Peptic ulcer: Rise and Fall. *Wellcome Witnesses to Twentieth Century Medicine* Vol 14 ed. Christie D. A., Tansey E. M. p9 (2, 69)

Doll R., Friedlander P. H., Pygott F. 1956 Dietetic treatment of peptic ulcer *Lancet* i: 5–9 (2, 150)

Doll R., Hill I. D., Hutton C., Underwood D. J. 1962 Clinical trial of a triterpenoid liquorice compound in gastric and duodenal ulcer. *Lancet* ii: 793–796 (2, 153)

Doll R., Jones F. A. 1951 *Occupational factors in the aetiology of gastric and duodenal ulcer. With an estimate of the incidence in the general population.* London: HMSO. MRC Special report series No 276 (2, 60)

Doll R., Pygott F. 1952 Factors influencing the rate of healing of gastric ulcers. *Lancet* i: 171–5 (2, 147)

Doll R., Pygott F. 1954 Clinical trial of Robaden and of cabbage juice in the treatment of gastric ulcer. *Lancet* ii:1200–04 (2, 151)

Doll R., Jones F. A., Buckatzsch M. M. 1951 *Occupational factors in the aetiology of gastric and duodenal ulcers.* Special Report Series. No 276 Medical Research Council, HMSO., London (5, 122)

Doniach I., Shiner M. 1957 Duodenal and jejunal biopsies II Histology. *Gastroenterology* 33: 71–76 (3, 87)

Dornhorst A. C., Kent Harrison. Pierce J. W., 1954 Observations on the normal oesophagus and cardia *Lancet* i 695–698 (1, 25)

Dossetor J. F. B., Gibson A. A. M., McNeish A. S. 1981 Childhood coeliac disease is disappearing. *Lancet* i: 322–3 (3, 205)

Douglas A. P., Booth C. C. 1970 Digestion of gluten peptides by normal human jejunal mucosa and by mucosa from patients with adult coeliac disease. *Clin. Sci.* 38: 11–25 (3, 135)

Douthwaite A. H. 1938 Some recent advances in medical diagnosis and treatment. *Brit. Med. J.* i: 1143–46 (2, 75)

Douthwaite A. H., Lintott G. A. M. 1938 Gastroscopic observation of the effect of aspirin and certain other substances on the stomach. *Lancet* ii 1222–25 (2, 76 and 6, 28)

Dowd B., Walker-Smith J. A. 1974 Samuel Gee, Aretaeus, and The Coeliac Affection. *Brit. Med. J* i 45–47 (3, 2)

Dragstedt L. R., Owens F. M. 1943 Supradiaphragmatic section of the vagus nerves in treatment of duodenal ulcer. *Proc. Soc. Exp. Biol.,* N. Y. 53:152 (2, 156)

Dragstedt Lester R. 1945 Vagotomy for gastroduodenal ulcer. *Annals of Surgery* 122: 973 -989 (2, 156)

Drossman D. A., Creed F. H., Olden, K. W., Svedlund J., Toner B. B. and Whitehead, W. E. 1999 Psychosocial aspects of the functional gastrointestinal disorders. *Gut,* 45 (Suppl. II): 25–30(5, 372)

Drossman D. A. 1993 Psychosocial and psychologic mechanisms in GI disease. In: Kirsner, J. B. ed. *The Growth of Gastroenterologic Knowledge in the 20th Century.* Philadelphia: Lea and Febiger, 419–432 (5, 362)

Drossman D. A., McKee D. C., Sandler R. S., Mitchell C. M., Cramer E. M., Lowman B. C. and Burger A. L. 1988 Psychosocial factors in the irritable bowel syndrome. A multivariate study of patients and non-patients with irritable bowel syndrome. *Gastroenterology*, 95, 701–708 (5, 349)

Dudrick S. J., Wilmore D. W., Vars H. M., Rhoads J. E. 1968 Long term total parenteral nutrition with growth, development and positive nitrogen balance. *Surgery* 64: 134–142 (4, 290)

Dukes C. 1932 The classification of cancer of the rectum. *J. Path. Bact.* 35: 323–332 (4, 124)

Dunlop S. P., Jenkins D., Neal K. R. and Spiller R. C. 2000 Relative importance of enterochromaffin cell hyperplasia, anxiety, and depression in postinfectious IBS. *Gastroentrology*, 125: 1651–59 (5, 314)

Durham A. E. 1881 Carcinoma of the oesophagus. Gastrostomy. *Lancet* ii 872. (1, 44)

Duthie G. S., Drew P. J., Hughes M. A., Farouk R., Hodson R., Wedgewood K. R. and Monson J. R. T. 1988 A UK training programme for nurse practitioner flexible sigmoidoscopy and a prospective evaluation of the practice of the first UK trained nurse flexible sigmoidoscopist. *Gut*, 43, 711–714 (6, 143)

Duthie H. L., Kwong N. K., Brown B. H. and Whittaker G. E. 1971 Pacesetter potential of the human gastroduodenal junction. *Gut*, 12, 250–256 (5, 207)

Eade O. E., Lloyd R. S., Lang Celia, Wright R. 1977 IgA and IgG reticulin antibodies in coeliac and non-coeliac patients. *Gut*, 18: 991–993 (3, 218)

Eaden J. A., Abrams K. R., Mayberry J. F. 2001 The risk of colorectal cancer in ulcerative colitis: a meta analysis. *Gut* 48: 526–535 (4, 273)

Eaden J. A., Mayberry J. F. 2002 Guidelines for screening and surveillance of asymptomatic colorectal cancer in patients with inflammatory bowel disease. *Gut* 51 Suppl. V v10–v12 (4, 274)

Eaden J. A., Ward B., Mayberry J. F. 2000 How British gastroenterologists screen for colonic cancer in ulcerative colitis: an analysis of performance. *Gastrointest. Endosc.* 52: 153–8 (4, 272)

Earlam R. 1991 An MRC prospective randomised trial of radiotherapy versus surgery for operable squamous cell carcinoma of the oesophagus. *Ann. Roy. Coll. Surg. (Eng.)* 73, 8–12 (1, 77)

Earlam R., Cunha-Melo J. R. 1980 Oesophageal squamous cell carcinoma. 1. A critical review of surgery. *Brit. J. Surg.* 67, 381–390 (1, 75)

Earlam R., Cunha-Melo J. R. 1980 Oesophageal squamous cell carcinoma. 2. A critical review of radiotherapy. *Brit. J. Surg.* 67 457–461 (1, 76)

Eastwood M. A. 1969 Dietary Fibre and serum-lipids. *Lancet*, ii, 1222–24 (5, 174)

Eastwood M. A. 1973 Vegetable fibre: its physical properties. In Symposium *on fibre in human nutrition* Proc. Nutr. Soc. 32, 137–143 (5, 176)

Editorial 1902 Chronic Dyspepsia. *Lancet* Aug 23rd (5, 89)

Edkins J. S. 1905 On the chemical mechanism of gastric secretion. *Proc. Roy. Soc. B.* 76:376 (2, 31)

Edwards F. C., Truelove S. C. 1963 The course and prognosis of ulcerative colitis. *Gut* 4: 299–315 (4, 86)

Edwards F. C., Truelove S. C. 1964 The course and prognosis of ulcerative colitis. Part IV Carcinoma of the colon. *Gut* 5: 15–22 (4, 251)

Edwards F. R. 1939 On the Neurogenic origin of duodenal ulceration. *Liverpool Med. Chir. J.* 46, 181–198 (2, 157)

Edwards H. 1936 Specimen of Crohn' disease. *Trans. Med. Soc. Lond.* 59: 87–88 (4, 53)

Edwards H. C. 1984 On the acquisition of a gastroscope. *Brit. Med. J.* 289, 1784–85 (6, 20)

Ehsanullah M., Filipe M. I., Gazzard B. 1982 Mucin secretion in inflammatory bowel disease: correlation with disease activity and dysplasia. *Gut* 23: 485–489 (4, 235)

Ekbom A., Wakefield A. J., Zack M., Adami H. O. 1994 Perinatal measles infection and subsequent Crohn's disease. *Lancet* ii 508–510 (4, 216)

Ellis H. J., Pollock E. L., Engel W., Fraser J. S., Rosen-Bronson S., Wieser H., Ciclitira P. J. 2003 Investigation of the putative immunodominant T cell epitopes in coeliac disease. *Gut* 52, 212–217 (3, 185)

Ellis R. 1980 The uneasy oesophagus. *Brit. Med. J.* vol 280 334 (L) (5, 197)

El-Omar E. M., Carrington M., Chow W. H., McKoll K. E., Bream J. H. et al. 2000 The role of interleukin-1 polymorphisms in the pathogenesis of gastric cancer. *Nature* 404: 398–402 (2, 116)

El-Omar E. M., Banerjee S., Wirz A. and McColl K. E. L. 1996 The Glasgow Dyspepsia Severity Score–a tool for the global measurement of dyspepsia. *Eur. J. Gastroenterol. & Hepatol.* 8, 967–971 (5, 319)

Espiner H. J., Salmon P. R., Yeague R. H. and Read A. E. 1973 Operative colonoscopy. *Brit. Med. J.* i, 453–454 (6, 72)

Erichsen J. E. 1873 University College Introductory address. *Lancet* ii, 489–490 (2, 17)

Evans A. 1933 A rubber oesophagus. *Brit. J. Surg.* 20; 388–392 (1, 54)

Evans D. J., Pollock D. J. 1972 In-situ and invasive carcinoma of the colon in patients with ulcerative colitis. *Gut* 13: 566–570 (4, 258)

Evans J. G., Acheson E. D. 1965 An epidemiological study of ulcerative colitis and regional ileitis in the Oxford area. *Gut* 6: 311–324 (4, 115)

Evans P. R. C. 1954 The value of strict dieting, drugs and Robaden in peptic ulceration. *Brit. Med. J.* i, 612 (2, 152)

Ewald C. A., Boas J. 1885 Beitrage zur Physiologie und Pathologie der Verdauung. *Arch. F. Path. Anat.*, 101: 325–375 (5, 68)

Eyre J. W. H. 1904 Asylum dysentery in relation to B. dysenteriae. *Brit. Med. J.* i 1002–04 (4, 11)

Fagge C. H. 1872 A case of simple stenosis of the oesophagus, followed by epithelioma. *Guy's Hosp. Reports* 17: 413– 421 (1, 80)

Fairley N. H., Mackie F. P. 1937 The clinical and biochemical syndrome in lymphadenoma and allied diseases involving the mesenteric lymph glands. *Brit. Med. J.* i: 375–380 (3, 111)

Farah D. A., Calder I., Benson L. and Mackenzie J. F. 1985 Specific food intolerance: its place as a cause of gastrointestinal symptoms. *Gut*, 26, 164–8 (5, 293)

Farrington P., Miller E. 1995 Measles vaccination as a risk factor for inflammatory bowel disease. *Lancet* i 1362 (4, 220)

Farthing M. J. G., et al. 1993 Nature and standards of gastrointestinal and liver services in the United Kingdom. Special report of BSG clinical services committee. *Gut*, 34, 1728–39 (6, 144)

Fayrer J. 1881 *Tropical Dysentery and Chronic Diarrhoea.* J & A Churchill, London 121–171 (3, 11)

Feeney M. A., Clegg A. J., Winwood P. J., Snook J. A. 1997 A case-control study of measles vaccination and inflammatory bowel disease. *Lancet* ii 764 -766 (4, 221)

Fellows I. W., Ogilvie A. L., Atkinson M. 1983 Pneumatic dilatation in achalasia. *Gut* 24, 1020–23 (1, 35)

Fenwick S. 1877 Lecture on atrophy of the stomach *Lancet* ii 1–4,39–41, 77–78 (2, 136)

Fenwick S. 1880 *On the Atrophy of the Stomach and on the Nervous Affections of the Digestive Organs.* Churchill, London (2, 137)

Ferguson A., Hutton M. M., Maxwell J. D. 1970 Adult coeliac disease in hyposplenic patients. *Lancet* i: 163–4 (3, 152)

Ferguson A., MacDonald T. T. 1977 Effects of local delayed hypersensitivity on the small intestine. In *Immunology of the Gut*. Ciba Foundation Symposium No 46 p322 (3, 158)

Ferguson A., MacDonald T. T., McClure J. P., Holden R. J. 1975 Cell-mediated immunity to gliadin within the small-intestinal mucosa in celiac disease. *Lancet* i: 895–897 (3, 160)

Ferguson A., Maxwell J. D., Carr K. E. 1969 Progressive changes in small intestinal villous pattern with increasing gestation. *J. Pathology* 99: 87–91 (3, 153)

Ferguson A., Murray D. 1971 Quantitation of intraepithelial lymphocytes in human jejunum. *Gut* 12: 988–994 (3, 155)

Ferguson A., Parrott D. M. V. 1972 The effect of antigen deprivation on thymus-dependent and thymus-independent lymphocytes in the small intestine of the mouse. *Clin. & Exp. Immunol.* 12 477–488 (3, 156)

Ferguson A., Parrott D. M. V. 1973 Histopathology and time course of rejection of allografts of foetal mouse intestine. *Transplantation* 15: 546–554 (3, 157)

Fielding J. F. 1985 "Inflammatory" bowel disease. *Brit. Med. J.* i 47–48 (4, 3)

Fielding J. F. 1986 The relative risk of inflammatory bowel disease among parents and siblings of Crohn's disease patients. *J. Clin. Gastroenterology* 8: 655–657 (4, 128)

Fielding J. F., Prior P., Waterhouse J. A. H., Cooke W. T. 1972 Malignancy in Crohn's disease. *Scand. J. Gastroenterol.* 7: 3–7 (4, 282)

Filipe M. I., Dawson. 1970 The diagnostic value of mucosubstances in rectal biopsies from patients with ulcerative colitis and Crohn's disease. *Gut* 11: 229–234 (4, 234)

Filipe M. I., Ramanchandra S. 1995 The histochemistry of intestinal mucins: changes in disease. In *Gastrintestinal and Oesophageal Pathology*. ed Whitehead R. 2nd edition, Churchill Livingstone, Edinburgh 73–95 (4, 236)

Finch E. 1960 *The Moynihan Chirurgical Club* (1909–59) Annals of the Roy. Coll. Surg. Eng. 26, 180–194 (2, 127)

Fitz R. H. 1886 Perforating inflammation of the vermiform appendix; with special reference to its early diagnosis and treatment. *Trans. Assoc. Am. Physicians* I; 107–144 (5, 80)

Fitzpatrick M. 2004 *MMR and Autism: What Parents Need to Know*. Routledge ISBN 0 415 32179 4 (4, 228)

Fletcher J., Hinton J. M. 1967 Tuberculin sensitivity in Crohn's disease. A controlled study. *Lancet* ii 753–754 (4, 169)

Fletcher P. 1633 *The Purple Island, or The Isle of Man: Together with Piscatorie Eclogs and Other Poeticall Miscellanies.* Cambridge, Universitie of Cambridge. (3, 3)

Flexible Gastroscope, the. 1933 Leading article. *Lancet,* ii, 813 (6, 19)

Florey H. M. 1955 Mucin and the protection of the body. *Proc. Roy. Soc. Lond.* 143: 144–8 (4, 230)

Flynn M., Hammond P., Darby, C., Hyland J. and Taylor I. 1981 Faecal bile acids and the irritable bowel syndrome. *Digestion,* 22: 144–9 (5, 254)

Fone D. J., Cooke W. T., Meynell M. J., Brewer D. B., Harris E. L., Cox EV. 1960 Jejunal biopsy in adult celiac disease and allied disorders. *Lancet* i: 933–938 (3, 89)

Food and the Gut. 1985 edited by Hunter J. O. & Alun Jones V. Addenbrooke's Hosp. Cambridge. Balliere Tindall, Eastbourne (4, 311)

Forbes A., Gabe S., Lennard-Jones J. E., Wilkinson K. 2003 Screening and surveillance for asymptomatic colorectal cancer in inflammatory bowel disease. *Gut* 52: 769 (L) (4, 275)

Ford A. C., Forman D., Bailey A. G., Axon A. T. R. and Moayyedi, P. 2005 A community screening program for Helicobacter pylori saves money: 10 year follow up of a randomised controlled trial. *Gastroenterology* 129, 1910–17 (5, 328)

Ford A. C., Talley N. J., Spiegel B. M. R., Foxx-Orenstein A. E., Schiller, L., Quigley, E. M. M. and Moayyedi, P. 2008 Effect of fibre, antispasmodics, and peppermint oil in the treatment of irritable bowel syndrome: systematic review and meta-analysis. *Brit. Med. J.* 337, 1388–92 (5, 401)

Ford M. J., McMiller P., Eastwood J. and Eastwood M. A. 1987 Life events, psychiatric illness and the irritable bowel syndrome. *Gut,* 28, 160–5 (5, 345)

Fordtran J. S., Santa Ana C. A., Morawski S. G., Bo-Linn G. W. and Schiller L. R. 1986 Pathophysiology of chronic diarrhoea: insights derived from intestinal perfusion studies in 31 patients. *Clinics in Gastroenterology* 15: 3, 477–490 (5, 248)

Forrest A. P. M. 1958 The treatment of duodenal ulcer by gastroenterostomy, gastroenterostomy and vagotomy, and partial gastrectomy. *Gastroenterology* 89: 307–311 (2, 161)

Fox J. A. and Kreel L. 1969 Technique of retrograde colonic intubation and its initial application to high colonic biopsy. *Gut*, 8, 77–82 (6, 67)

Fox J. A. 1969 A fibreoptic colonoscope. *Brit. Med. J.* iii, 50 (6, 68)

Fox J. A. 1971 Fibreoptic colonoscope. *Proceedings of the Royal Society of Medicine*. 64, 1191–92 (6, 69)

Frankel Eugene. 1970 Jacques Babinet. *Dict Scientific Biog*. 1, 357–358 Charles Scribner and Sons, N. Y. (6, 34)

Franklin A. W. 1954 Rickets, In *The History and Conquest of Common Diseases*. ed. by W. R. Bett, University of Oklahoma Press. (3, 27)

Franklin R. H. 1942 Two cases of successful removal of the thoracic oesophagus for carcinoma. *Brit. J. Surg*. 30, 141–6 (1, 60)

Fraser A. G., Orchard T. R., Jewell D. P. 2002 The efficacy of azathioprine for the treatment of inflammatory bowel disease: a 30 year review. *Gut* 50: 485–489 (4, 338)

Frazer A. C. 1951 *Fat Absorption* chapter 21 Steatorrhoea 528–546 (3, 52)

Frazer A. C. 1960 Pathogenetic concepts of the malabsorption syndrome. *Gastroenterology* 38: 389–398 (3, 133)

Frazer A. C., Fletcher R. F., Ross C. A. C., Shaw B., Sammons H. G., Schneider R. 1959 Gluten-induced enteropathy:the effect of partially digested gluten. *Lancet* ii: 252–255 (3, 132)

Frazer A. C., French J. M., Thompson M. D. 1949 Radiographic studies showing the induction of a segmentation pattern in the small intestine in normal human subjects. *Brit. J. Radiol*. 22, 123–136. (3,53)

Freezer C. R. E., Gibson C. S., Matthews E. 1928 Neutralisation of HCl by various alkalies *Guy's Hosp. Reports* lxxviii 191– 197 (2, 123)

French J. M., Hawkins C. F., Smith N. 1957 The effect of a wheat-gluten-free diet in adult idiopathic steatorrhoea. A study of 22 cases. *Quart. J. Med. n.s.* 26, 481–499 (3, 81)

Friend J. 1717 *Hippocratis de Morbis Popularibus* London (5, 9)

Fry L., Seah P. P., McMinn R. M. H., Hoffbrand A. V. 1972 Lymphocytic infiltration of epithelium in diagnosis of gluten-sensitive enteropathy. *Brit. Med. J.* iii: 371–374 (3, 162)

Fullerton G. M., Bell G., and the west of Scotland laparoscopic cholecystectomy audit group. 1994 Prospective audit of the introduction of laparoscopic cholecystectomy in the west of Scotland. *Gut* 35: 1121–26 (4, 350)

Funk C. 1914 *Die Vitamine*. Wiesbaden (3, 30)

Future requirements for colonoscopy in Britain. 1987 Report by the Endoscopy Section Committee of the British Society of Gastroenterology. *Gut,* 28, 772–775 (6, 116)

Fyke F. E., Code C. F., Schlegel J. F. 1956 The gastro-esophageal sphincter in healthy human beings *Gastroenterologia* Basel 86; 135–150 (1, 28)

Gabriel W. B. 1950 Chronic ulcerative colitis with pseudopolyposis terminating in diffuse colloid carcinoma of the colon. *Proceedings of the Royal Society of Medicine* 43: 680–682 (4, 247)

Garlock J. 1940 Surgical treatment of carcinoma of the esophagus. *Arch. Surg.* 41 1184–1214 (1, 59)

Gastroscopy as an established method. 1937 Leading article, *Lancet*, ii, 1200–01 (6, 26)

Gear M.W. L., Wilkinson S. P. 1989 Open access upper alimentary endoscopy. *Brit. J. Hosp. Med.* 41, 438–444 (1, 109)

Gear M.W. L. and Barnes R. J. 1980 Endoscopic studies of dyspepsia in a general *practice Brit. Med. J.* ii 1136–37 (5, 128)

Gear M.W. L., Ormiston M. C., Barnes R. J., Rocyn-Jones J. and Voss, G. C. 1980 Endoscopic studies of dyspepsia in the community: an "open-access" service. *Brit. Med. J.* i, 1135 (6, 90)

Gear M. W. L., Dent N. A., Colin-Jones D. G., Lennard-Jones J. L. and Colley J. R. T. 1990 Future needs for ERCP: incidence of conditions leading to bile duct obstruction and requirements for diagnostic and therapeutic biliary procedures. *Gut* 31, 1150–55 (6, 113)

Gee S. 1868 Rickets. *St. Bart. Hosp. Rep.* 4, 69 (3, 28)

Gee S. 1888 On the coeliac affection. *St. Bart. Hosp. Rep.* 2, 417–20 (3, 1)

Gemmell J. F. 1898 *Idiopathic Colitis (Dysentery).* Balliere, Tindall, and Cox, London ppviii- 140 (4, 9)

Gent A. E., Hellier M. D., Grace R. H., Swarbrick E. T., Coggon D. 1994 Inflammatory bowel disease and domestic hygiene in infancy. *Lancet* i 766–767 (4, 159)

Giaffer M. H., Cann P., Holdsworth C. D. 1991 Long-term effects of elemental and exclusion diets for Crohn's disease. *Alimentary Pharmacology and Therapeutics.* 5: 115–125 (4, 321)

Giaffer M. H., North G., Holdsworth C. D. 1990 Controlled trial of polymeric versus elemental diet in treatment of active Crohn's disease. *Lancet* i 816–818 (4, 319)

Gibbons R. A. 1889 The coeliac affection in children. *Edin. Med. J.* 35: 321–330 and 420–428 (3, 8)

Gibbs D. D. 2000 *John Hunter and the Stomach*. Delivered to the Trustees of the Hunterian Collection: The Royal College of Surgeons (unpublished) (5, 28)

Gibbs D. D. 1997 The Demon of Dyspepsia: Some Nineteenth-Century Perceptions of Disordered Digestion. In *Gastroenterology in Britain: Historical Essays* ed W F Bynum Wellcome Trust p37 (5, 53)

Gibbs D. D. 1968 *Exfoliative Cytology of the Stomach*. Butterworths, London (6, 50)

Gibbs D. D. 1967 Gastric endoscopy. *Hosp Med*, 2, 154–8 (6, 52)

Gibson P. R., Dow E. L., Selby W. S., Strickland R. S., Jewell D. P. 1984 Natural killer cells and spontaneous cell-mediated cytotoxicity in the human intestine. *Clin. Exp. Immunol.* 56: 438–444 (4, 195)

Gibson P. R., Hermanowicz A., Verhaar H. J. J., Ferguson D. P. J., Lopez Bernal A., Jewell D. P. 1985 Isolation of intestinal mononuclear cells: factors released which affect lymphocyte viability and function. *Gut* 26: 60–68 (4, 194)

Gibson P. R., Jewell D. P. 1986 Local immune mechanisms in Inflammatory bowel disease and colorectal carcinoma. Natural killer cells and their activity. *Gastroenterology* 90: 12–19 (4, 196)

Gilat T., Hacohen D., Lilos P., Langman M. J. S. 1987 Childhood factors in ulcerative colitis and Crohn's disease. An international cooperative study. *Scand. J. Gastroenterol.* 22: 1009–24 (4, 157)

Gilford H. 1893 A case of perforated gastric ulcer for which gastrorrhaphy was performed: death on the 31st day. *Brit. Med. J.* i, 944–946 (2, 18)

Gill A. M. 1947 Pain and the healing of peptic ulcers. *Lancet* i: 291 (2, 145)

Gill W. G. 1939 Regional ileitis (Crohn's disease) 5. Two cases of acute regional ileitis treated conservatively. *Guy's Hosp. Reports* 89: 77–79 (4, 55)

Gill R. C., Kellow, J. E., Browning, C. and Wingate, D. L. 1990 The use of intraluminal strain-gauges for recording ambulant small bowel motility. *Amer. J. Physiol.* 258; G 610–15 (5, 239)

Gillen C. D., Andrews H. A., Prior P., Allan R. N. 1994 Crohn's disease and colorectal cancer. *Gut* 35: 651–655 (4, 286)

Gillen C. D., Walmsley R. S., Prior P., Andrews H. A., Allan R. N. 1994 A comparison of the colorectal cancer risk in extensive colitis. *Gut* 35: 1590–92 (4, 287)

Gilvarry J., Buckley M. J. M., Hamilton H. and O'Morain C. A. 1997 Eradication of Helicobacter pylori affects symptoms in non-ulcer dyspepsia. *Scand. J. Gastroenterol.* 32: 535–540 (5, 318)

Ginzberg L. 1986 Regional enteritis: historical perspective. *Gastrenterology* 90: 1310–11 (4, 41)

Girdwood R. H., Delamore I. W., Williams A. W. 1961 Jejunal biopsy in malabsorptive disorders of the adult. *Brit. Med. J.* i; 319–323 (3, 98)

Glenard F. 1885 Application de la methode naturelle a l'analyse de la dyspepsie nerveuse; determination d'une espece. *Lyon Med.,* 48:449–464; 492–505; 532–543; 563–583 (5, 83)

Goldgraber M. B., Humphreys E. M., Kirsner J. B., Palmer W. L. 1958 Carcinoma and ulcerative colitis: a clinical-pathologic study II Statistical analysis. *Gastroenterology* 34: 840–846 (4, 246)

Goligher J. C., Pulvertaft C. N., de Dombal F. T.,Conyers J. H., Duthie H. L., Feather D. B., Latchmore A. J. C., Harrop Shoesmith J., Smiddy F. G., Willson-Pepper J. 1968 Five- to Eight-year results of Leeds/York controlled trial of elective surgery for duodenal ulcer. *Brit. Med. J.* i: 781–789 (2, 162)

Goligher J. C., Hoffmann D. C., deDombal F. T. 1970 Surgical treatment of severe attacks of ulcerative colitis, with special reference to the advantages of early operation. *Brit. Med. J.* ii 703–706 (4, 84)

Gomborone J. E., Dewsnap P. A., Libby G. W. and Farthing M. J. G. 1993 Community study reveals that dysfunctional illness attitudes in irritable bowel syndrome are not wholly a reflection of patient status. *Gastroenterology,* 104, A:153 (5, 356)

Gomborone J. E., Dewsnap P. A., Libby G. W. and Farthing M. J. G. 1995 Abnormal illness attitudes in irritable bowel syndrome. *J. Psychosom. Res.* 39, 227–230 (5, 357)

Gomborone J. E., Dewsnap P. A., Libby G. W. and Farthing M. J. G. 1993 Selective affective biasing in recognition memory in the irritable bowel syndrome. *Gut,* 34, 1230–33 (5, 358)

Gomez J. and Dally P. 1977 Psychologically mediated abdominal pain in surgical and medical outpatient clinics. *Brit. Med. J.* i 1451–53 (5, 338)

Goode A., Hawkins T., Feggetter J. G. W., Johnston I. D. A. 1976 Use of an elemental diet for long-term nutritional support in Crohn's disease. *Lancet* i 122–4 (4, 296)

Goodhart J. F. 1905 *The Diseases of Children.* ed by G. F. Still 8th edition J & A Churchill, London 111–2 (5, 335)

Gorard D. A., Gomborone J. E., Libby G. W. and Farthing M. J. G. 1996 Intestinal transit in anxiety and depression. *Gut,* 39,551–555 (5, 359)

Gorard D. A., Libby G. W. and Farthing M. J. G. 1994 Influence of antidepressants on whole gut and orocaecal transit times in health and irritable bowel syndrome. *Alimentary Pharmacology and Therapeutics* 8. 159–166 (5, 394)

Gordon-Taylor G., Hudson R. V., Dodds E. C., Warner J. L. and Whitby L. E. H. 1929 The remote results of gastrectomy. *Brit. J. Surg.* 16, 641–667 (2, 140)

Gordon-Taylor G. 1943 Leonard Braithwaite(O) *Brit. Med. J.* i 24 (2, 126)

Gore S., Healy C. J., Sutton R., Eyre-Brook I. A., Gear M. W. L., Shepherd N. A., Wilkinson S. P. 1993 Regression of columnar lined (Barrett's) oesophagus with continuous omeprazole therapy. *Alimentary Pharmacology and Therapeutics* 7 623–628 (1, 110)

Gore S., Gilmore I. T., Haigh C. G., Brownless S. M., Stockdale H. and Morris, A. I. 1990 Colonic transit in man is slowed by ondansetron (GR38032F), a selective 5-hydroxytryptamine receptor (type 3) antagonist. *Alimentary Pharmacology and Therapeutics* 4, 139–144 (5, 381)

Gough K. R., Read A. E., Naish J. M. 1962 Intestinal reticulosis as a complication of idiopathic steatorrhoea. *Gut* 3: 232–239 (3, 113)

Gould G. M. 1903 *Biographic Clinics: the Origin of the Ill-health of De Quincy, Carlyle, Darwin, Huxley and Browning*. Rebman Limited, London (5, 61 and 5, 63)

Grace P., Quereshi A., Darzi A., et al. 1991 Laparoscopic cholecystectomy: 100 consecutive cases. *Irish Med. J.* 84: 12–14 (4, 351)

Grant W. 1779 *Some Observations on the Origins, Progress, and Method of Treating the Atrabilious Temperament and Gout*. London Printed for T. Cadell in the Strand. (5, 30)

Graves R. J. 1824 An account of the chemical properties of an acid found in the human stomach, together with remarks upon the manner in which it is formed both in disease and in health. *Trans. Assoc. Fell. Licen. Kings Queens Coll. Phys. Ireland* 4, 316–331 (2, 8)

Green J. R. B., Lobo A. J., Holdsworth C. D., Leicester R. J., Gibson J. A., Kerr G. D., Hodgson J. H. F., Parkins K. J., Taylor M. D. and the Abacus Investigator Group. 1997 Balsalazide is more effective and better tolerated than mesalazine in the treatment of acute ulcerative colitis. *Gastroenterology* 114: 1–10 (4, 107)

Greenberg G. R., Fleming C. R., Jeejeebhoy K. N., Rosenberg I. H., Sales D., Tremaine W. J. 1988 Controlled trial of bowel rest and nutritional support in the management of Crohn's disease. *Gut* 29: 1309–15 (4, 209 and 295)

Gregory R. A.,Tracy H. J. 1959 *J. Physiol.* 149: 58P & 70P (2, 45)

Gregory R. A., Tracy H. J. 1961 *J. Physiol.* 156: 523 (2, 47)

Gregory R. A., Tracy H. J., French J. M., Sircus W. 1960 Extraction of a gastrin-like substance from a pancreatic tumour in a case of Zollinger-Ellison syndrome. *Lancet* i 1045–48 (2, 48)

Greig M. A., Neithercut W. D., Hossack M., MacDonald A. M. I., El Nujumi A. M., McColl K. E. L. 1990 Suicidal destruction of H. pylori mediated by its urease activity. *Gut* 31: A600 (2, 201)

Griffith G. H., Owen G. M., Kirkman S. And Shields R. 1966 Measurement of rate of gastric emptying using chromium-51. *Lancet*, i, 1244–45 (5, 199)

Gull W. 1855 Fatty stools from disease of the mesenteric glands. *Guy's Hosp. Reports.* i: 369 (3, 6)

Gully J. M. 1846 *The Water Cure in Chronic Disease.* John Churchill, London (5, 55)

Guthrie E., Creed F. H., Dawson D. and Tomenson B. 1993 A controlled trial of psychological treatment for the irritable bowel syndrome. *Br. J. Psychiatry*, 163, 315–321 (5, 367)

Gwee K. A., Collins S. M., Read N. W., Rajnakova A., Deng Y., Graham, J. C., McKendrick M. W. and Moochhala S. M. 2003 Increased rectal mucosal expression of interleukin 1B in recently acquired post-infectious irritable bowel syndrome. *Gut*, 52, 523–526 (5, 308)

Gwee K. A., Leong Y. L., Graham C., McKendrick M. W., Collins S. M., Walters S. J., Underwood J. E. and Read N. W. 1999 The role of psychological and biological factors in post-infective gut dysfunction. *Gut*, 44, 400–406 (5, 306)

Gwyn Williams, D., Truelove, S. C., Gear, M. W. L., Massarella, G. R. and Fitzgerald, N. W. 1968 Gastroscopy with biopsy and cytological sampling under direct vision. *Brit. Med. J.* i,535–539 (6, 54)

Gyde S. N. 1990 Screening for colorectal cancer in ulcerative colitis: dubious benefits and high costs. *Gut* 31: 1089–92 (4, 269)

Gyde S. N., Prior P., Allan R. N., Stevens A., Jewell D. P., Truelove S. C., Lofberg R., Brostrom O., Hellers G. 1988 Colorectal cancer in ulcerative colitis: a cohort study of primary referrals from three centres. *Gut* 29: 206–217 (4, 268)

Gyde S. N., Prior P., Macartney J. C., Thompson H., Waterhouse J. A. H., Allan R. N. 1980 Malignancy in Crohn's disease. *Gut* 21: 1024–29 (4, 285)

Gyde S. N., Prior P., Thompson H., Waterhouse J. A. H., Allan R. N. 1984 Survival of patients with colorectal cancer complicating ulcerative colitis. *Gut* 25: 228–231 (4, 266)

Haas S. V. 1924 The value of the banana in the treatment of celiac disease. *Amer J. Dis. Child* 24: 421–437 (3, 65)

Hadfield G. 1939 The primary histological lesion of regional ileitis. *Lancet* ii 773–775 (4, 57)

Hadley G. D. 1965 The gastrocamera. *Brit. Med. J.* ii,1209–12 (5, 124)

Hale-White W. 1888 On simple ulcerative colitis and other rare intestinal ulcers. *Guy's Hosp. Reports*. 14: 131–162. (4, 8)

Hale-White W. 1935 *Great Doctors of the Nineteenth Century*. E Arnold & Co. London p236 (4, 8)

Hamilton Bailey and Bishop W. J. 1946 *Notable Names in Medicine and Surgery* H. K. Lewis, London p10 (1, 8)

Hampson A. C., Shackle J. W. 1924 Megalocytic and non-mgalocytic anaemias. *Guy's Hosp. Reports* 74: 193–216 (3, 40)

Hannay A. J. 1833 An Extraordinary Dilatation (with hypertrophy?) of all the Thoracic Portions of the Oesophagus causing Dysphagia. *Edin. Med. and Surg. Journal* XL 65–72 (1, 11)

Hancock P. E. T. and Shiner M. 1958 Combined gastroscopy and gastric biopsy under direct vision. *Lancet*, i, 1204–05 (6, 32)

Hans Herlinger with Laurel Marshfield 2005 *A Dream Surpassing Every Impasse: Becoming a Doctor Against all the Odds: As an Austrian Jew, on the Eve of World War 2, a Memoir.* Blue Horizon Communications. (6, 92)

Hardcastle J. D., Chamberlain J. O., Robinson M. H. E., Moss S. M., Amar S. S., Balfour T. W., James P. D and Mangham C. M. 1996 Randomised controlled trial of faecal occult-blood-screening for colorectal cancer. *Lancet*, 348, 1472–77 (6, 150)

Hardwicke C. 1939 Prognosis in coeliac disease: a review of seventy-threee cases. *Arch. Dis. Child* 14: 279–294 (3, 77)

Hardy T. L., Brooke B. N., Hawkins C. F. 1949 Ileostomy and ucerative colitis. *Lancet* ii 5–9 (4, 74)

Hardy T. L., Bulmer E. 1933 Ulcerative colitis. A survey of ninety-five cases. *Brit. Med. J.* ii 812–815 (4,34) Harmer M., Bailey A. G. S. 1986 Crohn's disease: two fortunate young men. *Lancet* ii 94–96 (4, 56)

Harper A. A. 1946 The effect of extracts of gastric and intestinal mucosa on the secretion hydrochloric acid by the cat's stomach. *J. Physiol.* 105:31P (2, 46)

Harper P. H., Lee E. C. G., Kettlewell M. G. W., Bennett M. K., Jewell D. P. 1985 Role of the faecal stream in the maintenance of Crohn's colitis. *Gut* 26: 279–284 (4, 205)

Harper P. H., Truelove S. C. Lee E. C. G., Kettlewell M. G. W., Jewell D. P. 1983 Split ileostomy and ileocolostomy for Crohn's disease of the colon and ulcerative colitis: a 20 year survey. *Gut* 24: 106–113 (4, 204)

Harries A. D., Baird A., Rhodes J. 1982 Non-smoking: a feature of ulcerative colitis. *Brit. Med. J.* i 706 (4, 151)

Harris F. I., Bell G. H., Brunn H. 1933 Chronic cicatrizing enteritis. Regional ileitis (Crohn). A new surgical entity. *Surg. Gynae. Obstet.* 57: 637–645 (4, 43)

Harris O. D., Cooke W. T., Thompson H., Waterhouse J. A. H. 1967 Malignancy in Adult Coeliac Disease and Idiopathic Steatorrhoea. *Amer. J. Med.* 42: 899–912 (3, 116 and 3, 200)

Harvey R. F., Bradshaw J. M. 1980 A simple index of Crohn's disease activity. *Lancet* i 514–515 (4, 304)

Harvey R. F. and Read A. E. 1973 Effect of cholecystokinin on colonic motility and symptoms in patients with the irritable bowel syndrome. *Lancet*,i: 1–3 (5, 181 and 5, 213)

Harvey R. F., Brown N. J. G., Mackie D. B., Keeling D. H. and Davies W. T. 1970 Measurement of gastric emptying time with a gamma camera. *Lancet*, i, 16–18 (5, 200)

Harvey R. F., Pomare E. W. and Heaton K. W. 1973 Effects of increased dietary fibre on intestinal transit. *Lancet*, i: 1278–80 (5, 182)

Harvey R. F., Salih S. Y. and Read A. E. 1983 Organic and functional disorders in 2000 gastroenterological outpatients. *Lancet*, i, 632–634 (5, 133 and 5, 271)

Hawkey C. J., Hawthorne A. B., Hudson N., Cole A. T., Mahida Y. R., Daneshmend T. K. 1991 Separation of the impairment of haemostasis by asprin from mucosal injury in the human stomach. *Clin. Sci.* 81, 565–573 (2, 93)

Hawkins H. P. 1909 An address on the natural history of ulcerative colitis and its bearing on treatment. *Brit. Med. J.* i 765–770 (4, 17)

Hawkins H. P. 1906 The reality of enterospasm and its mimicry of appendicitis. *Brit. Med. J.* i, 65–69 (5, 96)

Hawthorne A. B., Logan R. F. A., Hawkey C. J. 1989 Azathioprine in resistant ulcerative colitis. *Gastroenterology* 96: A201 (4, 336)

Hawthorne A. B., Logan R. F. A., Hawkey C. J., Foster P. N., Axon A. T. R., Swarbrick E. T., Scott B. B., Lennard-Jones J. E. 1992 Randomised controlled trial of azathioprine withdrawal in ulcerative colitis. *Brit. Med. J.* ii 20–22 (4, 337)

Heading R. C., Tothill P., McLoughlin G. P. and Shearman D. J. C. 1976 Gastric emptying rate measurement in man. A double isotope scanning technique for simultaneous study of liquid and solid components of a meal. *Gastroenterology*, 71, 45–50 (5, 201)

Heaton K. W. 1969 Keeping bile salts in their place. *Gut* 10, 857–863 (5, 180)

Heaton K. W. 1981 Is bran useful in diverticular disease? *Brit. Med. J.* 283.1523–24 (5, 286)

Heaton K. W. 1989 The Rev Hubert Carey Trowell. *Monk's Roll* vol IX 533–536 (5, 165)

Heaton K. W., Ghosh S. and Braddon F. E. M. 1991 How bad are the symptoms and bowel dysfunction of patients with the irritable bowel syndrome? A prospective, controlled study with emphasis on stool form. *Gut*, 32, 73–79 (5, 267)

Heaton K. W., O'Donnell L. J., Braddon F. E., Mountford R. A., Hughes, A. O. and Cripps, P. J. 1992 Symptoms of irritable bowel syndrome in a British urban community: Consulters and non-consulters. *Gastroenterology*, 102, 1962–67 (5, 353)

Heller E. 1914 Extra-mukosa Cardioplastik beim chronischen Cardiospasmus etc *Mittheil A. d. Grenzgeb. D. Med. U. Chir.* Lvii s 141–9 (1, 19)

Van Helmont I. B. 1648 *Sextuplex Digestio Alimenti Humani*, Ortus Medicinae, Amsterdam p208 (5, 13)

Henning N. 1932 Erfahrungen mit dem flexible Gastroskop nach Wolf-Schindler. *Munchen med Weschr* 32, 1269–71 (6, 17)

Henry D. A. Sharpe G., Chaplain S., Cartwright S., Kitchingman G., Bell G. D. and Langman M. J. 1979 The (14c) – breath test. A comparison of different forms of analysis. *Br. J. Clin. Phar.* 8: 539–545 (2, 192)

Henson G. F., Rob C. G. 1955 Duodenal ulcer treated by vagotomy and gastro-enterostomy. Results of 100 consecutive cases. *Brit. Med. J.* ii: 588–589 (2, 160)

Hermon Taylor 1941 A new gastroscope with controllable flexibility. *Lancet*, ii, 276–277 (6, 29)

Hermon-Taylor J., Barnes N., Clarke C., Finlayson C. 1998 Mycobacterium paratuberculosis cervical lymphadenitis, followed five years later by terminal ileitis similar to Crohn's disease. *Brit. Med. J.* i 449–452 (4, 148)

Hern J. R. B. 1931 Ulcerative colitis. *Guy's Hosp. Reports* 81: 322–373 (4, 33)

Herodotus 1992 *The Histories* Book Two chap 77. The Folio Society, London (5, 71)

Herter C. A. 1908 *Infantilism From Chronic Intestinal Infection*. Macmillan New York (3, 13)

Heubner J. O. L. 1909 *Jahrb. f. Kinderheilk* Berlin 70 667 (3, 14)

Hill O. W. and Blendis L. M. 1967 Physical and psychological evaluation of "non-organic" abdominal pain. *Gut*, 8, 221–229 (5, 337)

Hill W. 1909 The gastroscope and its uses. *Brit. Med. J.* ii, 1096–97 (6, 12)

Hill W. 1912 *On Gastroscopy* John Bale, Sons and Danielsson, Ltd. Oxford House, London (6, 13)

Hin H., Bird G., Fisher P., Jewell D. P. 1999 Coeliac disease in primary care: a case finding study. *Brit. Med. J.* 318, 164–7 (3, 226)

Hinton J. M. 1966 Risk of malignant change in ulcerative colitis. *Gut* 7: 427–432 (4, 254)

Hinton J. M., Lennard-Jones J. E. & Young A. C. 1969 A new method for studying gut transit times using radiopaque markers. *Gut*, 10, 842–847 (5, 161 and 5, 205)

Hirschowitz B. I. 1961 Endoscopic examination of the stomach and duodenal cap with the fibrescope. *Lancet*, i, 1074–78 (6, 45)

Hirschowitz B. I. 1963 A fibre optic flexible oesophagoscope. *Lancet*, ii, 388 (6, 49)

Hirschowitz B. I. 1979 A personal history of the Fiberscope. *Gastroenterology* 76, 864–869 (6, 44)

Hoare A. M. 1975 Comparative study between endoscopy and radiology in acute upper gastrointestinal haemorrhage. *Brit. Med. J.* i, 27–30 (6, 104)

Hoare A. M. and Hawkins C. F. 1976 Upper gastrointestinal endoscopy with and without sedation: patients' opinions. *Brit. Med. J.* ii, 20 (6, 126)

Hobbs J. R., Hepner G. W. 1968 Deficiency of M-globulin in coeliac disease. *Lancet* i: 217–220 (3, 209)

Hobbs J. R., Hepner G. W., Douglas A. P., Crabbe P. A., Johansson S. G. O. 1969 Immunological mystery of coeliac disease. *Lancet* ii: 649–650 (3, 141)

Hobson A. R. and Aziz Q. 2004 Brain imaging and functional gastrointestinal disorders: has it helped our understanding? *Gut*, 53, 1198–1206 (5, 400)

Hodgson H. J. F., Potter B. J., Skinner J., Jewell D. P. 1978 Immune-complex mediated colitis in rabbits: an experimental model. *Gut* 19: 225–232 (4, 181)

Hodgson H. J. F., Wand J. R., Isselbacher. 1978 Decreased suppressor cell activity in inflammatory bowel disease. *Clin. Exp. Immunol.* 32: 451–458 (4, 189)

Holborow E. J., Weir D. M., Johnson G. D. 1957 A serum factor in Lupus Erythematosus with affinity for tissue nuclei. *Brit. Med. J.* ii: 732–734 (3, 214)

Holdstock D. J., Misiewicz J. J. and Waller S. L. 1969 Observations on the mechanism of abdominal pain. *Gut*, 10, 19–31 (5, 150 and 5, 340)

Holdstock G. 1978 Jejunal biopsy without the need for screening. *Lancet* i: 1236–37 (3, 189)

Holdstock G., Eade O. E., Isaacson P., Smith C. L. 1979 Endoscopic duodenal biopsies in coeliac disease and duodenitis. *Scand. J. Gastroenterology.* 14: 717–720 (3, 191)

Holdstock G., Wiseman M., Loehry C. A. 1979 Open-access endoscopy service for general practitioners. *Brit. Med. J.* i 457–459 (5, 129)

Holdsworth C. D. and Atkinson M. 1984 Gastroenterology services: a regional review. *Brit. Med. J.* i, 1245–47 (6, 117)

Holdsworth C. D. 1985 Drug treatment of irritable bowel syndrome. In *Irritable Bowel Syndrome* ed Read, N. W. Grune and Stratton, 223–232 (5, 270)

Holmes G. K. T., Prior P., Lane M.R., Pope D., Allan R. N. 1989 Malignancy in coeliac disease: effect of a gluten-free diet. *Gut* 30, 333–338 (3, 199)

Holmes G. K. T., Stokes P. L., Sorahan T. M., Prior P., Waterhouse J. A. H., Cooke W. T. 1976 Coeliac disease, gluten-free diet, and malignancy. *Gut* 17: 612–619 (3, 201)

Holmes R., Hourihane D. O'B., Booth C. C. 1961 Dissecting microscope appearance of jejunal biopsy specimens from patients with idiopathic steatorrhoea. *Lancet* i: 81–83 (3, 102)

Hopkins H. H. and Kapany N. 1954 A flexible fibrescope using static scanning. *Nature*, 173, 39–41 (6, 40)

Horrocks Jane C. & de Dombal F. T. 1975 Computer-aided diagnosis of "dyspepsia". *Dig. Dis. Sci.* 20, Number 5 397–406 (5, 132)

Horton R. 2004 *MMR: Science and Fiction. Exploring the Vaccine Crisis.* Granta books ISBN 1 86207 764 9 (4, 227)

Horton R. 2001 Lotronex and the FDA: a fatal erosion of integrity. *Lancet*, 357, 1544–45 (5, 390)

Hospital Doctors Training for the Future. 1993 Report of the Working Group on Specialist Medical Training. Calman Implementation Steering Group HMSO (6, 145)

Houghton E. A. W., Naish J. M. 1958 Familial ulcerative colitis and ileitis. *Gastroenterologia* (Basel) 89: 65–74 (4, 113)

Houghton L. A. and Whorwell P. J. 2005 Towards a better understanding of abdominal bloating and distension in functional bowel disorders. *Neurogastroenterol. Motil.* 17, 500–511 (5, 393)

Houghton, L. A., Atkinson, W., Whitaker, R. P., Whorwell, P. J. and Rimmer, M. J. 2003 Increased platelet depleted plasma 5-hydroxytryptamine concentration following meal ingestion in symptomatic female subjects with diarrhoea predominant irritable bowel syndrome. *Gut*, 52, 663–670 (5, 387)

Houghton L. A., Brown, H., Atkinson W., Morris, J., Fell C., Whorwell P. J., Lockhart S. and Keevil B. 2009 5-hydroxytryptamine signalling in irritable bowel syndrome with diarrhoea: effects of gender and menstrual status. *Alimentary Pharmacology and Therapeutics* 30, 919-929 (5, 388)

Houghton L. A., Calvert E. L., Jackson N. A., Cooper P. and Whorwell P. J. 2002 Visceral sensation and emotion: a study using hypnosis. *Gut*, 51, 701–704 (5, 361)

Houghton L. A., Heyman D. J. and Whorwell P. J. 1996 Symptomatology, quality of life and economic features of irritable bowel syndrome – the effect of hypnotherapy. *Alimentary Pharmacology and Therapeutics* 10, 91–95 (5, 297)

Howdle P. D., Ciclitira P. J., Simpson F. G., Losowsky M. S. 1981 Are all gliadins toxic in coeliac diseae? *Gut* 22: A 874 (3, 184)

Howdle P. D., Corazza G. R., Bullen A. W., Losowsky M. S. 1981 In-vitr diagnosis of coeliac disease: an assessment. *Gut* 22; 939–947 (3, 171)

Howdle P. D., Zajdel M. E., Smart C. J., Trejdosiewicz L. K., Blair G. E., Losowsky M. S. 1989 Lack of a serologic response to an EIB protein of adenovirus 12 in coeliac disease. *Scand. J. Gastroenterol.* 24: 282–6 (3, 179)

Howel-Evans W., McConnell R. B., Clarke C. A., Sheppard P. M. 1958 Carcinoma of the oesophagus with keratosis palmaris et plantaris (tylosis). A study of two families. *Quart. J. Med* 27 413– 429 (1, 79)

Howship, J. 1830 *Practical Remarks on the Discrimination and Successful Treatment of Spasmodic Stricture in the Colon Considered as an Occasional Cause of Habitual Confinement of the Bowels*. London (5, 73)

Hubble D. V. 1963 Diagnosis and management of coeliac disease in childhood. *Brit. Med. J.* ii: 701–6 (3, 93)

Hubble D. 1943 Charles Darwin and psychotherapy. *Lancet*, 30th Jan 129–33 (5, 57)

Hudson M., Chitolie A., Hutton R. A., Smith M. S. H., Pounder R. E., Wakefield A. J. 1996 Thrombotic vascular risk factors in inflammatory bowel disease. *Gut* 38: 733–737 (4, 215)

Hudson T. 2004 Thompson Hancock, P. E. (O) *Monk's Roll* XI 240 (6, 24)

Hugot J. P., Chamaillard M. et al 2000 Association of NOD 2 leucine-rich repeat variants in susceptibility to Crohn's disease. *Nature* 411: 599–603 (4, 145)

Hugot J. P., Laurent-Puig P. et al 1996 Mapping of a susceptibility locus for Crohn's disease on chromosome 16. *Nature* 379: 821–823 (4, 141)

Huibregstse J., Haverkamp H. J. and Tytgat G. T. 1981 Transpapillary positioning of a large 3.2 mm biliary endoprosthesis. *Endoscopy*, 13, 217–219 (6, 111)

Humphries H., Bourke S., Dooley C., McKenna D., Power B., Keane C. T., Sweeney E. C., O'Morain C. 1988 Effect of treatment on Campylobacter pylori in peptic ulcer disease: a randomised prospective trial. *Gut* 29: 279–283 (2, 190)

Hunt J. N. 1959 Gastric emptying and secretion in man. *Physiol. Rev.* 39: 491–533 (2, 37)

Hunt J. N and Spurrell, W. R. 1951 The pattern of emptying of the human stomach. *J. Physiol.* (Lond) 113; 151–168 (5, 198)

Hunt T. C. 1972 Symposium on carbenoloxone. *Br. Med. Week.* Tokyo (2, 154)

Hunter J. 1772 On the stomach itself being digested after death. *Phil. Trans. R. Soc.* 62: 447–454 (2, 6 and 5, 26)

Hunter J. O. 1991 Food allergy–or enterometabolic disorder? *Lancet* ii 495–496 (4, 315 and 5, 292)

Hunter J. O. 1985 Irritable bowel syndrome. *Proc. Nutr. Soc.* 44, 141–3 (5, 291)

Hurst A., Morton C. J., Cook F., Cox A. N., Gardiner N., Schlesinger E. G., Todd A. H. 1907 The passage of food along the human alimentary canal. *Guy's Hosp. Reports*, 61, 85–110 (1, 2) (5, 97)

Hurst A. F., Cook, F., Schlesinger E. G. 1908 The sensibility of the stomach and intestines in man. *J. Physiol.* (London) 37, 481–490 (5, 101)

Hurst A. 1909 Duodenal ulcer *Guy's Hosp.Gaz.* 23: 332–335 (2, 25)

Hurst A. F. 1910 A clinical lecture on muco-membranous colitis. *Clinical Journal* 36: 263–267 (4, 12 and 25) (5, 87 and 103 and 105)

Hurst A. F. 1911 *The Goulstonian Lectures on the Sensibility of the Alimentary Canal.* Oxford University Press, London (5, 102)

Hurst A. F. 1913 Bastedo's sign: a new symptom of chronic appendicitis. *Lancet,* i, 816–817 (5, 94)

Hurst A. F. 1913 Discussion following Jordan's paper. *Brit. Med. J.* Oct 11th 915–918 (1, 14)

Hurst A. F. 1915 Achalasia of the cardia. *Quart. J. Med.* 8, 300–308 (1, 3)

Hurst A. F. 1919 *Constipation and Allied Intestinal Disorders.* Oxford University Press 2nd edit. p101 (5, 99)

Hurst A. F. 1921 Ulcerative colitis. *Guy's Hosp. Reports* 71; 26–41 (4, 27)

Hurst A. F. 1922 An address on the sins and sorrows of the colon. (Delivered before the Harrogate Medical Society,November 26th, 1921.) *Brit. Med. J.,* i, 941–943 (5, 107)

Hurst A. F. 1922 Chronic appendicitis and appendicular dyspepsia. *Guy's Hosp. Reports.* 72, 386–399 (5, 92)

Hurst A. F., Rowlands R. P. 1924 Case of achalasia of the cardia relieved by operation. *Proceedings of the Royal Society of Medicine* (clin section) xvii No 1045 (1, 20)

Hurst A. F. 1924 *Essays and Addresses on Digestive and Nervous Diseases and on Addisons's Anaemia and Asthma.* Heinemann, London, p110. (1, 4)

Hurst A. F. 1925 Is medical or surgical treatment indicated for ulcerative colitis? *Guy's Hosp. Reports* 75: 48–50 (4, 29)

Hurst A. F. 1926 A discussion on the diagnosis and treatment of colitis. *Lancet* ii 1151–54 (4, 24 and 26 and 32) (6, 61)

Hurst A., Stewart M. J. 1929 *Gastric and Duodenal Ulcer.* Oxford Med. Pub p48 (2, 26)

Hurst A., Stewart M. J. 1929 *Gastric and Duodenal Ulcer.* Oxford Med Pub p59 (2, 29)

Hurst A. F., Stewart M. J. 1929 *Gastric and Duodenal Ulcer* Ox. Med Pub p387 (2, 121)

Hurst A. F., Stewart M. J. 1929 *Gastric and Duodenal Ulcer* p438 (2, 125 and 132)

Hurst A. F., Stewart M .J. 1929 *Gastric and Duodenal Ulcer.* Pp 69–70 (2, 71)

Hurst A. F. and Stewart M. J. 1929 Diagnosis from reflex dyspepsias. In: *Gastric and Duodenal Ulcer*. Oxford University Press 234–237 (5, 95)

Hurst A. H., Rake G. W. 1930 Achalasia of the cardia. *Quart. J. Med.* 23; 491–508 (1, 81)

Hurst A. F. 1930 "Mythical maladies." *Clinical Journal* 59: p282 (5, 116)

Hurst A. F. 1930 "Mythical maladies." *Clinical Journal* 59: 277–283 (5, 117)

Hurst A. F. 1935 Prognosis of ulcerative colitis. *Lancet* ii 1194–96 (4, 35)

Hurst A. F. 1935 Ulcerative colitis. *Guy's Hosp. Reports* 85: 317–355 (4, 37 and 244)

Hurst A. F. 1937 Observation and experiment and the physiology of the stomach. *Brit. Med. J.* ii, 785–789 (6, 25)

Hurst A. F., Lintott G. A. M. 1939 Aspirin as a cause of haematemesis: a clinical and gastroscopic study. *Guy's Hosp. Reports.* 89, 173–6 (2, 77)

Hurst A. F. 1941 Aspirin and Gastric Haemorrhage. *Brit. Med. J.* (L) i: 768 (2, 78)

Hurst A. F. 1942 Severe case of the sprue syndrome. *Guy's Hosp. Reports* 91: 22–24 (3, 48)

Hurst A. F. 1942 The pathogenesis of the sprue syndrome as seen in tropical sprue, non-tropical sprue and coeliac disease. *Guy's Hosp. Reports.* 91: 1–21 (3, 47)

Hurst A. F. 1949 *A Twentieth Century Physician, Being the Reminiscences of Sir Arthur Hurst*. E Arnold and Copp, London 120–1 (5, 100)

Hutchinson T., Wilks S. & Clark A. 1857 Tubular Exudation Casts of the Intestine. *Trans. Pathol. Soc.* Vol 9: 188–194 (5, 77)

Huxley L. (ed) 1900 *Life and Letters of Thomas Henry Huxley* 2 vols. Appleton and Company, New York (5, 62)

Hywel Jones J. 1969 Colonic cancer and Crohn's disease. *Gut* 10: 651–654 (4, 281)

Iftikhar S. Y., James P. D., Steele R. J. C., Hardcastle J. D., Atkinson M. 1992 Length of Barrett's oesophagus: an important factor in the development of dysplasia and adenocarcinoma. *Gut* 33 1155–58 (1, 105)

Illingworth C. F. W., Scott L. D. W., Jamieson R. A. 1944 Acute perforated peptic ulcer. *Brit. Med. J.* 2: 617–620 & 655–658 (2, 56)

Ireland A., Mason C. H., Jewell D. P. 1988 Controlled trial comparing olsalazine and sulphasalazine for the maintenance treatment of ulcerative colitis. *Gut* 29: 835–837 (4, 103)

Jackman W. A. 1934 Localised hypertrophic enteritis as a cause of intestinal obstruction with a report of two cases. *Brit. J. Surg.* 21: 112–3 (4, 51)

Jackson C. 1929 Peptic ulcer of the oesophagus *J.A.M.A.* 92; 369–372 (1, 84)

James A. H. 1951 Duodenal intubation with magnet-tipped tubes. *Lancet* i 209–10 (2, 38)

James A. H. 1977 Breakfast and Crohn's disease. *Brit. Med. J.* i 943–945 (4, 149)

James A. H., Pickering G. W. 1949 Role of gastric acidity in pathogenesis of peptic ulcer. *Clin. Sci.* 8: 181–210 (2, 39)

Jamieson R. A. 1955 Acute perforated peptic ulcer – frequency and incidence in West of Scotland. *Brit. Med. J.* 222–227 (2, 157)

Janossy G.,Tidman N., Selby W. S., Thomas J. A., Grainger. Kung, P. C.,Goldstein G. 1980 Human T-lymphocytes of inducer and suppressor type occupy different microenvironments. *Nature* 288: 81– 84 (3, 168) (4, 186)

Jewell D. P., MacLennan I. C. M. 1973 Immune complexes in inflammatory bowel disease. *Clin. Exp. Immunol.* 14: 219–226 (4, 167)

Jewell D. P., Truelove S. C. 1974 Azathioprine in ulcerative colitis: final report on controlled therapeutic trial. *Brit. Med. J.* ii 627–630 (4, 334)

Johnson J. 1827 *Essay on Morbid Sensibility of the Stomach and Bowels, as the Proximate Cause, or Characteristic Condition of Indigestion, Nervous Irritability, Mental Despondency, Hypochondriasis, etc. etc.* American edition published by Benjamin & Thomas Kite, Philadelphia. (5, 41)

Johnston D. 1975 Operative mortality and postoperative morbidity of highly selective vagotomy. *Brit. Med. J.* iv 545–547 (2, 167)

Johnston D., Goligher J. C., Pulvertaft C. N., Walker B. E., Amdrup E., Jensen H. E. 1972 The two- to four-year clinical results of highly selective vagotomy (parietal-cell vagotomy) without a drainage procedure for duodenal ulcer. *Gut* 13: 842–847 (2, 165)

Johnston G. W. and Rodgers H. W. 1973 A review of fifteen years experience in the use of sclerotherapy in the control of acute haemorrhage from oesophageal varices. *Brit. J. Surg.*, 60, 797–800 (6, 98)

Johnstone A. S. 1941 Annotation *Lancet* ii 18 (1, 90)

Jones B. J. M. 1986 Enteral feeding: techniques of administration. *Gut* 27: Suppl. 1: 47–50 (4, 301)

Jones F. A. and Pollak H. 1945 Civilian dyspepsia *Brit. Med. J.* i, 797– 800 (5, 121)

Jones F. A. 1947 Haematemesis and mealaena. *Brit. Med. J.* ii:441 & 477 (2, 79)

Jones F. A., Doll R., Fletcher C. and Rodgers H. W. 1951 The risks of gastroscopy. A survey of 49,000 examinations. *Lancet,* i, 647–651 (6, 30)

Jones F. A. and Gummer J. W. P. 1960 *Clinical Gastroenterology.* Blackwell Sci. Pub. Oxford. 54–64. (5, 334)

Jones F. A. & Godding E. W. 1972 *Management of Constipation.* Oxford, Blackwell. (5, 174)

Jones F. A. 1976 Foreword to *Modern Topics in Gastrointestinal Endoscopy* ed Schiller K. F. R. and Salmon P. R. William Heinemann Medical Books Ltd. London vii (6, 42)

Jones F. A. 1981 Are fibre supplements really necessary in diverticular disease of the colon? A controlled clinical trial. *Brit. Med. J.* 282: 1629 (L) (5, 285)

Jones F. A., Lennard-Jones J. E., Hinton J. M., Reeves W. G. 1986 Dangers of immunosuppressive drugs in ulcerative colitis. *Brit. Med. J.* i 1418 (4, 324)

Jones F. A. 1987 Gastroenterology in Britain before 1937:and the founding of the Gastro-Enterological Club. *Gut,* Jubilee Suppl. p4 (6, 27)

Jones F. A. 1992 *New concepts in human nutrition in the twentieth century: the special role of micronutrients.* The Caroline Walker Lecture, 1992 (3, 31)

Jones H., Cooper P., Miller V., Brooks N. and Whorwell P. J. 2006 Treatment of non-cardiac chest pain: a controlled trial of hypnotherapy. *Gut,* 55, 1403–08 (5, 366)

Jones H. W., Grogono J., Hoare A. M. 1988 Surveillance in ulcerative colitis: burdens and benefit. *Gut* 29: 325–331 (4, 264)

Jones J., Cann P., Gomborone J., Forbes A., Heaton K., Hungin P., Kumar D., Libby G., Spiller R., Read N., Silk D. and Whorwell P. 2000 Guidelines for the management of the irritable bowel syndrome. *Gut* 47 (Suppl. II): ii 1–ii 19 (5, 374)

Jones M., Crowell M., Olden K. and Creed F. H. 2007 Functional gastrointestinal disorders: an update for the psychiatrist. *Psychosomatics,* 48, 93–102 (5, 378)

Jones P. F., Munro A., Ewan S. W. B. 1977 Colectomy and ileo-rectal anastomosis: report on a personal series, with a critical review. *Brit. J. Surg.* 64: 615–623 (4, 340)

Jones P. F., Bevan G., Hawley P. R. 1978 Ileostomy or ileorectal anastomosis for ulcerative colitis? *Brit. Med. J.* i 1459–63 (4, 342)

Jones P. F., Keenan R. A. 1986 The place of colectomy with ileo-rectal anastomosis in inflammatory bowel disease. *Ann. Chir. et Gynae.* 75: 75–81 (4, 341)

Jones R. H., Lydeard S. E., Hobbs F. D. R., Kenkre J. E., Williams E. I., Jones S. J., Repper J. A., Caldow J. L., Dunwoodie W. M.B. and Bottomley J. M. 1990 Dyspepsia in England and Scotland. *Gut*, 31, 401–405 (5, 316)

Jones S. 1875 *St. Thos. Hosp. Reports.* Successful gastrostomy (1, 41)

Kagnoff M. F., Paterson Y. J., Kumar P. J., Kasarda D. D., Carbone F. R., Unsworth D. J., Austin R. K. 1987 Evidence for a role of a human intestinal adenovirus in the pathogenesis of coeliac disease. *Gut* 28 995–1001 (3, 177)

Kantor J. L. 1934 Regional (terminal) ileitis: its roentgen diagnosis. *J. Amer. Med. Assoc.* 103: 2016–2021 (4, 46)

Kay A. W. 1953 Effect of large doses of histamine on gastric secretion of HCl. *Brit. Med. J.* ii: 77–80 (2, 42)

Kellow J. E., Gill, R. C. and Wingate D. L. 1990 Prolonged ambulatory recordings of small bowel motility demonstrate abnormalities in the irritable bowel syndrome. *Gastroenterology* 98, 1208–18 (5, 240)

Kelly D. A., Phillips A. D., Elliott E. J., Dias J. A., Walker-Smith J. A. 1989 Rise and fall of coeliac disease 1960–85. *Arch. Dis. Child* 64 1157–60 (3, 207)

Kendall R. E. 1993 in *William Cullen and the Eighteenth Century World* ed Doig A., Ferguson J. P. S., Milne I. A. and Passmore R Edinburgh University Press 223–228 (5, 24)

Kennedy T., Johnston G. W., Macrae J. D., Anne Spencer E. F. 1975 Proximal gastric vagotomy: interim results of a randomised controlled trial. *Brit. Med. J.* ii 301–303 (2, 166)

Kenrick K. G., Walker-Smith J. A. 1970 Immunoglobulins and dietary protein antibodies in childhood coeliac disease. *Gut* 11: 635–640 (3, 210)

Kettell J., Jones R. H. and Lydiard S. 1992 Reasons for consultation in irritable bowel syndrome. *Br. J. Gen. Pract.* 42, 459–461 (5, 352)

King P. M., Blazeby J. M., Ewings P., Franks P. J., Longman R. J., Kendrick A. H., Kipling R. M., Evans L. B., Soulsby M. J., Kennedy R. H. 2006 Randomised clinical trial comparing laparoscopic and open surgery for colorectal cancer within an enhanced recovery programme. *Brit. J. Surg.* 93; 300–308 (4, 354)

Kingham, J. C. G. and Dawson, A. M. 1985 Origin of chronic right upper quadrant pain. *Gut*, 26, 783–788 (5, 224) (5, 341)

Kirby J., Fielding J. F. 1984 Very adult coeliac disease! The need for jejunal biopsy in the middle aged and elderly. *Irish Med. J.* 77: 263–267 (3, 127)

Kirk A. P., Lennard-Jones J. E. 1982 Controlled trial of azathioprine in chronic ulcerative colitis. *Brit. Med. J.* i 1291–92 (4, 335)

Kirsner J. B. 1985 Inflammatory bowel disease at the University of Chicago – the first 50 years: some personal reflections. *Amer. J. Gastroenterology.* 80: 219–228 (4, 36)

Kirsner J. B. 1985 *Amer. J. Gastroenterol.* 80: 221 (4, 58)

Kirsner J. B. 1985 *Amer. J. Gastroenterol.* 80: 222 (4, 66)

Kirsner J. B., Palmer W. L. 1951 Effect of corticotrophin (ACTH) in chronic ulcerative colitis. *J. Amer. Med. Assoc.* 147: 541–549 (4, 65)

Kirsner, J. B. and Palmer, W. L. 1958 The Irritable Colon, *Gastroenterology*, 34, 3, 491–500 (5, 138)

Kocher T. 1911 (trans. Styles) *Textbook of Operative Surgery*. London 5th edition (1, 57)

Kramer P., Ingelfinger F. J. 1949 Motility of the human esophagus in control subjects and patients with esophageal disorders. *Amer. J. Med.* 7; 168–174 (1, 26)

Kramer P., Ingelfinger F. J., Atkinson M 1956 The motility and pharmacology of the esophagus in cardiospasm *Gastroenterologia* Basel 86; 174–8 (1, 27)

Kramer P. 1989 Diagnostic value of esophageal balloon distension (letter). *Gastroenterology*, 96, 271–272 (5, 231)

Kumar P. J. 2003 Debate. European and North American populations should be screened for coeliac disease – Antagonist *Gut* 52: 170–1 (3, 229)

Kumar, D. And Wingate, D. L. 1985 The irritable bowel syndrome: a paroxysmal disorder. *Lancet*, ii, 973–977 (5, 241)

Kussmaul, A. 1868 Uber Magenspiegelung. Berichte uber die Verhandlungen der naturforschenden Gesellschaft *Freiberg I B* 5, 112 (6, 8)

Kussmaul, A. 1869 Ueber die Behandlung der Magenerweiterung durch eine neue Methode mittelst der Magenpumpe. *Dtsch. Arch. Klin. Med.* 6: 455–500 (Dec. 23) (5, 66)

Kwong N. K., Brown B. H., Whittaker G. E. and Duthie H. L. 1972 Effects of gastrin, secretin, and cholecystokinin-pancreozymin on the electrical activity, motor activity and acid output of the stomach in man. *Scand. J. Gastroenterol.* 7, 161–170 (5, 208)

Kyle J. 1992 Crohn's disease in the North-eastern and Northern Isles of Scotland: an epidemiological review. *Gastroenterology* 103: 392–399 (4, 120)

Labenz J., Borsch G. 1995 Towards an optimal treatment of Helicobacter pylori-positive peptic ulcers. *Amer. J. Gastroenterol.* 90: 692–694 (2, 206)

Lamm H. 1930 *Biegsame optische Gerate. Ztschr. f. Instrumentenk.*, 50: 579–581 (6, 37)

Lancaster-Smith M. J., Parveen Kumar, Marks R., Clark M. L. and Dawson A. M. 1974 Jejunal mucosal immunoglobulin-containing cells and jejuna fluid immunoglobulins in adult celiac disease and dermatitis herpetiformis. *Gut*, 15, 371–376 (3, 196)

Lander F. P. L., Maclagan N. F. 1934 One hundred histamine test meals on normal students. *Lancet* ii 1210–13 (2, 36)

Lane J. A., Murray L. J., Noble S., Egger M., Harvey I. M., Donovan J. L., Nair P. and Harvey R. F. 2006 Impact of Helicobacter pylori eradication on dyspepsia, health resource use, and quality of life in the Bristol helicobacter project: randomised controlled trial. *Brit. Med. J.* i 199–204 (5, 333)

Lane W. A. 1913 An address on chronic intestinal stasis. *Brit. Med. J.* ii: 1126 (5, 109)

Langman M. J. S. 1970 Epidemiological evidence for the association of aspirin and acute gastrointestinal bleeding. *Gut* 11: 627–634 (2, 82)

Langman M. J . S., McConwell T. H., Sigelhalter D. J., McConwell R. B. 1985 Changing patterns of coeliac disease frequency: an analysis of celiac society membership records. *Gut* 26: 275–278(3, 206)

Langmead F. 1913 Discussion on alimentary taxaemia; its sources, consequences and treatment. Proceedings of the Royal Society of Medicine 6: (Gen) 319–20 (3, 21)

Lauder Brunton T. 1886 *Lettsomian Lectures: In Disorders of Digestion, Their Consequences and Treatment.* Macmillan and Co., London 1–79 (5, 65)

Laurence B. H. and Cotton P. B. 1980 Decompression of malignant biliary obstruction by duodenoscopic intubation of bile duct. *Brit. Med. J.* i, 522–523 (6, 112)

Lawrence J. S. 1952 Dietetic and other methods in the treatment of peptic ulcer. *Lancet* i: 482–485 (2, 148)

Le Fanu J. 1999 *The Rise and Fall of Modern Medicine*. Little, Brown & Co. (UK) chap 12, 186 (2, 100)

Lee J. C. W., Lennard-Jones J. E. 1996 Inflammatory bowel disease in 67 families each with three or more affected first-degree relatives. *Gastroenterology* 111: 587–596 (4, 139)

Leigh R. J., Marsh M. M., Crowe P. J., Garner V., Gordon D. B. 1985 Studies of intestinal lymphoid tissue IX–Dose-dependent gluten-induced lymphoid infiltration of coeliac jejunal epithelium. *Scand. J. Gastroenterol.* 20; 715–719 (3, 165)

Lempriere J. 1788 *A Classical Dictionary*. Reading T. Cadell. London (3, 4)

Lennard-Jones J. E., Longmore A. J., Newall A. C., Wilson C. W. E., Jones F. A. 1960 An assessment of prednisone, salazopyrin and topical hydrocortisone hemisuccinate used as an out-patient treatment for ulcerative colitis. *Gut* 1: 217–222 (4, 88)

Lennard-Jones J. E., Vivian A. B. 1960 Fulminating ulcerative colitis: recent experience in management. *Brit. Med. J.* ii 96–102 (4, 85 and 289)

Lennard-Jones J. E., Misiewicz J. J., Parrish J. A., Ritchie J. K., Swarbrick E. T. 1966 Prospective study of outpatients with extensive colitis. *Lancet* i, 1065–67 (4, 256)

Lennard-Jones J. E., Fletcher J., Shaw D. G. 1968 Effect of different foods on the acidity of the gastric contents in patients with duodenal ulcer. *Gut* 9: 177–182 (2, 172)

Lennard-Jones J. E. 1986 Compliance, cost and common sense limit cancer control in colitis. *Gut*, 27, 1403–07 (6, 115)

Lennard-Jones J. E., Melville D. M., Morson B. C., Ritchie J. K., Williams C. B. 1990 Precancer and cancer in extensive ulcerative colitis: findings among 401 patients over 22 years. *Gut* 31; 800–806 (4, 257)

Lennard-Jones J. E. 1991 Screening for colorectal cancer in ulcerative colitis. *Gut* 32: 722–723 (4, 271)

Lennard-Jones J. E. 1997 Inflamed passions; an interview with T. T. MacDonald. *Gut* 40 (Suppl. 2) S17 (4, 78)

Leroy d'Etoilles. 1845 in *De Lavacherie "De l'Oesophagectomie"*, Bruxelles (1, 42)

Leube W. 1876 *Ziemssen's Handbuch der Speziellen Pathologie und Therapie*. Leipzig. (2, 52)

Leube, W. O. 1883 Beitrage zur Diagnostik der Magenkrankheiten *Dtsch. Arch. Klin. Med.* 33, 1–21 (5, 67)

Leukonia R. M., Schroder H., Price-Evans D. A. 1973 Pharmacokinetics and azo-link cleavage of salazopyrin in man. *Gut* 14: A426 (4, 98)

Levi A., Beardshall K., Haddad G., Playford R., Ghosh P., Calam J. 1989 Campylobacter pylori and duodenal ulcer: The gastrin link. *Lancet* i 1167–68 (2, 109)

Levy R. L., Olden K. W., Naliboff B. D., Bradley L. A., Francisconi C., Drossman D. A. and Creed F. H. 2006 Psychological aspects of the functional gastrointestinal disorders. *Gastroenterology*, 130, 1447–58 (5, 373)

Lewis I. 1946 The surgical treatment of carcinoma of the oesophagus. *Brit. J. Surg.* 34:18–31 (1, 68)

Linder G. C., Harris C. F. 1930 Calcium and phosphorus metabolism in chronic diarrhoea with tetany. *Quart. J. Med.* 23: 195–211 (3, 36)

Linder T. E., Simmen D. and Stool S. E. 1997 The history of endoscopy. In *Onary Inventions in the 20th Century. Arch. Otolaryngol, Head, Neck Surgery* 123, 1161–63 (6, 48)

Lindsay M. K. M., Nordin B. E. C., Norman A. P. 1956 Late prognosis in coeliac disease. *Brit. Med. J.* i: 14–18 (3, 117)

Lister J. 1867 On a new method of treating compound fractures. *Lancet* i 327 (2,16)

Littlewood J. M., Crollick A. J., Richards I. D. G. 1980 Childhood coeliac disease is disappearing. *Lancet* ii: 1359–60 (3, 203)

Litynski G. 1996 Erich Muhe – a surgeon ahead of his time. The first laparoscopic cholecystectomies. *Highlights in the History of Laparoscopy.* Bernert, Frankfurt (5; 347,348,349)

Lockhart-Mummery H. E., Morson B. C. 1960 Crohn's disease (regional enteritis) of the large intestine and its distinction from ulcerative colitis. *Gut* 1: 87–105 (4, 125)

Lockhart-Mummery J. P. 1904 The diagnosis of tumours in the upper rectum and sigmoid flexure by means of the electric sigmoidoscope. *Lancet* i 1781–83 (4, 14) (6, 59)

Lockhart-Mummery J. P. 1905 Remarks on the value of the sigmoidoscope in the diagnosis between primary and secondary colitis. *Brit. Med. J.* ii 1630–31 (4, 15)

Lockhart-Mummery, J. P. 1907 The causes of colitis with special reference to its surgical treatment. *Lancet*, i, 1638–43 (4, 16)

Lockhart-Mummery J. P. 1923 *Diseases of the Rectum and Colon.* Balliere, Tindall & Cox. London p429 (4, 28)

Logan R. F. A., Edmond M., Somerville K. W., Langman M. J. S. 1984 Smoking and ulcerative colitis. *Brit. Med. J.* i 751–753 (4, 153)

Logan R. F. A., Gillon J., Ferrington C., Ferguson A. 1981 Reduction of gastrointestinal protein loss by elemental diet in Crohn's disease of the small bowel. *Gut* 22: 383–387 (4, 208)

Logan R. F. A., Tucker G., Rifkind E. A., Heading R. C., Ferguson A. 1983 Changes in clinical features of celiac disease in adults in Edinburgh and the Lothians 1960–79. *Brit. Med. J.* i: 95–97 (3, 208)

Logan R. P. H., Polson R. J., Misiewicz J. J., Rao G., Karim N. Q., Newell D., Johnson P., Wadsworth J., Walker M. M., Baron J. H. 1991 Simplified single sample 13 Carbon urea breath test for Helicobacter pylori: comparison with histology, culture, and ELISA serology. *Gut* 32: 1461–64 (2, 195)

Lovell R. 1661 *PANZOORUKTOLOGIA Sive Panzoologico minealogia or a Compleat History of Animals and Minerals* Godwin, Oxford 366 (5, 2)

Low G. C. 1928 Sprue. An analytical study of 150 cases. *Quart. J. Med.* 21; 523–534 (3, 25)

Lucey M. R., Clark M. L., Lowndes Jo, and Dawson A. M. 1987 Is bran efficacious in irritable bowel syndrome? A double blind placebo controlled cross over study. *Gut,* 28, 221–225 (5, 288)

Lumsden K., Chaudhary N. A. & Truelove S. C. 1963 The irritable colon syndrome. *Clinical Radiology,* 14, 54–63 (5, 171)

Lyall A. 1937 Chronic peptic ulcer of the oesophagus: a report of 8 cases. *Brit. J. Surg.* 24: 534–547 (1, 86)

Lydeard S. and Jones R. 1989 factors affecting the decision to consult with dyspepsia: comparison of consulters and non-consulters. *J. R. Coll. Gen. Pract.* 39, 495–498 (5, 351)

Lynch D. A. F., Lobo A. J., Sobala G. M., Dixon M. F., Axon A. T. R. 1993 Failure of colonoscopic surveillance in ulcerative colitis. *Gut* 34: 1075–80 (4, 263)

MacDonald C. E., Wicks A. C., Playford R. J. 1997 Ten year experience of screening patients with Barrett's oesophagus in a University Teaching Hospital. *Gut* 41; 303–307 (1, 114)

MacDonald T. T., Ferguson A. 1976 Hypersensitivity reactions in the small intestine – 2 – effects of allograft rejection on mucosal architecture and lymphoid cell infiltrate. *Gut* 17; 81–91 (3, 159)

MacDonald T. T., Monteleone G. 2001 Interleukin-12 and Th1 immune responses in Peyers patches. *Trends Immunol.* 22: 244–247 (4, 199)

MacDonald T. T., Spencer J. M. 1988 Evidence that activated T cells play a role in the development of enteropathy in human small intestine. *J. Exp. Med.* 167: 1341–49 (3, 175)

MacDonald A. J. and Bouchier I. A. D. 1980 Non-organic gastrointestinal illness: a medical and psychiatric study. *Br. J. Psychiatry.* 136, 276–283 (5, 339)

MacDougall I. P. M. 1964 The cancer risk in ulcerative colitis. *Lancet* ii, 655–658 (4, 252)

MacFarlane B., Leicester R., Romaya C. and Epstein O. 1999 Colonoscopy services in the United Kingdom. *Endoscopy*, 31, 409–412 (6, 146)

Machella T. E., Hollan O. R. 1951 The effect of cortisone on the clinical course of chronic regional enteritis and chronic idiopathic ulcerative colitis. *Amer. J. Med. Sci.* 221: 501–507 (4, 64)

MacKay C. 1966 Perforated peptic ulcer in the West of Scotland: a survey of 5,343 cases during 1954 – 63. *Brit. Med. J.* i:701–705 (2, 58)

MacKay C., MacKay H. P. 1976 Perforated peptic ulcer in the West of Scotland 1964–73 *Proc. Surgical Research Society* 157–8 (2, 59)

Mackay H. M. M. 1923 Studies of rickets in Vienna 1919–22. *MRC Special Report series* No 77 (3, 37)

Mackay H. M. M. 1931 Nutritional anaemia in infancy. *MRC Special Report series* No 157 (3, 38)

Mackenzie M. 1881 On the use of the oesophagoscope in diseases of the gullet. *Med. Times & Gazette* July 16 (6, 7)

Mackintosh P., 1981 A critical analysis of HLA in coeliac family studies in Birmingham. In: *The Genetics of Coeliac Disease.* Ed R. B. McConnell MTP Press Ltd. Lancaster. 201–206 (3, 147)

Mackintosh P., Asquith p1978 HLA and Coeliac Disease. *British Medical Bulletin* 34: 291–294 (3, 148)

Mahida Y. R., Patel S., Gionchetti P., Vaux D., Jewell D. P. 1989 Macrophage subpopulations in lamina propria of normal and inflamed colon and terminal ileum. *Gut* 30: 826–834 (4, 193)

Mahida Y. R., Wu K., Jewell D. P. 1989 Enhanced production of interleukin 1-B by mononuclear cells isolated from the mucosa with active ulcerative colitis and Crohn's disease. *Gut* 30: 835–838 (4, 197)

Mahon J., Blair G. E., Wood G. M., Scott B. B., Losowsky M. S., Howdle P. D. 1991 Is persistent adenovirus 12 infection involved in coeliac disease? A search for viral DNA using the polymerase chain reaction. *Gut* 32 1114–16 (3, 180)

Malizia G., Trejdosiewicz L. K., Wood G. M., Howdle P. D., Janossy G., Losowsky M.S. 1985 The microenvironment of celiac disease: T cell phenocytes and expression of the T2 "T Blast" antigen by small bowel lymphocytes. *Clin. Exp. Immunol.* 60 437 (3, 172)

Mallas E. G., Williamson N., Cooper B. T., Cooke W. T. 1977 IgA class reticulin antibodies in relatives of patients with celiac disease. *Gut* 18: 647–650 (3, 219)

Management of Dyspepsia: Report of a Working Party. 1988 *Lancet* i, 576–579 (5, 134)

Manning A. P. and Heaton K. W. 1976 Bran and the irritable bowel. *Lancet*, i; 588 (5, 272)

Manning, A. P., Wyman, J. B. and Heaton, K. W. 1976 How trustworthy are bowel histories? *Brit. Med. J.* iii 213–214 (5, 185)

Manning, A. P., Heaton, K. W., Harvey, R. F. and Uglow, p1977 Wheat fibre and irritable bowel syndrome. *Lancet* ii 417–418 (5, 184)

Manning, A. P., Thompson, W. G., Heaton, K. W. and Morris, A. F. 1978 Towards positive diagnosis of the irritable bowel. *Brit. Med. J.* 2653–654 (5, 187)

Manousos, O. N., Truelove, S. C. & Lumsden, K. 1967 Transit time of food in patients with diverticulosis or irritable colon syndrome and normal subjects. *Brit. Med. J.* iii 760–762 (5, 172)

Mansfield J. C., Giaffer M. H., Holdsworth C. D. 1995 Controlled trial of oligopetide versus amino acid diet in treatment of active Crohn's disease. *Gut* 36: 60–66 (4, 320)

Manson P. 1880 China. *Imperial Maritime Customs. Medical Reports for the half-year ended 31st March 1880.* 19th Issue. Published by order of the Inspector General of Customs. Shanghai 33–37 (3, 10)

Manson-Bahr P. 1924 The morbid anatomy and pathology of sprue and their bearing upon aetiology. *Lancet* i 1148–51 (3, 60)

Mantzaris G. J., Karagiannis J. A., Priddle J. D., Jewell D. P. 1990 Cellular hypersensitivity to a synthetic dodecapeptide derived from human adenovirus 12 which resembles a sequence of A-gliadin in patients with coeliac disease. *Gut* 31; 668–673 (3, 178)

Marsden, C. A. 1981 Effect of L-tryptofan on mouse brain 5-hydroxytpryptamine: comparison of values obtained using a fluorimetric assay and liquid chromatographic assay with electrochemical detection. *J. Neurochem.* 36, 1621–26 (5, 384)

Marsh G. W., Stewart J. S. 1970 Splenic function in adult coeliac disease. *Brit. J. Haematol* 19: 445–57 (3, 151)

Marsh M. N., Swift J. A., Williams E. D. 1968 Studies of small-intestinal mucosa with the scanning electron microscope. *Brit. Med. J.* iv 95–96 (3, 164)

Marsh M. N., Bjarnason I., Shaw J., Ellis A., Baker R., Peters T. J. 1990 Studies of intestinal lymphoid tissue XIV- HLA status, mucosal morphology, permeability and epithelial lymphocyte populations in first degree relatives of patients with coeliac disease. *Gut* 31; 32–36 (3, 167)

Marsh M. N. 1990 Grains of truth: evolutionary changes in small intestinal mucosa in response to environmental antigen challenge. *Gut* 31; 111–4 (3, 166)

Marsh M. N. 1992 Gluten, Major Histocompatibility Complex, and the Small Intestine. A Molecular and Immunobiologic Approach to the Spectrum of Gluten Sensitivity ("Celiac Sprue") *Gastroenterology* 102; 337 (3, 163)

Marshall B. J., Warren J. R. 1984 Unidentified curved bacilli in the stomach of patients with gastritis and peptic ulceration. *Lancet* i 1311– (2, 97)

Marshall B. J., Royce H., Annear D. I., Goodwin C. S., Pearman J. W., Warren J. R., et al 1984 Original isolation of Campylobacter Pyloridis from human gastric mucosa. *Microbios Letters* 25 83–88 (2, 96)

Marshall B. J., Armstrong J. A., McGechie D. B., Glancy R. J. 1985 Attempt to fulfil Koch's postulates for pyloric campylobacter. *Med. J. Aus.* 142; 436 -439 (2, 99)

Marshall B. J., McGechie D. B., Rogers P. A., Glancy R. J. 1985 Pyloric campylobacter infection and gastroduodenal disease. *Med. J. Aus.* 142; 439 -444 (2, 98)

Marshall B. J., Goodwin C. S., Warren J. R., et al. 1988 Prospective double-blind trial of duodenal ulcer relapse after eradication of Campylobacter pylori. *Lancet* ii: 1437–42 (2, 191)

Marshall B. J. 1989 History of the discovery of Campylobacter pylori. In Blaser M. J. ed *Campylobacter Pylori in Gastritis and Peptic Ulcer Disease* New York. Igakushoin 7–23 (2, 95)

Martin D. F., May S. J., Tweedle D. E., Hollander D., Ravenscroft M. M., Miller J. P. 1981 Difference in relapse rates of duodenal ulcer after healing with cimetidine or tripotassium dicitrato bismuthate. *Lancet* i: 7–10 (2, 185)

Martin L. C., Lewis N. 1949 Peptic ulcer cases reviewed after ten years. Effect of medical treatment and indications for gastrectomy. *Lancet* ii: 1115–20 (2, 146)

Matsunaga F. 1959 Clinical studies in ulcerative colitis and its related diseases in Japan. Proc. *First World Congress Gastroenterol.* Washington 1958 Williams and Wilkins vol 2 Baltimore 955–963 (6, 63)

Matthews P. M. 2001 Developing the role of the nurse endoscopist. *Nursing Times*, 97, 56–57. (6, 139)

Maxton D. G., Morris J. and Whorwell P. J. 1996 Selective 5-hydroxytryptamine antagonism: a role in irritable bowel syndrome and functional dyspepsia? *Alimentary Pharmacology and Therapeutics* 10, 595–599 (5, 383)

Maxton D. G., Morris J. and Whorwell P. J. 1991 More accurate diagnosis of irritable bowel syndrome by the use of "non-colonic" symptomatology. *Gut*, 32, 784–786 (5, 355)

Mayberry J. F., Rhodes J., Newcombe R. G. 1978 Breakfast and dietary aspects of Crohn's disease. *Brit. Med. J.* ii 1401 (4, 150)

Mayberry J. F., Rhodes J., Newcombe R. G. 1980 Familial prevalence of inflammatory bowel disease in relatives of patients with Crohn's disease. *Brit. Med. J.* i: 84. (4, 129)

Mayberry J. F., Ballantyne K. C., Hardcastle J. D., Mangham C., Pye G. 1989 Epidemiolocal study of asymptomatic inflammatory bowel disease: the identification of cases during a screening programme for colorectal cancer. *Gut* 30; 481–483 (4, 119)

Mayo H. 1828 A case of Dilated Oesophagus. *Lond. Med. Gaz.* 3; 121(L) (1, 10)

Mayo Robson A. W. 1908 An address on some abdominal tumours simulating malignant disease and their treatment. *Brit. Med. J.* i 425–428 (4, 39)

Mayou R., Bryant B., Sanders D., Bass C., Klimes I. and Forfar C. 1997 A controlled trial of cognitive behaviour therapy for non-cardiac chest pain. *Psychol. Med.*, 27, 1021–31 (5, 364)

McCallion K., Mitchell R. M. S., Wilson R. H., Kee F., Watson R. G. P., Collins J. S. A. and Gardiner K. R. 2001 Flexible sigmoidoscopy and the changing distribution of colorectal cancer: implications for screening. *Gut*, 48, 522–525 (6, 153)

McCarthy C. F., Frazer I. D., Evans K. T., Read A. E. 1966 Lymphoreticular dysfunction in idiopathic steatorrhoea. *Gut* 7: 140 (3, 150)

McColl K. E. L., El Omar E. 1994 Effect of H. pylori infection on gastrin and gastric acid secretion. In Hunt R. H., Tytgat G. N. J., eds. *Helicobacter Pylori: Basic Mechanisms to Clinical Cure*. Boston; Kluwer Academic 245–256 (2, 107)

McColl K. E. L., El Omar E. 1995 Review article: gastrin releasing peptide and its value in assessing gastric secretory function. *Aliment. Phar.and Ther*. 9: 341–347 (2, 108)

McColl K., Murray L., El-Omar E., Dickson A.,El-Nujumi A., Wirz A.,Kelman A., Penny C., Knill-Jones R. and Hilditch T. 1998 Symptomatic benefit from eradicating Helicobacter pylori infection in patients with non-ulcer dyspepsia. *New England Journal of Medicine* 339; 1869–74 (5, 320)

McColl K. E. L.,Gillen D. and Dickson A. S. 1999 Eradication of Helicobacter pylori in functional dyspepsia *Brit. Med. J.* ii, 451 (L) (5, 323)

McColl K. E. L. 2001 Protagonist: Should we eradicate Helicobacter pylori in non-ulcer dyspepsia? *Gut* 48, 759 (5,330)

McColl K. E. L., Murray L. S., Gillen D., Walker A., Wirz A., Fletcher J., Mowat C., Henry E., Kelman A. and Dickson A. 2002 Randomised trial of endoscopy with testing for Helicobacter pylori compared with non-invasive H. pylori testing alone in the management of dyspepsia. *Brit. Med. J.* i 999–1002 (5, 331)

McCollum E. V. et al. 1922 An experimental demonstration of the existence of a vitamin which promotes calcium absorption. *J. Biol. Chem.* 53; 293 (3, 33)

McCombie, C. W. & Smith, J. C. 1998 Harold Hopkins 1918–94 *Biograph Memoirs Fell Roy Soc.* 44, 239–244 (6, 39)

McConnell R. B. 1983 Ulcerative colitis – genetic features. *Scand. J. Gastroenterol. Suppl.* 88: 18: 14–16 (4, 130 and 137)

McConnell R. B. 1990 Genetics of inflammatory bowel disease. In *Inflammatory Bowel Disease* ed Allan R. N., Keighley M. R. B., Alexander Williams J., Hawkins C. F. Edinburgh, Churchill Livingstone 11–13 (4, 138)

McConnell, A. A., Eastwood, M. A. and Mitchell, W. D. 1974 Physical characteristics of vegetable food stuffs that could influence bowel function. *J. Sci. Food Agric.* 25, 1457–64 (5, 275)

McCrae W. M. 1969 The inheritance of coeliac disease. *J. Med. Genet.* 6: 129–131 (3, 126)

McCrae W. M. 1970 The inheritance of coeliac disease. In *Coeliac Disease*, ed Booth C. C., Dowling R. H. Edinburgh & Churchill Livingstone, London 55–63 (3, 129)

McCrae W. M., Eastwood M. A., Martin M. R., Sircus W. 1975 Neglected celiac disease. *Lancet* i: 187–190 (3, 194)

McIntyre P. B., Powell-Tuck J., Wood S. R., Lennard-Jones J. E., Lerebours E., Hecketsweiler P., Galmiche J. P., Colin P. 1986 Controlled trial of bowel rest in the treatment of severe acute colitis. *Gut* 27: 481–485 (4, 294)

McIntyre P. B., Rodrigues L. A., Lennard-Jones J. E., Barrison I. G., Walker J. G., Baron J. H., Thornton P. C. 1988 Balsalazide in the maintenance treatment of patients in ulcerative colitis, a double-blind comparison study with sulphasalazine. *Alimentary Pharmacology and Therapeutics* 2: 237–243 (4, 106)

McIntyre P. B., Wood S. R., Powell-Tuck J., Lennard-Jones J. E. 1983 Nocturnal nasogastric tube feeding at home. *Gut* 24: A488 (4,300)

McIntyre A. S., Thompson D. G., Day, S., Burnham W. R. and Walker E. R. 1992 Modulation of human upper intestinal nutrient transit by a beta adrenoreceptor mediated pathway *Gut*, 33, 1062–70 (5, 246)

McKeown K. C. 1976 Total three-stage oesophagectomy for cancer of the oesophagus. *Brit. J. Surg.* 63; 259–262 (1, 73)

McKeown K. C. 1994 *A Tale of Two Citadels. Memoirs of a surgeon and his times*. The Pentland Press Ltd. Durham. ISBN 1–85821–208–1 (1, 74)

McKeown K. C. 1994 in *A Tale of Two Citadels*. Pentland Press Ltd. Durham p104 (1, 21)

McMichael H. B. 1979 Physiology of carbohydrate, electrolyte and water absorption. *Research & Clin. Forums*. I; 25–28 (4, 298)

McNeish A. S. 1967 Jejunal biopsy in infants and underweight children. *Arch. Dis. Child* 42 623– 625 (3, 121)

McNeish A. S., Harms H. K., Rey J., Shmerling D. H. Visacorpi J. K., Walker-Smith J. A. 1979 The diagnosis of coeliac disease. *Arch. Dis. Child*. 54: 783–786 (3, 124)

McNulty C. A. M., Dent J. C., Uff J. S., Gear M. W. L., Wilkinson S. P. 1989 Detection of Campylobacter pylori by the biopsy urease test: an assessment in 1445 patients *Gut* 30 1058–62 (2, 105)

McNulty C. A. M., Gearty J. C., Crump B. et al. et al 1986 Campylobacter pyloridis and associated gastritis: investigator blind placebo- controlled trial of bismuth salicylate and erythromycin ethylsuccinate. *Brit. Med. J*. 293; 645–649 (2, 106 and 187)

McNulty C. A. M., Watson D. M. 1984 Spiral bacteria of the gastric antrum. *Lancet* i 1068–69 (2, 103)

McNulty C. A. M., Wise R. 1985 Rapid diagnosis of Campylobacter-associated gastritis. *Lancet* I 1443–44(L) (2, 104)

McRae, S., Younger, K., Thompson, D. G. and Wingate, D. L. 1982 Sustained mental stress alters human jejunal motor activity. *Gut*, 23,404–409 (5, 238)

Meade T. W., Arie T. H. D., Brewis M., Bond D. J., Morris J. N. 1968 Recent history of ischaemic heart disease and duodenal ulcer in doctors. *Br.Med. J.* iii: 701–704 (2, 62)

Mearin, F., Cucala, M., Azpiroz, F. and Malagelada, J. R. 1991 The origin of symptoms on the brain-gut axis in functional dyspepsia. *Gastroenterology*, 101, 999–1006 (5, 300)

Medical Aspects of Dietary Fibre 1980 A report of the Royal College of Physicians Pitman Medical Limited, Tunbridge Wells. (5, 273)

Mee A. S., McLaughlin J. E., Hodgson H. J. F., Jewell D. P. 1979 Chronic immune colitis in rabbits. *Gut* 20: 1–5 (4, 182)

Mee A. S., Jewell D. P. 1980 Monocytes in inflammatory bowel disease: monocyte and serum lysosomal enzyme activity. *Clin. Sci.* 58: 295–300 (4, 184)

Mee A. S., Szawatakowski M., Jewell D. P. 1980 Monocytes in inflammatory bowel disease: phagocytosis and intracellular killing. *J. Clin. Pathol.* 33: 921–925 (4, 183)

Mee A. S., Burke M., Vallon A. G., Newman J., Cotton P. B. 1985 Small bowel biopsy for malabsorption: comparison of the diagnostic adequacy of endoscopic forceps and capsule biopsy specimens. *Brit. Med. J.* iii: 769–772 (3, 193)

Meeuwisse G. 1970 Diagnostic criteria in coeliac disease. *Acta. Paed. Scand.* 59: 461–464 (3, 123)

Mellanby E. 1919–20 Discussion on the importance of accessory food factors (vitamines) in the feeding of infants. *Proceedings of the Royal Society of Medicine.* Sect Dis Child. 13; 52 (3, 32)

Melville D. M., Ritchie J. K., Nicholls R. J., Hawley P. R. 1994 Surgery for ulcerative colitis in the era of the pouch: the St. Mark's Hospital experience *Gut* 35: 1076– 1080 (4, 345)

Memorandum on Future National Needs for Fibre-Optic Endoscopy of the Gastrointestinal tract 1973 British Society for Digestive Endoscopy. Samuel Walker Ltd., Hinckley, Leics. (6, 83)

Meulengract E. 1935 Treatment of haematemesis and melaena with food: the mortality. *Lancet* ii 1220–2 (2, 143)

Mikulicz-Radecki Johann von.,1882 uber Gastroskopie und Oesophagoskopie mit Demonstration am Lebenden. *Verhard, d. Dent. Gesellsch. F. Chir.* XI Cong. 30–38 (1, 17)

Miller D. S., Keighley A. C., Langman M. J. S. 1974 Changing patterns in epidemiology of Crohn's disease. *Lancet* ii 691–693 (4, 121)

Miller R. 1921 A fatal case of coeliac infantilism. *Lancet* i: 743–746 (3, 16)

Milton-Thompson G. J., Williams J. G., Jenkins D. J. A., Misiewicz J. J. 1974 Inhibition of nocturnal acid secretion in duodenal ulcer by one oral dose of metiamide. *Lancet* i: 693–694 (2, 173)

Milton-Thompson G. J. and Lewis, B. 1971 The breakdown of dietary cellulose in man. *Gut*, 12, 853–854 (5, 276)

Minot G. R., Murphy W. P. 1926 Treatment of pernicious anaemia by a special diet. *J.A.M.A.* 87: 470–476 (3, 41)

Misiewicz J. J., Lennard-Jones J. E., Connell A. M., Baron J. H., Jones F. A. 1965 Controlled trial of sulphasalazine in maintenance therapy for ulcerative colitis. *Lancet* i 185–9 (4, 91)

Misiewicz J. J. & Baron J. H. 1987 Gerard Crean, a mini-biography. *Gut*, Jubilee Suppl. 48 (5, 131)

Misiewicz J. J., Waller S. L. and Eisner M. 1966 Motor responses of human gastrointestinal tract to 5-hydroxytryptamine in vivo and in vitro. *Gut*, 7, 208–216 (5,379)

Misiewicz J. J., Waller S. L., Fox R. H., Goldsmith R. and Hunt T. J. 1968 The effect of elevated body temperature and of stress on the motility of the stomach and colon in man. *Clin. Sci.*, 34, 149–159 (5, 151)

Misiewicz J. J., Harris A. W., Bardhan K. D., Levi S., O'Morain C., Cooper B. T., Kerr G. D., Dixon M. F., Langworthy H., Piper D. Lansoprazole Study Group. 1997 One week triple therapy for Helicobacter pylori: a multicentre comparative study. *Gut* 41:735–739 (2, 205)

Mitchell D. N., Cannon P., Dyer N. H., Hinson K. F. W., Willoughby J. M.T. 1969 The kveim test in Crohn's disease. *Lancet* ii 571–573 (4, 171)

Moayyedi P., Duffett S., Braunholtz D., Mason S., Richards I. D. G., Dowell, A. C. and Axon, A. T. R. 1998 The Leeds Dyspepsia Questionnaire: a valid tool for measuring the presence and severity of dyspepsia. *Alimentary Pharmacology and Therapeutics*. 12, 1257–62 (5, 325)

Moayyedi,P., Braunholtz, D., Duffett, S., Mason,S., Richards, I. D. G., Dowell, A. C. and Axon, A. T. R. 1998 What proportion of dyspepsia in the general population is attributable to Helicobacter pylori? *Gut*,42 (Suppl. 1) A75 (5, 326)

Moayyedi, P., Feltbower, R., Brown, J., Mason,S., Mason, J., Nathan, J., Richards, I. D. G., Dowell, A. C. and Axon A. T. R. 2000 The effect of population H. pylori screening and treatment on dyspepsia and quality of life in the community: results of a randomised controlled trial. *Lancet*, 355, 1665–69 (5, 327)

Moayyedi, P., Soo, S., Deeks, J., Forman, D., Mason, J., Innes, M. and Delaney, B. 2000 Systematic review and economic evaluation of Helicobacter pylori eradication treatment for non-ulcer dyspepsia. *Brit. Med. J.* ii 659–664 (5, 329)

Molberg O., McAdam S. N., Korner R., Sollid L. M., Lundin K. E. A. 1998 Tissue transglutaminase selectivity modifies gliadin peptides that are recognised by gut derived T cells. *Nat. Med.* 4; 713–717 (3, 225)

Molesworth H. W. L. 1933 Granuloma of intestine. Stenosis of ileo-caecal valve. *Brit. J. Surg.* 21: 370–372 (4, 50)

Montgomery A. M. P.,Goka A. K. J.,Kumar P. J.,Farthing M. J. G., Clark M. L. 1988 Low gluten diet in the treatment of adult coeliac disease: effect on jejunal morphology and serum anti-gluten antibodies. *Gut* 29; 1564–68 (3, 197)

Montgomery S. M., Pounder R. E., Wakefield A. J. 1997 Infant mortality and the incidence of inflammatory bowel disease. *Lancet* i 472–473 (4, 224)

Moore N. 1882 Stricture of intestine at the ileo-caecal valve. *Trans. Pathol. Soc.* 34: 112–3 (4, 49)

Moore N. 1918 *The History of St. Bartholemew's Hospital.* C. Arthur Pearson Ltd. London vol 2; 733 (3, 5)

Moriarty K. J. and Dawson, A. M. 1982 Functional abdominal pain: further evidence that whole gut affected. *Brit. Med. J.* 284; 1670–72 (5, 223)

Morley J. S., Tracy H. J., Gregory R. A. 1965 Structure-function relationships in the active C-terminal tetrapeptide sequence of gastrins. *Nature* 207: 1356–59 (2, 49)

Morrice A. A. G. 2004 Sir William Arbuthnot Lane. *Oxf. Dict. Nat. Biog.* Article 34394 (5, 110)

Morris P. J. 1965 Familial ulcerative colitis. *Gut* 6: 176–8 (4, 133)

Morris T., Rhodes J. 1984 Incidence of ulcerative colitis in the Cardiff region. 1968–77 *Gut* 26: 846–848 (4, 117)

Morse T. H. 1894 Ruptured gastric ulcer treated by laparotomy, gastric suture, and washing out of the peritoneum; Recovery. *Med. Chir. Trans.* 77,187–191 (2, 19)

Morson B. C., Belcher J. R. 1952 Adenocarcinoma of the oesophagus and ectopic gastric mucosa. *Brit. J. Cancer* 6; 127–130 (1, 102)

Morson B. C., Pang L. S. C. 1967 Rectal biopsy as an aid to cancer control in ulcerative colitis. *Gut* 8: 423–434 (4, 255)

Morson B. C. 1971 *Interpretation of rectal biopsies in inflammatory bowel disease.* Sir Arthur Hurst Lecture to Brit Soc. Gastroenterology. (6, 62)

Mortimer P. 1970 quoted by Booth C. C. in *Coeliac Disease.* Ed. Booth C. C., Dowling R. H. Churchill Livingstone, Edinburgh & London p62 (3, 128)

Mortimer P. E., Stewart J. S., Norman A. P., Booth C. C. 1968 Follow-up Study of Coeliac Disease. *Brit. Med. J.* ii: 7–9 (3, 118)

Moschcowitz E., Wilensky A. O. 1923 Non-specific granulomata of the intestine. *Amer. J. Med. Sci.* 66: 48–66 (4, 40)

Moss S. F., Calam J. 1993 Acid secretion and sensitivity to gastrin in patients with duodenal ulcer: effect of eradication of Helicobacter pylori. *Gut,* 34, 888–892 (2, 110)

Motson R. W., Kadirkamanathan S. S., Gallegos N. 2002 Minimally invasive surgery for ileo-colic Crohn's disease. *Colorectal Dis.*4 (2): 127–131 (4, 353)

Mousseau M., Barbin J. et al. 1956 *Arch. Mal. Appar. Digest.*45 208 (1, 47)

Moynahan E. J. 1973 Coeliac disease in the West of Ireland. *Brit. Med. J.* i: 484 (3, 131)

Moynihan B. G. 1910 *Duodenal Ulcer* Philadelphia: Saunders (2, 24) (5, 90 and 91)

Moynihan B. G. 1907 An address on the pathology of the living. *Br. Med.J.* ii 1381–84. (2; 20,22,119)

Moynihan B. G. 1901 On duodenal ulcer and its surgical treatment. *Lancet* ii 1656 (2, 21)

Moynihan B. G. 1907 Mimicry of malignant disease in the large intestine. *Edin. Med. J.* 21: 228–236 (4, 38)

Moynihan B. G. 1913 The gifts of surgery to medicine. *Brit. Med. J.* ii, 169–175 (2, 23) (5, 179)

Moynihan B. G.1928 Lloyd Roberts Lecture on some problems in gastric surgery. *Brit. Med. J.* ii 1021 (2, 128)

Moynihan, B. G. 1928 Some problems in gastric surgery. *Brit. Med. J.* ii, 1021–26 (2, 128 and 133)

Moynihan B. G. 1932 Lecture on the prognosis of gastric and duodenal ulcer *Brit. Med. J.* i 1–3 (2, 129)

Moynihan R. 2002 Alosetron: a case study in regulatory capture, or a victory for patient's rights? *Brit. Med. J.* 325, 592–595 (5, 391)

Mylotte M., Egan-Mitchell B., McCarthy C.F., McNicholl B. 1973 Incidence of coeliac disease in the West of Ireland. *Brit. Med. J.* i: 703–706 (3, 130)

Naish J. M. 2003 Personal communication (4, 112)

Nanda R., James, R., Smith H., Dudley, C. R. K. and Jewell D. P. 1989 Food intolerance and the irritable bowel syndrome. *Gut*, 30, 1099–1104 (5, 294)

Naomi I., Lee J. et al. 1996 Analysis of the contribution of HLA genes to genetic predisposition in inflammatory bowel disease. *Amer. J. Hum. Genet.* 59: 226–233 (4, 140)

Nathanson L. K., Shimi S. and Cuschieri A. 1991 Laparoscopic cholecystectomy: the Dundee technique *Brit. J. Surg.* 78, 155–9 (6, 155)

Neal K. R., Barker L. and Spiller R. C. 2002 Prognosis in post-infective irritable bowel syndrome: a six year follow up study. *Gut*, 51: 410–413 (5, 312)

Neal K. R., Hebden J. and Spiller R. C. 1997 Prevalence of gastrointestinal symptoms six months after bacterial gastroenteritis and risk factors for development of the irritable bowel syndrome: postal survey of patients. *Brit. Med. J.* 314: 779–782 (5, 311)

Neoptolemos J. P., Carr-Locke D. L. and Fossard D. P. 1984 The management of common bile duct calculi by endoscopic sphincterotomy in patients with gall bladders in situ. *Brit. J. Surg.* 71, 69–71 (6, 108)

Newton H. A. S., Hurst A. F. 1913 The normal movements of the colon in man. *J. Physiol.* (London) 47, 57–65 (5, 98)

NIH Consensus Conference. 1994 Helicobacter pylori in peptic ulcer disease. *J.A.M.A.* 272: 65–69 (2, 204)

Nissen R. 1961 Gastropexy and "Fundoplication" in surgical treatment of hiatus hernia. *Amer. J. Dig. Dis.* 6: 954– 961 (1, 96)

Niwa H. 1965 Endoscopy of the colon *Gastroenterol. Endosc.* (Tokyo) 7, 402–408 (6, 64)

Nurse endoscopist, The. 1994 Report of a British Society of Gastroenterology Working Party. Summary, *Gut*, 36, 795 (6, 140)

Obituary 1855 The late Mr. Avery. *Lancet*, i, 331–332 (6, 4)

O'Donnell L. J., Virgee J. and Heaton K. W. 1988 Pseudo-diarrhoea in the irritable bowel syndrome: patients' records of stool form reflect transit time while stool frequency does not. *Gut*, 29, A 1455 (5, 259)

O'Donoghue D. P., Dawson A. M., Powell-Tuck J., Bown R. L., Lennard-Jones J. E. 1978 Double-blind withdrawal trial of azathioprineas maintenance treatment for Crohn's disease. *Lancet* ii 955–957 (4, 331)

O'Morain C., Segal A. W., Levi A. J. 1984 Elemental diet as primary treatment of acute Crohn's disease: a controlled clinical trial. *Brit. Med. J.* i 1859–62 (4, 206 and 303)

Observations on the Dissection of Daniel Coates, who was executed at Tyburn, *1710*, B. M. MS. Sloane 2039, ff130–5 (5, 8)

Oettle G. J. and Heaton K. W. 1986 "Rectal dissatisfaction" in the irritable bowel syndrome. A manometric and radiological study. *Int. J. Colorect. Dis.* 1, 183–5 (5, 256)

Oettle G. J. and Heaton K. W. 1987 Is there a relationship between symptoms of the irritable bowel syndrome and objective measurements of large bowel function? A longitudinal study. *Gut*, 28, 146–9 (5, 257)

Ogilvie A. L. Dronfield M.W., Ferguson R., Atkinson M. 1982 Palliative intubation of oesophago-gastric neoplasms at fibreoptic endoscopy. *Gut* 23 1060–67 (1, 53)

Ogilvie W. H. 1938 The approach to gastric surgery. II – Ulcer of the stomach. *Lancet* ii 295–299 (2, 138)

Ogilvie W. H. 1951 The Large Bowel and Its Functions. *Proceedings of the Royal Society of Medicine* 44, 200–206 (4, 111)

Ogilvie W. H. 1951 The Large Bowel and Its Functions. *Proceedings of the Royal Society of Medicine* 44, 6–12 (4, 118)

Ohsawa T. 1933 The surgery of the esophagus *Arch. Jap. Surg.* 10, 605–700 (1, 61)

Oi I., Kobayashi S. and Kondo T. 1970 Endoscopic pancreatocholangiography. *Endoscopy*, 2, 103–6 (6, 77)

Organisation of a gastrointestinal service. 1975 Standing Committee on Gastroenterology, RCP. The College, London (6, 85)

Ornstein M. H., Littlewood E. R., Baird I. M., Fowler J., North W. R. S. and Cox, A. G. 1981 Are fibre supplements really necessary in diverticular disease of the colon? A controlled clinical trial. *Brit. Med. J.* 282: 1353–56 (5, 284)

Orr I. M., Johnson H. D. 1947 Vagal resection in the treatment of duodenal ulcer. *Lancet* ii: 84–89 (2, 158)

Osler W. 1901 *The Principle and Practice of Medicine.* Young J. Pentland 4th ed. 485–486 (2, 118)

Osler W. 1901 *The Principle and Practice of Medicine.* Young J. Pentland 4th ed 478 (2, 15)

Osler W. 1901 *The Principle and Practice of Medicine.* Young J Pentland 4th ed 544 (5, 104)

Osler W. 1901 *The Principle and Practice of Medicine.* Young J Pentland 4th ed 541–543 (5, 85)

Osler W. 1901 *The Principle and Practice of Medicine.* Young J Pentland 4th ed 497–505 (5, 69)

Osler W. 1959 *William Beaumont* Dover Publications, Inc. New York pxi (5, 42)

Overholt B. 1968 Clinical experience with the fibersigmoidoscope. *Gastrointest. Endosc.* 15, 27 (6, 65)

Painter N. S., Truelove S. C., Ardran G. M. & Tuckey M. 1965 Segmentation and the localisation of intraluminal pressures in the human colon, with special reference to the pathogenesis of colonic diverticula. *Gastroenterology,* 49, 169–177 (5, 155)

Painter N. S. 1967 Diverticulosis of the Colon–Fact or Speculation. *Amer. J. Dig. Dis.*12, 222 -227 (5, 156)

Painter N. S. & Burkitt D. P. 1971 Diverticular disease of the colon: a deficiency disease of western civilisation. *Brit. Med. J.* ii 450–454 (5, 159)

Painter N. S. 1972 Irritable or irritated bowel? *Brit. Med. J.* ii, 46 (L) (5, 173)

Painter N. S., Almeida A. Z. & Colebourne K. W. 1972 Unprocessed bran in the treatment of diverticular disease of the colon. *Brit. Med. J.* ii, 137–140 (5, 157)

Painter N. S. 1975 *Diverticular Disease of the Colon: A Deficiency Disease of Western Civilisation.* Heinemann, London (5, 170)

Palmer R. L., Stonehill E., Crisp, A. H., Waller S. L. and Misiewicz J. J. 1974 Psychological characteristics of patients with the irritable bowel syndrome. *Postgrad. Med. J.* 50, 416–419 (5, 343)

Paris, J. A. 1825 *Pharmacologia*, 6th edition, London p48 (5, 6)

Parkes M., Satsangi J., Lathrop G. M., Bell J. I., Jewell D. P. 1996 Susceptibility loci in inflammatory bowel disease. *Lancet* ii 1588 (L) (4, 144)

Parkinson J. W. K. Ed. 1833 *Hunterian Reminiscences, Being the Substance of a Course of Lectures on the Principles and Practice of Surgery, Delivered by the Late Mr. John Hunter in the Year 1785; Taken in Short-Hand and Afterwards Fairly Transcribed by the Late Mr. James Parkinson*. Sherwood, Gilbert and Piper, London (5, 25)

Parks A. G., Nicholls R. J. 1978 Proctocolectomy without ileostomy for ulcerative colitis. *Brit. Med. J.* ii 85–88 (4, 344)

Parry L. A. 1928 Dr. Smethurst's lucky escape. In *Some Famous Medical Trials*, reprinted 2000 by Beard Books, Washington DC 193–207 (4, 1)

Parsons L. G 1913 Intestinal infantilism – discussion. *Birmingham Med. Review*. 74:33 (3, 34)

Parsons L. G. 1927 The bone changes occurring in renal and coeliac infantilism and their relationship to rickets. *Arch. Dis. Child.* ii 1 & 98 (3, 35)

Paterson H. J. 1909 Jejunal and gastrojejunal ulcer following gastroenterostomy. *Annals of Surgery* 50: 367–440 (2, 130)

Paull A., Trier J. S., Dalton M. D., Camp R. C., Loeb P., Goyal R. K. 1976 The histologic spectrum of Barrett's oesophagus. *New England Journal of Medicine* 295; 476–480 (1, 103)

Paulley J. W. 1948 Regional ileitis. *Lancet* i 923 (3, 57)

Paulley J. W. 1949 Chronic diarrhoea symposium *Proceedings of the Royal Society of Medicine* 42: 241–244 (3, 58 and 61)

Paulley J. W. 1950 Ulcerative colitis–a study of 173 patients. *Gastroenterology* 16 566 (3, 56)

Paulley J. W. 1951 Discussion on the aetiology of the sprue syndrome *Gastroenterologia* 78 Fasc 6 361 (3, 62)

Paulley J. W. 1952 *Transactions of the Roy. Soc. Trop. Med. & Hyg.* 46: 594–595 (3, 63)

Paulley J. W. 1954 Observations on the aetiology of idiopathic steatorrhoea; Jejunal and lymph node biopsies. *Brit. Med. J.* ii 1318–29 (3, 64)

Paulley J. W. 1959 Emotion and personality in the aetiology of steatorrhoea. *Amer. J. Dig. Dis.* 4, 352–360 (3, 55 and 59)

Pavey F. 1869 *A Treatise on the Function of Digestion*. 2nd edition John Churchill & Son (2, 9)

Payler D. K., Pomare E. W., Heaton K. W. and Harvey R. F. 1975 The effect of wheat bran on intestinal transit. *Gut*, 16, 209–213 (5, 183)

Payne R. T. and Newman C. E. 1940 Interim Report on dyspepsia in the Army. *Brit. Med. J.* ii, 819–821 (5, 120)

Payne W. W. and Poulton E. P. 1927 Experiments on visceral sensation: Part 1, The relation of pain to activity in the human oesophagus. *J. Physiol.* lxiii 217–241 (5, 189)

Payne-James J. J., Silk D. B. A. 1990 Use of elemental diets in the treatment of Crohn's disease by gastroenterologists. *Gut* 31: 1424 (4, 310)

Penston J. G. 1996 Review article: clinical aspects of Helicobacter pylori eradication therapy in peptic ulcer disease. *Alimentary Pharmacology and Therapeutics* 10: 469–486 (2, 207)

Penston J. G. and Pounder R. E. 1996 A survey of dyspepsia in Great Britain. *Alimentary Pharmacology and Therapeutics* 10, 83–89 (5, 317)

Peppercorn M. A., Goldman P. 1973 Distribution studies of salicyl-azo-sulfapyridine and its metabolites. *Gastroenterology* 64: 240–245 (4, 94)

Percival T. 1789 *Essays Medical, Philosophical and Experimental*, 4th ed., vol 2 (3, 26)

Perrett A. D., Truelove S. C., Massarella G. R. 1968 Crohn's disease and cancer of the colon. *Brit. Med. J.* i 464–468 (4, 280)

Peters T. J., Bjarnason I. 1984 Coeliac syndrome: biochemical mechanisms and the missing peptidase hypothesis revisited. *Gut* 25: 913–918 (3, 137)

Peters G. A. and Bargen J. A. 1944 The irritable bowel syndrome. *Gastroenterology*, 3, 399–402 (5, 136)

Pettigrew T. J. 1838–40 *Medical Portraits Gallery, 4 volumes "John Abernethy FRS"* Fisher and Son, London II, 10 (5, 39)

Philip A. P. W. 1824 *A Treatise on Indigestion and its Consequences Called Nervous and Bilious Complaints; With Observations on the Organic Diseases in Which They Sometimes Terminate*. 4th edition. Thomas and George Underwood, London (5, 40)

Pickering G. 1974 *Creative Malady* George Allen and Unwin, London, (5, 58)

Pink I. J., Creamer B. 1967 Response to a gluten-free diet of patients with the coeliac syndrome. *Lancet* i: 300–304 (3, 110)

Pink I. J., Croft D. N., Creamer B. 1970 Cell loss from the small intestinal mucosa: a morphological study. *Gut* 11; 217–222 (3, 108)

Plague, Pox & Pestilence 1997 edited by Kiple K. F. Weidenfeld and Nicolson 160–5 (2, 4)

Plummer H. S. 1908 Cardiospasm; with a report of forty cases. *J.A.M.A.* 51; 549–554 (1, 16)

Pollock A. V. 1952 Vagotomy in the treatment of peptic ulceration: review of 1524 cases. *Lancet* ii: 795–802 (2, 159)

Porter R. 1999 in *The Greatest Benefit to Mankind*. Fontana Press. London 3: p49 (4, 18)

Poulter L. W., Campbell D. A., Munro C., Janossy G. 1986 Discrimination of human macrophages and dendritic cells in chronic inflammatory bowel disease. *Scand. J. Immunol.* 21: 401–407 (4, 190)

Pounder R. E., Williams J. G., Milton-Thompson G. J. 1975 Effect of metiamide on duodenal ulcer: a controlled trial. *Brit. Med. J.* ii 307–309 (2, 176)

Pounder R. E., Williams J. G., Milton-Thompson G. J., Misiewicz J. J. 1975 24–hour control of intragastric acidity by cimetidine in duodenal ulcer patients. *Lancet* ii: 1069–72 (2, 180)

Powell-Tuck J., Nielson T., Farwell J. A., Lennard-Jones J. E. 1978 Team approach to long term intravenous feeding in patients with gastrointestinal disorders. *Lancet* ii, 825–828 (4, 293)

Power Sir Darcy 1930 My Book by John Abernethy, XI Epoch-making Books in British Surgery. *Brit. J. Surg.*, 17, 369–372 (5, 38)

Price W. 1956 *Textbook of the Practice of Medicine*. 9th edition p577 (2, 3)

Prior P., Gyde S. N., Macartney J. C., Thompson H., Waterhouse J. A. H., Allan R. N. 1982 Cancer morbidity in ulcerative colitis. *Gut* 23: 490–497 (4, 265)

Prior A. and Read N. 1993 Reduction of rectal sensitivity and post-prandial motility by granisetron, a 5 HT3–receptor antagonist, in patients with irritable bowel syndrome. *Alimentary Pharmacology and Therapeutics* 7, 175–180 (5, 382)

Prior A., Colgan, S. M. and Whorwell P. J. 1990 Changes in rectal sensitivity after hypnotherapy in patients with irritable bowel syndrome. *Gut*, 31, 896–898 (5, 298)

Prior A., Maxton, D. and Whorwell P. J. 1990 Anorectal manometry in irritable bowel syndrome: differences between diarrhoea and constipation-predominant subjects. *Gut*, 31, 458–462 (5, 262)

Prior A., Sorial, E., Sun W. M., and Read, N. W. 1993 Irritable bowel syndrome: differences between patients who show rectal sensitivity and those who do not. *Eur. J. Gastroenterol Hepatol* 5, 342–349 (5, 263)

Prior A., Wilson, K., Whorwell P. J. and Faragher E. B. 1989 Irritable bowel syndrome in the gynaecological clinic. Survey of 798 new referrals. *Dig. Dis. Sci.* 34, 1820–24 (5, 354)

Probert C. S. J., Jayanthi V., Pinder D., Wicks A. C., Mayberry J. F. 1992 Epidemiologicqal study of ulcerative proctocolitis in Indian migrants and the indigenous population of Leicestershire. *Gut* 33: 687–693 (4, 147 and 239)

Probert C. S. J., Warren B. F., Perry T., Mackay E. H., Mayberry J. F., Corfield A. P. 1995 South Asian and European colitics show characteristic differences in colonic mucus glycoprotein type and turnover. *Gut* 36: 696–702 (4, 240)

Prout B. J. 1974 A rapid method of obtaining a jejunal biopsy using a Crosby capsule and gastrointestinal fibrescope. *Gut* 15: 571–572 (3, 188)

Prout W. 1824 On the nature of acid and saline matters usually existing in the stomach of animals. *Phil. Trans. R. Soc.* 1:45–49 (2, 7)

Provenzale I. and Revignas A. 1969 An original method for guided intubation of the colon. *Gastrointest. Endosc.* 16, 73–76 (6, 66)

Provision of a gastroenterological service in the District General Hospital 1979 Working Party of the Gastroenterological Liaison Committee with the DHSS. HMSO booklet and BSG (6, 88)

Provision of gastrointestinal endoscopy and related services for a district general hospital. 1991 Report of a Working Party of the Clinical Services Committee of the British Society of Gastroenterology. *Gut*, 32, 95–105 (6, 131)

Pullan R. D., Thomas G. A. O., Rhodes M., Newcombe R. G., Williams G. T., Allen A., Rhodes J. 1994 Thickness of adherent mucus gel on colonic mucosa in humans and its relevance to colitis. *Gut* 35: 353–359 (4, 237)

Pulvertaft C. N. 1968 Comments on the incidence and natural history of gastric and duodenal ulcer *Postgrad. Med. J.* 44: 597–602 (2, 61)

Purton T. 1821 An extraordinary Case of Distension of the Oesophagus, forming a sac, extending from two inches below the Pharynx to the Cardiac Orifice of the Stomach. *London Med. and Physical Journal* XLV, 1540–542 (1, 9)

Quain R. 1895 Some Clinical Observations and Professional Reminiscences. *Brit. Med. J.* ii, 1147 (5, 64)

Quine M. A., Bell D. G., McCloy, R. F., Charlton J. E., Devlin H. B. and Hopkins, A. 1995 Prospective audit of upper gastrointestinal endoscopy in two regions of England: safety, staffing and sedation methods. *Gut*, 36, 462–467 (6, 133)

Rae J. W., Allison R. S. 1953 The effect of diet and regular living conditions on the natural history of peptic ulcer. *Quart. J. Med.* 22: 439– 455 (2, 149)

Rake G. W. 1926 A case of annular muscular hypertrophy of the oesophagus. *Guy's Hosp. Reports* 76; 145–152 (1, 5)

Rake G. W. 1927 On the pathology of achalasia of the cardia. *Guy's Hosp. Reports.* 77 141–150 (1, 6)

Raouf A. H., Hildrey V., Daniel J., Walker R. J., Krasner N., Elias E., Rhodes J. M. 1991 Enteral feeding as the sole treatment for Crohn's disease: controlled trial of whole protein v amino acid based feed and a case study of dietary challenge. *Gut* 32: 702–707 (4, 210)

Read N. W. 1986 Diarrhee motrice *Clinics in gastroenterology* 15:3, 657–686 (5, 249)

Read N. W. 1991 The neurotic bowel: a paradigm for the irritable bowel syndrome. in *Irritable Bowel Syndrome, New Ideas and Insights Into Pathophysiology*. ed Read, N. W. Blackwell Scientific publications, Oxford (5, 265)

Read N. W. and Brown, N. J. 1991 The small intestine and the ileal brake. in: *Gastrointestinal Transit: Pathophysiology and Pharmacology*. Ed Kamm M. A. and Lennard-Jones, J. E. Wrightson Biomedical Publishing Ltd. Petersfield (5, 251)

Read, N. W., McFarlane, A., Kinsman, R. I., Bates, T. E., Blackhall, N. W., Farrar, G. B. J., Hall, J. C., Moss, G., Morris, A. P., O'Neil, B., Welch, I. Mcl., Lee, Y. and Bloom, S. R. 1984 The effect of infusion of nutrient solutions into the ileum on gastrointestinal transit and plasma levels of neurotensin and enteroglucagon. *Gastroenterology*, 86: 274–280 (5, 250)

Reaumur R. A. F. de, 1752 *Sur la digestion des oiseaux. Memoires de mathematiques et de physique* Premier memoire, 461 Paris (5, 17)

Recommendations for Training in Gastrointestinal Endoscopy. 1999 Joint Advisory Group. Royal College of Physicians, London (6, 132 & 149 & 157)

Rees R. G. P., Hare W. R., Grimble G. K., Frost P. G., Silk D. B. A. 1992 Do patients with moderately impaired gastrointestinal function requiring enteral nutrition need a pre-digested nitrogen source? A prospective crossover controlled clinical trial. *Gut* 33: 877–881 (4, 302)

Rees G. 1810 *Practical Observations on Disorders of the Stomach with Remarks on the Use of Bile in Promoting Digestion* Allen, London (5, 34) *Registrar General's Annual Reports* (1905–35) (2, 53)

Regula J. et al 1995 Photosensitisation and photodynamic therapy of oesophageal, duodenal, and colorectal tumours using 5 aminolaevulinic acid induced protoporphyrin 1X- a pilot study *Gut* 36; 67–75 (1, 115)

Rhodes J. M., Bartholemew T. C., Jewell D. P. 1981 Inhibition of leucocyte motility by drugs used in ulcerative colitis. *Gut* 22: 642–647 (4, 185)

Rhodes J. M. 1996 Unifying hypothesis for inflammatory bowel disease and associated colon cancer: sticking the pieces together with sugar. *Lancet* i, 40–44 (4, 241)

Rhodes J. M. 2000 Colorectal cancer screening in the UK: Joint Position Statement by the British Society of Gastroenterology, the Royal College of Physicians, and the Association of Coloproctology of Great Britain and Ireland. *Gut*, 46, 746–748 (6, 154)

Rice-Oxley J. M., Truelove S. C. 1950 Ulcerative colitis: course and prognosis. *Lancet* i 663–666 (4, 68)

Richmond T. 1909 The gastroscope and its uses. *Brit. Med. J.* ii, 1195–96 (6, 5)

Riddell R. H., Goldman H., Ransohoff D. F., et al. 1983 Dysplasia in inflammatory bowel disease: standardised classification with provisional clinical applications. *Hum. Pathol.* 14: 931–968 (4, 260)

Riddell R. H., Morson B. C. 1979 Value of sigmoidoscopy and biopsy in detection of carcinoma and premalignant change in ulcerative colitis. *Gut* 20: 575–580 (4, 259)

Riecken E. O., Stewart J. S., Booth C. C., Pearse A. G. E. 1966 A histochemical study on the role of lysosymes in idiopathic steatorrhoea before and during a gluten-free diet. *Gut* 7 317–332 (3, 134)

Riordan A. M., Hunter J. O., Cowan R. E., Crampton J. R., Davidson J. R., Dickinson R. J., Dronfield M. W., Fellows I. W., Hishon S., Kerrigan G. N. W., Kennedy H. J., McGouran R. C. M., Neale G., Saunders J. H. B. 1993 Treatment of active Crohn's disease by exclusion diet. East Anglian Multicentre Controlled Trial. *Lancet* ii, 1131–34 (4, 316)

Ritchie J. K., Hawley P. R., Lennard-Jones J. E. 1981 Prognosis of cancer in ulcerative colitis. *Gut* 22: 752–755 (4, 267)

Ritchie H. D., Thompson D. G. and Wingate D. L. 1980 Diurnal variation in human jejunal fasting motor activity. *J. Physiol.* 305, 54–55P (5, 237)

Ritchie J. A. 1973 Pain from distension of the pelvic colon by inflating a balloon in the irritable colon syndrome. *Gut*, 14,125–32 (5, 143 and 253)

Ritchie J. A. 1985 Mechanisms of Pain in the Irritable Bowel Syndrome. 163–171 In: *Irritable Bowel Syndrome* ed Read, N. W. Grune and Stratton, London (5, 221)

Ritchie J. A., Ardran G. M. & Truelove S. C. 1962 Motor activity of the sigmoid colon of humans. *Gastroenterology*, 43,642–668 (5, 142)

Ritchie J. A. 1968 Colonic motor activity and bowel function. Part 1. Normal movement of contents. *Gut.* 9, 442–456 (5, 141)

Ritchie J. A. and Truelove S. C. 1980 Comparison of various treatments for irritable bowel syndrome. *Brit. Med. J.* ii: 1317–19 (5, 217)

Roberts C. J., Digger R. 1982 Non-smoking: a feature of ulcerative colitis. *Brit. Med. J.* ii 440 (4, 152)

Robertson C. R., Langlois K., Martin C. G., Slezak G., Grossman M. I. 1950 Release of gastrin in response to bathing the pyloric mucosa with acetylcholine. *Amer. J. Physiol.* 163: 27–33 (2, 33)

Rodgers, H. W. 1937 *Textbook of Gastroscopy by N. Henning* (trans). OUP, London (6, 21)

Rollason T. P., Stone J., Rhodes J. M. 1984 Spiral organisms in endoscopic biopsies of the human stomach. *J. Clin. Pathol.* 37: 23–26 (2, 188)

Root H. K. 1856 *The People's Medical Lighthouse.* Ranney, New York, p114 (5, 108)

Rothery G. A., Patterson J. E., Stoddard C. J., Day D. W. 1986 Histological and histochemical changes in columnar lined (Barrett's) oesophagus *Gut* 27; 1062–68 (1, 104)

Rowlands, E. N. & Wolff, H. S. 1960 The radio pill. Telemetering from the digestive tract. *Brit. Commun. Electron.* 7, 598–701 (5, 144)

Russel J. C. 1898 Diagnosis and treatment of spasmodic stricture of the oesophagus. *Brit. Med. J.* June 4th 1450 -1451 (1, 15)

Rutter M. D., Saunders B. P., Schofield G., Forbes A., Price A. B., Talbot I. C. 2004 Pancolonic indigo carmine dye spraying for the detection of dysplasia in ulcerative colitis. *Gut* 53: 256–260 (4, 277)

Rutter M. D., Wilkinson K. H., Rumbles S., Forbes A., Saunders B. P. 2003 How effective is cancer surveillance in ulcerative colitis? *Gut*, 52; Suppl. 1A66 (4, 276)

Ryan F. P., Smart R. C., Holdsworth C. D., Preston F. E. 1978 Hyposplenism in inflammatory bowel disease. *Gut* 19: 50–55 (4, 318)

Ryle J. A. 1921 Inhibition of gastric secretion by butter and cream *Guy's Hosp.Rep*.lxxi 54 (2, 122)

Ryle J. A. 1924 Fatty stools from obstruction of the lacteals. *Guy's Hosp. Reports* lxxiv: 1–8 (3, 17)

Ryle J. A. 1928 Chronic Spasmodic Affections of the Colon and the Diseases which they Simulate. *Lancet*, ii, 1115–17 (5, 114)

Ryle J. A. 1932 The natural history of duodenal ulcer. *Lancet* i: 327–334 (2, 67 and 72)

Ryle J. A. 1936 *The Natural History of Disease*. Oxford University Press (5, 115)

Sachar D. B. 2002 Appendix redux. *Gut* 51: 764–765 (4, 158)

Sakula J., Shiner M. 1957 Coeliac disease with atrophy of the small-intestine mucosa. *Lancet* i: 876–877 (3, 90)

Salmon P. R., Branch R. A., Collins C., Espiner H. and Read A. E. 1971 Clinical evaluation of fibreoptic sigmoidoscopy employing the Olympus CF-SB colonoscope *Gut*, 12, 729–735 (6, 71)

Salmon P. R., Brown P., Htut T. & Read A. E. 1972 Endoscopic examination of the duodenal bulb: clinical evaluation of forward- and side-viewing fibreoptic systems in 200 cases. *Gut* 13, 170–5 (6, 56)

Salmon P. R., Brown P., Williams R., Read A. E. 1974 Evaluation of colloidal bismuth (De-Nol) in the treatment of duodenal ulcer employing endoscopic selection and follow up. *Gut* 15: 189–193 (2, 184)

Sand G. 1855 *Histoire de ma Vie*. Vol xviii. p295 Paris (5, 88)

Sanderson I. R., Boulton P., Menzies I. S., Walker-Smith J. A. 1987 Improvement of abnormal lactulose/rhamnose permeability in active Crohn's disease of the small bowel by an elemental diet. *Gut* 28: 1073–76 (4, 305)

Sanderson I. R., Udeen S., Davies P. J. W., Savage M. O., Walker-Smith J. A. 1987 Remission induced by an elemental diet in small bowel Crohn's disease. *Arch. Dis. Child* 61: 123–7 (4, 211)

Sarkar S., Aziz, Q., Woolf C. J., Hobson A. R. and Thompson D. G. 2000 Contribution of central sensitisation to the development of non-cardiac chest pain *Lancet*, ii, 1154–59 (5, 303 & 399)

Satsangi J., Parkes M., Louis E. et al 1996 Two stage genome-wide search in inflammatory bowel disease provides evidence for susceptibility loci on chromosomes 3,7 and 12. *Nat. Genet.* 14: 199–202 (4, 146)

Satsangi J., Welsh K. I., Bunce M., Julien C., Farrant J. M., Bell J. I., Jewell D. P. 1996 Contribution of genes of the major histocompatibility complex to susceptibility and disease phenotype in inflammatory bowel disease. *Lancet* i, 1212–17 (4, 143)

Sauer W. G., Bargen J. A. 1949 Chronic ulcerative colitis and carcinoma. *J. Amer. Med. Assoc.* 141: 982–985 (4, 245)

Saunders B. P., Bell G. D., Williams C. B., Bladen J. S. and Anderson, A. P. 1995 First clinical results with a real time, electronic imager as an aid to colonoscopy. *Gut*, 36, 913–917 (6, 147)

Saverymuttu S. H., Camilleri M., Rees H., Lavender J. P., Hodgson H. J. F., Chadwick V. S. 1986 Indium-111 granulocyte scanning in the assessment of disease extent and disease activity in inflammatory bowel disease. *Gastroenterology* 90: 1121–28 (4, 202)

Saverymuttu S. H., Hodgson H. J. F., Chadwick V. S. 1985 Controlled trial comparing prednisolone with an elemental diet plus non-absorbable antibiotics in active Crohn's disease. *Gut* 26: 994–998 (4, 207)

Schiller K. F. R., Truelove S. C. and Williams D. G. 1970 Haematemesis and melaena, with special reference to factors influencing the outcome. *Brit. Med. J.* i, 7–14 (6, 80)

Schiller K. F. R. 2003 Sidney Truelove and gastrointestinal endoscopy. A look at the contribution of Sidney Truelove to gastrointestinal medicine and the history of the endoscope. *Oxford Med School Gazette* Issue 54, vol 1 (6, 82)

Schiller K. F. R., Axon A. T. R., Carr-Locke D. L., Cockel R., Donovan I. A., Edmondstone W. M, Ellis A., Gilmore I. T., Harvey R. F., Linaker B. D., Morris A. I., Wastell C., Williams J. G., Gillon K. R. W. 1989 Duodenal ulcer recurrence after healing with omeprazole or cimetidine treatment: a multicentre study in the UK. *Gut* 30: A1490 (2, 198)

Schiller L. R., Davis D. R., Santa Ana C. A., Morawski S. G. and Fordtran J. S. 1982 Studies of the mechanism of the antidiarrheal effect of codeine. *J. Clin. Invest.* 70: 999–1008 (5, 247)

Schindler R. 1922 Bericht uber 120 Falle von Gastroskopie. Arztl. Verein Munchen, 25. Reported in *Deutsche Med. Wehnschr.* 48, 310 (6, 14)

Schindler R. 1923 *Lehrbuch und Atlas der Gastroskopie.* Munich, I. F. Lehmann (6, 15)

Schindler R. 1932 Ein vollig ungerfahrliches, flexible Gastroskop. *München Med. Wsch.* 32, 1268–69 (6, 16)

Schindler R. 1937 *Gastroscopy: the Endoscopic Study of Gastric Pathology.* Univ. of Chicago Press, Chicago, Illinois (6, 18 & 36)

Schrager J., Oates M. D. G. 1978 Relation of human intestinal mucus to disease states. *British Medical Bulletin* 34: 79–82 (4, 231)

Schroder H., Campbell D. E. S. 1972 Absorption, metabolism and excretion of salicyl-azo-sulfapyridine in man. *Clin Pharmacol Therap.* 13: 539–551 (4, 93)

Schroder H., Price-Evans D. A. 1972 Acetylator phenotype and adverse effects of sulphasalazine in healthy subjects. *Gut* 13: 278–284 (4, 95)

Scoping our Practice; the 2004 Report of the National Confidential Enquiry into Patient Outcome and Deaths. London. NCEPOD <www.ncepod. org.uk/2004> (6, 161)

Scott B. B., Losowsky M. S. 1976 Peroral small-intestinal biopsy: experience with the hydraulic multiple biopsy instrument in routine clinical practice. *Gut* 17: 740–743 (3, 187)

Scott B. B., Losowsky M. S. 1976 Patchiness and duodenal-jejunal variation of the mucosal abnormality in coeliac disease and dermatitis herpetiformis. *Gut* 17: 984–992 (3, 186)

Scott B. B., Jenkins D. 1981 Endoscopic small-intestinal biopsy. *Gastrointestinal Endoscopy* 27, 162–7 (3, 192)

Scott B. B., Goodall A., Stephenson P., Jenkins D. 1984 Small intestinal plasma cells in coeliac disease. *Gut* 25; 41–46 (3, 173)

Scott H. H. 1923 The nature and treatment of sprue. *Brit. Med. J.* ii, 1135–37 (3, 24)

Scott Harden W. G. 1960 *Mod Trends in Diagnostic Radiology.* Ed. J. W. McLaren Butterworths (5, 123)

Seah P. P., Fry Lionel, Hoffbrand A. V., Holborow E. J. 1971 Tissue antibodies in dermatitis herpetiformis and adult coeliac disease. *Lancet* i: 834–836 (3, 215)

Seah P. P., Fry Lionel, Rossiter M. A., Hoffbrand A. V., Holborow E. J. 1971 Antireticulin antibodies in childhood celiac disease. *Lancet* ii: 681–682 (3, 216)

Seah P. P., Fry Lionel, Holborow E. J., Rossiter M. A., Doe W. F., Magalhaes A. F., Hoffbrand A. V. 1973 Antireticulin antibody: Incidence and diagnostic significance. *Gut* 14: 311–315 (3, 217)

Segal A. W. 2005 How neutrophils kill microbes. *Ann. Rev. Immunol.* 23: 197–223 (4, 200)

Segal A. W., Loewi G. 1976 Neutrophil dysfunction in Crohn's disease. *Lancet* ii 219–221. (4, 178 and 201)

Segal A. W., Peters T. J. 1975 The nylon column dye test: a possible screening test of phagocytic function. *Clin. Sci. Mol. Med.* 49: 591–596 (4, 176)

Selby W. S., Janossy G., Jewell D. P. 1981 Immunohistological characterisation of intraepithelial lymphocytes of the human gastrointestinal tract. *Gut* 22: 169–176 (3, 169) (4, 187)

Selby W. S., Poulter L. W., Hobbs S., Jewell D. P. 1983 Heterogeneity of HLA-DR positive histiocytes in human intestinal lamina propria: a combined histochemical and immunohistological analysis. *J. Clin. Pathol.* 36: 379–384 (4, 192)

Selby W. S., Janossy G., Bofill M., Jewell D. P. 1983 Lymphocyte subpopulations in the human small intestine. The findings in normal mucosa and in the mucosa of patients with coeliac disease. *Clin. Exp. Immunol* 52: 219 (3, 170)

Selby W. S., Janossy G., Bofill, Jewell D. P. 1984 Intestinal lymphocyte subpopulations in inflammatory bowel disease: an analysis by immunohistological and cell isolation techniques. *Gut* 25: 32–40 (4, 188)

Selby W. S., Barr G. D., Ireland A., Mason C. H., Jewell D. P. 1985 Olsalazine in active ulcerative colitis. *Brit. Med. J.* 291; 1373–75 (4, 102)

Senn H. 1972 *Fektalswehr bei Homoblastosen*. p36 Berlin (4, 179)

Shanahan F. 2000 Mechanisms of immunologic sensation of intestinal contents. *Amer. J. Physiol.* 278: G191–G196 (4, 198)

Shanahan F. 2002 Crohn's disease. *Lancet* i p65 (4, 212)

Sharma B. K., Walt R. P., Pounder R. E., Gomes M. de F. A., Wood E. C., Logan L. H. 1984 Optimal dose of oral omeprazole for maximal 24 hour decrease of gastric acidity. *Gut* 25: 957–964 (2, 197)

Shearman D. J. C., Warwick, R. R. G., MacLeod, I. B. and Dean, A. C. B. 1971 Clinical evaluation of the Olympus duodenoscope. *Lancet*, i, 726–729 (6, 55)

Sheil F. O'M., Clark C. G., Goligher J. C. 1968 Adenocarcinoma associated with Crohn's disease. *Brit. J. Surg.* 55: 53–58 (4, 279)

Sheldon W. 1949 Coeliac disease: a relation between dietary starch and fat absorption. *Arch. Dis. Child*. 24: 81–87 (3, 67)

Sheldon W. 1955 *Diseases of Infancy and Childhood*. p217 Churchill, London (3, 78)

Sheldon W. 1969 Prognosis in Early Adult Life of Coeliac Children Treated with a Gluten-free Diet. *Brit. Med. J.* i;401–404 (3, 95)

Sheldon W., Tempany E. 1966 Small intestine peroral biopsy in coeliac children. *Gut* 7: 481–489 (3, 94 and 120)

Sherren J. 1912 On the early recognition of, and prevention of carcinoma of the stomach. Quoted by Hill, in: *On Gastroscopy*. John Bale Sons & Danielson, Oxford St. London p1 (6, 10)

Shiner M. 1956 Duodenal biopsy. *Lancet* i: 17–19 (3, 83)

Shiner M. 1956 Jejunal-biopsy tube *Lancet* i: 85 (3, 84)

Shiner M. 1957 Duodenal and jejunal biopsies. I. A discussion of the method, its difficulties and applications. *Gastroenterology* 33: 64–70 (3, 85)

Shiner M. 1960 Coeliac disease: Histopathological findings in the small intestinal mucosa studied by a peroral biopsy technique. *Gut*, 1,48–54 (3, 91)

Shiner M., Doniach I. 1960 Histopathologic studies in steatorrhoea. *Gastroenterology* 38: 419–440 (3, 86)

Shiner M., Ballard J. 1972 Antigen-antibody reactions in jejunal mucosa in childhood coeliac disease after gluten challenge. *Lancet* i: 1202–05 (3, 143)

Shiner M. 1973 Ultrastructural changes suggestive of immune reactions in the jejunal mucosa of coeliac children following gluten challenge. *Gut*,14: 1–12 (3, 154)

Shoemaker G. E. 1898 The Importance of Chronic Irritability of the Colon, with Mucous Stools as a Symptom of Appendicitis. *Ann.Surg*. 6; 733–740 (5, 82)

Shorter R. G., Cardoza M., ReMine S. G., Spencer R. S., Huizenga K. A. 1970 Modification of in-vitro cytotoxicity of lymphocytes from patients with chronic ulcerative colitis or granulomatous colitis for allogenic colonic epithelial cells. *Gastroenterology* 58: 692–698 (4, 173)

Shorter R. G., Huizenga K. A., Spencer J. 1972 A working hypothesis for the aetiology and pathogenesis of non-specific inflammatory bowel disease. *Dig. Dis*. 17: 1024–32 (4, 174)

Shuster S., Marks J. 1965 Dermatogenic enteropathy. *Lancet* i, 1361–63 (3, 161)

Sippy B. W. 1915 Gastric and duodenal ulcer: Medical cure by an efficient removal of gastric juice corrosion. *Trans. Assoc. Am. Physicians* 30: 129–148 (2, 120)

Sircus W 1984 Medical-surgical collaboration and practice of gastroenterology. *Postgrad. Med. J.* 60: 725–732 (4, 69)

Sircus W 2003 Milestones in the evolution of endoscopy; a short history. *J Roy Coll Phys Edin* 33, 124–134 (6, 31)

Skinner D. B., Belsey R. H. R. 1967 Surgical management of esophageal reflux and hiatus hernia: Long term results with 1,030 patients. *J. Thorac. Cardiovasc. Surg.* 53: 33– 54 (1, 95)

Skirrow M.B. 1977 Campylobacter enteritis: a "new" disease. *Brit. Med. J.* ii, 9–11 (2, 101)

Skirrow M.B. 2001 Personal communication. (2, 102)

Sladen G. E. 1987 in *History of the British Society of Gastroenterology 1937–87* ed J. H. Baron *Gut*, 28, Jubilee supplement p16 (4, 76)

Slaney G., Brooke B. N. 1959 Cancer in ulcerative colitis. *Lancet* ii, 694–698 (4, 250)

Smale S., Bjarnason I., Forgacs I., Prasad P., Mukhood M., Wong M., Ng A. and Mulcahy H. E. 2003 Upper gastrointestinal endoscopy performed by nurses: scope for the future? *Gut*, 52, 1090–94 (6, 141)

Smith A. C., Price A. B., Borriello P., Levi A. J. 1988 A comparison of ranitidine and tripotassium dicitratobismuth (TDB) in relapse rates of duodenal ulcer. The role of campylobacter pylori (CP) *Gut* 29: A 711 (2, 189)

Smith P. M., Brian Jones D. and Rose J. D. R. 1982 Simplified fibre endoscopic sclerotherapy for oesophageal varices. *J. Roy. Coll. Phys.* 16, 4, 236–238 (6, 101)

Smith, P. M. and Williams, R. 1992 A comparison of workloads of physician-gastroenterologists and other consultant physicians. *J. Roy. Coll. Phys.* 26, 2, 167–8 (6, 120)

Smith P. M., Kerr G. D., Cockel R. et al 1994 A comparison of omeprazole and ranitidine in the prevention of recurrence of benign oesophageal stricture. *Gastroenterology* 107, 1312–18 (1, 108)

Smith T. S. 1835–37 *The Philosophy of Health, or an Exposition of the Physical and Mental Constitution of Man: With a View to the Promotion of Human Longevity and Happiness.* 2 vols Knight, London II p642–644 (5, 44)

Smithers D. W. 1955 Radiotherapy for carcinoma of the oesophagus *Brit. J. Radiol. n.s.* 28: 554–564 (1, 71)

Snook J. A. and Shepherd H. A. 1994 Bran supplementation in the treatment of irritable bowel syndrome. *Alimentary Pharmacology and Therapeutics* 8, 511–514 (5, 289)

Soehendra N. and Reynders-Frederix V. 1980 Palliative bile duct drainage – a new endoscopic method of introducing a transpapillary drain. *Endoscopy*, 12, 8–11 (6, 110)

Somerville K., Faulkner G., Langman M. J. S. 1986 Non-steroidal anti-inflammatory drugs and bleeding peptic ulcer. *Lancet* i 462–464 (2, 90)

Somerville K. W., Logan R. F. A., Edmond M., Langman M. J. S. 1984 Smoking and Crohn's disease. *Brit. Med. J.* ii, 954–956 (4, 154)

Sonnenberg A. 1995 Temporal trends and geographical variations of peptic ulcer disease. *Alimentary Pharmacology and Therapeutics*9 (Suppl.)3–12 (2, 111)

Southgate D. A. T. 1978 The definition, analysis and properties of dietary fibre.In *Dietary Fibre: Current Developments of Importance to Health*. ed K W Heaton, Newman Publishing, London 9 -19 (5, 175)

Southgate D. A. T. and Durnin J. V. G. A. 1970 Colonic conversion factors. An experimental reassessment of the factors used in the calculation of the energy value of human diets. *Br. J. Nut.* 24, 517–535 (5, 277)

Souttar H. S. and Thompson T. 1909 The gastroscope and its uses. *Brit. Med. J.* ii, 843–846 (6, 11)

Souttar H. S. 1927 Treatment of carcinoma of the oesophagus: based on 100 personal cases and 18 post-mortem reports. *Brit. J. Surg.* 15, 76–94 (1, 46)

Spallanzani L. 1783 *Experiences de Digestion de l'Homme et de Differentes Especes d'Animaux*. Translated by J. Senebier, Barthélemy Chirol, Geneva (5, 18)

Spencer J. M., MacDonald T. T., Diss T. C., Walker-Smith J. A., Ciclitira P. J., Isaacson P. G. 1989 Changes in intraepithelial lymphocyte subpopulations in coeliac disease and enteropathy associated T cell lymphoma (malignant histiocytosis of the intestine). *Gut* 30; 339–346 (3, 176)

Spiller R. C., Trotman I. F., Higgins B. E., Ghatel M. A., Grimble, G. K., Lee, Y. C., Bloom, S. R., Misiewicz, J. J. and Silk, D. B. A. 1984 The ileal brake–inhibition of jejunal motility after ileal fat infusion in man. *Gut*, 25, 365–374 (5, 309)

Spiller R. C., Brown M. L. and Phillips S. F. 1986 Decreased fluid tolerance, accelerated transit, and abnormal motility of the human colon induced by oleic acid. *Gastroenterology*, 91, 100–7 (5, 310)

Spiller R. C., Jenkins, D., Thornley J. P., Hebden J. M., Wright T., Skinner M. and Neal, K. R. 2000 Increased rectal mucosal enteroendocrine cells, T lymphocytes, and increased gut permeability following acute Campylobacter enteritis and in post-dysenteric irritable bowel syndrome. *Gut*, 47, 804–811 (5, 313)

Spiller R., Aziz, Q., Creed F., Emmanuel A., Houghton L., Hungin P., Jones R., Kumar D., Rubin G., Trudgill N. and Whorwell P. 2007 Guidelines on the irritable bowel syndrome: mechanisms and practical management. *Gut*, 56; 1770–98 (5, 315 and 375)

Spriggs E. I. 1931 Functional disorders of the colon. *Quart. J. Med.* 24, 533–541 (5, 135 and 304)

Srivastava E. D., Mayberry J. F., Morris T. J., Smith P. M., Williams G. T., Roberts G. M., Newcombe R. G., Rhodes J. 1992 Incidence of ulcerative colitis in Cardiff over 20 years: 1968–87. *Gut* 33: 256–258 (4, 118)

Stack W. A., Williams D., Stevenson M. et al. 1999 Immunosuppressive therapy for ulcerative colitis: results of a nation-wide survey among consultant physician members of the British Society of Gastroenterology. *Alimentary Pharmacology and Therapeutics*. 5: 569–575 (4, 332)

Staffing of endoscopy units. 1987 Report of a Working Party. *Gut*, 28, 1682–85 (6, 122)

Stanciu C. and Bennett J. R. 1975 The general pattern of gastro-duodenal motility: 24 hour recordings in normal subjects. *Rev. Med. Chir. Soc. Med. Nat. Iasi;* 79, 31–36 (5, 204)

Steele G. H. 1943 Excision of oesophagus and oesophago gastrostomy *Lancet* ii, 797– 798 (1, 65)

Steer H. W., Colin-Jones D. G. 1975 Mucosal changes in gastric ulceration and their response to carbenoloxone sodium. *Gut* 16: 590–597 (2, 186)

Stephen A. M. and Cummings J. H. 1979 Water holding by dietary fibre and its relationship to faecal output in man. *Gut*, 20, 722–729 (5, 278)

Stephen A. M. and Cummings J. H. 1980 The microbial contribution to the human faecal mass. *J. Med. Microbiol.* 13, 45–52 (5, 279)

Stevens F. M., Lloyd R. S., Egan-Mitchell B., Mylotte M. J., Fottrell P. F., Wright R., McNicholl B., McCarthy C. F. 1975 Reticulin antibodies in patients with celiac disease and their relatives. *Gut* 16: 598–602 (3, 220)

Stevens F. M., McCarthy C. F. 1976 The endoscopic demonstration of celiac disease. *Endoscopy* 8, 177–180 (3, 190)

Stewart J. S., Pollock D. J., Hoffbrand A. V., Mollin D. L., Booth C. C. 1967 A study of proximal and distal intestinal structure and absorptive function in idiopathic steatorrhoea. *Quart J. Med. n.s.* 36: 425–444 (3, 103)

Stewart M. J. 1923 The pathology of gastric ulcer. *Brit. Med. J.* ii 955 & 1021 (2, 27)

Stewart M. J., Hartfall S. J. 1929 Chronic peptic ulcer of the oesophagus. *J. Path. Bact.* 329–14 (1, 85)

Still G. F. 1918 The Lumleian Lectures on coeliac disease. *Lancet* ii:163, 193, 227 (3, 15)

Stokes P. L., Asquith P., Holmes G. K. T., Mackintosh P., Cooke W. T. 1972 Histocompatibility antigens associated with adult coeliac disease. *Lancet* ii: 162–4 (3, 146)

Strauss A. A., Strauss S. F. 1944 Surgical treatment of ulcerative colitis. *Surg. Clin. N. Amer.* 24: 211–224 (4, 72)

Strauss H. 1903 Zur Methodik der Rectoskopie. *Berlin Klin. Wschr.* 48, 1100–04 (4, 13) (6, 58)

Summers J. E. 1905 Surgical treatment of chronic muco-membranous colitis and ulcerative colitis. *Annals of Surgery* 42(1) 97–109 (5, 70 and 86)

Susser M. & Stein Z. 1962 Civilisation and peptic ulcer. *Lancet* i:115–9 (2, 65)

Svartz N. 1942 Salazopyrin, a new sulphanilamide preparation B. Therapeutic results in ulcerative colitis. *Acta. Med. Scand.* 110: fasc 6, 580–598 (4, 59)

Svartz N. 1948 The treatment of 124 cases of ulcerative colitis with salazopyrine and attempts at desensitisation in cases of hypersentiveness to sulfa. *Act. Med. Scand. Suppl.* 206 465 (4, 60)

Svartz N. 1956 The treatment of ulcerative colitis. *Gastroenterologia*, Basel. 86: 683–688 (4, 62)

Swain C. P., Bown S. G., Storey D. W., Kirkham J. S., Salmon P. R. and Northfield T. C. 1981 Controlled trial of argon laser photocoagulation in bleeding peptic ulcer. *Lancet*, ii, 1313–16 (6, 106)

Swarbrick E. T., Bat, L., Hegarty J. E., Williams C. B. and Dawson A. M. 1980 Site of pain from the irritable bowel. *Lancet* ii: 443–446 (5, 222)

Swinson C. M., Levi A. J. 1980 Is coeliac disease underdiagnosed? *Brit. Med. J.* iv 1258–60 (3, 195)

Swinson C. M., Slavin G., Coles E. C., Booth C. C. 1983 Coeliac disease and malignancy *Lancet* i: 111–5 (3, 198)

Sydenham T. 1681–2 Epistolary Dissertation to Dr. Cole The Works of Thomas Sydenham vol 2 R. G. Latham *Sydenham Society,* London 1850 56–118 (5, 4 and 5)

Sydenham T. 1683 A Treatise on Gout and Dropsy. The Works of Thomas Sydenham vol 2 R. G. Latham,. *Sydenham Society,* London 1850 129 (5, 3)

Sylvius F. D. 1679 *De Alimentorum Fermentatione in Ventriculi Caesa.* Opera Medica Praxeos Medicae Idea Nova, lib. 1, cap. Vii, 166.Amsterdam (5,14)

Symonds C. J. 1887 The treatment of malignant stricture of the oesophagus by tubage or permanent catheterism. *Brit. Med. J.* i, 870–873 (1, 45)

Szurszeski J. H. 1969 A migrating electric complex of the canine small intestine. *Amer. J. Physiol.* 217, 1757–63 (5, 152)

Talley N. J., Janssens J., Lauritsen K., Racz I, and Bolling-Sternevald E. 1999 Eradication of Helicobacter pylori in functional dyspepsia: randomised double blind placebo controlled trial with 12 months' follow up. *Brit. Med. J.* i 833–837 (5, 322)

Talley N. J., Lauritsen K. and Bolling-Sterneveld E. 1999 Eradication of Helicobacter pylori in functional dyspepsia. *Brit. Med. J.* ii 451 (L) (5, 324)

Talley N. J., Phillips S. F., Melton L. J., Wiltgen D., Mulvihill C. and Zinsmeister, A. R. 1990 Diagnostic value of the Manning criteria in irritable bowel syndrome. *Gut,* 31: 77–81 (5, 188)

Tanner A. R. 1996 ERCP: present practice in a single region. Suggested standards for monitoring performance. *Eur J. Gastroenterol Hepatol* 8, 145–8 (6, 156)

Tanner N. 1947 The present position of carcinoma of the oesophagus. *Postgrad. Med. J.* 23, 109–139 (1, 69)

Taylor K. B., Roitt I. M., Doniach D., Couchman K. G., Shapland C. 1962 Autoimmune phenomena in pernicious anaemia: gastric antibodies. *Brit. Med. J.* ii 1347–52 (4, 162)

Taylor K. B., Thompson D. L., Truelove S. C., Wright R. 1961 An immunological study of coeliac disease and idiopathic steatorrhoea *Brit. Med. J.* ii 1727–31 (3, 138)

Taylor K. B., Truelove S. C. 1961 Circulating antibodies to milk protein in ulcerative colitis. *Brit. Med. J.* ii 924–929 (4, 161)

Taylor K. B., Truelove S. C., Wright R. 1964 Serological reaction to gluten and cow's milk proteins in gastrointestinal disease. *Gastroenterology* 46: 99–108 (3, 139)

Taylor I. 1984 Colonic motility in the irritable colon syndrome. In Read, N. W. (ed) *Irritable Bowel Syndrome.* pp89–104, Grune & Stratton, London (5, 212)

Taylor I., Darby, C. F., Hammond P. and Basu P. 1978 Is there a myoelectrical abnormality in the irritable bowel syndrome? *Gut,* 19, 391–395 (5, 210)

Taylor I., Duthie, H. L., Smallwood R. and Linkens D 1975 Large bowel myoelectrical activity in man. *Gut,* 16, 808–814 (5, 209)

Teague R. H., Fraser D., Clamp J. R. 1973 Changes in monosaccharide content of mucus glycoproteins in ulcerative colitis. *Brit. Med. J.* i, 645–646 (4, 233)

Teague R. H., Salmon P. R. and Read A. E. 1973 Fibreoptic examination of the colon: a review of 255 cases. *Gut,* 14, 139–142 (6, 73)

Teahon K., Bjarnason I., Pearson M., Levi A. J. 1990 Ten years experience with an elemental diet in the management of Crohn's disease. *Gut* 31: 1133–37 (4, 317)

Teahon K., Smethurst P., Levi A. J., Menzies I. S., Bjarnason I. 1992 Intestinal permeability in patients with Crohn's disease and their first degree relatives. *Gut* 33: 320–323 (4, 308)

Thaysen T. E. H. 1929 The " Coeliac Affection" – idiopathic steatorrhoeas. *Lancet* i 1086–89 (3, 46)

Thaysen T. E. H. 1932 *Non-tropcal Sprue: a Study of Idiopathic Steatorrhoea.* Oxford University Press (3, 49)

Thjodleifsson B., Wormsley K. G. 1974 Gastric response to metiamide *Brit. Med. J.* ii: 304–306 (2, 174)

Thomas G. A. O., Millar-Jones D., Rhodes J., Roberts G. M., Williams G. T., Mayberry J. F. 1995 Incidence of Crohn's disease in Cardiff over 60 years: 1986–90 an update.*Eur. J. Gastroenterol. & Hepatol.* 7: 401–405 (4, 127)

Thomas G. A. O., Rhodes J., Green J. T. 1998 Inflammatory bowel disease and smoking – a review. *Amer. J. Gastroenterol.* 93: 144–9 (4, 155)

Thompson M. R. 1980 Indomethacin and perforated duodenal ulcer. *Brit. Med. J.* i, 448 (2, 84)

Thompson M. R. 1981 The unnatural history of drug-associated gastric ulcers. *Gut* 22: A877 (2, 85)

Thompson N., Driscoll R., Pounder R. E., Wakefield A. J. 1996 Genetics versus environment in inflammatory bowel disease: results of a British twin study. *Brit. Med. J.,* 312: 95–96 (4, 132)

Thompson N. P., Montgomery S. M., Pounder R. E., Wakefield A. J. 1995 Is measles vaccination a risk factor for inflammatory bowel disease? *Lancet* i, 1071–74 (4, 219)

Thompson N. P., Pounder R. E., Wakefield A. J. 1995 Perinatal and childhood risk factors for inflammatory bowel disease: a case control study. *Eur. J. Gastroenterol. & Hepatol.* 7: 385–390 (4, 218)

Thompson N. P., Wakefield A. J., Pounder R. E. 1995 Inherited disorders of coagulation appear to protect against inflammatory bowel disease. *Gastroenterology* 108: 1011–15 (4, 214)

Thompson V. C. 1945 Successful resection for carcinoma of the lower end of the oesophagus with immediate oesophagogastrostomy. *Brit. J. Surg.* 32; 377–380 (1, 63)

Thompson D. G., Laidlow, J. and Wingate D. L. 1979 Abnormal small bowel motility demonstrated by radiotelemetry in a patient with irritable colon. *Lancet* ii 1321–23 (5, 232)

Thompson D. G., Wingate D. L., Archer, L., Benson M. J., Green W. J. and Hardy R. J. 1980 Normal patterns of human upper small bowel motor activity recorded by prolonged radiotelemetry. *Gut,* 21, 500–506 (5, 233)

Thompson D. G., Archer, L., Green W. G. and Wingate D. L. 1981 Fasting motor activity occurs during a day of normal meals in healthy subjects. *Gut,* 22, 489–492 (5, 234)

Thompson D. G., Richelsen E. and Malagelada J. R. 1982 Perturbation of gastric emptying and duodenal motility via the central nervous system. *Gastroenterology* 73; 1200–06 (5, 243)

Thompson D. G., Richelson E. and Malagelada J. R. 1983 Perturbation of upper gastrointestinal function by cold stress *Gut* 24; 277–283 (5, 244)

Thompson D. G., Binfield P., De Belder A., O'Brien, J., Warren S, and Wilson, M. 1985 Extraintestinal influences on exhaled breath hydrogen measurement during the investigation of gastrointestinal disease. *Gut,* 26, 1349–52 (5, 245)

Thompson W. G. and Heaton K. G. 1980 Functional bowel disorders in apparently healthy people. *Gastroenterology,*79: 283–288 (5, 219)

Thompson W. G., Dotevall G., Drossman D. A., Heaton K. W. and Kruis W. 1989 Irritable bowel syndrome: guidelines for the diagnosis. *Gastroenterology Int.* 2, 92–95 (5, 266)

Thomson J. 1854 *An Account of the Life, Lectures and Writings of William Cullen MD* William Blackwood and Sons, Edinburgh: Vol Methodicae 125 (5, 22)

Thornton J. L. 1953 *John Abernethy a Biography.* Distributed by Simpkin Marshall Ltd, London (5, 35)

Tibble J., Teahon K., Thjodleifsson B., Roseth A., Sigthorsson G., Bridger S., Foster R., Sherwood R., Fagerhol M., Bjarnason B. 2000 A simple method for assessing intestinal inflammation in Crohn's disease. *Gut* 47: 506–513 (4, 309)

Tidy H. L. 1920 in discussion of paper by Fletcher, H. M., Case of Renal Infantilism, *Proceedings of the Royal Society of Medicine* (Sec. Child. Dis.) xiii, 123 (3, 40)

Tidy H. L. 1941 Discussion of dyspepsia in the forces. *Proc. Roy. Soc. Med.* XXXIV 411–426 (5, 119)

Tilestone W. 1906 Peptic ulcer of the oesophagus. *Amer. J. Med. Sci.* 132, 240–265 (1, 83)

Torek F. 1913 The first successful case of resection of the thoracic portion of the Esophagus for carcinoma. *Surg. Gynae. Obstet.* 16; 614–617 (1, 55)

Training in Gastroenterology 1974 British Society of Gastroenterology Report C. Nicholls and Company Ltd. Manchester (6, 87)

Travers B. 1816 Rupture of the stomach and escape of its contents into the cavity of the abdomen. *Medico-Chir Trans.* 8; 231–240 (2, 51)

Travis S. P. L., Tysk C., deSilva H. J., Sandberg-Gertzen H., Jewell D. P., Jarnerot G. 1992 Optimum dose of olsalazine for maintening remission in ulcerative colitis. *Gut 35*; 1282–86 (4, 104)

Trimble K. C., Pryde A. and Heading R. C. 1995 Lowered oesophageal sensory thresholds in patients with symptomatic but not excess gastro-oesophageal reflux: evidence for a spectrum of visceral hypersensitivity in GORD. *Gut*, 37, 7–12 (5, 301)

Trotter T. 1807 *A View of the Nervous Temperament; Being a Practical Enquiry into the Increasing Prevalence, Prevention, and Treatment of Those Diseases Commonly Called Nervous, Bilious, Stomach, and Liver*

Complaints; Indigestion; Low Spirits; Gout, etc. Second edition, Printed by Edward Walker, Newcastle for Longman, Hurst, Rees, and Orme, London. (5, 33)

Trounce J. R., Deuchar D. C., Kauntze R., Stevenson J. J., Thomas G. A. 1956 Observations on achalasia of the cardia. *Gastroenterologia* Basel 86:178. (1, 29)

Trounce J. R., Deuchar D. C., Kauntze R., Stevenson J. J., Thomas G. A. 1957 Observations on achalasia of the cardia. *Quart.J. Med. n.s.* 26, 433– 443 (1, 30)

Trousseau A. 1862 *Clinique Medicale de l'Hotel Dieu de Paris*, 2, 112–4 (3, 19)

Trousseau A. 1867 *Lectures on clinical medicine.* New Sydenham Soc., London 35: 370 (3, 20)

Trowell J. E., Yoong A. K. H., Saul K. J., Gant P. W., Bell G. D. 1987 A simple half-gram stain for demonstrating Campylobacter pyloridis in sections. *J. Clin. Pathol.* 40: 702 (2, 193)

Trowell H. C. 1960 *Non-infective Disease in Africa.* Edward Arnold. London (5, 164)

Trowell H. C. 1972 Crude fibre, dietary fibre and atherosclerosis. *Atherosclerosis,*16, 138–140 (5, 166)

Trowell H. C. 1981 Editor, *Western Diseases: Their Emergence and Prevention* Edward Arnold, London (5, 169)

Truelove S. C., Witts L. J. 1955 Cortisone in ulcerative colitis. Final report on a therapeutic trial. *Brit. Med. J.* ii, 1041–48 (4, 70)

Truelove S. C., Richards W. C. D. 1956 Biopsy studies in ulcerative colitis. *Brit. Med. J.* i 1315–18 (4, 71)

Truelove S. C. 1958 Treatment of ulcerative colitis with local hydrocortisone hemisuccinate sodium. A report of a controlled therapeutic trial. *Brit. Med. J.* ii, 1072–77 (4, 80)

Truelove S. C. 1960 Stilboestrol, phenobarbitone and diet in chronic duodenal ulcer. *Br.Med.J.* ii: 559–566 (2, 155)

Truelove S. C. 1961 Ulcerative colitis provoked by milk. *Brit. Med. J.* i, 154–160 (4, 160)

Truelove S. C., Watkinson G., Draper G. 1962 Comparison of corticosteroid and sulphasalazine therapy in ulcerative colitis. *Brit. Med. J.* ii, 1708–11 (4, 82)

Truelove S. C., Ellis H., Webster C. U. 1965 Place of a double barrelled ileostomy in ulcerative colitis and Crohn's disease of the colon: a preliminary report. *Brit. Med. J.* i, 150–3 (4, 203)

Truelove S. C., Reynell P. C. 1965 in *Diseases of the Digestive System*. Blackwell, Oxford 2nd ed p216 (2, 81)

Truelove S. C., Willoughby C. P., Lee E. C. G., Kettlewell M. G. W. 1978 Further experience in the treatment of severe attacks of ulcerative colitis. *Lancet* ii, 1086–88 (4, 291)

Truelove S. C. 1987 British Society for Digestive Endoscopy. *Gut*, Jubilee Suppl. BSG (6, 81)

Tudor Edwards A., Lee E. S. 1936 Extirpation of the oesophagus for carcinoma. *J. Laryngol. Otol.* 51 281–292 (1, 66)

Turner G. Grey. 1946 *Injuries and Diseases of the Oesophagus*. Cassell & Co. Ltd, p65 (1, 13)

Turner G. Grey. 1946 *Injuries and Diseases of the Oesophagus*. Cassell & Co. Ltd. p73 (1, 23)

Turner G. Grey. 1946 *Injuries and Diseases of the Oesophagus*. Cassell & Co. Ltd. p91 (1, 58)

Turner G. Grey. 1931 Some experiences in the surgery of the oesophagus. Bigelow Memorial Lecture *New England Journal of Medicine* 205: 657–674 (1, 22)

Turner G. Grey. 1933 Excision of the thoracic oesophagus for carcinoma – with construction of an extrathoracic gullet. *Lancet* ii, 1315–16 (1, 56)

Turner G. Grey. 1944–45 The George Haliburton Hume Memorial Lectures *Newcastle Medical J.* XXII (1, 36)

Tweedsmuir 1982 *John Buchan a Memoir*. Iola (2, 117)

Tysk C., Lindberg E., Jarnerot G., Floderus-Myrhed B. 1988 Ulcerative colitis and Crohn's disease in an unselected population of monozygotic and dizygotic twins. A study of heritability and the influence of smoking. *Gut* 29: 990–996 (4, 131)

Uhlmann V., Martin C. M., Sheil S. O., Pilkington L., Silva I., Killalea A., Murch S. B., Walker-Smith J. A., Thomson M., O'Leary J. J. 2002 Potential viral pathogenic mechanism for new variant inflammatory bowel disease. *J. Mol. Pathol.* 55: 84–90 (4, 226)

UK Colorectal cancer Screening Pilot Group 2004 Results of the first round of a demonstration pilot of screening for colorectal cancer in the United Kingdom. *Brit. Med. J.* 329 133–5 (6, 151)

UK Flexible Sigmoidoscopy Screening Trial Investigators 2002 Single flexible sigmoidoscopy screening to prevent colorectal cancer: base line findings of a UK multicentre randomised trial. *Lancet*, 359, 1291–1300 (6, 152)

Ulcer Wars. Broadcast on 16 May 1994. *Horizon*, BBC 2. (2, 203)

Ulcerative colitis 1909 Symposium and discussion. *Proceedings of the Royal Society of Medicine. vol 2, part 2, medical section*, 59– 151 (4, 23)(6, 60)

Unsworth D. J., Johnson G. D., Haffenden G., Fry L., Holborow E. J. 1981 Binding of wheat gliadin in vitro to reticulin in normal and dermatitis herpetiformis skin. *J. Invest. Dermatol.* 76: 88–93 (3, 221)

Unsworth D. J., Manuel P. D., Walker-Smith J. A., Campbell C. A., Johnson D. G., Holborow E. D. 1981 New immunofluorescent blood test for gluten sensitivity. *Arch. Dis. Child* 56: 864–868 (3.222)

Vallon A. G., Cotton P. B., Lawrence B. H., Armengol Miro J. R. and Salord Oses J. C. 1981 Randomised trial of endoscopic argon laser photocoagulation in bleeding peptic ulcers. *Gut,* 22, 228–233 (6, 105)

Van Berge-Henegouwen G. P., Mulder C. J. J. 1993 History of Dicke's discovery of the gluten-free diet for coeliac sprue. In *Gastro-intestinal Disease* Ed M. H. Sleisenger and J. S. Fordtran W. B. Saunders 5th ed chap 50, 1072–77 (3, 68)

Van de Kamer J. H. 1974 Coeliac disease: a Historical Review. *J. Irish Med. Assoc.* 67, 405–406 (3, 71)

Van de Kamer J. H., Ten Bokkel Huinink H., Weijers H. A. 1949 Rapid method for the determination of fat in faeces. *J. Biol. Chem.* 177: 347 (3, 75)

Vane J. 1971 Inhibition of prostaglandin synthesis as a mechanism of action for aspirin-like drugs *Nature (New Biology)* 231–232 (2, 92)

Vantrappen G. and Hellemans J. 1976 Diffuse Muscle Spasm of the Oesophagus and the Lower Oesophageal Sphincter. *Clinics in Gastroenterology* vol 5, No 1, 59–72 (5, 193)

Vantrappen G., Janssens J., Hellemans J. and Ghoos Y. 1977 The interdigestive motor complex of normal subjects and patients with bacterial overgrowth. *J. Clin. Invest.* 59; 1158–66 (5, 203)

Vantrappen G., Janssens J., Peeters T. L., Bloom S. R. and Christofides N. D. 1979 Motility and the interdigestive migrating motor complex in man. *Dig. Dis. Sci.* 2, 4497–500 (5, 215)

Vaughan J. M., Hunter D. 1932 The treatment by Marmite of megalocytic hyperchromic anaemia occurring in idiopathic steatorrhoea. *Lancet* i, 829–834 (3, 44)

Vedder E. B., Duval C. W. 1902 The etiology of acute dysentery in the United States. *J. Exp. Med.* 6: 181–205 (4, 10)

Verzar F., McDougall E. J. 1936 *Absorption From the Intestine.* Longmans, Green & Co., London (3, 50)

Vilardell F. 2006 *Digestive Endoscopy in the Second Millenium.* Grupo Aula Medica, S. L. ISBN: 1–58890–420–2 (TNY) (6, 2 & 43)

Viridet J. 1692 *Tractatus Novus Medico-Physicus de Prima Coctione Praecipuque de Ventriculi Fermento.* Geneva pp90, 93, 95, 224 (5, 16)

Visick A. H. 1948 A study of the failures after gastrectomy. Hunterian Lecture. *Ann. Roy. Coll. Surg. (Eng.)* 3: 266–284 (2, 134)

Von Bergmann G. 1932 *Funktionelle Pathologie.* Berlin p68 (1, 89)

Von Haller A. 1759–66 *Experimenta Physiologiae Corporis Humani.* Lausannae (5, 20)

Vorhaus M. G. 1934 Modern aspects of gastroenterology: book review. *Amer. J. Dig. Dis.,* vol 1, 211 (6, 22)

Wakefield A. J., Murch S. H., Anthony A., Linnell J., Casson D. M., Malik M., Berelowitz M., Dhillon A. P., Thompson M. A., Harvey P., Valentine A., Davies S. E., Walker-Smith J. A. 1998 Ileal-lymphoid-nodular hyperplasia, non-specific colitis, and pervasive developmental disorder in children. *Lancet* i, 637– 641 (4, 225)

Wakefield A. J., Pittilo R. M., Sim R., Cosby S. L., Stephenson J. R., Dhillon A. P., Pounder R. E. 1993 Evidence of persistent measles virus infection in Crohn's disease. *J. Med. Virol.* 39: 345–353 (4, 217)

Wakefield A. J., Sawyer A. M., Dhillon A. P., Pittilo R. M., Rowles P. M., Lewis A. A. M., Pounder R. E. 1989 Pathogenesis of Crohn's disease: multifocal gastrointestinal infarction. *Lancet* ii, 1057–62 (4, 213)

Walk, L. 1966 The history of gastroscopy. *Clio Medica,* 1, 209–222 (6, 9)

Walker A. J., Dewar E. P. 1985 Emergency peptic ulcer surgery – an association with NSAIDs *Gut,* 26 A1118 (2, 89)

Walker A. R. P., Walker B. F. & Richardson B. D. 1970 Bowel transit times in Bantu populations. *Brit. Med. J.* iii 48–49 (L) (5, 162)

Wall A. J., Douglas A. P., Booth C. C., Pearse A. G. F. 1970 Response of the jejunal mucosa in adult coeliac disease to oral prednisolone. *Gut* 1, 17–14 (3, 140)

Waller B. K., Schumacher, K. A., Weidenmaier W. and Friedrich J. M. 1991 Dilated biliary tree: evaluation with MR cholangiography with T-2 weighted contrast-enhanced fast sequence. *Radiology,* 181, 805–808 (6, 160)

Waller S. L. and Misiewicz J. J. 1969 Prognosis in the irritable bowel syndrome. *Lancet,* ii; 753– 756 (5, 220)

Wallis F. C. 1909 The surgery of colitis. *Brit. Med. J.* i,10–13 (4, 21)

Walt R., Katchinski B., Logan R., Ashley J., Langman M. J. S. 1986 Rising frequency of ulcer perforation in elderly people in the United Kingdom. *Lancet* i 489–492 (2, 83)

Walton A. J. 1925 The surgical treatment of cardiospasm. *Brit. J. Surg.* 13, 701–737 (1, 18)

Walton A. J. 1944 Discussion on treatment of duodenal ulcer. *Proceedings of the Royal Society of Medicine* 38: 91 (2, 135)

Ward M. 1977 The pathogenesis of Crohn's disease. *Lancet* ii, 903–905 (4, 180)

Warren J. R., Marshall B. J. 1983 Unidentified curved bacilli on gastric epithelium in active chronic gastritis. *Lancet* i, 1273–75 (2, 94)

Warren S., Sommers S. C. 1948 Cicatrizing enteritis (regional enteritis) as a pathological entity. *Amer. J. Pathol.* 24: 475–501 (4, 278)

Watkinson G. W. 1951 A study of the changes in pH of gastric contents in peptic ulcer using the 24–hour test meal. *Gastroenterology* 18, 377–390 (2, 40)

Watkinson G. 1958 Treatment of ulcerative colitis with topical hydrocortisone hemisuccinate sodium. A controlled trial employing restricted sequential analysis. *Brit. Med. J.* ii 1077– 1082 (4, 81)

Watkinson G. 1960 The incidence of chronic peptic ulcer found at necropsy. *Gut* 1: 14–30 (2, 54 & 55)

Watkinson G. 1961 Medical management of ulcerative colitis. *Brit. Med. J.* i, 147–151 (4, 79 & 87)

Watkinson G., de Dombal F. T. 1968 The management of ulcerative colitis. *Scot. Med. J.* 13: 133–143 (4, 325)

Watson T. 1848 *Lectures on the Principles and Practice of Physic.* London 3rd ed. vol 1 p160 and 184 (5, 76)

Watson T. 1848 *Lectures on the Principles and Practice of Physic.* London 3rd ed vol 2 343–350. (1, 39)

Watson T. 1848 *Lectures on the Principles and Practice of Physic;* London 3rd ed. vol 2 437–454. (5, 47 & 49)

Webster A. D. B., Slavin G., Shiner., Platts-Mills T. A. E., Asherson G. L. 1981 Coeliac disease with severe hypogammaglobulinaemia. *Gut* 22: 153–7 (3, 145)

Weedon D. D., Shorter R. G., Ilstrup D. M., Huizenga K. A., Taylor W. F. 1973 Crohn's disease and cancer. *New England Journal of Medicine* 289: 1099–1103 (4, 284)

Weijers H. A. 1950 *Fat Absorption in Normal and Diseased Neonates and*

Children, Especially in Patients with Coeliac Disease. Thesis. Univ. of Utrecht. The Netherlands (in Dutch). (3, 74)

Weil J., Bell G. D., Powell K., Morden A., Harrison G., Gant P. W., Jones P. H., Trowell J,E. 1991 Omeprazole and Helicobacter pylori: temporary suppression rather than true eradication. *Alimentary Pharmacology and Therapeutics* 5: 309–313 (2, 200)

Weil J., Langman M. J. S. 1991 Screening for gastrointestinal cancer: an epidemiological review. *Gut* 32: 220–224 (4, 270)

Weir R. 1902 A new use for the useless appendix in the surgical treatment of obstinate colitis. *Med. Rec.* 62: 201–202 (4, 20)

Weiser M. M., Douglas A. P. 1976 An alternative mechanism for gluten toxicity in coeliac disease. *Lancet* i: 567–569 (3, 136)

Wells C. 1952 Ulcerative colitis and Crohn's disease. *Ann. Roy. Coll. Surg. (Eng.)* 11:105–120 (4, 122)

Wells C. A. 1957 Duodenal ulcer: a study in the development of method. *Irish J. Med. Sci.* 7; 32–41 (2, 139)

West J., Logan R. F. A., Hill P. G., Lloyd A., Lewis S., Hubbard R., Reader R., Holmes G. K. T., Khaw K-T. 2003 Seroprevalence, correlates,and characteristics of undetected celiac disease in England. *Gut* 52: 960–965 (3, 227)

Westaby D., Macdougall B. R. D. and Williams R 1985 Improved survival following injection sclerotherapy for oesophageal varices: final analysis of a controlled trial. *Hepatology* 5, 827–830 (6, 100)

Whitehead W. E., Bosmajian L., Zonderman A. B., Costa P. T. Jr. And Shuster, M. M. 1988 Symptoms of psychological distress associated with irritable bowel syndrome. Comparison of community and medical clinic samples. *Gastroenterology*, 95, 709–714 (5, 350)

Whitehead W. E., Engel B. T. and Schuster M. M. 1980 Irritable bowel syndrome. Physiological and psychological differences between diarrhoea-predominant and constipation-predominant patients. *Dig. Dis. Sci.* 25, 404–413 (5, 255)

Whitehead W. E., Holtcotter B., Enck P., Hoelzl R., Holmes K. D., Anthony J., Shabsin H. S. and Shuster M. M. 1990 Tolerance for recto-sigmoid distension in irritable bowel syndrome *Gastroenterology*, 98, 1187–92 (5, 299)

Whitfield P. F., Hobsley M. 1987 Comparison of maximal gastric secretion in smokers and non-smokers with and without duodenal ulcer. *Gut* 28, 557–560 (2, 74)

Whorwell P. J., Prior A., and Faragher E. B. 1984 Controlled trial of hypnotherapy in the treatment of severe refractory irritable-bowel syndrome. *Lancet*, ii 1232–34 (5, 295)

Whorwell P. J., Lupton E. W., Erduran D. and Wilson K. 1986 Bladder smooth muscle dysfunction in patients with irritable bowel syndrome. *Gut*, 27, 1014–17 (5, 261)

Whorwell P. J., McCallum M., Creed F. H. and Roberts C. T. 1986 Non-colonic features of irritable bowel syndrome. *Gut*, 27, 37–40 (5, 260)

Whorwell P. J., Prior A. and Colgan S. M. 1987 Hypnotherapy in severe irritable bowel syndrome: further experience. *Gut*, 28, 423–425 (5, 296)

Whorwell P. J., Houghton L. A., Taylor E. E. et al. 1992 Physiological effects of emotion: assessment via hypnosis. *Lancet*, 340, 69–72 (5, 360)

Whorwell P. J., Ruegg P., Earnest D., Dunger-Baldauf C. 2004 Tegaserod significantly improves bloating in female irritable bowel syndrome patients with constipation. *Gastroenterology* 126, A-643. W1470 (5, 392)

Whytt R. 1764 *Observations on the Nature, Causes and Cures of Those Disorders Which Have Been Commonly Called Nervous, Hypochondriac or Hysteric*; Balfour, Edinburgh (5, 21)

Wicks A. C. B., Robertson G. S. M. and Veitch P. S. 1999 Structured training and assessment in ERCP has become essential for the Calman era. *Gut*, 45, 154–6 (6, 158)

Wilkinson S. P., Biddlestone L., Gore S., Shepherd N. A. 1999 Regression of columnar lined (Barrett's) oesophagus with omeprazole 40mg daily: results of 5 years of continuous therapy. *Alimentary Pharmacology and Therapeutics* 13, 1205–09 (1, 111)

Wilks S. 1859 *Lectures on Pathological Anatomy delivered at Guy's Hospital during the summer sessions 1857–58* Longmans, Brown, Green, Longmans, Roberts, London (4, 6) (5, 78)

Wilks S. 1859 Morbid appearance in the intestines of Miss Bankes. *Med. Times & Gazette* 19, 2, 264–265 (4, 4)

Wilks S. 1866 Dilatation of the oesophagus. *Trans. Path. Soc. London* 17, 138–9 (1, 12)

Wilks S. & Moxon W. 1875 *Lectures on Pathological Anatomy* Second edition J. & A. Churchill, London pp409–410 (5, 79)

Williams C. B. and Muto T. 1972 Examination of the whole colon with the fibreoptic colonoscope. *Brit. Med. J.* iii, 278–281 (6, 74)

Williams C. B. and Muto, T. and Rutter K. R. P. 1973 Removal of polyps with fibreoptic colonoscope: a new approach to colonic polypectomy. *Brit. Med. J.* i, 451–452 (6, 75)

Williams C. B. 1979 Colonoscopy- a new view. *J. Roy. Soc. Med.* 72, 483–484 (6, 95)

Williams E. J., Taylor, S., Fairclough P., Hamlyn A., Logan R. F., Martin D., Riley S. A., Veitch P., Wilkinson M., Williamson P. R. and Lombard M. 2007 Are we meeting the standards set for endoscopy? Results of a large-scale prospective survey of endoscopic retrograde cholangio-pancreatograph practice. *Gut*, 56, 821–829 (6, 162)

Williams J., Russell, R., Durai D., Cheung W. Y., Farrin A., Bloor K., Coulton S. and Richardson G. 2009 Effectiveness of nurse delivered endoscopy: findings from randomised multi-institution nurse endoscopy trial. (MINuET) *Brit. Med. J.* 338, 231 (6, 142)

Williams K. D. G. and Dawson J. L. 1979 Fibreoptic injection of oesophageal varices. *Brit. Med. J.* ii, 766–767 (6, 99)

Williams W. A., Edwards Felicity, Lewis T. H. C. and Coghill N. F. 1957 Investigation of non-ulcer dyspepsia by gastric biopsy. *Brit. Med. J.* i, 372–377 (5, 127)

Willis T. 1674 *Pharmaceutice Rationalis*. First English Translation London 1679 p23 (1, 7)

Willoughby C. P., Aronson J. K., Agback H., Bodin N. O., Truelove S. C. 1982 Distribution and metabolism in healthy volunteers of disodium azodisalicylate, a potential therapeutic agent for ulcerative colitis. *Gut* 23:1081–87 (4, 101)

Willoughby J. M. T., Kumar P. J., Beckett J., Dawson A. M. 1971 Controlled trial of azathioprine in Crohn's disease. *Lancet* ii, 944–947 (4, 330)

Willoughby J. M. T., Mitchell D. N. 1971 In-vitro inhibition of leucocyte migration in Crohn's disease by a sarcoid spleen suspension. *Brit. Med. J.* ii, 155–7 (4, 172)

Willoughby J. M. T., Mitchell D. N., Wilson J. D. 1971 Sarcoidosis and Crohn's disease in siblings. *Amer. Rev. Resp. Dis.* 104: 249–254 (4, 170)

Willoughby Lyle H. 1935 The case of Dr. Smethurst in *King's and Some King's Men*. Oxford Union Press, London 64–66 (4, 2)

Wills L 1931 Treatment of "pernicious anaemia of pregnancy" and "tropical anaemia". *Brit. Med. J.* i: 1059–64 (3, 42)

Wilson T. S. 1922 A physiological explanation of pain due to functional disturbance of the muscles of colon. *Brit. Med. J.* i, 944–946 (5, 112)

Wilson T. S. 1927 *Tonic Hardening of the Colon.* Humphrey Milford Oxford University Press (5, 113)

Wingate D. L. 1976 The eupeptide system: a general theory of gastrointestinal hormones. *Lancet,* i, 529–532 (5, 216)

Wingate D. L. 1981 Backwards and forwards with the migrating motor complex. *Dig. Dis. Sci.* 26; 641–666 (5, 235)

Wingate D. L. 1983 Complex clocks. *Dig. Dis. Sci.* 28, 1133–40 (5, 236)

Wingate D. L. 1991 Small Bowel Motor Activity: A Key to Understanding Functional Disorders of the Bowel. In *Irritable Bowel Syndrome.* ed. N. W. Read 24–28 Blackwell Scientific Publications (5, 242)

Wingate D. L. 2008 A 20–year perspective–from *Journal of Gastrointestinal Motility to Neurogastroenterology and Motility. Neurogastroenterol. Motil.* 20 (Suppl. 1), 1–7 (5, 214)

Witts L. J. 1966 *The stomach and anaemia* Athlone Press, London (2, 141)

Witts L. J. 1937 Haematemesis and melaena. *Br. Med. J.* i, 847–852 (2, 144)

Witts L. J. 1960 in *Controlled Clinical Trials* (edited by Bradford Hill) Oxford p10 (4, 89)

Wollman M. R., David D. S., Brennan B. L., Lewy J. E., Stenzel K. H., Rubin A. L., Miller D. R. 1972 The nitroblue tetrazolium test. *Lancet* ii, 289–291 (4, 175)

Wood G. M., Shires S., Howdle P. D., Losowsky M. S. 1986 Immunoglobulin production by celiac biopsies in organ culture. *Gut* 27, 1151–60 (3, 174)

Wood I. J., Doig R. K., Motteram R., Hughes A. 1949 Gastric biopsy *Lancet* i, 18–21 (3, 82)

Wood J. 2002 in: Peptic Ulcer: Rise and Fall. *Wellcome Witnesses to Twentieth Century Medicine* vol 14 eds. Christie D. A., Tansey E. M. 73–76 (2, 183)

Woodward J. 1718 *State of Physick and of Diseases* London (5, 10)

Woodward J. 1710–11 *Of the Body of Man; Of Health, of Diseases, and of Remedies; Three Physico-Mechanical Lectures Read in the Theater of the College of Physitians.* Gulstonian Lectures. B. M. MSSloane 2039, ff. 115–29 (5, 7)

Wright A. D. 1935 Two cases of Crohn's disease. *Trans. Med. Soc. Lond.* 58: 94–96 (4, 52)

Wright G. 1919 Secondary jejunal and gastro-jejunal ulceration. *Brit. J. Surg.* 6: 390–401 (2, 131)

Wright R., McCollum R. W., Klatskin G. 1969 Australia antigen in acute and chronic liver disease. *Lancet* ii, 117–121 (4, 166)

Wright R., Truelove S. C. 1965 A controlled therapeutic trial of various diets in ulcerative colitis. *Brit. Med. J.* ii, 138–141 (4, 163)

Wright R., Truelove S. C. 1965 Circulating antibodies to dietary proteins in ulcerative colitis. *Brit. Med. J.* ii, 142–4 (4, 164)

Wright R., Truelove S. C. 1966 Autoimmune reactions in ulcerative colitis. *Gut* 7: 32–40 (4, 165)

Wright T. A., Gray M. R., Morris A. I., Gilmore I. T. et al 1996 Cost effectiveness of detecting Barrett's cancer. *Gut* 39, 574–579 (1, 113)

Wyllie J. H., Hesselbro T., Black J. W. 1972 Effects in man of histamine H2–receptor blockade by burimamide. *Lancet* ii: 1117–20 (2, 171)

Wyman J. B., Heaton, K. W., Manning A. P. and Wicks A. C. B. 1978 Variability of colonic function in healthy subjects *Gut* 19, 146–150 (5, 186 & 218)

Yearsley, J. 1862 Introduction to the art of laryngoscopy *Med. Circ.* Vol XX (6, 3)

Young W. F., Pringle E. M. 1971 110 Children with Coeliac Disease, 1950–69 *Arch. Dis. Child.* 46: 421–436 (3, 119)